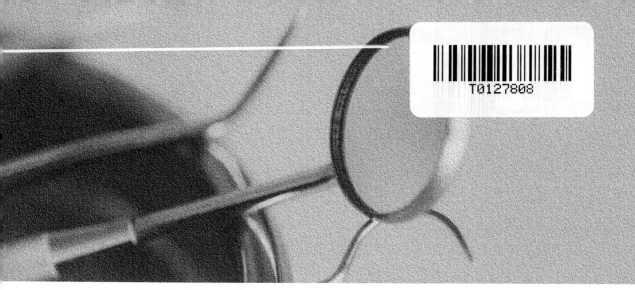

Mosby's
Review for the NBDE
Part One

SECOND EDITION

edited by

Frank Dowd, DDS, PhD
Professor Emeritus
Department of Pharmacology
School of Medicine
School of Dentistry
Creighton University
Omaha, Nebraska

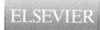

3251 Riverport Lane
St. Louis, Missouri 63043

MOSBY'S REVIEW FOR THE NBDE, PART I, SECOND EDITION   ISBN: 978-0-323-22561-8
Copyright © 2015 by Mosby, an imprint of Elsevier Inc.
Copyright © 2007 by Mosby, Inc., an affiliate of Elsevier Inc.

Notices

Knowledge and best practice in this field are constantly changing. As new research and experience broaden our understanding, changes in research methods, professional practices, or medical treatment may become necessary.

Practitioners and researchers must always rely on their own experience and knowledge in evaluating and using any information, methods, compounds, or experiments described herein. In using such information or methods they should be mindful of their own safety and the safety of others, including parties for whom they have a professional responsibility.

With respect to any drug or pharmaceutical products identified, readers are advised to check the most current information provided (i) on procedures featured or (ii) by the manufacturer of each product to be administered, to verify the recommended dose or formula, the method and duration of administration, and contraindications. It is the responsibility of practitioners, relying on their own experience and knowledge of their patients, to make diagnoses, to determine dosages and the best treatment for each individual patient, and to take all appropriate safety precautions.

To the fullest extent of the law, neither the Publisher nor the authors, contributors, or editors, assume any liability for any injury and/or damage to persons or property as a matter of products liability, negligence or otherwise, or from any use or operation of any methods, products, instructions, or ideas contained in the material herein.

International Standard Book Number: 978-0-323-22561-8

Executive Content Strategist: Kathy Falk
Senior Content Development Specialist: Brian Loehr
Publishing Services Manager: Julie Eddy
Senior Project Manager: Marquita Parker
Design Direction: Brian Salisbury

Printed in the United States

Last digit is the print number: 9 8 7 6 5

 Working together
to grow libraries in
developing countries

www.elsevier.com • www.bookaid.org

Section Editors

Nisha J. D'Silva, BDS, MSD, PhD
Associate Chair, Division of Oral Pathology/Medicine/
  Radiology
School of Dentistry
University of Michigan
Ann Arbor, Michigan

Katherine M. Howard, PhD
Assistant Professor
Department of Biomedical Sciences
School of Dental Medicine
University of Nevada, Las Vegas
Las Vegas, Nevada

Stanley J. Nelson, DDS, MS
Professor and Co-Chair
Department of Clinical Sciences
School of Dental Medicine
University of Nevada, Las Vegas
Las Vegas, Nevada

Joseph W. Robertson, DDS, BS
Faculty
Department of Nursing and Health Professions
Oakland Community College
Bloomfield Hills, Michigan

Michael G. Schmidt, PhD
Professor of Microbiology and Immunology
Department of Microbiology and Immunology
Medical University of South Carolina
Charleston, South Carolina

Preface

How to Use This Text

This review book is the compiled work by experts in each of the relevant disciplines represented on the National Board Dental Exam (NBDE). This second edition includes recent updates and important changes from the first edition for each NBDE subject. This text is a tool to help prepare students for taking the NBDE and to help identify strengths and weaknesses so students can better utilize their study time. This text is not meant to replace years of professional training or to simply provide questions so that students may pass the exams if they memorize the answers. Instead, this book will help direct students to the topic areas they may need to further review and will strengthen students' knowledge and exam-taking skills.

Dental schools generally do well in preparing their students for practice and for board exams. Usually, there is a good correlation between students who do well in their dental courses and those who score well on their board exams. Therefore to best prepare for board exams, students should focus on doing well in their course work. It is in the students' best interest to focus more board exam study time on the areas in which they have not performed as well in their dental coursework. Most students are aware of their areas of weakness and therefore will have the opportunity to focus more resources on these areas when studying for boards.

Helpful Hints for Preparing to Take Your Board Examinations

1. Pace yourself and make a study schedule. As when taking a course, it is always better to give yourself sufficient assimilation time rather than "cramming" over a short period of time, and if you start studying early enough, you should not have to make major changes in your daily schedule.
2. Study in a quiet environment similar to that in which the test is given. Stick to your schedule and minimize distractions to avoid last minute panic and the urge to "cram."
3. Know your weaknesses and focus more of your resources on strengthening these areas. Look back at your grades from the courses that relate to the exam topics. These will indicate areas that need more attention. Also, use this book as a trial run to help point to content areas that may need more review.
4. Many find practice exams useful. You can employ practice exams in several ways: study with others by asking each other questions; test yourself with flashcards or notes that are partially covered from view; or answer questions from this text. In each case, be sure to check your answer to find out whether you achieved the correct answer. Each section of this review book has practice exam questions. There is also a sample exam with questions from each discipline. This book also contains explanations as to why an answer is a correct answer and why the distracters are not. See if these explanations agree with the reasons for making your selections. The questions are written in the formats used on the National Boards including the new formats of matching, ordering, and multiple correct/multiple responses.
5. Block off time for practice examinations, such as the review questions and sample exam in this text. Time yourself and practice your test speed; then compare your time to the estimated time needed to complete each section of the NBDE.
6. If your school offers board reviews, we highly recommend taking them. These may assist you with building your confidence with what material you have already mastered and may help you focus on material that you need to spend more time studying.
7. Stay positive about the board exam. If you prepare well, you should do well on the exam. Besides, think of all the people who have preceded you and have passed the exam. What has been done can be done. Consider making a study group composed of people who will be good study partners and who are able to help the other members in the group review and build confidence in taking the exam.
8. Exams are administered by the Joint National Commission on Dental Education (JNCDE) contracting with Prometric, Inc. (Prometric.com) at various testing centers. Exams are taken electronically. Students seeking to take the National Board Exam must be approved by their Dean, who recommends eligibility for the exam to JNCDE. More information on the exam is available at the American Dental Association (ADA) website.

Helpful Hints During the Taking of Examinations

1. It is important to note that questions that are considered "good" questions by examination standards will have incorrect choices in their answer bank that are very close to the correct answer. These wrong choices are called "distracters:" they are meant to determine

those who have the best knowledge of the subject. The present NBDE review questions should be used to help the test taker better discriminate similar choices, as an impetus to review a subject more intensively. (Distractors in questions on the actual board exam help determine which students have the best knowledge of the subject.) Most test takers do better by reading the question and trying to determine the answer before looking at the answer bank. Therefore consider trying to answer questions without looking at the answer bank.

2. Eliminate answers that are obviously wrong. This will allow a better chance of picking the correct answer and reduce distraction from the wrong answers.

3. Only go back and change an answer if you are absolutely certain you were wrong with your previous choice, or if a different question in the same exam provides you with the correct answer.

4. Read questions carefully. Note carefully any negative words in questions, such as "except," "not," and "false." If these words are missed when reading the question, it is nearly impossible to get the correct answer; noting these key words will make sure you do not miss them.

5. If you are stuck on one question, consider treating the answer bank like a series of true/false items relevant to the question. Most people consider true/false questions easier than multiple choice. At least if you can eliminate a few choices, you will have a better chance at selecting the correct answer from whatever is left.

6. Never leave blanks, unless the specific exam has a penalty for wrong answers. It is better to choose incorrectly than leave an item blank. Check with those giving the examination to find out whether there are penalties for marking the wrong answer.

7. Some people do better on exams by going through the exam and answering known questions first, and then returning to the more difficult questions later. This helps to build confidence during the exam. This also helps the test taker avoid spending too much time on a few questions and running out of time on less difficult questions that may be at the end. In addition, you may find additional insight to the correct answer in other exam questions later in the exam.

8. Pace yourself during the exam. Determine ahead of time how much time each question will take to answer. Do not rush, but do not spend too much time on one question. Sometimes it is better to move to the next question and come back to the difficult ones later, since a fresh look is sometimes helpful.

9. Bring appropriate supplies to the exam, such as reading glasses, appropriate for a computer screen. If you get distracted by noise, consider bringing ear plugs. It is inevitable that someone will take the exam next to the person in the squeaky chair, or the one with the sniffling runny nose. Most exams will provide you with instructions as to what you may or may not bring to the exam. Be sure to read these instructions in advance.

10. Make sure that once you have completed the exam all questions are appropriately answered. Review before you submit your answers electronically.

11. Presently, the part I exam is constructed as follows;

Description	# of Items	Time
Optional Tutorial	NA	15 minutes
Discipline-based, multiple-choice test items with 3-5 testlets (Testlets contain patient cases with related questions.)	~200	3.5 hours
Optional scheduled break	NA	One hour max.
Discipline-based, multiple-choice test items with 3-5 testlets	~200	3.5 hours
Optional Post-examination Survey	NA	15 minutes

Helpful Hints for the Post-Examination Period

It may be a good idea to think about what you will be doing after the exam.

1. Most people are exhausted after taking board exams. Some reasons for this exhaustion may be the number of hours, the mental focus, and the anxiety that exams cause some people. Be aware that you may be tired, so avoid planning anything that one should not do when exhausted, such as driving across the country, operating heavy machinery or power tools, or studying for final exams. Instead, plan a day or two to recuperate before you tackle any heavier physical or mental tasks.

2. Consider a debriefing or "detoxification" meeting with your positive study partners after the exam. Talking about the exam afterwards may help reduce stress. However, remember that the feelings one has after an exam may not always match the exam score (e.g., students who feel they did poorly may have done well, or students who feel they did well may not have.)

3. Consider doing something nice for yourself. After all, you will have just completed a major exam. It is important to celebrate this accomplishment.

We wish you the very best with taking your exams and trust that this text will provide you with an excellent training tool for your preparations.

Additional Resources

This review text is intended to aid the study and retention of dental sciences in preparation for the National Board Dental Examination. It is not intended to be a substitute for a complete dental education curriculum. For a truly comprehensive understanding of the basic dental sciences, please consult these supplemental texts.

Anatomical Basis of Dentistry, Third Edition
Bernard Liebgott

Anatomy of Orofacial Structures, Seventh Edition
Richard W. Brand, Donald E. Isselhard

Rapid Review Gross and Developmental Anatomy, Third Edition
N. Anthony Moore, William A. Roy

Berne & Levy Physiology, Sixth Edition
Bruce M. Koeppen, Bruce A. Stanton

Medical Biochemistry, Third Edition
John W Baynes, Marek H Dominiczak

Illustrated Anatomy of the Head and Neck, Fourth Edition
Margaret J. Fehrenbach, Susan W. Herring

Illustrated Dental Embryology, Histology, and Anatomy, Third Edition
Mary Bath-Balogh, Margaret J. Fehrenbach

Molecular Cell Biology, Seventh Edition
Harvey Lodish, Arnold Berk, Chris A. Kaiser, Monty Krieger

Oral Anatomy, Histology & Embryology, Fourth Edition
Barry K. B. Berkovitz, G. R. Holland, Bernard. J. Moxham

Guyton and Hall Textbook of Medical Physiology, Eleventh Edition
John E. Hall

Wheeler's Dental Anatomy, Physiology, and Occlusion, Ninth Edition
Stanley J. Nelson, Major M. Ash Jr.

Management of Temporomandibular Disorders and Occlusion, Seventh Edition
Jeffery P. Okeson

Medical Microbiology, Seventh Edition
Patrick Murray, Ken Rosenthal, and Michael Pfaller

Robins and Cotran Pathologic Basis of Disease, Eighth Edition
Vinay Kumar, Abul K. Abbas, Nelson Fausto, Jon C. Astor

Oral and Maxillofacial Pathology
Brad W. Neville, Douglas D. Damm, Carl C. Allen, Jerry E. Bouquot

Contents

Anatomic Sciences

JOSEPH W. ROBERTSON

OUTLINE

The anatomic sciences portion of the National Dental Boards tests the following: gross anatomy, histology, and embryology. Gross anatomy encompasses a wide range of topics, including bones, muscles, fasciae, nerves, circulation, spaces, and cavities. Details and diagrams focus on topics emphasized on the National Dental Boards. Because it is outside the scope of this book to cover every detail, it is recommended that you refer to class notes, anatomy texts and atlases, and previous examinations for a more thorough understanding of the information presented. A limited number of figures and diagrams are included in this text. It will be helpful to you to refer to other anatomy texts and atlases for additional figures and diagrams.

1.0 Gross Anatomy

1.1 Head and Neck

1.1.1 Oral Cavity

Vascular Supply

The main blood supply to the head and neck is from the subclavian and common carotid arteries. The origins of these arteries differs for the right and left sides. On the right side, the brachiocephalic trunk branches off and bifurcates into the right subclavian artery and right common carotid artery. On the left side, the left common carotid artery and left subclavian artery branch off separately from the arch of the aorta.

A. Subclavian artery.
  1. Origin: the right subclavian artery arises from the brachiocephalic trunk. The left subclavian artery arises directly from the arch of the aorta.

2. Important divisions.
  a. Vertebral artery—supplies the brain (refer to Internal Carotid section).
  b. Internal thoracic artery—descends to supply the diaphragm and terminates as the superior epigastric artery, which helps supply the abdominal wall.
  c. Thyrocervical or cervicothyroid trunk—divides into three arteries: suprascapular artery, transverse cervical artery, and inferior thyroid artery.
  d. Costocervical trunk—divides into two branches, superior intercostals and deep cervical arteries, which supply muscles of intercostal spaces.
  e. Dorsal scapular artery—supplies the muscles of the scapular region.
B. Common carotid artery.
  1. Origin: the right common carotid branches from the brachiocephalic trunk. The left common carotid branches from the arch of the aorta.
  2. The common carotid ascends within a fibrous sheath in the neck, known as the *carotid sheath*. This sheath also contains the internal jugular vein and the vagus nerve (CN X).
  3. Major branches.
    a. Both the right and the left common carotid arteries bifurcate into the internal and external carotid arteries.
    b. Note: the carotid sinus baroreceptors are located at this bifurcation. These baroreceptors help monitor systemic blood pressure and are innervated by the glossopharyngeal nerve (CN IX).
C. External carotid artery (Figure 1-1, *A*).
  1. Branches of the external carotid artery supply tissues of the head and neck, including the oral cavity.
  2. Origin: the external carotid artery branches from the common carotid artery.
  3. Major branches.
    a. Superior thyroid artery.
      (1) Origin: branches from the anterior side of the external carotid artery, just above the carotid bifurcation.

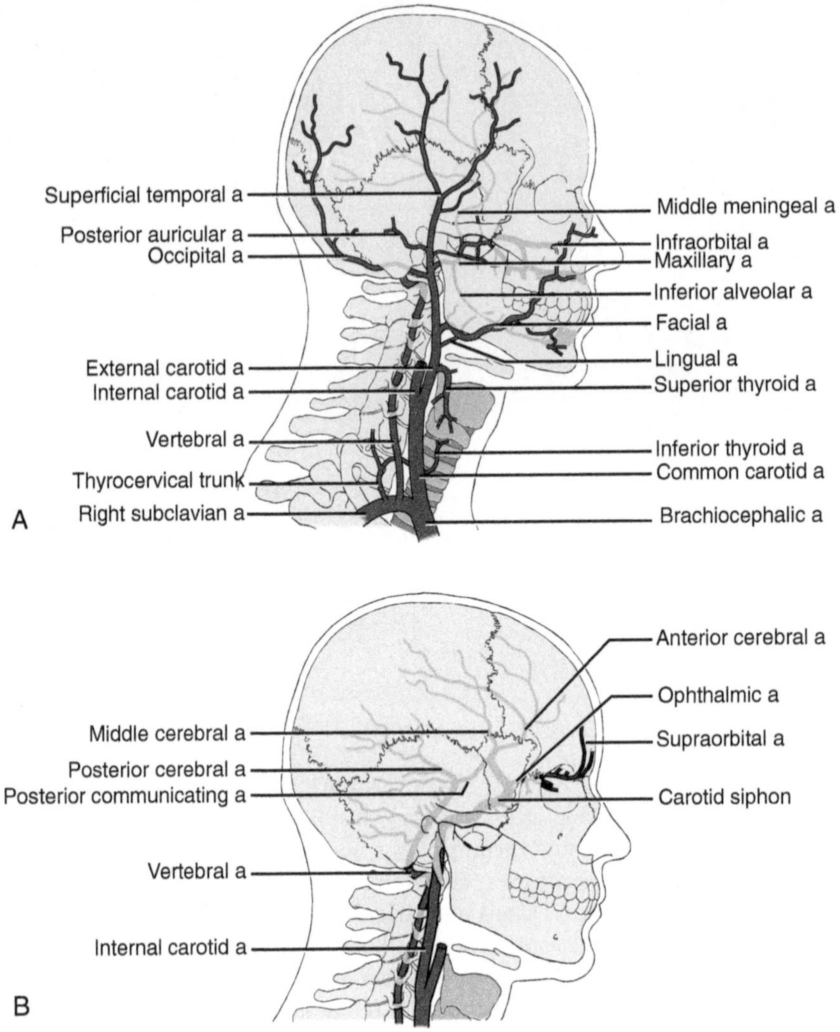

Figure 1-1 Arteries of the head and neck. **A,** Right external carotid artery and its branches. **B,** Right internal carotid and vertebral arteries and their branches within the skull. *(From Liebgott B: The Anatomical Basis of Dentistry, ed 3, St. Louis, Mosby, 2011.)*

(2) Major branches.
  (a) Infrahyoid artery—supplies the infrahyoid muscles.
  (b) Sternocleidomastoid (SCM) artery—supplies a portion of the SCM muscle.
  (c) Superior laryngeal artery—pierces through the thyrohyoid membrane, with the internal laryngeal nerve, as it travels to supply the muscles of the larynx.
  (d) Cricothyroid artery—supplies the thyroid gland.
b. Lingual artery.
  (1) Origin: branches from the anterior side of the external carotid artery, near the hyoid bone. It often arises along with the facial artery, forming the linguofacial trunk. It travels anteriorly between the hyoglossus and middle pharyngeal constrictor muscles.
  (2) Major branches.
  (a) Suprahyoid artery—supplies the suprahyoid muscles.
  (b) Dorsal lingual artery—supplies the tongue, tonsils, and soft palate.
  (c) Sublingual artery—supplies the floor of the mouth, mylohyoid muscle, and sublingual gland.
  (d) Deep lingual artery—supplies the tongue.
c. Facial artery.
  (1) Origin: branches from the anterior side of the external carotid, just above the lingual artery.
  (2) Major branches and the structures they supply are listed in Table 1-1.
d. Ascending pharyngeal artery.
  (1) Origin: branches from the anterior side of the external carotid artery, just above the superior thyroid artery.
  (2) Branches supply the pharynx, soft palate, and meninges.
e. Occipital artery.
  (1) Origin: branches from the posterior side of the external carotid, close to the hypoglossal nerve (CN XII).

(2) Branches supply the SCM and suprahyoid muscles, dura mater, meninges, and occipital portion of the scalp.

f. Posterior auricular artery.

(1) Origin: branches from the posterior side of the external carotid, near the level of the styloid process and superior to the stylohyoid muscle.

(2) Branches supply the mastoid air cells, stapedius muscle, and internal ear.

g. Maxillary artery.

(1) Origin: branches from the external carotid in the parotid gland and travels between the mandibular ramus and sphenomandibular ligament before reaching the infratemporal and pterygopalatine fossa. From there, the artery divides around the lateral pterygoid muscle into three major branches—mandibular, pterygoid, and pterygopalatine divisions (Figure 1-2, Table 1-2).

(2) Branches of the mandibular division.

(a) Deep auricular artery and anterior tympanic artery—supply the tympanic membrane.

(b) Inferior alveolar artery (IAA)—the IAA has the same branches and anatomic pathway as its corresponding nerve, the inferior alveolar nerve (IAN), a branch of CN V_3 (refer to the IAN sensory pathway in the Cranial Nerves section) and terminates as the mental artery.

(c) Middle meningeal and accessory arteries—the middle meningeal artery travels through the foramen spinosum to supply the meninges of the brain and dural lining of bones in the skull.

(3) Branches of the pterygoid division.

(a) Deep temporal arteries—supply the temporalis muscle.

(b) Pterygoid arteries—supply the medial and lateral pterygoid muscles.

(c) Masseteric artery—supplies the masseter.

(d) Buccal artery—supplies the buccinator and buccal mucosa.

(4) Branches of the pterygopalatine division.

(a) The pterygopalatine division follows the pterygomaxillary fissure into the pterygopalatine fossa, where the artery divides. Its major divisions include the posterior

Table 1-1	
Major Branches of the Facial Artery and the Structures They Supply	
BRANCHES	**STRUCTURES SUPPLIED**
Ascending palatine artery	Soft palate, tonsils, pharynx
Tonsillar artery	Tonsils, tongue
Glandular artery	Submandibular gland
Submental artery	Submandibular gland, mylohyoid and anterior digastric muscle
Inferior labial artery	Lower lip
Superior labial artery	Upper lip
Lateral nasal artery	Nose
Angular artery	Eyelids, nose

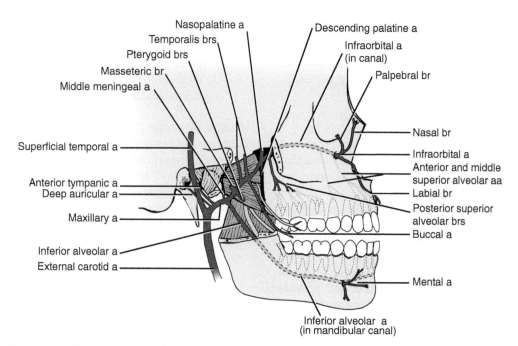

Figure 1-2 Branches of the maxillary artery. *(From Liebgott B: The Anatomical Basis of Dentistry, ed 3, St. Louis, Mosby, 2011.)*

Table 1-2

Branches of Three Major Divisions of the Maxillary Artery and the Structures They Supply

BRANCHES OF THREE MAJOR DIVISIONS	STRUCTURES SUPPLIED
Mandibular Division	
Inferior alveolar artery (IAA) branches	
Deep auricular artery	Tympanic membrane
Anterior tympanic artery	Tympanic membrane
IAA (dental branches)	Mandibular posterior teeth and surrounding tissues
Mylohyoid artery	Mylohyoid muscle, floor of mouth
Incisive artery	Anterior teeth and surrounding tissues
Mental artery	Chin, lower lip
Middle meningeal artery	Meninges of the brain, dura of bones in the skull
Pterygoid division	
Deep temporal arteries	Temporalis muscle
Pterygoid arteries	Pterygoid muscles
Masseteric artery	Masseter
Buccal artery	Buccinator, buccal mucosa
Pterygopalatine division	
Posterior superior alveolar artery	Maxillary posterior teeth, maxillary sinus
Infraorbital artery, including anterior and middle superior alveolar, orbital, and facial branches	Maxillary anterior teeth, orbital area, and lacrimal gland
Greater palatine artery	Hard palate, lingual gingiva of maxillary posterior teeth
Lesser palatine artery	Soft palate, tonsils
Sphenopalatine artery	Nasal cavity

superior alveolar artery, the greater and lesser palatine arteries, and the infraorbital artery. All of these branches travel and divide with their corresponding nerves to the structures they vascularize. For their anatomic pathways, refer to the sensory pathways of their corresponding nerves in the Cranial Nerves section.

(b) Posterior superior alveolar artery—supplies the maxillary sinus, molar, and premolar teeth as well as the neighboring gingiva.

(c) Descending palatine artery—drops inferiorly and divides into the greater palatine artery and lesser palatine artery.

(d) Sphenopalatine artery—branches in the pterygopalatine fossa and travels to the nasal cavity, where it branches to supply surrounding structures. Note: it is most commonly associated with serious nosebleeds in the posterior nasal cavity.

(e) Infraorbital artery—terminates as nasal and palpebral branches of the maxillary artery. Its branches supply the orbital region, facial tissues, and maxillary sinus and maxillary anterior teeth (via the anterior superior alveolar artery).

(f) Superficial temporal artery—terminal branch of the external carotid artery.

D. Internal carotid artery (see Figure 1-1, *B*).
　1. Origin: the internal carotid divides from the common carotid artery and continues in the carotid sheath into the cranium. In contrast to the external carotid artery, it has no branches in the neck.
　2. Branches of the internal carotid artery as well as the vertebral arteries serve as the major blood supply for the brain.
　3. Major branches.
　　a. Anterior and middle cerebral arteries: the internal carotid terminates into these two arteries. These arteries anastomose with the posterior and anterior communicating arteries to form the circle of Willis. The circle of Willis also communicates with the vertebral arteries via the basilar and posterior cerebral arteries.
　　b. Pathology notes: berry aneurysms most commonly occur in the circle of Willis, particularly in the anterior communicating and anterior cerebral arteries. Strokes often occur from a diseased middle cerebral artery.
　　c. Supraorbital artery—leaves the orbit through the supraorbital notch. Branches supply the upper eyelid, forehead, and scalp.
　　d. Ophthalmic artery—supplies the orbital area and lacrimal gland.

Venous Drainage

Deoxygenated blood from the head and neck is drained by a network of veins that eventually terminate in the jugular veins. The blood from the jugular veins is ultimately returned to the heart via the subclavian and brachiocephalic veins, which join to form the superior vena cava.

A. Veins of the neck: jugular veins.
　1. Internal jugular vein.
　　a. The internal jugular vein serves as the major source of venous drainage of deoxygenated blood from the head and neck region. This region consists of both extracranial tissues and intracranial structures, including the brain.
　　b. Termination: the internal jugular vein travels down within the carotid sheath and joins the subclavian

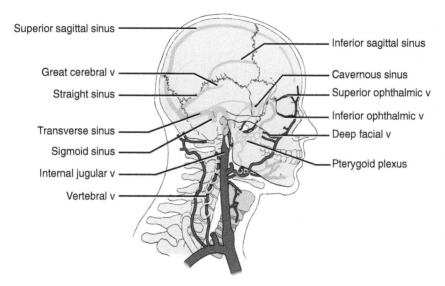

Superior sagittal sinus
Great cerebral v
Straight sinus
Transverse sinus
Sigmoid sinus
Internal jugular v
Vertebral v

Inferior sagittal sinus
Cavernous sinus
Superior ophthalmic v
Inferior ophthalmic v
Deep facial v
Pterygoid plexus

Figure 1-3 Deep veins of the head and neck and communications with the facial vein. *(From Liebgott B: The Anatomical Basis of Dentistry, ed 3, St. Louis, Mosby, 2011.)*

vein to form the brachiocephalic vein and its tributaries, including the intracranial venous sinuses, lingual vein, pharyngeal vein, occipital vein, common facial vein, superior thyroid vein, and middle thyroid vein. The brachiocephalic vein terminates in the superior vena cava, which empties into the right atrium of the heart.

2. External jugular vein.
   a. The external jugular vein drains extracranial tissues from the head and face.
   b. Termination: the external jugular vein terminates into the subclavian vein and its tributaries, including the posterior division of the retromandibular vein, posterior auricular vein, transverse cervical vein, suprascapular vein, and anterior jugular vein.
B. Veins of the cranium: venous drainage of the brain.
   1. Deoxygenated blood drains from the brain through a series of dural sinuses.
   2. Pathways of deoxygenated blood: blood from the superior sagittal sinus, inferior sagittal sinus (via the straight sinus), and occipital sinuses drains at the confluence of sinuses, which is located in the posterior cranium. From here, the blood flows through the transverse sinuses to the sigmoid sinuses, which ultimately empty into the internal jugular vein (Figure 1-3).
   3. Note: cerebrospinal fluid is drained via reabsorption into the superior sagittal sinus.
C. Veins of the face: venous drainage of the face and oral cavity.
   1. Facial vein.
      a. Serves as the major source of venous drainage for superficial facial structures, or the same areas that are supplied by the facial artery.

   b. Termination: the facial vein joins with the retromandibular vein to form the common facial vein, which drains into the internal jugular vein.
   c. Tributaries: supratrochlear, supraorbital, nasal, superior and inferior labial, muscular, submental, tonsillar, and submandibular veins.
   d. Dental significance: because the facial vein has no valves to maintain the direction of blood flow and it communicates with the cavernous sinus via the superior ophthalmic and deep facial vein, infection from the facial vein can travel to the cavernous sinus and cause severe medical problems.
2. Superior and inferior ophthalmic veins.
   a. Drain tissues of the orbit.
   b. Communicate with the facial vein via the supraorbital vein.
   c. Termination: facial vein and cavernous sinus.
3. Retromandibular veins.
   a. Formed by the joining of the maxillary and superficial temporal veins in the parotid gland.
   b. Termination: the retromandibular vein bifurcates into an anterior and posterior division. The anterior division descends and joins the facial vein to become the common facial vein, which terminates into the internal jugular vein. The posterior division terminates into the external jugular vein.
4. Pterygoid plexus.
   a. A network of veins located at the level of the pterygoid muscles that drains deoxygenated blood from deep facial tissues, including the intraoral cavity, and the meninges.
   b. Termination: drains into the retromandibular vein via the maxillary veins.

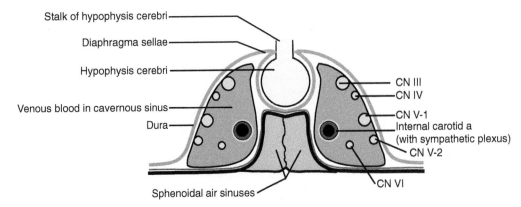

Stalk of hypophysis cerebri
Diaphragma sellae
Hypophysis cerebri
Venous blood in cavernous sinus
Dura
Sphenoidal air sinuses
CN III
CN IV
CN V-1
Internal carotid a (with sympathetic plexus)
CN V-2
CN VI

Figure 1-4 Coronal section through cavernous sinuses to show their content and relationships. *CN,* Cranial nerve. *(From Liebgott B: The Anatomical Basis of Dentistry, ed 3, St. Louis, Mosby, 2011.)*

c. Tributaries: middle meningeal, infraorbital, sphenopalatine, muscular, buccal, palatine, inferior alveolar, and deep facial veins.

5. Cavernous sinuses.
   a. Located on both sides of the sella turcica of the sphenoid bone. The right and left cavernous sinuses are joined by the intercavernous sinuses.
   b. Tributaries: ophthalmic and external cerebral veins, sphenoparietal sinuses, and pterygoid plexuses.
   c. Structures running through the cavernous sinus include CN III, CN IV, CN V_1, CN V_2, CN VI, and the internal carotid artery (Figure 1-4). Note: these nerves and the structures they innervate can be affected by a cavernous sinus infection.
   d. Termination: the superior and inferior petrosal sinuses. The petrosal sinuses ultimately drain into the internal jugular vein.
   e. Cavernous sinus thrombosis: because blood flow in the cavernous sinus is slow moving, dental or eye infections that spread to the cavernous sinuses can result in an infective blood clot, called *cavernous sinus thrombosis.* This condition can result in an urgent, possibly fatal, medical emergency. The infection has the potential to spread as a result of certain venous communications with the cavernous sinus.
      (1) Superior ophthalmic vein—drains into the cavernous sinus. The superior ophthalmic vein can also act as a passageway for infection to spread from the facial vein to the cavernous sinus because they are joined via the angular vein.
      (2) Deep facial vein—drains into the pterygoid plexus of veins, which drains into the cavernous sinus. The deep facial vein is a tributary of the facial vein.

Lymphatic Drainage

A. Lymphatic drainage of the head and neck is accomplished through a series of lymphatic vessels and lymph nodes. Lymph from a region is first drained into a primary lymph node and then a secondary lymph node and ultimately ends up in the venous circulation (Figure 1-5).

1. Superficial lymph nodes (Table 1-3).
   a. Submandibular nodes.
      (1) Located beneath the angle of the mandible.
      (2) Secondary node: the submandibular nodes drain into the deep cervical lymph nodes.
      (3) Tissues drained include the lower eyelids, nose, cheek, maxillary sinus, upper lip, palate, sublingual and submandibular glands, tongue body, all of the maxillary teeth except the third molar, and all of the mandibular teeth except the incisors.
   b. Submental nodes.
      (1) Located beneath the chin.
      (2) Secondary node: lymph from the submental lymph nodes drains into the submandibular or deep cervical lymph nodes.
      (3) Tissues drained include the lower lip, mandibular incisors, anterior floor of the mouth, tip of the tongue, and the chin.
   c. Parotid (preauricular) nodes.
      (1) Located on the surface of the parotid gland.
      (2) Secondary node: deep cervical lymph nodes.
      (3) Tissues drained include the scalp, eyelids, external ear, and lacrimal gland.
   d. Mastoid (postauricular) nodes.
      (1) Located adjacent to the mastoid process.
      (2) Secondary node: deep cervical nodes.
      (3) Tissues drained include the scalp and external ear.
   e. Occipital nodes.
      (1) Located at the occipital region of the skull.
      (2) Secondary node: deep cervical nodes.
      (3) Tissues drained include the scalp.
2. Deep lymph nodes (Table 1-4).
   a. Retropharyngeal nodes.
      (1) Located within the retropharyngeal space.
      (2) Secondary node: superior deep cervical nodes.

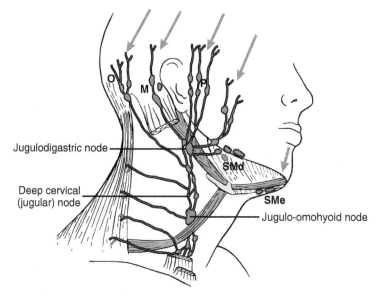

Figure 1-5 Lymphatic drainage of the face. *M,* Mastoid (postauricular) nodes; *O,* occipital nodes; *P,* parotid (preauricular) nodes; *SMd,* submandibular nodes; *SMe,* submental nodes. *(From Liebgott B: The Anatomical Basis of Dentistry, ed 3, St. Louis, Mosby, 2011.)*

Table 1-3		
Superficial Lymph Nodes		
PRIMARY NODE	**TISSUES DRAINED**	**SECONDARY NODE**
Submandibular nodes	Lower eyelids Nose Cheek Maxillary sinus Upper lip Palate Sublingual gland Submandibular gland Maxillary teeth except third molar Mandibular teeth except incisors Tongue body	Deep cervical nodes
Submental nodes	Lower lip Mandibular incisors Floor of the mouth Tip of the tongue Chin	Submandibular or deep cervical nodes
Parotid (preauricular) nodes	Scalp Eyelids External ear Lacrimal gland	Deep cervical nodes
Postauricular nodes	Scalp External ear	Deep cervical nodes
Occipital nodes	Scalp	Deep cervical nodes

---

(3) Tissues drained include the hard and soft palate, middle ear, external auditory meatus, paranasal sinuses, nasopharynx, and posterior nasal cavity.

3. Deep parotid nodes.
   a. Located within the parotid gland.
   b. Secondary node: deep cervical nodes.
   c. Tissues drained include the parotid gland and middle ear.

4. Deep cervical nodes.
   a. The chain of deep cervical nodes extends vertically down the entire length of the neck. They receive lymph from both superficial and deep lymph nodes.
   b. Termination.
      (1) The left deep cervical chains form the left jugular lymph trunk, which terminates in the thoracic duct.

Table 1-4

Deep Lymph Nodes

	LOCATION	STRUCTURES DRAINED
Superior deep cervical lymph nodes	Inferior to anterior border of sternocleidomastoid muscles	Maxillary third molars Nasal cavity Palate Tongue
Deep parotid nodes	Middle ear Parotid gland	Deep cervical nodes
Retropharyngeal lymph nodes	Posterior pharynx, at level of C1 vertebrae	Nasal cavity Palate Sinuses Pharynx

---

Table 1-5

Cranial Nerves

	NERVE	SENSORY	MOTOR	PARASYMPATHETIC
CN I	Olfactory	X	—	—
CN II	Optic	X	—	—
CN III	Oculomotor	—	X	X
CN IV	Trochlear	—	X	—
CN V	Trigeminal	X	X	—
CN VI	Abducens	—	X	—
CN VII	Facial	X	X	X
CN VIII	Vestibulocochlear	X	—	—
CN IX	Glossopharyngeal	X	X	X
CN X	Vagus	X	X	X
CN XI	Accessory	—	X	—
CN XII	Hypoglossal	—	X	—

CN, Cranial nerve.

---

(2) The right deep cervical chains form the right jugular lymph trunk, which terminates in the right lymphatic duct.

1.1.2 Cranial Nerves

Basic Principles and Definitions

A. Basic principles and definitions.
1. There are 12 cranial nerves (Table 1-5).
2. Function: cranial nerves function as sensory or motor neurons, or both. Four cranial nerves (CN III, CN VII, CN IX, and CN X) also have parasympathetic functions (see Table 1-5).
3. Foramen: a hole in bone. In this context, it specifically refers to the opening where a particular nerve passes through a hole in the skull.
4. Ganglion: group of nerve cell bodies found outside the central nervous system (CNS).
5. Reflexes: cranial nerves also serve as afferent and efferent nerves for certain reflexes associated with the

Table 1-6

Reflexes

	AFFERENT	EFFERENT
Corneal (blink) reflex	CN V_1	CN VII
Gag reflex	CN IX	CN X
Jaw jerk	CN V_3	CN V_3
Oculocardiac reflex	CN V_1	CN X

CN, Cranial nerve.

head and neck. These nerve reflexes are summarized in Table 1-6.

B. Cranial nerve mnemonics.
1. Cranial nerves: "Oh, Oh, Oh, To Touch and Feel Very Good, Very Awesome Humps."
2. Function: "Some Say Marry Money, But My Brother Says Big Brains Matter More." CN I is Sensory, CN II

is *Sensory*, CN III is *Motor*, CN IV is *Motor*, CN V is *Both* sensory and motor, and so forth.

Cranial Nerve Nuclei

A. Cranial nerve nuclei.
   1. Nucleus: a group of nerve cell bodies in the CNS.
   2. Brainstem organization.
      a. The brainstem plays a major role in transmitting information from the cranial nerves to and from the brain. The brainstem can be divided into three parts: midbrain, pons, and medulla.
      b. Cell bodies of cranial nerves that share common functions are grouped into different clusters or nuclei. These motor and sensory nuclei are scattered throughout the brainstem and cervical spinal cord.
      c. The cranial nerve nuclei are listed in Tables 1-7 and 1-8.

Table 1-7

Cranial Nerve Motor Nuclei

	CRANIAL NERVES	MIDBRAIN	PONS	MEDULLA	FUNCTION
Oculomotor nuclei	III	X	—	—	Motor
Edinger-Westphal nucleus	III	X	—	—	Autonomic (parasympathetic)
Trochlear nucleus	IV	X	—	—	Motor
Trigeminal motor nucleus	V	—	X	—	Motor
Abducens nucleus	VI	—	X	—	Motor
Facial (motor) nucleus	VII	—	X	—	Motor
Superior salivatory nucleus	VII	—	X	—	Motor (secretory)
Nucleus ambiguus	IX, X, and XI	—	—	X	Motor
Dorsal motor nucleus of the vagus	X	—	—	X	Motor and autonomic (parasympathetic)
Hypoglossal nucleus	XII	—	—	X	Motor
Accessory nucleus	XI	*Located in the cervical spinal cord*			Motor

Table 1-8

Cranial Nerve Sensory Nuclei

	CRANIAL NERVES	MIDBRAIN	PONS	MEDULLA	FUNCTION
Mesencephalic nucleus	V	X	X	—	Proprioception, jaw jerk reflex, including periodontal ligament fibers involved in the reflex
Trigeminal main (chief) sensory nuclei, or descending tract of CN V	V	—	X	—	Sensory function of CN V, including touch on the face Blink reflex
Cochlear nucleus	VIII	—	X	—	Sensory function of CN VIII, including hearing
Vestibular nucleus	VIII	—	X	X	Sensory function of CN VIII, including body positioning and equilibrium
Spinal trigeminal nucleus	V	—	X	X	Sensory of CN V, including pain and temperature. Contains fibers of primary sensory neurons
Nucleus of solitary tract, or solitary nucleus	VII, IX and X	—	X	X	Sensory of CN VII, IX, and X, including taste

CN, Cranial nerve.

Cranial Nerves
A. CN I: olfactory nerve.
  1. Foramen: cribriform plate of ethmoid bone.
  2. Sensory distribution: smell.
  3. Anatomic pathway: from the nasal epithelium, olfactory nerves cross the cribriform plate to join the olfactory bulb in the brain.
B. CN II: optic nerve.
  1. Foramen: optic canal.
  2. Sensory distribution: vision.
  3. Anatomic pathway: there are two optic nerves. Each optic nerve consists of medial (nasal) and lateral (temporal) processes. When the right optic nerve leaves the retina, its medial process crosses over the midline at the optic chiasma and joins the lateral process from the left side, forming the left optic tract. The right lateral process remains on the right side and together with the left medial process forms the right optic tract. The optic tract continues to the lateral geniculate body of the thalamus.
  4. Note: the central artery of the retina, a branch of the ophthalmic artery, courses through the optic nerve.
C. CN III: oculomotor nerve.
  1. Foramen: superior orbital fissure.
  2. Somatic efferent motor distribution: superior, medial, and inferior rectus muscles; inferior oblique muscle; and levator palpebrae superioris, which raises the eyelid.
  3. Motor pathway: oculomotor nerve fibers run through the oculomotor nucleus in the midbrain to the extrinsic eye muscles.
  4. Visceral efferent parasympathetic distribution: lacrimal gland, sphincter pupillae, and ciliary lens muscles. The last two control the pupillary light reflex (constricts pupil) and shape of the lens (constricts for near vision), respectively.
  5. Parasympathetic pathway: preganglionic nerve fibers originate at the Edinger-Westphal nucleus in the midbrain and are carried by the oculomotor nerve to the ciliary ganglion, where postganglionic neurons extend to the lacrimal gland and eye.
  6. Mnemonic: all eye muscles are innervated by CN III (oculomotor) except SO_4 and LR_6 (i.e., the superior oblique is innervated by CN IV, and lateral rectus is innervated by CN VI).
D. CN IV: trochlear nerve.
  1. Foramen: superior orbital fissure.
  2. Motor distribution: superior oblique muscle, which moves the eyeball laterally and downward.
E. CN V: trigeminal nerve.
  1. Three divisions: ophthalmic, maxillary, and mandibular.
  2. V_1—ophthalmic nerve.
    a. Foramen: superior orbital fissure.
    b. Sensory distribution: cornea, eyes, nose, forehead, and paranasal sinuses.
    c. Sensory pathway: the ophthalmic nerve branches from the trigeminal ganglion and exits the skull via the superior orbital fissure. It divides into three major nerves: frontal, lacrimal, and nasociliary nerves.
  3. V_2—maxillary nerve.
    a. Foramen: foramen rotundum.
    b. Sensory distribution: cheek, lower eyelid, upper lip, nasopharynx, tonsils, palate, and maxillary teeth.
    c. Sensory pathway: the maxillary nerve branches from the trigeminal ganglion and exits the skull through the foramen rotundum. It passes through the pterygopalatine fossa, where it communicates with the pterygopalatine ganglion and terminates as the infraorbital and zygomatic nerves (Figure 1-6, Table 1-9).
    d. Pterygopalatine ganglion: communicating branches suspend from the maxillary nerve. Branches consist of sensory, sympathetic, and parasympathetic fibers and include nerves traveling to the lacrimal gland, oral cavity, upper pharynx, and nasal cavity.
    e. Infraorbital nerve: the posterior superior alveolar nerve branches off the infraorbital nerve in the pterygopalatine fossa. The infraorbital nerve passes through the inferior orbital fissure to enter the orbit floor, coursing along the infraorbital groove toward the infraorbital canal. In the canal, the middle superior and anterior superior alveolar nerves branch off. The infraorbital nerve exits the maxilla via the infraorbital foramen and divides into inferior palpebral, lateral nasal, and superior labial branches.
    f. Zygomatic nerve: after branching from the maxillary nerve, the zygomatic nerve passes through the orbit after entering from the superior orbital fissure. A nerve branches off to the lacrimal gland, carrying with it parasympathetic fibers from the pterygopalatine ganglion (CN VII). The zygomatic nerve continues into the zygomatic canal, where it divides into the zygomaticofacial and zygomaticotemporal nerves. It also travels to the lacrimal gland.
    g. Greater and lesser palatine nerves: the palatine nerves branch from the pterygopalatine ganglion and descend down the pterygopalatine canal toward the posterior palate.
    h. Nasal branches: lateral nasal branches divide from the pterygopalatine ganglion toward the posterior nasal cavity. One of these branches, the nasopalatine nerve, extends past the septum, through the nasopalatine canal, and enters through the palate via the nasopalatine foramen. It also connects with the greater palatine nerve near the canine region.

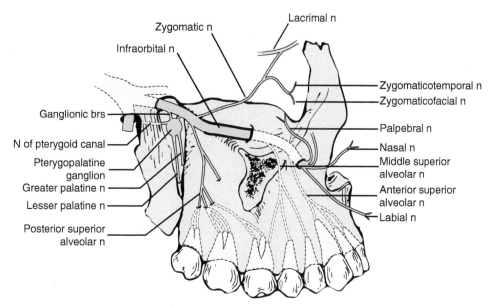

Figure 1-6 The maxillary nerve and its branches. *(From Liebgott B: The Anatomical Basis of Dentistry, ed 3, St. Louis, Mosby, 2011.)*

Table 1-9

Branches of the Maxillary Nerve (Cranial Nerve V₂)

V₂ BRANCH	FUNCTION	DISTRIBUTION
Posterior superior alveolar nerve	Sensory	Maxillary second and third molars Maxillary first molar: palatal and distobuccal root Maxillary sinus
Middle superior alveolar nerve	Sensory	Maxillary first and second premolars Maxillary first molar: mesiobuccal root
Anterior superior alveolar nerve	Sensory	Maxillary anterior teeth
Greater palatine nerve	Sensory	Posterior hard palate Lingual gingiva of maxillary posterior teeth
Lesser palatine nerve	Sensory	Soft palate Tonsils
Nasopalatine nerve	Sensory	Anterior hard palate Lingual gingiva of maxillary anterior teeth

4. V₃—mandibular nerve.
   a. Foramen: foramen ovale.
   b. Sensory distribution: lower cheek, external auditory meatus, temporomandibular joint (TMJ), chin, lower lip, tongue, floor of the mouth, and mandibular teeth.
   c. Motor distribution: muscles of mastication (temporalis, masseter, internal and external pterygoid muscles), anterior belly of the digastric, tensor tympani, tensor veli palatini, and mylohyoid muscle.
   d. Note: the mandibular nerve (V₃) is the largest division of the trigeminal nerve and is the only one with motor function.
   e. Anatomic pathway: both motor and sensory fibers of the mandibular nerve exit the skull through the foramen ovale, where they form the mandibular trunk. The trunk divides into anterior and posterior divisions in the infratemporal fossa. The anterior trunk further divides into the buccal (or long buccal), masseteric, lateral pterygoid, and deep temporal nerves. Divisions of the posterior trunk include the lingual, inferior alveolar (IAN), and auriculotemporal nerves (Figure 1-7, Table 1-10).
   f. IAN: the IAN descends lateral to the lingual nerve and medial pterygoid muscle toward the mandibular foramen. It stays medial to the sphenomandibular ligament and lateral to the neck of the mandible within the pterygomandibular space. Before entering the foramen, the mylohyoid nerve branches off. The IAN passes through the mandibular foramen into the mandibular canal, where it travels with the

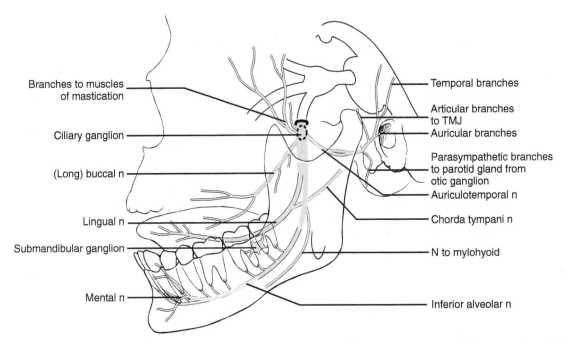

Figure 1-7 Mandibular division of the trigeminal nerve (cranial nerve V₃). *TMJ,* Temporomandibular joint. *(From Liebgott B: The Anatomical Basis of Dentistry, ed 3, St. Louis, Mosby, 2011.)*

IAA and inferior alveolar vein and forms a dental plexus, providing innervation to the mandibular posterior teeth. The IAN then divides into the mental nerve and the incisive nerve. The mental nerve exits the mandible via the mental foramen, which is usually located around the apex of the second mandibular premolar. The incisive nerve continues toward the mandibular anterior teeth.

g. Lingual nerve: the lingual nerve descends toward the base of the tongue, coursing between the medial pterygoid muscle and the mandible. It remains medial to the IAN. The chorda tympani (a branch from CN VII, containing parasympathetic fibers) joins it before it meets the submandibular ganglion, where it continues toward the submandibular and sublingual glands. The lingual nerve continues toward the tip of the tongue, crossing medially under the submandibular duct.

h. Auriculotemporal nerve: the auriculotemporal nerve travels posteriorly and encircles the middle meningeal artery remaining posterior and medial to the condyle. It continues up toward the TMJ, external ear, and temporal region, passing through the parotid gland and traveling with the superficial temporal artery and vein. Postganglionic parasympathetic nervous system fibers from the lesser petrosal branch, a branch from CN IX, join the auriculotemporal nerve to the parotid gland.

F. CN VI: abducens nerve.
 1. Foramen: superior orbital fissure.
 2. Motor distribution: lateral rectus muscle, which moves the eyeball laterally (i.e., abducts the eye).

Table 1-10
Branches of the Mandibular Division of the Trigeminal Nerve (Cranial Nerve V₃)

V₃ BRANCH	FUNCTION	DISTRIBUTION
Long buccal nerve	Sensory	Cheek Buccal gingiva of posterior mandibular teeth Posterior buccal mucosa
Lingual nerve	Sensory	Lingual gingiva of mandibular teeth Floor of mouth
Inferior alveolar nerve	Sensory	Mandibular posterior teeth
Mental nerve	Sensory	Chin Lower lip Anterior labial mucosa
Incisive nerve	Sensory	Mandibular anterior teeth
Auriculotemporal nerve	Sensory	TMJ External auditory meatus Auricle
Deep temporal nerves, anterior and posterior	Motor	Temporalis muscle
Masseteric nerve	Motor	Masseter muscle
Lateral pterygoid nerve	Motor	Lateral pterygoid muscle

TMJ, Temporomandibular joint.

G. CN VII: facial nerve.
   1. Sensory distribution: taste for the anterior two thirds of the tongue.
   2. Motor distribution: muscles of facial expression.
   3. Parasympathetic distribution: sublingual, submandibular, and lacrimal glands.
   4. Anatomic pathway: the facial nerve enters the internal acoustic meatus, located in the temporal bone. In the bone, the facial nerve communicates with the geniculate ganglion, and the chorda tympani nerve branches off. The facial nerve continues and descends to exit the skull via the stylomastoid foramen. The auricular nerve and nerves to the posterior belly of the digastric and stylohyoid muscles branch off before the facial nerve divides into five main branches: temporal, zygomatic, buccal, mandibular, and cervical branches. These nerves innervate the muscles of facial expression.
   5. Greater petrosal nerve: the greater petrosal nerve branches from the geniculate ganglion, carrying preganglionic parasympathetic fibers in it, and travels through the foramen lacerum. It is joined by the deep petrosal nerve (which contains sympathetic fibers from the carotid plexus) before it enters the pterygoid canal. It emerges as the nerve of the pterygoid canal. The nerve of the pterygoid canal continues toward the pterygopalatine fossa in the sphenoid bone, where it meets the pterygopalatine ganglion (Figure 1-8). Postganglionic parasympathetic fibers emerge from the ganglion and continue toward the lacrimal gland (along the zygomatic nerve, a branch of CN V_2)

and smaller glands in the nasal cavity, upper pharynx, and palate.
   6. Chorda tympani: the chorda tympani branches from the facial nerve, carrying both sensory fibers for taste and preganglionic parasympathetic fibers. It exits from the temporal bone via the petrotympanic fissure and joins the lingual nerve (a branch of CN V_3) as it courses inferiorly toward the submandibular ganglion (see Figure 1-8). Postganglionic parasympathetic fibers emerge from the ganglion and continue toward the sublingual and submandibular glands and minor glands of the floor of the mouth. Sensory fibers also branch from the nerve and provide taste sensation to the anterior two thirds of the tongue.

H. CN VIII: vestibulocochlear nerve.
   1. Foramen: internal auditory meatus.
   2. Sensory distribution: equilibrium, balance, and hearing.

I. CN IX: glossopharyngeal nerve.
   1. Foramen: jugular foramen.
   2. Sensory distribution: posterior one third of the tongue (taste), pharynx, tonsils, middle ear, carotid sinus.
   3. Parasympathetic distribution: parotid gland.
   4. Motor and sensory pathways: the glossopharyngeal nerve exits the skull via the jugular foramen. It descends to the superior and inferior ganglion of CN IX, where the tympanic nerve of Jacobson (or tympanic nerve) branches off. Both ganglia contain sensory and motor cell bodies. The glossopharyngeal nerve continues inferiorly to provide sensory and

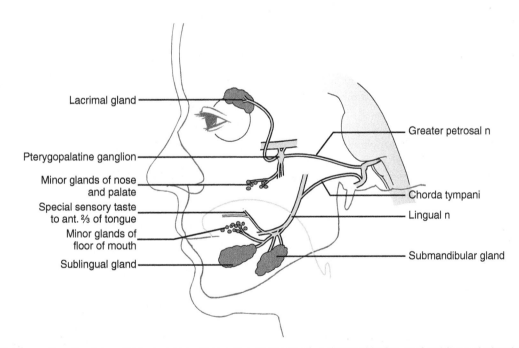

Figure 1-8 Visceral motor branches via trigeminal nerve to lacrimal, submandibular, and sublingual glands and minor glands of the nasal and oral cavities. *(From Liebgott B: The Anatomical Basis of Dentistry, ed 3, St. Louis, Mosby, 2011.)*

motor function to the posterior tongue, middle ear, pharynx, stylopharyngeus muscle, and carotid sinus.

5. Parasympathetic pathway: the tympanic nerve carries preganglionic parasympathetic fibers toward the tympanic cavity and plexus. It continues from there as the lesser petrosal nerve toward the otic ganglion, located behind the mandibular nerve (CN V₃). Postganglionic parasympathetic fibers emerge from the ganglion and travel along the auriculotemporal branch from CN V₃ to the parotid gland.

J. CN X: vagus nerve.
  1. Foramen: jugular foramen.
  2. Motor distribution (with fibers from CN XI): the laryngeal muscles (phonation, swallowing), all muscles of the pharynx except the stylopharyngeus (CN IX), and all muscles of the palate except the tensor veli palatini (CN V₃).
  3. Sensory distribution: posterior one third of the tongue (taste), heart, lungs, and abdominal organs.
  4. Parasympathetic distribution: heart, lungs, abdominal organs.
  5. Anatomic pathway: the vagus nerve exits the skull via the jugular foramen at the medulla. It descends through the superior and inferior ganglion of the vagus nerve, giving off branches in the pharynx and larynx. The vagus nerve descends and is accompanied by the carotid artery and jugular vein within the carotid sheath as it enters the thoracic area. In the thorax, the right and left vagus nerves give off the right and left recurrent laryngeal nerves, respectively, which both travel back up into the neck. The two vagus nerves meet to form the esophageal plexus. Past the diaphragm, the joined vagus nerves (esophageal plexus) divide into the anterior and posterior vagal trunks.
  6. Pharyngeal branches: the pharyngeal nerves branch from the inferior ganglion of the vagus nerve and travel to provide motor function to muscles of the pharynx.
  7. Superior laryngeal branches: branch from the vagus nerve just below the inferior ganglion. They divide into external and internal laryngeal branches.
    a. The external laryngeal nerve provides motor innervation to the cricothyroid muscle and inferior pharyngeal constrictor muscles.
    b. The internal laryngeal nerve travels with the superior laryngeal artery and pierces through the thyrohyoid membrane to provide sensory innervation to mucous membranes from the base of the tongue to the vocal folds. The internal laryngeal nerve also carries parasympathetic fibers.
  8. Recurrent laryngeal branches: the right recurrent laryngeal nerve ascends back to the neck around the subclavian artery. The left recurrent laryngeal nerve passes around the arch of the aorta or ligamentum

arteriosum before traveling up between the trachea and esophagus. As they ascend, the nerves provide sensory and parasympathetic innervation to mucous membranes and structures up to the vocal cords. The nerves continue as the inferior laryngeal nerves in the larynx, providing motor innervation to all the muscles of the larynx except the cricothyroid muscle. A motor branch also provides innervation to the inferior pharyngeal constrictor muscle.

K. CN XI: accessory nerve.
  1. Foramen: jugular foramen.
  2. Sensory distribution: the spinal portion supplies SCM and trapezius muscles. The cranial portion joins with the vagus nerve (CN X) in supplying motor function to palatal, laryngeal, and pharyngeal muscles.

L. CN XII: hypoglossal nerve.
  1. Foramen: hypoglossal canal.
  2. Motor distribution: intrinsic muscles of the tongue, genioglossus, hyoglossus, and styloglossus muscles.

Spaces and Cavities of the Head and Neck

It is important for a dentist to know the spaces and cavities of the head and neck because many of these spaces communicate with the oral cavity, and odontogenic infections can spread through them (Figure 1-9).

A. Spaces of the maxillary region.
  1. Vestibular space of the maxilla.
    a. Location: between the buccinator muscle and oral mucosa. It is inferior to the alveolar process.
    b. Potential odontogenic source of infection: maxillary molars.
  2. Canine fossa.
    a. Location: positioned just posteriorly and superiorly to the roots of the maxillary canines. It remains inferior to the orbicularis oculi muscle, posterior to the levator muscles, and anterior to the buccinator muscle.
    b. Potential odontogenic source of infection: maxillary canines and first premolars.
  3. Canine space.
    a. Location: situated within the superficial fascia over the canine fossa. It is posterior to the orbicularis oris muscle and anterior to the levator anguli oris muscle.
    b. Communications: buccal space.
  4. Superficial (buccal) space.
    a. Location: between the buccinator and masseter muscles.
    b. Consists of the buccal fat pad.
    c. Communications: canine and pterygomandibular spaces and space of the body of the mandible.

B. Spaces of the mandibular region.
  1. Vestibular space of the mandible.
    a. Location: between the buccinator muscle and oral mucosa. It is inferior to the alveolar process.

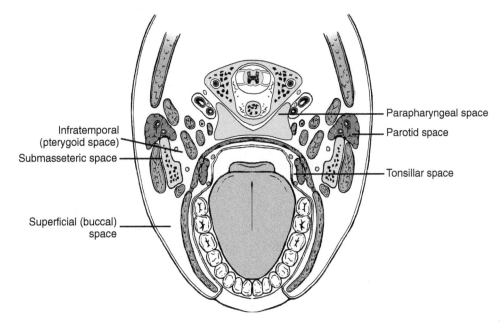

Figure 1-9 Horizontal section through the oral cavity to demonstrate parapharyngeal, tonsillar, and masticator regions. The submasseteric and infratemporal (pterygoid) regions of the masticator region are also shown. *(From Liebgott B: The Anatomical Basis of Dentistry, ed 3, St. Louis, Mosby, 2011.)*

b. Potential odontogenic source of infection: mandibular posterior teeth and canines.
2. Space of the body of the mandible.
   a. Location: between the body of the mandible and its periosteum.
   b. Potential odontogenic source of infection: all mandibular teeth.
   c. Communications: buccal, submental, submandibular, and sublingual spaces and the vestibular space of the mandible.
3. Masticator space—includes four spaces.
   a. Temporal space.
      (1) Location: between the temporalis muscle and its fascia.
      (2) Communications: infratemporal and submasseteric spaces.
   b. Infratemporal (pterygoid) space.
      (1) Location: laterally, it is bordered by the mandible and temporalis muscle. Medially, it is bordered by the lateral pterygoid plate and pharynx. It is inferior to the greater wing of the sphenoid bone.
      (2) Contents: maxillary artery and its branches, mandibular nerve and its branches, and the pterygoid plexus.
      (3) Infections of the infratemporal space are considered dangerous because of the potential of spread of infection to the cavernous sinus via the pterygoid plexus.
      (4) Potential odontogenic source of infection: maxillary third molars and infectious anesthetic needles.

c. Submasseteric space.
   (1) Location: between the masseter muscle and mandibular ramus.
   (2) Potential odontogenic source of infection: mandibular third molars (rare).
   (3) Communications: temporal and infratemporal spaces.
d. Pterygomandibular space.
   (1) Location: between the medial pterygoid muscle and mandibular ramus. It is inferior to the lateral pterygoid muscle.
   (2) Contents: IAN and inferior alveolar artery, lingual nerve, and chorda tympani.
   (3) This is the site for the IAN anesthetic block.
   (4) Potential odontogenic source of infection: mandibular second and third molars. Also consider contaminated anesthetic needles.
4. Submental space.
   a. Location: between the anterior bellies of the digastric muscles. It is superior to the suprahyoid muscles and inferior to the mylohyoid muscle.
   b. Contents: submental lymph nodes and anterior jugular vein.
   c. Potential odontogenic source of infection: mandibular central incisor, if the apex of the incisor lies below the mylohyoid line. Note: infection in this space causes swelling of the chin. If the infection spreads bilaterally to involve the sublingual and submandibular spaces, it is referred to as Ludwig's angina.
   d. Communications: space of the body of the mandible and submandibular and sublingual spaces.

5. Submandibular space.
   a. Location: between the mylohyoid and platysma muscle. It is medial to the mandible and lateral to the anterior and posterior bellies of the digastric muscles.
   b. Contents: submandibular lymph nodes, submandibular salivary gland, and facial artery.
   c. Potential odontogenic source of infection: mandibular second and third molars.
   d. Communications: infratemporal, submental, sublingual, and parapharyngeal spaces.
6. Sublingual space.
   a. Location: between the tongue and its intrinsic muscles and the mandible. It is superior to the mylohyoid muscle and inferior to the sublingual oral mucosa.
   b. Contents: sublingual salivary gland, submandibular salivary gland duct, lingual nerve and artery, and CN XII.
   c. Potential odontogenic source of infection: mandibular anterior teeth, premolars, and mesial roots of the first molars, presuming that the apices of these teeth lie above the mylohyoid line.
   d. Communications: submental and submandibular spaces and the space of the body of the mandible.
C. Spaces of the neck.
   1. Parapharyngeal space.
      a. Location: fascial space between the pharynx and medial pterygoid muscle, adjacent to the carotid sheath. It extends to the pterygomandibular raphe anteriorly and around the pharynx posteriorly.
      b. Communications: masticator, submandibular, retropharyngeal, and previsceral spaces.
   2. Retropharyngeal space.
      a. Location: between the vertebral and visceral fasciae, just posterior to the pharynx. It extends from the base of the skull, posterior to the superior pharyngeal constrictor muscle, and to the thorax.
      b. Because odontogenic infections can quickly spread down this space into the thorax, it is known as the *danger space*. For example, an untreated infection of a mandibular incisor, with an apex above the mylohyoid muscle, may spread along the following pathway: sublingual space → submandibular space → lateral pharyngeal or parapharyngeal space → retropharyngeal space → posterior mediastinum → possible death.
   3. Pterygomandibular space.
      a. Location: between the medial pterygoid muscle and mandibular ramus. It is inferior to the lateral pterygoid muscle.
      b. Contents: IAN and inferior alveolar artery, lingual nerve, and chorda tympani.
      c. This is the site for the IAN anesthetic block.
      d. Potential odontogenic source of infection: mandibular third molars.
      e. Communications: parapharyngeal space.

1.1.3 Extraoral Structures
Ear
A. External ear.
   1. Includes the auricle and external auditory meatus (Figure 1-10).
   2. The external auditory meatus (external ear) and tympanic cavity (middle ear) are separated by the tympanic membrane.
   3. Tympanic membrane (eardrum).
      a. The external surface is covered by epidermis (skin); the internal surface consists of a mucous membrane.

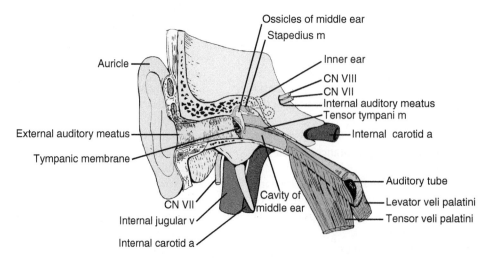

Figure 1-10 Coronal section through the skull to show the external, middle, and internal ear. *CN,* Cranial nerve. *(From Liebgott B: The Anatomical Basis of Dentistry, ed 3, St. Louis, Mosby, 2011.)*

b. It is crossed by the chorda tympani.

c. Transfers sound vibrations from air to auditory ossicles.

B. Middle ear.

1. Ossicles: malleus, incus, and stapes (see Figure 1-10).

2. Loud sounds cause the tensor tympani (which attaches to the malleus) to contract, pulling the malleus and tympanic membrane inward to reduce vibrations and prevent damage.

C. Internal ear.

1. Cochlea.

a. Senses hearing.

b. Receptors (hair cells) for hearing are located in the organ of Corti. This spiral organ lies along the cochlear duct, over the basilar membrane.

2. Vestibule.

a. Senses equilibrium.

b. Consists of the utricle and saccule.

3. Semicircular canals—sense balance and body position (see Figure 1-10).

Eye

The eye is comprised of concentric layers or coats (Figure 1-11) and the lens.

A. Fibrous layer.

1. Sclera—fibrous covering of the posterior five sixths of the eyeball.

2. Cornea—transparent, avascular layer that covers the center one sixth of the eyeball. It is more convex than the sclera and sticks out as a small lump.

B. Vascular coat.

1. Lies just behind the fibrous layer.

2. Consists of the choroids, ciliary body, and iris.

3. The iris separates the anterior and posterior chambers that are filled with aqueous humor. The center opening of the iris is the pupil. The size of the pupil is controlled by two muscles.

a. Constrictor pupillae muscle—constricts the pupil. It is innervated by PNS fibers from CN III via the ciliary ganglion.

b. Dilator pupillae muscle—dilates the pupil. It is innervated by sympathetic fibers.

C. Retina.

1. The inner lining of the eyeball is filled with vitreous humor.

2. Photosensitive region.

a. Includes area posterior to the ora serrata.

b. Optic disc.

(1) Where the optic nerve and central artery of the retina exit.

(2) Void of photoreceptors (blind spot).

c. Fovea centralis.

(1) Located approximately 2.5 mm lateral to the optic disc in a yellow-pigmented area (macula luna).

(2) Contains only cones. Vision is most acute from this area.

(3) Note: there is a decreasing number of cones and an increasing number of rods moving peripherally from this area (see Figure 1-11).

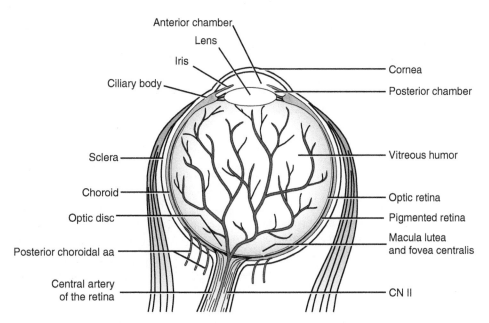

Figure 1-11 Horizontal section through the right eyeball to demonstrate three concentric coats, three refractive media, and blood supply. *CN,* Cranial nerve. *(From Liebgott B: The Anatomical Basis of Dentistry, ed 3, St. Louis, Mosby, 2011.)*

3. Cells of the retina.
  a. Epithelial cells.
    (1) Comprise the pigment epithelium.
    (2) Change every 12 days.
  b. Photoreceptors—two types.
    (1) Rods.
      (a) For nondiscriminative vision (low resolution). They are used for seeing in the dark and detecting motion.
      (b) Are highly convergent, making them very sensitive to light.
      (c) The density of rods increases toward the periphery of the eye. Density decreases toward the center of the eye (macula lutea and fovea centralis), where there are a greater number of cones.
    (2) Cones.
      (a) For acute vision (high resolution). They are also used for color vision.
      (b) Are less convergent, which gives them higher resolution abilities.
      (c) Three types of cones: red, green, and blue.
      (d) The greatest concentration of cones is at the fovea. This area contains only cones and is the area with the highest visual acuity.

	Cones	Rods
Photopigment	Opsin	Rhodopsin
Convergence	Low	High
Sensitivity to light	Low	High
Resolution	High	Low

    (3) Photoreceptor membrane potentials.
      (a) Low light (dark): a constant amount of cyclic guanosine monophosphate (cGMP) is released, causing sodium channels to open. This causes depolarization of the photoreceptor membrane, which results in the release of glutamate.
      (b) High light: causes decreased release of cGMP. This results in the closing of sodium channels, and the photoreceptor membrane hyperpolarizes.
  c. Bipolar cells—synapse with rods and cones.
  d. Ganglion cells—the axons of ganglion cells combine to form the optic nerve.
  e. Amacrine cells.
    (1) Interneurons that connect bipolar and ganglion cells. May contribute to bidirectional communication between these two cells.
    (2) May also play a role in detecting motion.
  f. Horizontal cells.
    (1) Interneurons that connect rods and cones with each other and with bipolar cells.
    (2) Axons aid in bidirectional communication between adjacent bipolar cells.
    (3) Communication is via changes in membrane potential. No action potential is created.

D. Lens.
  1. The lens, by virtue of its shape, controls focusing for near or distant vision. The shape is controlled by ciliary muscles. Stimulation of the parasympathetic nerve to the eye, leads to contraction of the ciliary muscles, resulting in relaxation of fibers that suspend the lens, allowing the lens to become fatter and accommodating for near vision.

1.1.4 Osteology

Bones

A. Skull.
  1. There are 22 cranial and facial bones in the skull (Figure 1-12). Note: some texts include the ossicles of the ears (6 bones) in the total bone count, for 28 bones in the skull.
    a. Cranial bones: ethmoid (1), frontal (1), occipital (1), parietal (2), sphenoid (1), temporal (2).
    b. Facial bones: inferior concha (2), lacrimal (2), mandible (1), maxilla (2), nasal (2), palatine (2), vomer (1), zygoma (2).
    c. Ossicles of the ears: malleus (2), incus (2), stapes (2).

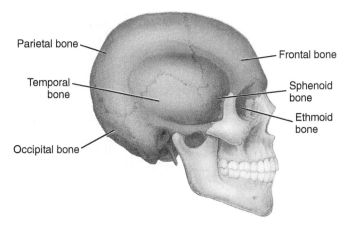

Figure 1-12 Lateral view of the external skull with the cranial bones highlighted. *(From Fehrenbach M, Herring S: Illustrated Anatomy of the Head and Neck, ed 4, Philadelphia, Saunders, 2012.)*

2. Cranial sutures.
    a. Coronal suture—joins the frontal and parietal bones.
    b. Sagittal suture—joins the left and right parietal bones.
    c. Lambdoidal suture—joins the parietal and occipital bones.
    d. Squamosal suture—joins the parietal and temporal bones.
    e. Temporozygomatic suture—joins the zygomatic and temporal bones.
    f. Medial palatine suture—joins the left and right palatine bones.
    g. Transverse palatine suture—joins the maxilla and palatine bones.
3. Sphenoid bone.
    a. The sphenoid bone is located along the midline of the cranium. It articulates with all the cranial bones and four facial bones—maxilla, palatine bones, vomer, and zygomatic.
    b. The sphenoid bone consists of a body, greater and lesser wings, and paired pterygoid processes.
        (1) The body contains the sphenoid sinuses.
        (2) The greater wing contributes to the roof of the infratemporal fossa and floor of the middle cranial fossa.
        (3) The lesser wing contains the optic canal, anterior clinoid process, and part of the superior orbital fissure.
        (4) The pterygoid process is composed of two thin plates, the medial and lateral pterygoid plates. The space between these two plates is the pterygoid fossa.
        (5) There is a space that forms between the pterygoid process and maxillae that is inferior and posterior to the orbit, called the *pterygopalatine fossa*.
    c. The sphenoid bone contains many foramina and fissures, including the foramen ovale, foramen rotundum, foramen spinosum, and superior orbital fissure.
    d. Sella turcica—a cradle at the center of the bone that houses the pituitary gland.
4. Ethmoid bone.
    a. The ethmoid bone is also located along the midline of the cranium. It articulates with the frontal, sphenoid, palatine, inferior concha, and lacrimal bones and the maxilla and vomer.
    b. Structures include the cribriform plate, perpendicular plate, and crista galli.
        (1) The cribriform plate serves as the roof of the nasal cavity and is pierced by branches of the olfactory nerve (CN I).
        (2) The perpendicular plate, the vomer, and the nasal septal cartilage form the nasal septum.

(3) The crista galli peaks upward into the anterior cranial fossa and is the attachment of the falx cerebri.
    c. The ethmoid bone houses the ethmoid sinuses and forms the superior and middle nasal conchae.
5. Temporal bone.
    a. The temporal bone forms the lower lateral walls of the skull. It articulates with the parietal, occipital, sphenoid, and zygomatic bones and the mandible through the TMJ.
    b. The temporal bone consists of three portions.
        (1) Squamous portion—includes the zygomatic process of the temporal bone. The inferior surface of the zygomatic process is the articular fossa. Anterior to this fossa is the articular eminence. This is where the TMJ articulates.
        (2) Petromastoid portion—includes the mastoid and styloid processes, jugular and mastoid notches, inner and middle ear, and carotid canal. Foramina include the stylomastoid foramen and the internal acoustic meatus.
        (3) Tympanic portion—includes the floor and anterior wall of the external acoustic meatus. It is separated from the petrous portion of the temporal bone via the petrotympanic fissure.
6. Maxilla.
    a. The left and right maxilla fuse to form the maxillae. The maxillae articulates with the frontal, lacrimal, nasal, inferior nasal concha, vomer, zygoma, sphenoid, ethmoid, and palatine bones (Figure 1-13).
    b. Each maxilla consists of a body and four processes: frontal, zygomatic, alveolar, and palatine processes.
        (1) The body contains the maxillary sinuses.
        (2) The frontal process.
            (a) Contains an orbital surface that is part of the inferior wall or floor of the orbit.
            (b) It also forms the medial orbital rim with the lacrimal bone.
            (c) A groove, or the infraorbital sulcus, is present on the floor of the orbit. It becomes the infraorbital canal and terminates at the infraorbital foramen.
            (d) The inferior orbital fissure separates the orbital surface from the sphenoid bone.
        (3) The zygomatic process, along with the zygoma, forms the infraorbital rim.
        (4) The alveolar process houses roots of the maxillary teeth and is divided into left and right halves at the midline by the intermaxillary suture. A bony prominence observed behind the upper third molar is known as the *maxillary tuberosity*.
        (5) The right and left palatal processes, along with the palatine bones, fuse to form the hard palate (Figure 1-14). These two processes are

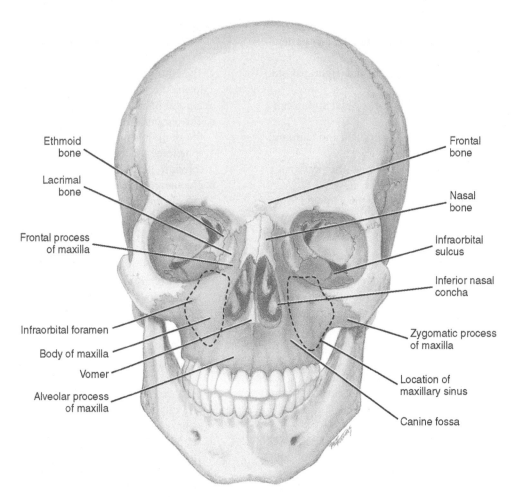

Figure 1-13 Anterior view of the skull with the maxilla and its associated landmarks highlighted. *(From Fehrenbach M, Herring S: Illustrated Anatomy of the Head and Neck, ed 4, Philadelphia, Saunders, 2012.)*

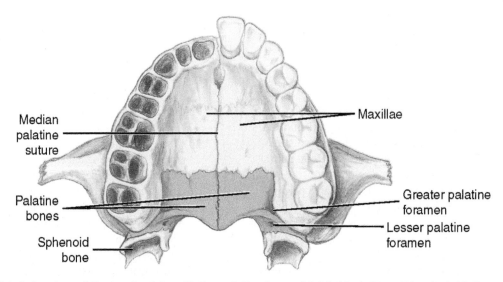

Figure 1-14 Inferior view of the hard palate with the palatine bones highlighted. *(From Fehrenbach M, Herring S: Illustrated Anatomy of the Head and Neck, ed 4, Philadelphia, Saunders, 2012.)*

separated by the median palatine suture. Anterior to this suture is the incisive foramen. This foramen is a landmark for the nasopalatine injection.

(6) Note: the posterior hard palate is covered by a fibrous, tendinous sheet called the *palatine aponeurosis*. The midline forms a ridge that is known as the *median palatine raphe*. The greater palatine foramen is a landmark for the greater palatine injection. The lesser palatine foramen transmits lesser palatine nerves and blood vessels to the soft palate and tonsils.

7. Mandible.
  a. The mandible is a single bone that consists of two vertical rami, a horizontal body, and an alveolar process (see Figure 1-13).
    (1) Each ramus includes a condyle and coronoid process.
      (a) Condyle—articulates with the mandibular fossa of the temporal bone to form the TMJ.
      (b) Coronoid process—serves as an attachment for the temporal muscle.
    (2) The anterior border of the ramus descends from the coronoid process to the external oblique line.
    (3) The horizontal portion of the mandible consists of the body and alveolar process, which contain the roots of the mandibular teeth. If an imaginary horizontal line were drawn around the level of the mental foramen, it would separate the body from the alveolar process.

  b. The mandible provides many surface landmarks.
    (1) From the lateral aspect, important landmarks include the mental protuberance, mental foramen, external oblique line, coronoid process, and condyle.
    (2) From the medial aspect, important landmarks include the mandibular foramen, lingula, mylohyoid line and groove, submandibular and sublingual fossa, and retromolar triangle.
  c. Mandibular growth takes place in several areas.
    (1) The alveolar process and body increase in width and height.
    (2) The mandibular arch is lengthened by adding bone to its posterior border of the ramus and removing bone from its anterior border.
B. Cranial openings.
  1. Cranial openings include foramina, canals, and meatus.
  2. Important cranial openings are summarized in Table 1-11.
C. Orbit.
  1. The orbit is the cavity in the skull that houses and safeguards the eyeball. Seven cranial and facial bones make up the walls of each orbit—the frontal, sphenoid, zygomatic, palatine, ethmoid, maxilla, and lacrimal bones (Table 1-12).
  2. Bony openings of the orbit.
    a. Optic canal—found at the apex of the orbit.
    b. Inferior orbital fissure—separates the floor of the orbit from its lateral wall.
    c. Superior orbital fissure—lies between the greater and lesser wings of the sphenoid bone.

Table 1-11

Cranial Openings, Their Location, and Contents

FORAMEN	BONE	CONTENTS
Cribriform plate	Ethmoid	CN I
Foramen magnum	Occipital	CN XI and brainstem (medulla); vertebral and spinal arteries
Foramen ovale	Sphenoid	CN V_3
Foramen rotundum	Sphenoid	CN V_2
Foramen spinosum	Sphenoid	Middle meningeal vessels
Hypoglossal canal	Occipital bone	CN XII
Incisive foramen	Maxilla	Nasopalatine nerve
Inferior orbital fissure	Sphenoid, maxilla	CN V_2 (or infraorbital nerve) and zygomatic nerve; infraorbital artery, ophthalmic vein
Internal acoustic meatus	Temporal	CN VII and VIII
Jugular foramen	Occipital, temporal	CN IX, X, and XI; internal jugular vein
Optic canal	Sphenoid	CN II; ophthalmic artery
Stylomastoid foramen	Temporal	CN VII
Superior orbital fissure	Sphenoid	CN III, IV, V_1, and VI; ophthalmic veins

CN, Cranial nerve.

Table 1-12

Cranial and Facial Bones That Form the Orbit

ORBITAL STRUCTURE	BONES	COMMUNICATIONS
Roof or superior wall	Frontal bone—orbital plate Sphenoid bone—lesser wing	
Medial wall	Ethmoid bone—orbital plate	
Superior-medial wall	Lacrimal bone	
Inferior-medial wall	Frontal bone—orbital plates Maxilla—orbital plate	
Lateral wall	Zygomatic bone—frontal process Sphenoid bone—greater wing	Superior orbital fissure
Floor or inferior wall	Maxilla—orbital plate Zygomatic bone Palatine bone—orbital process	Inferior orbital fissure
Apex	Sphenoid bone—lesser wing Palatine bone	Optic canal

Table 1-13

Boundaries and Communications of the Pterygopalatine Fossa

AREA	BONES	COMMUNICATIONS
Roof	Sphenoid bone—body	—
Floor	Pterygopalatine canal	—
Anterior	Maxilla—tuberosity	Orbit via the inferior orbital fissure
Posterior	Sphenoid bone—pterygoid process	Pterygoid canal, foramen rotundum, and pharyngeal canal
Medial	Palatine bone—vertical plate	Nasal cavity via the sphenopalatine foramen
Lateral	Pterygomaxillary fissure	Infratemporal fossa via the pterygomaxillary fissure

---

D. Nasal cavity.
   1. The nasal cavity is divided into two parts by the nasal septum. Each side contains three conchae. The superior and middle conchae are located in the ethmoid bone. The inferior conchae is a separate bone.
   2. Between the conchae are small slitlike openings, or meatus, which allow communication between the nasal cavity and paranasal sinuses or the nasolacrimal duct.
      a. Superior meatus—opens into the posterior ethmoid sinus.
      b. Middle meatus—consists of several openings.
         (1) Semilunar hiatus—opens into the frontal, anterior ethmoid, and maxillary sinuses.
         (2) Ethmoid bulla—opens into the middle ethmoid sinus.
      c. Inferior meatus—communicates with the nasolacrimal duct, which drains tears from the eye.
      d. Sphenoid sinus—directly communicates with the nasal cavity.
      e. Sphenopalatine foramen—opens into the pterygopalatine fossa.

E. Fossa.
   1. Pterygopalatine fossa.
      a. Boundaries and communications of the pterygopalatine fossa are listed in Table 1-13.
      b. Communicates with the infratemporal fossa via the pterygomaxillary fissure.
      c. Contents: branches of the maxillary artery, branches of the maxillary trigeminal nerve (CN V_2), and pterygopalatine ganglion.
   2. Infratemporal fossa.
      a. Boundaries and communications of the infratemporal fossa are listed in Table 1-14.
      b. Contents: branches of the mandibular nerve (CN V_3), chorda tympani, otic ganglion, branches of the maxillary artery, pterygoid venous plexus, temporalis, and lateral and medial pterygoid muscles.

1.1.5 Muscles

A. Muscles of facial expression: major muscles and their actions (Figure 1-15).
   1. Eyes and eyebrows.
      a. Occipitofrontalis (epicranius) muscle—raises the eyebrows and forehead.

Table 1-14

Boundaries and Communications of the Infratemporal Fossa

AREA	BONES	COMMUNICATIONS
Roof	Sphenoid bone—greater wing	Temporal fossa, foramen ovale, foramen spinosum
Floor	*Open*	—
Anterior	Maxilla—tuberosity	Orbit via the inferior orbital fissure
Posterior	*Open*	—
Medial	Sphenoid bone—lateral pterygoid plate	Pterygopalatine fossa via pterygomaxillary fissure
Lateral	Mandible—ramus, coronoid process	—

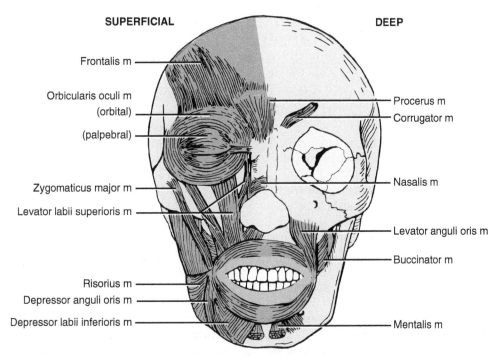

SUPERFICIAL   DEEP

Frontalis m

Orbicularis oculi m
(orbital)

(palpebral)

Procerus m
Corrugator m

Zygomaticus major m

Levator labii superioris m

Nasalis m

Levator anguli oris m

Buccinator m

Risorius m
Depressor anguli oris m
Depressor labii inferioris m

Mentalis m

Figure 1-15 Muscles of facial expression. Anterior view. Superficial muscles are shown on the right; deeper muscles are shown on the left. *(From Liebgott B: The Anatomical Basis of Dentistry, ed 3, St. Louis, Mosby, 2011.)*

  b. Orbicularis oculi—closes the eyelids, blinking.
  c. Corrugator—depresses the eyebrows.
 2. Cheek.
  a. Buccinator muscle—compresses the cheek against the teeth and aids in chewing.
   (1) Origin: buccal surface of the maxillary and mandibular alveolar processes and pterygomandibular raphe.
   (2) Insertion: angle of the mouth or lip.
 3. Mouth.
  a. Orbicularis oris—closes and protrudes upper and lower lips.
  b. Depressor anguli oris—depresses angle of mouth.

  c. Levator anguli oris—lifts the corner of the mouth.
  d. Zygomaticus major—draws angle of the mouth up and back.
  e. Risorius—draws angle of the mouth laterally.
 4. Lips.
  a. Levator labii superioris—pulls lip up.
  b. Depressor labii inferioris—depresses lower lip.
 5. Chin.
  a. Mentalis—puckers skin of chin, protrudes lower lip.
 6. Nose.
  a. Nasalis—compressor nares compresses nostrils, dilator nares dilates or flares nostrils.

Table 1-15

Origins and Insertions of the Muscles of Mastication

MUSCLE	ORIGIN	INSERTION
Temporalis	Temporal fossa	Coronoid process of mandible
Masseter		
Superficial head	Anterior two thirds of inferior border of zygomatic arch	Angle of mandible—lateral surface
Deep head	Posterior one third of inferior border of zygomatic arch	Ramus and body of mandible
Medial pterygoid		
Superficial fibers	Pyramidal process of palatine bone, pterygoid fossa of sphenoid bone, and maxillary tuberosity	Angle of mandible—medial surface
Deep fibers	Pyramidal process of palatine bone and medial surface of lateral pterygoid plate of sphenoid bone	
Lateral pterygoid		
Superior head	Infratemporal crest of greater wing of sphenoid bone	Condyle of mandible—anterior surface A few fibers insert into anterior portion of TMJ articular capsule
Inferior head	Lateral pterygoid plate of sphenoid bone	Condyle of the mandible—anterior surface

TMJ, Temporomandibular joint.

B. Muscles of mastication.
   1. There are four primary muscles of mastication—temporalis, masseter, and medial and lateral pterygoid muscles.
      a. In general, the temporalis, masseter, and medial pterygoid muscles elevate the mandible or close the mouth.
      b. The lateral pterygoid muscle is involved in protrusion, depression, and contralateral excursion of the mandible.
      c. The origins and insertions of these muscles are described in Table 1-15.
   2. The hyoid muscles assist the muscles of mastication in retruding and depressing the mandible.
   3. The muscles of mastication and hyoid muscles are involved in coordinating mandibular movements).
      a. Closing the mouth.
         (1) Temporalis—anterior (vertical) and posterior horizontal fibers.
         (2) Masseter—superficial head.
         (3) Medial pterygoid.
      b. Opening the mouth.
         (1) Lateral pterygoid.
         (2) Assisting muscles.
            (a) Infrahyoid muscles—these muscles and the posterior belly of the digastric muscle aid in depressing and stabilizing the hyoid bone, allowing the suprahyoid muscles to help pull down the mandible.
            (b) Suprahyoid muscles—especially the anterior belly of the digastric muscle.
      c. Protrusion.
         (1) Medial pterygoid.
         (2) Lateral pterygoid—inferior head.
      d. Retrusion.
         (1) Temporalis—posterior fibers.
         (2) Assisting muscles.
            (a) Suprahyoid muscles—especially both bellies of the digastric muscle.
            (b) Lateral pterygoid.
      e. Lateral excursion.
         (1) Lateral pterygoid—on the nonworking side (i.e., the opposite side of the direction of movement). Note: an injured lateral pterygoid causes the jaw to shift to the same side of the injury.
         (2) Assisting muscle: temporalis, which acts as a stabilizer.
C. Hyoid muscles.
   1. The hyoid muscles are divided into two groups, depending on their location above or below the hyoid bone.
      a. The suprahyoid muscles are superior to the hyoid bone and include the anterior and posterior digastric muscles—mylohyoid, geniohyoid, and stylohyoid (Figure 1-16). The mylohyoid muscle forms the floor of the mouth.
      b. The infrahyoid muscles are inferior to the hyoid bone and include the sternothyroid, sternohyoid, omohyoid, and thyrohyoid. These muscles are summarized in Table 1-16.
   2. Infrahyoid muscles.
      a. Innervation: cervical nerves (C1–C3) via the cervical plexus and of ansa cervicalis.
      b. Major actions.
         (1) Assist the muscles of mastication in depressing or retruding the mandible.
         (2) Depress the hyoid bone and larynx when swallowing.

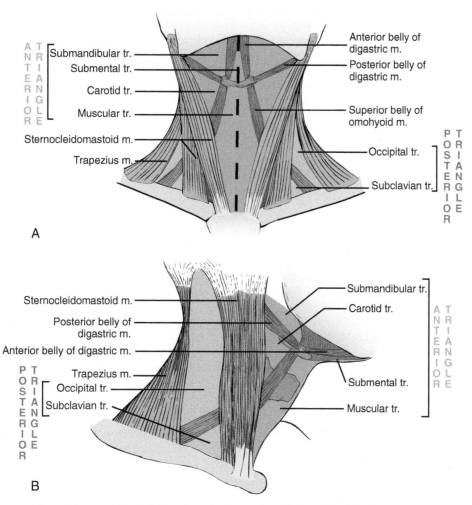

Figure 1-16 Key muscles of the neck that delineate anterior and posterior triangles. **A,** Anterior view. **B,** Right lateral view. *(From Liebgott B: The Anatomical Basis of Dentistry, ed 3, St. Louis, Mosby, 2011.)*

Table 1-16			
Origins, Insertions, and Innervation of the Hyoid Muscles			
	INNERVATION	**ORIGIN**	**INSERTION**
Suprahyoid			
Digastric muscle			
Anterior belly	CN V₃	Digastric fossa	Intermediate tendon
Posterior belly	CN VII	Mastoid notch of temporal bone	Intermediate tendon
Mylohyoid	CN V₃	Mylohyoid line	Hyoid bone
Geniohyoid	C1 via CN XII	Genial tubercles	Hyoid bone
Stylohyoid	CN VII	Styloid process	Hyoid bone
Infrahyoid			
Omohyoid			
Superior belly	C1–C3	Intermediate tendon	Hyoid bone
Inferior belly	C1–C3	Scapula	Intermediate tendon
Sternohyoid	C1–C3	Sternum	Hyoid bone
Sternothyroid	C2–C3	Sternum	Thyroid cartilage
Thyrohyoid	C1 via CN XII	Thyroid cartilage	Hyoid bone

CN, Cranial nerve.

Table 1-17

Origins, Insertions, and Innervation of the Neck Muscles

	INNERVATION	ORIGIN	INSERTION
Platysma	CN VII	Fascia of the deltoids and pectoralis	Mandible
Sternocleidomastoid	CN XI	Clavicle and sternum	Mastoid process of temporal bone
Trapezius	CN XI, C3–C4	Extends from occipital bone to cervical and thoracic vertebral column	Clavicle and spine of the scapula

CN, Cranial nerve.

3. Suprahyoid muscles.
   a. Innervation (see Table 1-16).
   b. Major actions.
      (1) Assist in pulling the mandible down during mouth opening.
      (2) Raise the hyoid bone and larynx when swallowing.
D. Neck muscles.
   1. The muscles in the neck include the platysma, SCM, and trapezius. These muscles are summarized in Table 1-17.
   2. Platysma—a thin layer of muscle found in the superficial fascia of the neck.
   3. SCM.
      a. A major landmark in the neck, dividing each side of the neck into anterior and posterior triangles (see Figure 1-16). The anterior triangle can be divided further into the submandibular triangle, submental triangle, carotid triangle and muscular triangle. The posterior triangle can be divided into the occipital and subclavian triangle.
      b. Actions: contraction of one SCM tilts the head laterally to that same side, while turning the face toward the opposite side. Contraction of both SCMs flexes the neck.
      c. The carotid pulse can be felt at the anterior-superior border of the SCM muscle, just posterior to the thyroid cartilage.
   4. Trapezius.
      a. Action: contraction of the trapezius elevates the clavicle and scapula (i.e., shrugging shoulders).
E. Muscles of the soft palate.
   1. Muscles of the soft palate include the palatoglossus, palatopharyngeus, levator veli palatini, tensor veli palatini, and uvula (Figure 1-17).
      a. The palatoglossus forms the anterior tonsillar pillar.
      b. The palatopharyngeus forms the posterior tonsillar pillar and closes off the nasopharynx and larynx during swallowing.
      c. The tensor veli palatini wraps around the lateral side of the pterygoid hamulus and tenses the soft palate.
      d. These muscles are summarized in Table 1-18.

   2. Innervation: refer to the next list item, (Muscles of the pharynx) for innervation of muscles of the soft palate.
F. Muscles of the pharynx.
   1. The muscles of the pharynx include the superior, middle, and inferior constrictor muscles; the stylopharyngeus; and the salpingopharyngeus. The major action of these muscles is to move the pharynx and larynx during swallowing. The origins, insertions, and actions of these muscles are presented in Table 1-19.
   2. Innervation.
      a. Muscles of the soft palate and pharynx all are innervated via the pharyngeal plexus (CN IX, CN X, and CN XI), with three exceptions.
         (1) Tensor veli palatini—innervated by CN V_3.
         (2) Stylopharyngeus—innervated by a motor branch of CN IX.
         (3) Mucous membranes of the pharynx—innervated by CN V_2.
      b. Motor function: CN XI via CN X nerve fibers.
      c. Sensory function: CN IX.
G. Muscles of the larynx.
   1. The muscles of the larynx include the cricothyroid, oblique and transverse arytenoids, thyroarytenoid, and lateral and posterior cricoarytenoids. A summary of these muscles and their actions is presented in Table 1-20.
   2. Innervation: all muscles of the larynx are innervated by CN X via the recurrent laryngeal nerve except the cricothyroid, which is innervated by CN X via the external laryngeal nerve.

Tongue

A. Surface anatomy (Figure 1-18).
   1. Dorsum of tongue—divided into two parts. The anterior two thirds of the tongue from apex to sulcus terminalis lies relatively freely in the oral cavity, and the posterior one third of the tongue covers the oral cavity and lies in the pharynx.
   2. Sulcus terminalis—a V-shaped depression that is an embryologic remnant resulting from the fusion between the first and second pharyngeal arches.
   3. Foramen cecum—a small pit located at the intersection of the tip of the "V" of the sulcus terminalis and

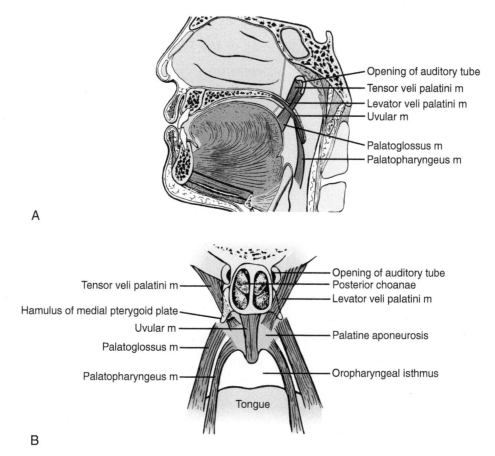

Figure 1-17 Muscles of the soft palate. **A,** Lateral aspect. **B,** Posterior aspect. The left veli palatini muscle has been cut to reveal the tensor veli palatini muscle. *(From Liebgott B: The Anatomical Basis of Dentistry, ed 3, St. Louis, Mosby, 2011.)*

Table 1-18

Origins, Insertions, and Actions of the Muscles of the Soft Palate

	ORIGIN	INSERTION	ACTION
Palatoglossus	Fascia of the soft palate	Tongue	Raises tongue, depresses soft palate
Palatopharyngeus	Soft palate	Thyroid cartilage, lateral wall of the pharynx	Moves palate down and back, moves pharynx up and forward, and raises and folds posterior wall of the larynx
Levator veli palatini	Petrous portion of temporal bone	Palatine aponeurosis	Raises soft palate
Tensor veli palatini	Medial pterygoid plate	Palatine aponeurosis	Tenses soft palate, opens auditory tube and eustachian tube
Uvular	Posterior nasal spine of the palatine bone and palatine aponeurosis	Uvula	Contracts uvula

median lingual sulcus. It is an embryologic remnant of the proximal opening of the thyroglossal duct.
4. Lingual papillae—elevated structures found on the surface of the tongue. There are four types.
   a. Filiform papillae.
      (1) Thin, pointy projections that comprise the most numerous papillae and give the tongue's dorsal surface its characteristic rough texture.
      (2) Arrangement: in rows parallel with the sulcus terminalis.
      (3) Histologically show more keratinization than the other papillae.
      (4) Do not contain taste buds.
      (5) Note: an overgrowth of these papillae results in hairy tongue. A loss of filiform papillae results in glossitis.

Table 1-19

Origins, Insertions, and Actions of the Muscles of the Pharynx

	ORIGIN	INSERTION	ACTION
Superior constrictor	Medial pterygoid plate, pterygoid hamulus, pterygomandibular raphe, mylohyoid line	Median pharyngeal raphe, Pharyngeal tubercle on base of skull	Constricts pharynx to help push food down into esophagus during swallowing; also raises larynx
Middle constrictor	Hyoid bone, stylohyoid ligament	Median pharyngeal raphe	—
Inferior constrictor	Thyroid and cricoid cartilages	Median pharyngeal raphe	—
Stylopharyngeus	Styloid process	Thyroid cartilage, lateral wall of pharynx	Raises and dilates pharynx, helping food move through; also raises larynx
Salpingopharyngeus	Eustachian tube	Lateral wall of pharynx	Raise and dilates pharynx, helping food move through

Table 1-20

Origins, Insertions, and Actions of the Muscles of the Larynx

	ORIGIN	INSERTION	ACTION
Cricothyroid	Cricoid cartilage	Thyroid cartilage	Raises cricoid cartilage, tenses vocal cords
Oblique arytenoid	Arytenoid cartilage	Arytenoid cartilage on opposite side	Adducts vocal cords
Transverse arytenoid	Arytenoid cartilage	Arytenoid cartilage on opposite side	Adducts vocal cords
Thyroarytenoid	Thyroid cartilage	Arytenoid cartilage	Adducts vocal cords
Lateral cricoarytenoid	Cricoid cartilage	Arytenoid cartilage	Adducts vocal cords
Posterior cricoarytenoid	Cricoid cartilage	Arytenoid cartilage	Adducts vocal cords

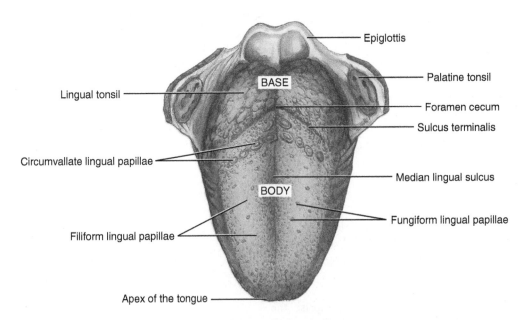

Figure 1-18 Dorsal view of the tongue with its landmarks noted. *(Modified from Fehrenbach M, Herring S: Illustrated Anatomy of the Head and Neck, ed 4, Philadelphia, Saunders, 2012.)*

b. Fungiform papillae.
  (1) Round, red spots that are less numerous than filiform papillae.
  (2) Histologically, they have a characteristic mushroom shape.
  (3) Contain taste buds.
c. Circumvallate (vallate) papillae.
  (1) The largest papillae and are about 12 in number.
  (2) Arrangement: in a row parallel and just anterior to the sulcus terminalis.
  (3) Contain taste buds and small salivary glands known as *von Ebner's glands.*
d. Foliate papillae.
  (1) Vertical folds found posteriorly on the side of the tongue.
  (2) Contain rudimentary taste buds in humans.
e. Note about taste buds: taste buds contain neuroepithelial (taste) cells. They can discriminate five taste sensations—salty, sweet, sour, bitter, and the more recently described umami taste (taste of L-glutamate).
B. Muscles of the tongue.
  1. Intrinsic muscles of the tongue—muscles found entirely within the tongue. Although they are not considered to be separate muscles, they can be divided into longitudinal, transverse, and vertical muscles. Their main function is to change the shape of the tongue.
  2. Extrinsic muscles of the tongue—three extrinsic muscles of the tongue include the genioglossus, styloglossus, and hyoglossus (some texts also include the palatoglossus). Although they all insert into the tongue, they originate from surrounding structures. A summary of their origins, insertions, and actions is presented in Table 1-21.
  3. Innervation.
    a. Motor function: motor innervation for all intrinsic and extrinsic muscles is from CN XII.
    b. Sensory function.
      (1) Anterior two thirds of the tongue.
        (a) General sensory—CN V_3 via the lingual nerve.
        (b) Special sensory (taste)—CN VII via the chorda tympani.
      (2) Posterior one third of the tongue: general and special sensation is innervated by CN IX.
      (3) Area around the epiglottis: innervated by CN X via the internal laryngeal nerve.
  4. Vascular supply—the blood supply is from branches of the lingual artery, including its terminal end, the deep lingual artery.

Triangles of the Neck

The SCM divides each side of the neck into anterior and posterior triangles. These triangles can be subdivided into smaller triangles (see Figure 1-16).
A. Anterior triangle.
  1. Borders: anterior margin of the SCM, midline of the neck, and inferior border of the mandible.
  2. Subdivisions.
    a. Submandibular (digastric) triangles.
      (1) Borders: upper margin of the anterior and posterior bellies of the digastric muscle, inferior border of the mandible.
      (2) Floor: mylohyoid and hyoglossus muscles.
      (3) Contents: submandibular gland, submandibular lymph nodes, lingual and facial arteries, CN XII, lingual nerve, and nerve to the mylohyoid muscle.
    b. Submental triangle.
      (1) Borders: between the right and left anterior bellies of the digastric muscle (beneath the chin) and body of the hyoid bone.
      (2) Floor: mylohyoid muscle.
      (3) Contents: submental lymph nodes.
    c. Muscular triangles.
      (1) Borders: inferior border of the superior belly of the omohyoid muscle, anterior border of the SCM, and anterior midline of the neck.
      (2) Floor: sternohyoid and sternothyroid (infrahyoid) muscles.
      (3) Contents: anterior branches of the ansa cervicalis, infrahyoid strap muscles, and lymph nodes.
    d. Carotid triangles.
      (1) Borders: superior border of the superior belly of the omohyoid muscle, inferior border of the posterior belly of the digastric muscle, and anterior border of the SCM.

Table 1-21

Origins, Insertions, and Actions of the Extrinsic Muscles of the Tongue

	ORIGIN	INSERTION	ACTION
Genioglossus	Genial tubercles on mandible	Tongue, hyoid bone	Protrudes and depresses tongue
Styloglossus	Styloid process of temporal bone	Tongue	Retracts tongue, curls up sides of tongue
Hyoglossus	Greater horn and body of hyoid bone	Tongue	Depresses tongue

(2) Floor: inferior pharyngeal constrictor and thyrohyoid muscles.

(3) Contents: common carotid artery (which bifurcates near the upper border of the thyroid cartilage) and its branches, internal jugular vein and its tributaries, vagus nerve (CN X) including external and internal laryngeal nerves, CN IX (branch to carotid sinus), CN XI, CN XII, and branches of the cervical plexus.

B. Posterior triangle.
  1. Borders: posterior border of the SCM, anterior border of the trapezius and the clavicle.
  2. Floor: splenius capitis, levator scapulae, posterior and middle scalene muscles.
  3. Contents: external jugular and subclavian vein and their tributaries, subclavian artery and its branches (C3, C4), branches of the cervical plexus, CN XI, suprascapular artery and vein, nerves to the upper limb and muscles of the triangle floor, phrenic nerve, and brachial plexus.
  4. It is subdivided by the omohyoid muscle into the occipital triangle (above the omohyoid) and subclavian (supraclavicular) triangle (below the omohyoid).
    a. Subclavian (supraclavicular) triangle.
      (1) Borders: inferior border of the inferior belly of the omohyoid, middle one third of the clavicle, and posterior border of the SCM.
      (2) Contents: subclavian artery and vein, branchial plexus, cervical artery and vein, external jugular vein, and scapular vein
    b. Occipital triangle.
      (1) Borders: superior border of the inferior belly of the omohyoid, posterior border of the SCM, and anterior border of the trapezius.
      (2) Contents: accessory nerve.

1.2 Axilla, Shoulders, and Upper Extremities

The axilla is a space described as a pyramid, with a base composed of the skin and superficial fascia of the armpit. The apex rises to the level of the midclavicle. It contains the nerves and blood vessels supplying the upper limbs.

A. Axilla.
  1. Boundaries: the axilla is bounded by three skeletal and muscular walls.
    a. Anterior wall.
      (1) Contains the clavicle superiorly and the pectoralis major and pectoralis minor muscles.
    b. Medial wall.
      (1) The lateral thoracic wall covered by the serratus anterior muscle.
    c. Posterior wall.
      (1) Formed primarily by the scapula and subscapularis muscle.

(2) Teres major and latissimus dorsi muscles contribute to the inferior aspect of the posterior wall.
  2. Contents.
    a. The axilla.
      (1) Brachial nerve plexus.
      (2) Axillary artery.
      (3) Axillary vein.
    b. The axillary sheath encloses the artery, vein, and nerve as they pass through the axilla from the posterior triangle of the neck to the arm.
    c. Axillary lymph nodes receiving lymph from the arm and breast travel through the axilla.

B. Shoulders and upper extremities.
  Limbs develop from outgrowths of the axial skeleton (Figure 1-19). The upper limb develops from body wall segments of the lower four cervical and first thoracic levels. Muscle, nerve, blood vessels, and lymphatic drainage arise concomitantly. The upper limb has four skeletal components: shoulder girdle, arm, forearm, and hand. Additional components include muscles, nerves, arterial supply and venous return, and lymphatic drainage.
  1. The shoulder girdle consists of the scapula and clavicle.
    a. The scapula is a broad, flat, thin, triangular-shaped bone.
      (1) The concave anterior surface is anchored by muscles to the posterior surface of ribs two through seven.
      (2) Three sides.
        (a) Vertebral medial border paralleling the vertebral column.
        (b) Axillary lateral border facing the axilla.
        (c) Suprascapular superior border.
      (3) The spine of the scapula runs horizontally across the convex posterior surface and divides it into two fossae for muscle attachments.
        (a) Supraspinous fossa above the spine.
        (b) Infraspinous fossa below the spine.
      (4) The acromion articulates with the clavicle at the acromioclavicular joint. The suprascapular notch, on the superior border of the spine, is the site of transmission of the suprascapular nerve and vessels.
      (5) The coracoid process projects laterally and anteriorly from the superolateral border.
      (6) The glenoid fossa, just below the base of the coracoid process, articulates with the head of the humerus at the joint of the shoulder.
      (7) The subscapular fossa on the concave anterior surface fits against the convex surface of the adjacent ribs.
    b. The clavicle is an S-shaped bone commonly known as the *collarbone*.

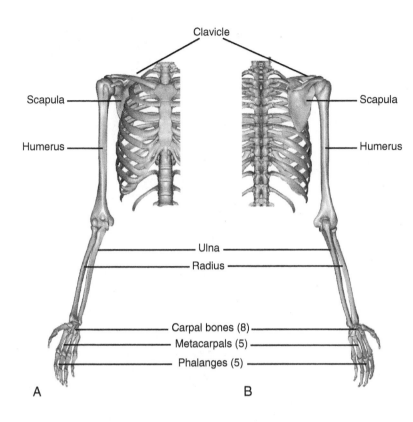

Clavicle

Scapula

Humerus

Scapula

Humerus

Ulna
Radius

Carpal bones (8)
Metacarpals (5)
Phalanges (5)

A   B

Figure 1-19 Skeleton of the upper right limb. **A,** Anterior view. **B,** Posterior view. *(From Liebgott B: The Anatomical Basis of Dentistry, ed 3, St. Louis, Mosby, 2011.)*

(1) The lateral end articulates at the acromioclavicular joint with the acromion of the scapula.
(2) The medial end articulates at the sternoclavicular joint with the manubrium.
(3) The medial half of the clavicle bends anteriorly, and the lateral half bends posteriorly.
(4) The inferior surface serves as the attachment for two ligaments.
   (a) The coraclavicular ligament binds the clavicle to the coracoid process.
   (b) The costoclavicular ligament binds the clavicle to the first rib.
2. The arm consists of the humerus bone (see Figure 1-19).
a. The humerus is the only bone of the arm.
   (1) The humerus articulates superiorly with the scapula and inferiorly with the radius and ulna of the forearm.
   (2) The rounded head on the superomedial aspect articulates with the glenoid fossa of the scapula.
   (3) The greater and lesser tubercles are on the anterior surface just below the head of the humerus and serve as attachments for muscles.
      (a) The greater tubercle is in the more lateral position.
      (b) The lesser tubercle is in the more anterior position.

(4) The anatomical neck lies just below the head; a surgical neck where the shaft meets the upper portion of the humerus is often the site of fractures.
(5) The intertubercular sulcus is occupied by the tendon of the long head of the biceps muscle; other muscles attach to the sides of the groove.
(6) The deltoid tuberosity, an elevation located anterolaterally on the midshaft of the humerus, is the site of attachment of the deltoid muscle.
(7) The trochlea, a spool-shaped process on the inferior surface, articulates with the ulna of the forearm.
(8) The capitulum, a round area located laterally to the trochlea, articulates with the radius of the forearm.
(9) The lateral epicondyle above the capitulum and medial epicondyle above the trochlea are prominences that serve as attachment sites for muscles.
(10) The medial and lateral supracondylar ridges are located above the medial and lateral epicondyles and are attachments for muscles.
(11) The coronoid fossa, on the anterior surface just superior to the trochlea, fits the coronoid process of the ulna of the forearm.
(12) The olecranon fossa, on the posterior surface just superior to the trochlea, fits the olecranon of the ulna of the forearm.

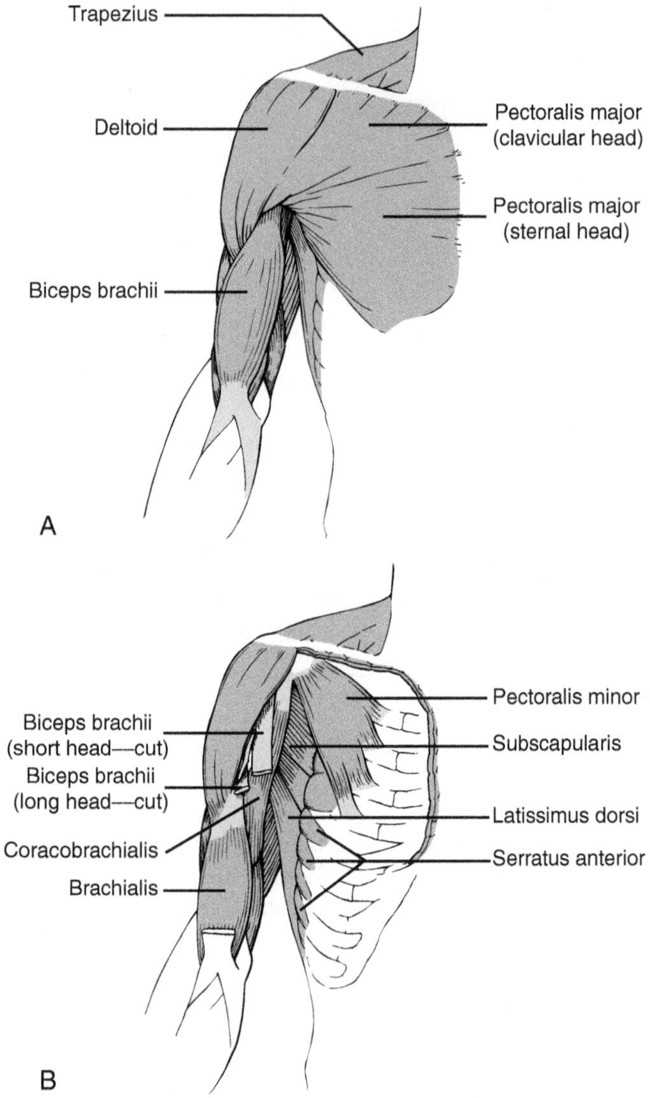

Figure 1-20 Muscles of the pectoral region and anterior right arm. **A,** Superficial. **B,** Deep. *(From Liebgott B: The Anatomical Basis of Dentistry, ed 3, St. Louis, Mosby, 2011.)*

3. The forearm consists of the radius and ulna (Figure 1-19).
   a. The radius is lateral to the ulna when in the anatomic position with palms facing forward or in the supine position.
      (1) The head of the radius is disc-shaped at the proximal end; it articulates superiorly with the capitulum of the humerus and medially with the radial notch of the ulna.
      (2) The radial tuberosity, a projection just below the head on the medial surface, is a site of muscle attachment.
      (3) The lateral styloid process is the pointed, distal portion of the radius.
      (4) The ulnar notch, a shallow depression on the inferomedial aspect of the radius, serves as the articulation with the distal end of the ulna.
   b. The ulna is lateral to the radius when in the pronated position with palms facing posteriorly.

      (1) The trochlear notch on the proximal end of the ulna curves around and articulates with the trochlea of the humerus.
      (2) The coronoid process extends in an anterior-inferior direction from the trochlear notch.
      (3) The olecranon is formed from the superior-posterior portion of the trochlear notch.
      (4) The medial styloid process is the distal projection of the ulna.
4. The wrist and hand consist of carpal bones, metacarpal bones, and phalanges.
   a. Carpal bones.
      (1) There are eight short, cuboidal carpal bones in the wrist, each arranged in a proximal and distal row with four bones in each row.
         (a) Proximal bones—scaphoid, lunate, triquetral, pisiform.
         (b) Distal bones—trapezium, trapezoid, capitate, hamate.

b. Metacarpal bones.

   (1) These bones form the skeleton of the palm of the hand; each base articulates superiorly with the distal row of carpals and inferiorly with the phalanges.

c. Phalanges.

   (1) Each finger has three phalanges—proximal, middle, and distal.

   (2) The thumb lacks a middle phalanx.

5. Muscles are grouped by region: pectoral, superficial back, shoulder, arm, forearm, and hand.

a. Pectoral (see Figure 1-20).

   (1) The pectoralis major muscle is a large, triangular muscle on the anterior chest wall arising from two heads (one from the clavicle and another from the sternum) and inserting into the humerus.

      (a) Can flex, medially rotate, and adduct the arm.

      (b) Supplied by the lateral and medial pectoral nerves.

   (2) The pectoralis minor muscle is a small, triangular muscle arising from the anterior chest wall deep to the pectoralis major muscle and inserting on the coracoid process of the scapula.

      (a) Protracts, depresses, and rotates the scapula laterally.

      (b) Supplied by the medial pectoral nerve.

   (3) The subclavius is a small muscle located below the clavicle.

      (a) Probably insignificant function.

      (b) Supplied by the nerve to subclavius.

   (4) The serratus anterior originates from the anterior chest wall and inserts into the vertebral border of the scapula.

      (a) Protracts the scapula and rotates it medially.

      (b) Supplied by the long thoracic nerve.

b. Superficial back (Figure 1-21, Table 1-22).

   (1) The trapezius muscle is large, thin, flat, and triangular; it covers the back of the neck and upper half of the trunk.

      (a) Superior fibers elevate and laterally rotate the scapula, inferior fibers depress the scapula, and middle fibers help to retract the scapula.

      (b) Supplied mainly by CN XI with a small supply from branches of the cervical plexus of nerves in the neck.

   (2) The latissimus dorsi is large, thin, and flat; it covers the lower half of the back, inserting into the humerus.

      (a) Adducts, extends, and medially rotates the arm.

      (b) Supplied by the thoracodorsal nerve.

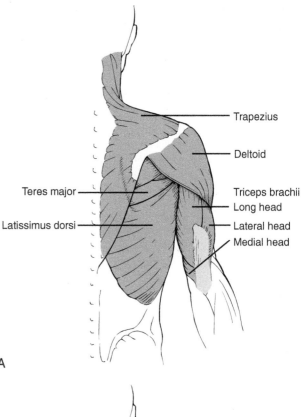

A

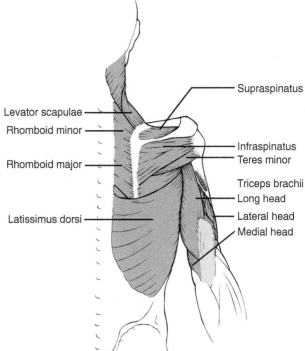

B

Figure 1-21 Posterior muscles of the right shoulder and arm. **A,** Superficial. **B,** Deep. *(From Liebgott B: The Anatomical Basis of Dentistry, ed 3, St. Louis, Mosby, 2011.)*

Table 1-22

Muscles of the Superficial Back

MUSCLE	ORIGIN	INSERTION	ACTION(S)	NERVE
Trapezius	Vertebrae: all thoracic and cervical spines Ligamentum nuchae (membranous extension of cervical spines) Skull: superior nuchal line and inion	Scapula: spine and acromion Clavicle: superior lateral third	1. Upper fibers elevate scapula 2. Lower fibers depress scapula 3. Middle fibers retract scapula 4. Rotates laterally (glenoid fossa points up)	CN XI: spinal accessory APR of C3–C4
Latissimus dorsi	Vertebrae: spines of T6–T12 Os coxae: iliac crest Lumbodorsal fascia Ribs: lower three to four	Humerus: floor of intertubercular sulcus	1. Adducts arm 2. Extends arm 3. Rotates arm medially	Thoracodorsal nerve
Levator scapulae	Vertebrae: transverse processes of C1–C4	Scapula: superior aspect of vertebral border	1. Elevates scapula 2. Rotates scapula medially (glenoid fossa down)	Dorsal scapular
Rhomboids	Vertebrae: spinous processes of C7–T5	Scapula: vertebral border	1. Retracts scapula 2. Rotates scapula medially (glenoid fossa down)	Dorsal scapular

From Liebgott B: The Anatomical Basis of Dentistry, ed 2, St. Louis, Mosby, 2001, p 439.

APR, Anterior primary rami; *CN,* cranial nerve.

(3) The levator scapulae originates from the vertebrae to insert on the superior border of the scapula.
  (a) Elevates and medially rotates the scapula.
  (b) Supplied by the dorsal scapular nerve.
(4) The major and minor rhomboid muscles originate from the vertebrae to insert into the vertebral border of the scapula.
  (a) Retract and medially rotate the scapula.
  (b) Supplied by the dorsal scapular nerve.
c. Shoulder (Table 1-23; see Figures 1-20 and 1-21).
(1) The deltoid muscle originates from bones of the pectoral girdle and inserts into the humerus, wrapping over the shoulder.
  (a) Anterior fibers flex and medially rotate the posterior fibers and extend and laterally rotate the arm at the shoulder; middle fibers abduct the arm.
  (b) Supplied by the axillary nerve.
(2) The teres major muscle originates from the scapula and inserts on the humerus.
  (a) Extends, medially rotates, and adducts the arm.
  (b) Supplied by the lower subscapular nerve.
(3) The rotator cuff muscles are four muscles—supraspinatus, infraspinatus, teres minor, and subscapularis—that originate from the scapula and insert into the upper humerus and joint capsule to hold the head of the humerus in the glenoid fossa.

  (a) Supraspinatus muscle.
    (i) An abductor of the arm at the shoulder.
    (ii) Supplied by the suprascapular nerve.
  (b) Infraspinatus muscle.
    (i) Laterally rotates and slightly adducts the arm.
    (ii) Supplied by the suprascapular nerve.
  (c) Teres minor muscle.
    (i) Laterally rotates, extends, and adducts the arm.
    (ii) Supplied by the axillary nerve.
  (d) Subscapularis muscle.
    (i) Medially rotates the arm.
    (ii) Supplied by both the upper and the lower subscapular nerves.
d. Arm muscles are divided into anterior flexors (biceps brachii, coracobrachialis, and brachialis) and posterior extensors (triceps brachii and anconeus) (Table 1-24; see Figures 1-20 and 1-21).
(1) Biceps brachii originates (the tendon of the long head) from the supraglenoid tubercle of the scapula and from the coracoid process of the scapula (the short head) and, along with the coracobrachialis, inserts into the upper forearm.
  (a) Flexes the elbow.
  (b) Supplied by the musculocutaneous nerve.
(2) Coracobrachialis originates from the coracoid process of the scapula and inserts on the humerus.
  (a) Flexes and adducts the arm.
  (b) Supplied by the musculocutaneous nerve.

Table 1-23

Muscles of the Shoulder

MUSCLE	ORIGIN	INSERTION	ACTION(S)	NERVE
Deltoid	Clavicle: inferior lateral third Scapula: acromion and spine	Humerus: deltoid tuberosity	1. Abducts arm 2. Flexes arm 3. Rotates arm medially (anterior fibers) 4. Extends arm (posterior fibers) 5. Rotates arm laterally (posterior fibers)	Axillary
Teres major	Scapula: inferior angle	Humerus: medial lip of intertubercular sulcus	1. Extends arm 2. Medially rotates arm 3. Adducts arm	Lower subscapular
Rotator cuff muscles				
Supraspinatus	Scapula: supraspinous fossa	Humerus: greater tubercle	1. Abducts arm 2. Stabilizes shoulder joint	Suprascapular
Infraspinatus	Scapula: infraspinous fossa	Humerus: greater tubercle	1. Rotates arm laterally 2. Adduction (slight) 3. Stabilizes shoulder joint	Suprascapular
Teres minor	Scapula: inferior lateral border	Humerus: greater tubercle	1. Rotates arm laterally 2. Extends arm 3. Adducts arm 4. Stabilizes arm at shoulder	Axillary
Subscapularis		Humerus: lesser tubercle Scapula: subscapular fossa	1. Rotates arm medially 2. Stabilizes shoulder joint	Upper and lower subscapular

From Liebgott B: The Anatomical Basis of Dentistry, ed 2, St. Louis, Mosby, 2001, p 439.

Table 1-24

Muscles of the Arm

MUSCLE	ORIGIN	INSERTION	ACTION(S)	NERVE
Anterior (Flexors)				
Biceps brachii	Scapula (short head): coracoid process Scapula (long head): supraglenoid tubercle	Radius: both heads blend into common tendon that inserts into radial tuberosity	1. Major flexor of forearm at elbow 2. Strong supinator of forearm at superior radioulnar joint 3. Weak flexor of arm at shoulder	Musculocutaneous
Coracobrachialis	Scapula: coracoid process	Humerus: medial aspect of midshaft	1. Flexes arm 2. Adducts arm	Musculocutaneous
Brachialis	Humerus: anterior distal aspect	Ulna coronoid process	1. Major flexor of forearm at elbow	Musculocutaneous
Posterior (Extensors)				
Triceps brachii	Scapula (long head): infraglenoid tubercle Humerus (lateral head): posterolateral surface Humerus (medial head): posterior surface below the radial groove	Ulna: all three heads blend into a single tendon that inserts into the olecranon	1. Extends forearm at elbow	Radial
Anconeus	Humerus: lateral epicondyle	Ulna: olecranon along with triceps	1. Extends forearm at elbow 2. Aids in pronation of forearm	Radial

From Liebgott B: The Anatomical Basis of Dentistry, ed 2, St. Louis, Mosby, 2001, p 440.

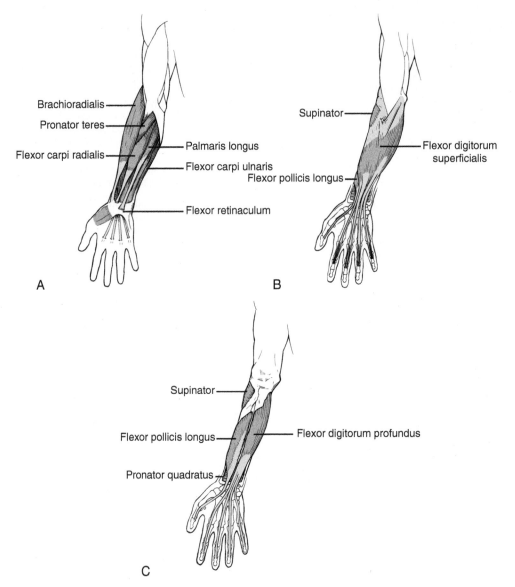

Brachioradialis

Pronator teres

Flexor carpi radialis

Palmaris longus

Flexor carpi ulnaris

Flexor retinaculum

A

Supinator

Flexor pollicis longus

Flexor digitorum superficialis

B

Supinator

Flexor pollicis longus

Flexor digitorum profundus

Pronator quadratus

C

Figure 1-22 Anterior muscles of the right forearm. **A,** Superficial. **B,** Intermediate. **C,** Deep. *(From Liebgott B: The Anatomical Basis of Dentistry, ed 3, St. Louis, Mosby, 2011.)*

(3) Brachialis originates from the humerus and inserts on the coronoid process of the ulna.
  (a) Flexes the elbow.
  (b) Supplied by the musculocutaneous nerve.
(4) Triceps brachii originates from three heads (one originates on the scapula and the other two on the humerus) and inserts into the ulna.
  (a) Extends the arm.
  (b) Supplied by the radial nerve.
(5) Anconeus arises from the lateral epicondyle of the humerus and inserts along with the triceps brachii on the olecranon of the ulna.
  (a) Considered by some to be a portion of triceps brachii.
  (b) Supplied by the radial nerve.

e. Forearm (and hand) muscles are divided into anterior (Figure 1-22, Table 1-25) and posterior (Figure 1-23, Table 1-26) groups and subdivided further into superficial, intermediate, and deep groups for anterior muscles and superficial and deep groups for posterior muscles.
(1) Anterior superficial group.
  (a) Pronator teres originates from the humerus and ulna to insert on the radius.
    (i) Pronates the forearm.
    (ii) Supplied by the median nerve.
  (b) Palmaris longus originates from the medial epicondyle of the humerus and inserts into the palmar aponeurosis of the hand.
    (i) Flexes the hand at the wrist.
    (ii) Supplied by the median nerve.

Table 1-25

Muscles of the Anterior Forearm Compartment

MUSCLE	ORIGIN	INSERTION	ACTION(S)	NERVE
Superficial				
Palmaris longus	Humerus: medial epicondyle via tendon	Palmar aponeurosis of hand Flexor retinaculum	1. Flexes hand at wrist	Median
Flexor carpi radialis	Humerus: medial epicondyle via common flexor tendon	Metacarpals: bases of second and third	1. Flexes hand at wrist 2. Abducts hand at wrist	Median
Flexor carpi ulnaris	Humerus: medial epicondyle via common flexor tendon Ulna: coronoid process	Fifth metacarpal, pisiform, and hamate bones	1. Flexes hand at wrist 2. Abducts hand at wrist	Ulnar
Pronator teres	Humeral head: medial epicondyle Ulnar head: coronoid process and medial aspect	Radius: lateral aspect of midshaft	1. Pronates forearm	Median
Intermediate				
Flexor digitorum superficialis	Humerus: medial epicondyle via common flexor tendon Radius: upper half of anterior shaft	Middle phalanges of all digits except thumb: palmar aspects	1. Flexes middle phalanges at proximal interphalangeal joints	Median
Deep				
Flexor pollicis longus	Ulna: coronoid process Interosseous membrane Radius: anterior surface of shaft	Distal phalanx of thumb: palmar side of base	1. Flexes thumb	Median
Pronator quadratus	Ulna: anterior distal surface of shaft	Radius: anterior distal aspect	1. Pronates forearm and provides power when pronating against resistance	Median
Flexor digitorum profundus	Ulna: medial and anterior aspect and adjacent interosseous membrane	Distal phalanges of all digits except thumb: bases	1. Flexes distal phalanges at distal interphalangeal joints	Ulnar and median

From Liebgott B: The Anatomical Basis of Dentistry, ed 2, St. Louis, Mosby, 2001, p 443.

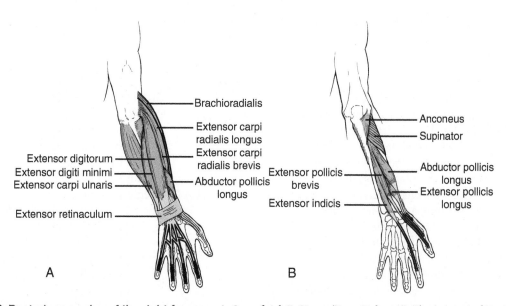

Figure 1-23 Posterior muscles of the right forearm. **A,** Superficial. **B,** Deep. *(From Liebgott B: The Anatomical Basis of Dentistry, ed 3, St. Louis, Mosby, 2011.)*

Table 1-26

Muscles of the Posterior Forearm Compartment

MUSCLE	ORIGIN	INSERTION	ACTION(S)	NERVE
Superficial				
Brachioradialis	Humerus: lateral epicondyle	Radius: styloid process	1. Flexes forearm at elbow: an exception	Radial
Extensor carpi radialis longus	Humerus: lateral supracondylar ridge and lateral epicondyle via common extensor tendon	Second metacarpal: base	1. Extends hand at wrist 2. Abducts hand at wrist	Radial
Extensor carpi radialis brevis	Humerus: lateral epicondyle via common extensor tendon	Third metacarpal: base	1. Extends hand at wrist 2. Abducts hand at wrist	Radial
Extensor carpi ulnaris	Humerus: lateral epicondyle via common extensor tendon Ulna: posterior border	Fifth metacarpal: base	1. Extends hand at wrist 2. Abducts hand at wrist	Radial
Extensor digitorum	Humerus: lateral epicondyle via common extensor tendon	Phalanges: lateral and dorsal aspects via extensor expansions	1. Extends fingers 2. Aids in extending wrist	Radial
Extensor digiti minimi	Humerus: lateral epicondyle via common extensor tendon	Proximal phalanx of fifth (little) finger: dorsal aspect	1. Extends little finger	Radial
Deep				
Supinator	Humerus: lateral epicondyle Ulna: proximal aspect below radial notch	Radius: lateral aspect of proximal end	1. Supinates forearm and turns palm forward in anatomic position, or up, as in accepting change when shoulder and elbow are flexed	Radial
Abductor pollicis longus	Ulna: middle third of posterior aspect Radius: middle third of posterior aspect Interosseous membrane	First metacarpal: radial side of base	1. Abducts thumb 2. Abducts wrist	Radial
Extensor pollicis longus	Ulna: middle third of posterior aspect Interosseous membrane	Distal phalanx of thumb: base	1. Extends distal phalanx of thumb	Radial
Extensor pollicis brevis	Radius: posterior aspect Interosseous membrane	Proximal phalanx of thumb: base	1. Extends proximal phalanx of thumb	Radial
Extensor indicis	Ulna: posterior aspect Interosseous membrane	Proximal phalanx of first (index) finger: dorsal aspect	1. Extends index finger	Radial

From Liebgott B: The Anatomical Basis of Dentistry, ed 2, St. Louis, Mosby, 2001, p 445.

(c) Flexor carpi radialis originates from the humerus and inserts into the bases of the second and third metacarpals.
  (i) Flexor and abductor of the wrist.
  (ii) Supplied by the median nerve.
(d) Flexor carpi ulnaris originates from the humerus and inserts into the fifth metacarpal, pisiform, and hamate bones.
  (i) Flexes and adducts the wrist.
  (ii) Supplied by the ulnar nerve.
(2) Anterior intermediate group.
  (a) Flexor digitorum superficialis originates from the common flexor tendon of the medial epicondyle of the humerus and the upper one half of the radius and inserts into the middle phalanges of all four digits.
  (i) It is a flexor of proximal interphalangeal joints, metacarpophalangeal joints, and the wrist joint.
  (ii) Supplied by the median nerve.
(3) Deep anterior group.
  (a) Flexor digitorum profundus originates from the anterior of the ulna and passes over the wrist as four tendons that insert into distal phalanges of the fingers.
  (i) Flexes the distal phalanges and the wrist.
  (ii) Supplied by the medial nerve on the radial aspect and the ulnar nerve on the ulnar aspect.

(b) Flexor pollicis longus originates from both the ulna and the radius and inserts into the distal phalanx of the thumb.
    (i) Flexes the thumb.
    (ii) Supplied by the median nerve.
(c) Pronator quadratus muscle arises from the ulna and inserts on the radius.
    (i) Pronates the forearm.
    (ii) Supplied by the median nerve.
(4) Posterior superficial group (see Figure 1-23, *A*).
  (a) Brachioradialis arises from the lateral epicondyle of the humerus and inserts into the styloid process of the radius.
    (i) Flexes the forearm at the elbow.
    (ii) Supplied by the radial nerve.
  (b) Extensor carpi radialis longus muscle.
  (c) Extensor carpi radialis brevis muscle.
  (d) Extensor carpi ulnaris.
  (e) Extensor digitorum muscles.
  (f) Extensor digiti minimi.
(5) Posterior deep group (see Figure 1-23, *B*).
  (a) Supinator.
  (b) Abductor pollicis longus.
  (c) Extensor pollicis longus.
  (d) Extensor pollicis brevis.
  (e) Extensor indicis.

6. Nerve supply.
  a. The brachial plexus of nerves arises in the neck (Figure 1-24).
    (1) It passes downward over the first rib and under the clavicle to the axilla and then to the upper limb.

  b. The brachial plexus of nerves provides the entire motor and sensory nerve supply to the upper limb.
    (1) The plexus arises from five roots from the anterior primary rami of spinal nerves C5, C6, C7, C8, and T1.
    (2) The five roots unite to form three trunks.
      (a) The upper trunk forms from the roots of C5 and C6.
      (b) The middle trunk forms from C7.
      (c) The lower trunk forms from C8 and T1.
    (3) Each of the three trunks divides in two to form six divisions.
    (4) The divisions reunite to form three cords.
      (a) Lateral cord.
      (b) Medial cord.
      (c) Posterior cord.
    (5) The cords divide to form five terminal branches.
  c. The roots, trunks, and cords of the brachial plexus lead to several collateral branches; these supply some of the muscles of the neck, upper limb girdle, and arm; there also is a cutaneous nerve supply to the arm and forearm.
    (1) The long thoracic nerve forms from the three upper roots of the anterior primary rami (C5, C6, and C7), runs inferiorly along the rib cage, and supplies the serratus anterior muscle.
    (2) The dorsal scapular nerve forms from the most superior root of the anterior primary rami (C5) to supply the rhomboid muscles.
    (3) The suprascapular nerve forms from the upper trunk, passes through the suprascapular notch of the scapula, supplies the subclavius muscle

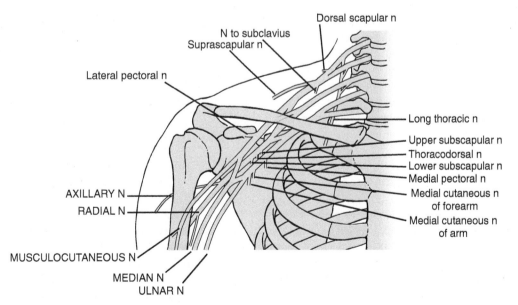

Figure 1-24 Branches of the right brachial plexus. Collateral branches are labeled in lowercase; terminal branches are labeled in uppercase. *(From Liebgott B: The Anatomical Basis of Dentistry, ed 3, St. Louis, Mosby, 2011.)*

and infraspinatus muscle, and is sensory to the shoulder joint.

(4) The lateral pectoral nerve forms from the lateral cord and supplies most of the pectoralis major muscle.

(5) The medial pectoral nerve forms from the medial cord, supplies the pectoralis minor muscle, and helps supply the pectoralis major muscle.

(6) Three motor branches leave the posterior cord to supply muscles of the pectoral girdle; the upper subscapular nerve to the subscapularis muscle, the lower subscapular nerve to the subscapularis muscle and teres major muscle, and the thoracodorsal nerve to the latissimus dorsi muscle.

(7) The medial cutaneous nerves of the arm and forearm leave the distal end of the medial cord.

d. The six divisions of the brachial plexus join to form five terminal branches.

(1) The musculoskeletal nerve supplies the three large flexor muscles located on the anterior arm (biceps brachii, coracobrachialis, and brachialis) and continues into the forearm as the lateral cutaneous nerve of the forearm.

(2) The median nerve supplies the flexors and pronators, which overlie the anterior of the forearm, and ends as cutaneous fibers to the lateral portion of the palm and palmar aspects of the thumb, first finger, second finger, and lateral portion of the third finger.

(3) The ulnar nerve supplies smaller intrinsic muscles of the hand responsible for fine movement and flexors and ends as cutaneous branches to the medial aspect of the hand.

(4) The radial nerve supplies all the extensor muscles of the upper limb and cutaneous branches to the skin of the posterior aspect of the arm and forearm and the lateral aspect of the dorsum of the hand.

(5) The axillary nerve supplies the shoulder joint and the area of the deltoid muscle.

e. Cutaneous nerves of the upper limb form from both collateral and terminal branches of the brachial plexus (Figure 1-25).

7. Arterial supply (Figure 1-26).

a. The subclavian artery supplies blood to the entire upper limb.

(1) The right subclavian artery arises from the brachiocephalic artery, and the left subclavian artery arises from the aortic arch; both loop upward and laterally through the root of the neck and descend over the first rib into the axilla.

(2) After crossing the first rib, the subclavian artery becomes the axillary artery.

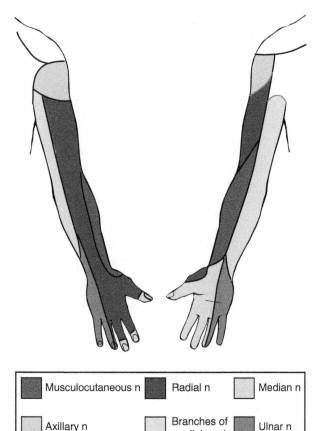

■ Musculocutaneous n	■ Radial n	□ Median n
□ Axillary n	□ Branches of medial cord	■ Ulnar n

Figure 1-25 Cutaneous innervation of the upper limb. *(From Liebgott B: The Anatomical Basis of Dentistry, ed 3, St. Louis, Mosby, 2011.)*

(3) The axillary artery passes through the axilla and provides several collateral branches that follow collateral branches of the brachial plexus of nerves.

(a) The axillary artery crosses over the tendon of the teres major muscle and enters the arm; at this point, it is called the *brachial artery*.

(4) The brachial artery is positioned on the anterior aspect of the humerus at midlength after entering the arm from the medial aspect.

(a) It provides several branches to muscles of the upper arm.

(b) It descends to the cubital fossa on the anterior aspect of the elbow.

(5) The brachial artery splits into the radial and ulnar arteries below the elbow.

(6) The radial artery descends on the lateral surface of the front of the forearm; this is where the pulse is located on the wrist.

(a) The radial artery enters the hand and loops medially as the deep palmar arch.

(b) The deep palmar arch anastomoses medially with a branch of the ulnar artery.

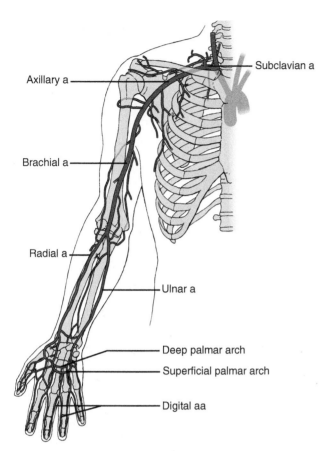

Axillary a

Subclavian a

Brachial a

Radial a

Ulnar a

Deep palmar arch

Superficial palmar arch

Digital aa

Figure 1-26 Arterial supply to the right upper limb. *(From Liebgott B: The Anatomical Basis of Dentistry, ed 3, St. Louis, Mosby, 2011.)*

(7) The ulnar artery descends on the medial surface of the front of the forearm.

  (a) The ulnar artery enters the hand and loops laterally as the superficial palmar arch.

  (b) The superficial palmar arch anastomoses medially with a branch of the radial artery.

(8) Digital arteries arise from the palmar arches to supply the medial and lateral aspects of each finger.

8. Venous return (Figure 1-27).

  a. Deep veins.

    (1) Deep veins of the upper limb share the names of and parallel the deep arteries.

    (2) Deep veins collect as the axillary vein.

    (3) The axillary vein ascends over the first rib and is then called the *subclavian vein.*

  b. Superficial veins.

    (1) The dorsal venous vein lies below the skin of the dorsum of the hand and receives tributaries from the fingers.

    (2) The cephalic vein drains the lateral aspect of the dorsal venous arch, spirals anteriorly at the wrist, and ascends on the lateral side of the arm and forearm.

(3) The basilic vein drains the medial aspect of the dorsal venous arch and ascends on the medial side of the arm and forearm.

  (a) As the basilic vein traverses the cubital fossa, it receives blood from the cephalic vein through the median cubital vein and the median antebrachial vein.

(4) Near the midpoint of the arm, the basilic vein curves deeply and joins the axillary vein.

9. Lymphatic drainage (Figure 1-28).

  a. Deep lymph vessels.

    (1) Deep lymph vessels follow radial, ulnar, brachial, and axillary veins to drain into axillary lymph nodes.

    (2) The axillary lymph nodes merge as the subclavian trunk.

    (3) The subclavian trunk drains upper limb lymph back into circulation at the confluence of the internal jugular and subclavian veins.

1.3 Thoracic Cavity

The thoracic cavity is surrounded by the thorax, a wall of muscle and bone. It extends from just superior to the first rib to the diaphragm. The diaphragm separates the thoracic cavity from the abdominal cavity.

A. The thoracic skeleton and its divisions: the thoracic skeleton is a round, cagelike structure consisting of the sternum, 12 pairs of ribs and associated costal cartilages, and 12 thoracic vertebrae.

1. Sternum—composed of three portions.

  a. Manubrium.

    (1) The midline jugular or suprasternal notch is palpated at the base of the anterior neck.

    (2) The lateral notches attach to the clavicles.

    (3) The lateral borders articulate with the costal cartilages of the first ribs.

  b. Body.

    (1) Joins the manubrium through a symphysis at the sternal angle.

    (2) Costal cartilages of the second ribs articulate with the sternum at the junction of the manubrium and body.

  c. Xiphoid process.

    (1) A small, inferior portion.

2. Ribs—features.

  a. Head, which articulates with the body of a thoracic vertebra.

  b. Neck.

  c. Tubercle, which articulates with the transverse process of a thoracic vertebra.

  d. Shaft.

  e. Angle where the rib turns inferiorly and anteriorly.

  f. Subcostal groove on the inferior internal surface that shelters the intercostal nerve and vessels.

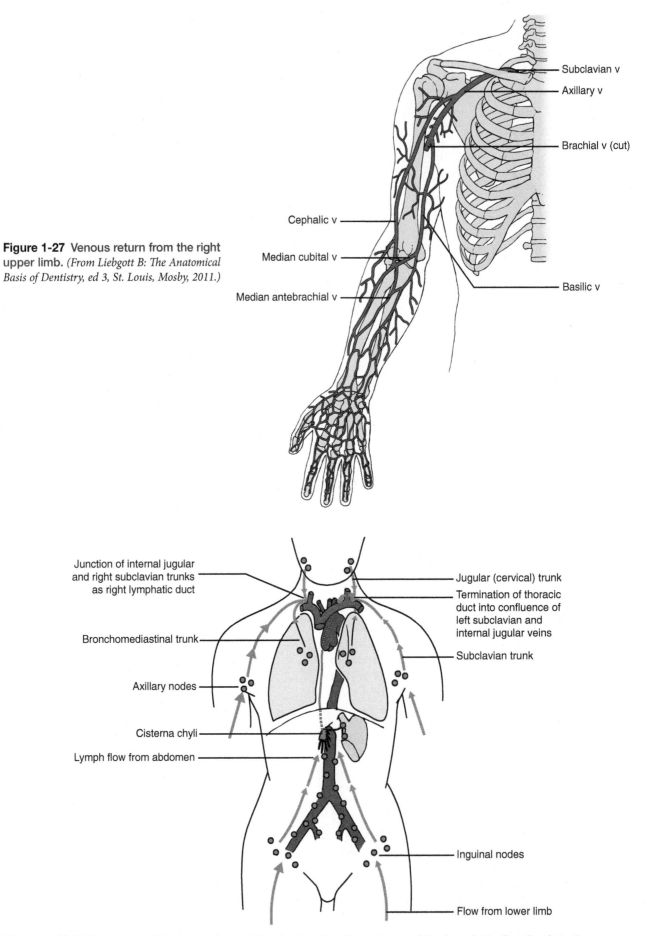

Figure 1-27 Venous return from the right upper limb. *(From Liebgott B: The Anatomical Basis of Dentistry, ed 3, St. Louis, Mosby, 2011.)*

Subclavian v

Axillary v

Brachial v (cut)

Cephalic v

Median cubital v

Median antebrachial v

Basilic v

Junction of internal jugular and right subclavian trunks as right lymphatic duct

Jugular (cervical) trunk

Termination of thoracic duct into confluence of left subclavian and internal jugular veins

Bronchomediastinal trunk

Subclavian trunk

Axillary nodes

Cisterna chyli

Lymph flow from abdomen

Inguinal nodes

Flow from lower limb

Figure 1-28 Major groups of lymph nodes and trunks showing the scheme of the lymphatic flow back to the venous system. *(From Liebgott B: The Anatomical Basis of Dentistry, ed 3, St. Louis, Mosby, 2011.)*

3. Ribs—types.
   a. True ribs are the upper seven pairs that attach directly to the sternum via costal cartilages.
   b. False ribs are the lower five pairs of ribs that attach indirectly to the sternum via costal cartilages or, in the case of the last pair, not at all.
   c. The first rib has some unique features on the superior aspect area.
      (1) Groove for the subclavian vein.
      (2) Scalene tubercle for attachment of the scalenus anterior muscle.
      (3) Roughened area for attachment of the scalenus medius muscle.
4. Thoracic vertebrae—unique features.
   a. Heart-shaped body.
   b. Long, slender spinous processes.
   c. The bodies and transverse processes have facets for articulation with ribs.
   d. Ribs 1, 10, 11, and 12 articulate with only a single vertebra.
   e. The other ribs articulate with the body of their own vertebra and that of the vertebra above.
5. Joints.
   a. In addition to joints between thoracic vertebrae, the remaining three types of joints allow for movement during inspiration.
      (1) Costovertebral joints are synovial joints between the heads of the ribs and vertebral bodies and between the tubercles of the ribs and transverse processes. They permit elevation and depression of the ribs.
      (2) Sternocostal joints are synovial joints between the costal cartilages of true ribs (exclusive of the costal cartilage of the first rib, which joins the first rib to the manubrium as a synchondrosis).
      (3) Costochondral joints are synchondroses between distal ends of ribs and their corresponding costal cartilages.
B. The thoracic wall—the thoracic (chest) wall includes surface features such as the breast and skeletal landmarks, muscles, and intercostal blood vessels and nerves.
   1. Breast.
      a. Arises as a modified sweat gland covered by skin within superficial fascia of the anterior chest wall.
      b. In women, the breast overlies the pectoralis muscle at the level of ribs two through six. An axillary tail extends laterally and superiorly to the axillary region.
      c. Within the breast are 15 to 20 lobules of glandular tissue lying within fat of the superficial fascia.
      d. The ducts of the glands empty to the surface through the nipple. The nipple is surrounded by an areola containing areolar glands.
      e. The breast is supported through suspensory ligaments (of Cooper) that anchor it to underlying deep fascia.
      f. Arterial blood is supplied by mammary branches of the axillary artery, the internal thoracic artery, and intercostal arteries.
      g. The breast may be divided into quadrants. The two lateral quadrants drain to the superior nodes of the axilla. The two medial quadrants drain to the axillary nodes, the anterior chest wall, and the interior abdominal wall. They may even drain to the opposite breast across the midline. Malignancies may spread along lymphatic routes.
   2. Skeletal landmarks.
      a. The suprasternal or jugular notch at the base of the neck is important in locating the trachea.
      b. The costal margin, formed by the inferior aspects of costal cartilages 7 through 10, meets in the midline at the xiphoid process. This landmark may be used to help determine the correct position on the sternum for external compressions during cardiopulmonary resuscitation (CPR).
      c. The sternal angle between the manubrium and sternum marks the position of the second rib. From this location, ribs can be counted externally because the first rib cannot be palpated.
   3. Muscles of the thorax—thoracic muscles stabilize the upper and lower ribs and elevate the remaining ribs during quiet inspiration. During forced inspiration, accessory muscles elevate the upper ribs to increase thoracic volume further.
      a. The diaphragm is the most important muscle of respiration. When it contracts, it increases the size of the thorax by pulling the central tendon inferiorly. It is supplied by the right and left phrenic nerves, which are the anterior primary rami of C3, C4, and C5.
      b. Extrinsic thoracic muscles are superficial muscles covering the chest wall that belong to other regions.
         (1) Upper limb muscles that originate from the thoracic skeleton include pectoralis major, pectoralis minor, serratus anterior, latissimus dorsi, rhomboid major, rhomboid minor, levator scapulae, and trapezius.
         (2) Muscles of the abdominal wall that attach to the thoracic skeleton include rectus abdominis, external oblique, internal oblique, and transversus abdominis.
         (3) Posterior muscles that attach to the thoracic skeleton include erector spinae and muscles of the back.
      c. Accessory extrinsic muscles of respiration insert into the skeleton of the upper thorax and elevate the sternum and ribs during forced inspiration. These muscles of the neck region include SCM,

scalenus anterior, scalenus medius, and scalenus posterior.

d. Intercostal muscles of the thorax extend in several directions—from rib to rib, sternum to rib, and vertebra to rib. They are listed from the surface inward and are involved in the process of breathing. Intercostal nerves supply these muscles.

   (1) The external intercostal muscle runs from rib to rib in an anterior-inferior direction. They elevate the ribs during inspiration.

   (2) The internal intercostal muscle extends from rib to rib in a posterior-inferior direction perpendicular to the external intercostal muscle. It depresses the ribs during expiration.

   (3) The innermost intercostal muscles run parallel to the internal intercostal muscles. The intercostal nerves and vessels course between these two layers. Posterior fibers are called *subcostals*, and anterior fibers are called *transversus thoracis*. They are thought to depress ribs during expiration.

e. Levator costarum muscles are back muscles that participate in respiration. They originate from transverse processes C7 to T11, run down and laterally, and insert into an area between the tubercle and angle of the rib below. These muscles elevate ribs during inspiration. They are innervated by the posterior primary rami of thoracic spinal nerves.

f. The serratus posterior superior and inferior muscles are located on the posterior thoracic wall.

   (1) The superior muscle runs downward and laterally from the lower cervical and upper thoracic vertebral spines to the upper ribs. It elevates the ribs during inspiration.

   (2) The inferior muscle runs upward and laterally from the upper lumbar and lower thoracic vertebral spines and inserts into the lower ribs. It depresses or stabilizes the lower ribs.

4. Intercostal blood vessels and nerves are located between the internal and innermost intercostal muscles found between pairs of ribs. They run under the subcostal groove of the superior rib of the pair.

a. Posterior intercostal arteries arise from the thoracic aorta in paired, segmented branches. They run laterally and anteriorly and supply the body wall.

b. Anterior intercostal arteries arise from the internal thoracic artery. These supply the anterior body wall and anastomose with the posterior intercostal arteries. The internal thoracic artery divides into two terminal branches, the superior epigastric artery of the anterior abdominal wall and the musculophrenic artery of the diaphragm.

c. Intercostal veins parallel the arteries. Anterior intercostal veins empty into the internal thoracic

veins. Posterior intercostal veins empty into the azygos and hemiazygos veins. The superior intercostal veins empty into the brachiocephalic veins.

d. Spinal nerves arise from the spinal cord in a paired, segmented manner. The anterior primary rami travel laterally and anteriorly along with the intercostal arteries and veins as intercostal nerves. Lateral cutaneous branches are given off laterally. As the nerves reach the midline, anterior cutaneous branches are given off to the anterior chest wall.

C. Pleural cavities (Figure 1-29).

  The pleural cavities contain the lungs. The pleural cavity is lined with pleura, a serous membrane.

1. Parietal pleura lines the pleural cavity itself. Parietal pleura is subdivided by region.

a. Costal pleura lines the inner aspect of the rib cage.

b. Diaphragmatic pleura lines the superior aspect of the diaphragm.

c. Mediastinal pleura covers the mediastinum.

d. Cervical pleura (cupola) extends into the neck.

2. Visceral pleura lines the lungs.

a. Both parietal and visceral pleura are continuous at the root of the lung.

3. Pleural recesses are areas of space between reflected areas of pleura.

a. The costodiaphragmatic recess is located laterally and inferiorly, and the costomediastinal recess is located medially and anteriorly.

D. Lungs.

  The pleural cavities contain the lungs. The alveoli are the functional site of the lungs, where the exchange of oxygen and carbon dioxide take place. The alveoli are supported by elastic tissue that tends to collapse and shrink the lung during expiration.

1. Surfaces of the lung.

a. The rounded, superior apex that bulges up through the thoracic inlet.

b. The mediastinal surface that contacts the mediastinum.

c. The convex costal surface that fits the ribs.

d. The concave base or diaphragmatic surface resting on the diaphragm.

2. Borders of the lung.

a. The anterior border separates the costal surface from the mediastinal surface.

b. The posterior border separates the costal surface from the mediastinal surface posteriorly.

c. The lower circumferential border separates the diaphragmatic surface from the costal and mediastinal surfaces.

3. Fissures and lobes of the lung.

a. The lungs are divided into lobes by fissures. The right lung has three lobes, and the left lung has two lobes. Although both lungs have an oblique fissure dividing them into upper and lower lobes, the right

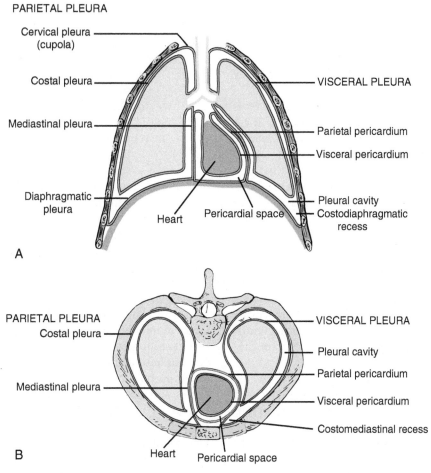

PARIETAL PLEURA

Cervical pleura (cupola)

Costal pleura

Mediastinal pleura

VISCERAL PLEURA

Parietal pericardium

Visceral pericardium

Diaphragmatic pleura

Heart

Pericardial space

Pleural cavity

Costodiaphragmatic recess

A

PARIETAL PLEURA

Costal pleura

Mediastinal pleura

VISCERAL PLEURA

Pleural cavity

Parietal pericardium

Visceral pericardium

Costomediastinal recess

B

Heart

Pericardial space

Figure 1-29 Sections through the thorax to show pleural cavities, mediastinum, and coverings. **A,** Coronal section. **B,** Transverse section. *(From Liebgott B: The Anatomical Basis of Dentistry, ed 3, St. Louis, Mosby, 2011.)*

lung has a second horizontal fissure that creates an additional middle lobe.

b. The cardiac notch on the left lobe is a feature substituting for the lack of a third, middle lobe.

4. The hilum of the lung is the entrance and exit for the air tubes and blood vessels.

a. The pulmonary artery carries unoxygenated blood from the right ventricle to the lungs, and the pulmonary vein carries oxygenated blood from the lungs.

b. The bronchi arise from the midline trachea. They carry air to the lung through the hilum during inspiration and from the lung during expiration.

c. The bronchial artery arises from the thoracic descending aorta and travels to the hilum to supply the lung.

d. Autonomic nerves enter the lungs through the hilum.

e. Lymphatic vessels enter and leave the lungs through the hilum.

E. Bronchi.

The trachea is composed of cartilaginous rings connected with fibroelastic tissue. The rings are incomplete;

the posterior portion that lacks cartilage is covered with fibrous tissue and involuntary muscle.

The trachea descends along with, but anterior to, the esophagus from the neck. The isthmus of the thyroid gland crosses the second or third tracheal ring. The trachea enters the inlet of the thorax, deep to the sternum; at vertebral level T5, it bifurcates at a midline cartilaginous ring called the *carina* into the right and left primary bronchus. The right primary bronchus is wider, shorter, and more directly in line with the trachea.

1. Right bronchus.

a. The right primary bronchus divides into three secondary bronchi, corresponding to the three lobes of the right lung. The secondary bronchus to the upper lobe separates before the primary bronchus passes through the hilum of the lung. The primary bronchus within the lobe divides and supplies secondary bronchi to the middle and lower lobes.

b. Each secondary bronchus further divides into tertiary bronchi that continue to divide until they lose cartilaginous support.

c. At this point, the walls of the tubes are lined with smooth muscle and are called *bronchioles*. Bronchioles end as terminal bronchioles, with ductules that lead into alveoli.

d. Alveoli are blind sacs that are one cell thick. They are the site of gas exchange.

e. Surrounding each alveolus are capillaries from arterioles supplied by pulmonary arteries. These capillaries anastomose with venules that course and unite as pulmonary veins.

2. Left bronchus.

a. The structure of the left bronchial tree is similar to the right, with two exceptions. Because there are only two lobes in the left lung, there are only two rather than three bronchi that divide to create tertiary bronchi.

F. Blood supply.

1. Bronchial arteries supply blood to the lungs. They branch from the descending aorta and course along with the bronchi and bronchioles to the parenchyma of the lung. Lymph vessels parallel the arterial vessels but drain in the opposite direction to the bronchomediastinal trunk.

G. Nerve supply.

1. The lungs are controlled by the sympathetic and parasympathetic divisions of the autonomic nervous system.

a. Pulmonary branches of the vagus nerve (CN X) function as parasympathetic efferent nerves. They are bronchoconstrictors and secretomotors.

b. Sympathetic efferents are derived mainly from the second, third, and fourth ganglia of the sympathetic trunk. They function as bronchodilators.

2. Both divisions form a pulmonary nerve plexus around the pulmonary vessels at the hilum of the lung. They surround and follow the vessels as they pass into the lung.

3. The phrenic nerve supplies pleura adjacent to the diaphragm and mediastinum. Costal pleura is supplied by intercostal nerves.

H. Mechanics of breathing.

1. Air is inhaled during inspiration and exhaled during expiration.

a. Inspiration: the muscles involved in breathing enlarge the pleural cavity in three planes to increase the volume and decrease the pressure within the lungs.

(1) The transverse diameter increases when intercostal muscles raise the ribs at the costovertebral and costosternal joints and move them laterally.

(2) The anterior-posterior diameter increases when the right and left rib pairs raise around the costovertebral joints and move the sternum anteriorly.

(3) The size of the vertical plane increases when the diaphragm contracts downward.

(4) During forced inspiration, additional muscles are called into action.

(a) Scalene muscles of the neck raise the first two ribs.

(b) The sternomastoid muscle raises the manubrium.

(c) Extremely labored breathing may include the pectoral muscles and the serratus anterior muscle.

b. Expiration: normal expiration is passive. Elastic recoil of the lungs forces air out when the muscles of respiration are relaxed.

(1) During forced expiration, abdominal muscles contract and raise intraabdominal pressure while the diaphragm relaxes.

Mediastinum

The mediastinum separates the pleural cavities. It is a group of midline structures covered on the left and right surfaces with mediastinal pleura. The mediastinum contains the heart and associated great vessels, thoracic trachea and bronchi, thoracic esophagus, vagus nerves, phrenic nerves, and thoracic duct. The mediastinum is divided into four areas: middle mediastinum, anterior mediastinum, superior mediastinum, and posterior mediastinum (see Figure 1-29).

I. Middle mediastinum.

1. Contains the pericardial sac and enclosed heart.

a. Pericardial sac.

(1) Pericardium comprises a tough outer layer of fibrous tissue and an inner layer of serous membrane called *visceral pericardium* or *epicardium*. The pericardial space between the visceral and parietal pericardium contains serous fluid.

(2) The outer layer is adherent to the diaphragm.

2. Heart.

a. Shape and position—the heart is within the thorax, behind the sternum, and above the diaphragm. It is located closer to the anterior chest wall than the posterior chest wall.

(1) The superior border is at the level of the sternal angle.

(2) The inferior border passes to the left above the xiphoid process to a point 10 cm left of the midline. The inferior border ends to the left as the apex of the heart, at the fifth intercostal space or the sixth rib.

(3) The left border runs obliquely upward toward the sternal angle.

(4) The right border runs parallel to the right of the sternum inferiorly to the level of the fifth intercostal space.

b. Chambers.
  (1) The right atrium forms the entire right surface and border of the heart and about one quarter of the anterior surface. The right auricle is an extension of the right atrium; it encircles the base of the aorta.
  (2) The left atrium is on the posterior surface of the heart. The left auricle encircles the base of the pulmonary trunk.
  (3) The right ventricle forms two thirds of the inferior border of the heart and most of the anterior surface.
  (4) The left ventricle forms almost all of the left border of the heart and the apex, which is a small piece of the left inferior border.
c. Surface of the heart: the heart has three surfaces and an apex.
  (1) The sternocostal surface is on the anterior surface of the heart. It is almost completely overlapped by the lungs.
  (2) The diaphragmatic surface rests on the diaphragm.
  (3) The posterior surface consists mostly of the left atrium and left ventricle.
  (4) The apex of the heart may be observed beating in the left fifth intercostal space, about 10 cm from the midline.
d. Features of the heart—two grooves on the surface of the heart delineate underlying septa between chambers.
  (1) The atrioventricular sulcus represents the septum separating the atria from ventricles.
  (2) The interventricular sulcus represents the septum separating the right ventricle from left ventricle.
e. Heart wall—the heart consists of three layers.
  (1) The epicardium (visceral pericardium) is a serous layer covering the external heart.
  (2) The myocardium is a layer of cardiac involuntary muscle with the property of automaticity.
  (3) The endocardium is an inner endothelial lining.
f. Entrances to and exits from the heart.
  (1) The superior and inferior venae cavae enter the right atrium carrying deoxygenated blood from veins of the circulatory system. The superior vena cava carries returning blood from the head, upper limb, and thorax. The inferior vena cava carries returning blood from the lower limbs and abdomen.
g. Internal features of the right atrium—the right atrium of the heart receives blood from the superior and inferior venae cavae.
  (1) The orifice of the superior vena cava lies superior to the orifice of the inferior vena cava. It does not have a valve.
  (2) The orifice of the inferior vena cava lies inferior to the orifice of the superior vena cava. It has a small, albeit rudimentary, crescent-shaped valve.
  (3) The crista terminalis is a ridge that runs vertically between orifices of the superior and inferior venae cavae. It represents the junction between the sinus venosus and the heart in the developing heart of the embryo.
  (4) The pectinate muscles radiate out from the crista terminalis at right angles.
  (5) The fossa ovalis, an oval depression above the valve of the inferior vena cava, represents the remnant of foramen ovale, the prenatal shunt from the right to the left atrium.
  (6) The right auricle is an appendage of the right atrium.
  (7) The left auricle is an appendage of the left atrium.
  (8) The right atrioventricular valve leads to the right ventricle. It is called the *tricuspid valve* because it has three leaflets.
  (9) The coronary sinus opens into the right atrium just above the atrioventricular orifice. It returns blood from the heart walls.
  (10) The sinoatrial and atrioventricular nodes are not visible on gross inspection of the heart. The sinoatrial node is located at the junction of the superior vena cava and the right atrium. It is the pacemaker of the heart. The atrioventricular node is located above the opening of the coronary sinus. It relays the signal from the sinoatrial node.
h. Internal features of the left atrium—the left atrium receives blood from pulmonary veins from the lungs.
  (1) The two right and two left pulmonary veins enter the heart through four separate orifices.
  (2) The left atrium is drained through the left atrioventricular valve. This valve is called the *bicuspid* or *mitral valve* because it has two leaflets.
i. Internal features of the right ventricle—the right ventricle receives blood from the right atrium through the right atrioventricular valve. It has a thicker, more muscular wall than the right atrium because it is a pumping chamber.
  (1) Ridges of cardiac muscle called *trabeculae carneae* give the internal surface a roughened appearance.
  (2) The right atrioventricular or tricuspid valve has three leaflets. The bases of these are anchored to a tendinous ring around the orifice of the valve.

(3) The chordae tendineae extend from the free edges of the cusps of the tricuspid valve to papillary muscles.

(4) Papillary muscles anchor the chordae tendineae and cusps to the heart wall. These muscles contract as the ventricles contract, ensuring that the cusps of the valve seal the orifice but are not pushed back into the right atrium.

(5) The pulmonary valve is a three-pocket valve. After the right ventricle contracts, the pockets of this valve fill with blood and prevent further backflow of blood into the right ventricle.

(6) The septomarginal trabecula contains cardiac fibers that conduct impulses from the interventricular septum to the anterior papillary muscle.

j. Internal features of the left ventricle—the left ventricle pumps blood to the whole body. The walls are thick and muscular.

(1) The trabeculae carneae are ridges of cardiac muscle that roughen the surface as they do in the right ventricle.

(2) The left atrioventricular valve has two valves. It is also known as the *mitral valve*.

(3) The chordae tendineae prevent the valves from extending into the left atrium during ventricular contraction.

(4) The aortic valve has three pockets. It prevents backflow of blood from the aorta back into the left ventricle following contraction.

k. Blood vessels—the right and left coronary arteries supply the heart muscle with oxygenated blood (Figure 1-30, *A*). They are the first pair of arteries to leave the aorta. They arise just above the aortic

valve. The various cardiac veins of the heart drain into the coronary sinus, which is a single, large vein that enters the right atrium of the heart.

(1) The right coronary artery passes inferiorly in the anterior atrioventricular sulcus and supplies blood to cardiac tissue. At the inferior margin of the heart, it gives off the right marginal branch, then turns posteriorly and ascends into the posterior atrioventricular sulcus until it reaches the posterior interventricular groove. It divides into two branches, one of which continues posteriorly in the atrioventricular sulcus to anastomose with the circumflex artery. The other branch turns down toward the apex of the heart to anastomose with the anterior interventricular branch of the left coronary artery.

(2) The left coronary artery, traveling between the left atrium and pulmonary trunk, reaches the atrioventricular or coronary sulcus. Here it gives off a left marginal artery and two terminal branches. The anterior interventricular branch descends in the sulcus toward the apex of the heart. It curves posteriorly and anastomoses with the posterior interventricular branch of the right coronary artery. The circumflex branch travels around in the atrioventricular sulcus to the posterior of the heart. It descends obliquely to anastomose with the terminal part of the right coronary artery.

(3) The great cardiac vein travels up the anterior interventricular sulcus and receives venous blood. It turns posterior and to the right as the coronary sinus (Figure 1-30, *B*). It receives

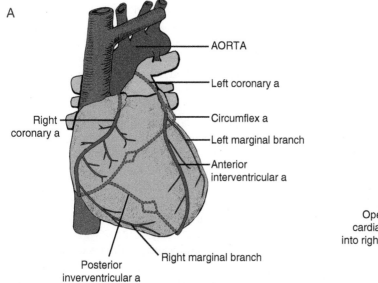
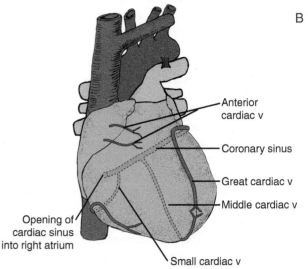

Figure 1-30 Blood vessels of the heart. A, Arterial supply. **B,** Venous drainage. *(From Liebgott B: The Anatomical Basis of Dentistry, ed 3, St. Louis, Mosby, 2011.)*

two tributaries, the oblique vein from the left atrium and the posterior vein of the left ventricle. As the coronary sinus approaches the right atrium, it receives the middle cardiac vein and small cardiac veins. Small anterior cardiac veins of the right ventricle drain directly into the right atrium. A small amount of blood passes to and from the heart wall via small venae cordis minimae.

l. Innervation—intrinsic control of heartbeat. A specialized conduction system initiates the heartbeat and conducts the impulse to cardiac muscle.

(1) The sinoatrial node initiates the heartbeat. It is located in the superior aspect of the crista terminalis at the junction of the superior vena cava and the right atrium. The initial impulse spreads out over atrial walls and causes them to contract and fill the ventricle.

(2) The atrioventricular node is located in the atrioventricular septum just above the opening of the coronary sinus. It relays impulses from the atrial walls and relays them to the interventricular septum via the bundle of His.

(3) The bundle of His divides into right and left segments, which descend in the interventricular septum to the right and left ventricular walls and cause them to contract.

m. Innervation—extrinsic modification of heartbeat.

(1) Parasympathetic fibers from the vagus nerve (CN X) slow the heart rate.

(2) Sympathetic fibers from the sympathetic trunk speed up the heart rate.

(3) The cardiac plexus is found on the inferior aortic arch border anterior to the bifurcation of the trachea. It receives preganglionic vagal fibers and postganglionic sympathetic fibers; it has both parasympathetic and sympathetic input. Efferent fibers from the cardiac plexus pass to the heart to modify the heartbeat.

n. Innervation—afferent or sensory cardiac nerves.

(1) Afferent nerve fibers accompany sympathetic nerves and carry feedback from the viscera to the CNS. When cardiac muscle lacks oxygen, impulses may rise to a conscious, painful level as angina pectoris.

J. Anterior mediastinum.

The anterior mediastinum contains connective tissue and fat, a small portion of the thymus gland, and a few lymph nodes.

K. Superior and posterior mediastinum.

1. The trachea and bronchi are described in the previous list item, (E. Bronchi)

2. The esophagus extends from the pharynx at vertebral level C6 to the abdomen at level T11 (Figure 1-31).

a. The esophagus has three components: a cervical, thoracic, and abdominal portion.

b. The esophagus has four constrictions: the origin or pharyngeal end; where it passes the aortic arch; the superior mediastinum, at the bifurcation of the trachea; and where it passes through the diaphragm.

c. The esophagus has a sphincter at both ends; the cricopharyngeus muscle prevents swallowing air at the pharyngeal end, and the cardiac sphincter prevents regurgitation of stomach contents at the abdominal end.

d. The esophagus enters the thorax and superior mediastinum through the thoracic inlet. It is anterior to the vertebrae and posterior to the trachea. It descends into the posterior mediastinum. The aortic arch and descending aorta intervene between the vertebrae and the esophagus below the level of the heart. The esophagus turns anteriorly and slightly to the left as it passes through the diaphragm.

e. In the cervical region, the esophagus receives branches from laryngeal arteries. In the thorax, it receives visceral branches from the aorta. In the abdomen, it receives branches from the short and left gastric arteries.

f. The esophagus acquires autonomic nerves as it descends. In the cervical region, it receives sympathetic fibers from the cervical sympathetic ganglia and parasympathetic fibers from recurrent laryngeal branches of the vagus nerve. In the thorax and abdomen, it picks up sympathetic fibers from the sympathetic trunk. The parasympathetic supply is from the vagus nerves. In the superior mediastinum, the right and left vagus nerves form a plexus around the esophagus and follow the esophagus into the posterior mediastinum and through the diaphragm. In the abdomen, the vagus nerves reconstitute as anterior and posterior vagal trunks.

3. Within the thorax, the aorta is divided into three parts: ascending aorta, aortic arch, and descending aorta.

a. The ascending aorta originates at the aortic orifice. It passes superiorly to the level of the second costal cartilage. Above the aortic valves, the ascending aorta bulges as the aortic sinus. The right and left coronary arteries arise from the right and left coronary sinuses.

b. The aortic arch begins at the level of the second costal cartilage. It arches to the left, and its superior border lies at about the midpoint of the manubrium. It descends to level T4 and continues inferiorly as the descending aorta.

(1) The brachiocephalic artery is the first branch arising from the aortic arch. It arches up to the right sternoclavicular joint. At this level, it divides into the right common carotid artery and the right subclavian artery.

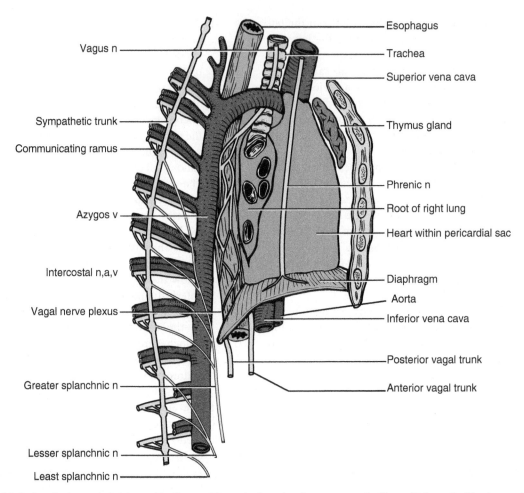

Figure 1-31 Lateral view of right mediastinum. The right lung has been removed. *(From Liebgott B: The Anatomical Basis of Dentistry, ed 3, St. Louis, Mosby, 2011.)*

(2) The left common carotid artery rises from the apex of the aortic arch posterior to the left sternoclavicular joint. It ascends through the left side of the neck.

(3) The left subclavian artery arises immediately distal to the left common carotid artery and passes to the left upper limb.

c. The descending aorta descends from vertebral level T4. It descends through the posterior mediastinum and provides branches to thoracic viscera and the thoracic wall. It ends by passing through the diaphragm to become the abdominal aorta at vertebral level T12.

(1) Visceral branches supply the lungs, esophagus, pericardium, and diaphragm.

(2) Somatic branches consist of the lower nine posterior intercostal arteries and the subcostal artery.

d. There are three main veins within the thorax: inferior vena cava, superior vena cava, and azygos and hemiazygos systems of veins.

(1) The inferior vena cava drains the lower limbs and the abdomen. It pierces the diaphragm, rises in the thorax, and ends in the inferior aspect of the right atrium of the heart.

(2) The superior vena cava is formed by the right and left brachiocephalic veins at the level of the first costal cartilage behind the manubrium. It drains the upper limbs and the head and neck. It then descends behind the sternum and enters the right atrium of the heart at the level of the third costal cartilage. The brachiocephalic veins are formed by a union of the internal jugular veins and the subclavian veins at the root of the neck behind the sternoclavicular joints.

(3) The azygos and hemiazygos system of veins drains the thoracic wall. The right and left ascending lumbar veins ascend from the abdomen to the thorax.

(a) The right ascending lumbar vein passes through the diaphragm and continues to rise as the azygos vein. The azygos vein empties into the superior vena cava.

(b) The left ascending lumbar vein continues up into the thorax as the inferior hemiazygos vein and drains the lower intercostal veins. It ascends to approximately vertebral level T8 and crosses the midline to join the azygos vein on the right side.

(c) An accessory, or superior, hemiazygos vein drains the fourth, fifth, sixth, and seventh intercostal veins as it descends to the level of T8. At T8, it enters the azygos vein. The upper three intercostal veins join to form the superior intercostal vein, which ascends to drain to the left brachiocephalic vein.

e. The thoracic duct begins in the abdomen as a small sac called *cisterna chyli*. Lymphatics drain into it from the lower extremities. Arising from cisterna chyli is the thoracic duct. It enters the thorax through the aortic opening in the diaphragm. Within the thorax, it acquires lymphatic drainage through the bronchomediastinal trunk. As the duct approaches the neck, it empties its contents into the confluence of the left internal jugular and left subclavian veins.

f. Four types of nerves are found in the thorax: intercostal nerves, sympathetic trunk and its branches, phrenic nerve and its branches, and vagus nerve.

(1) The intercostal nerves arise from the spinal cord as anterior primary rami of spinal nerves T1 through T12. These nerves supply the musculature of the thoracic walls and return cutaneous sensation from the skin of the chest wall and the upper abdominal wall.

(2) The sympathetic trunk and its branches run laterally to the thoracic vertebral bodies. Incoming white rami communicantes run from intercostal nerves in the ganglia of the sympathetic trunk. Outgoing postganglionic gray rami communicantes pass back to the intercostal nerves to be distributed along with the intercostal nerves.

(a) Splanchnic nerves do not synapse in the sympathetic chain of ganglia.

(3) The phrenic nerve arises from the neck from anterior primary rami of spinal nerves C3, C4, and C5. It descends along the anterior surface of the scalenus anterior muscle, entering the thoracic inlet anterior to the subclavian artery. It descends along the lateral mediastinum to the diaphragm. It carries efferent and afferent fibers to and from the diaphragm.

(4) The vagus nerve exits the skull through the jugular foramina. It descends and enters the thoracic inlet anterior to the subclavian arteries. The right vagus nerve gives rise to the right recurrent laryngeal nerve. The left vagus nerve gives rise to the left recurrent laryngeal nerve. Both vagus nerves descend posteriorly to the root of the lung, where they provide pulmonary branches to the pulmonary plexus and branches to the cardiac plexus. The nerves descend through the thorax as a nerve plexus surrounding the esophagus and then form again as anterior and posterior vagal trunks within the abdomen.

(5) The cardiac plexus is found below the aortic arch and anterior to the tracheal bifurcation. It receives sympathetic postganglionic fibers from the cervical sympathetic ganglia. It receives preganglionic parasympathetic fibers from the vagus nerves. Efferent fibers go to the heart.

(6) The pulmonary plexus surrounds pulmonary vessels at the root of the lungs. Sympathetic fibers come from the cardiac plexus. Parasympathetic fibers come from vagal nerves. Outgoing fibers go to the lung.

(7) The thymus gland is composed of lymphoid tissue; it produces T lymphocytes. The gland shrinks after puberty and is replaced by adipose tissue.

1.4 Abdominopelvic Cavity

The abdominopelvic cavity extends from the floor of the pelvis and rises to the level of the fifth intercostal space within the thoracic cage. The abdominal cavity is enclosed by the pelvic diaphragm below, the muscular anterolateral abdominal wall on the sides, and a muscular and bony posterior wall and the thoracic diaphragm above. The abdomen contains most of the digestive tract and the viscera of the genitourinary system.

A. Skeleton of the abdomen: the skeleton of the abdomen is divided into thoracic, vertebral, and pelvic components.

1. Thoracic component: the abdominal cavity extends into the thoracic cage between the fifth intercostal space above and the costal margin below. The thoracic cavity has been discussed in Section 1.3.

2. Vertebral component: the lower thoracic vertebrae, lumbar vertebrae, sacrum, and coccyx compose the vertebrae located in the abdomen.

a. Thoracic vertebrae: there are 12 thoracic vertebrae. They have numerous features that distinguish them from the rest of the vertebrae in the spinal column.

(1) The body is heart-shaped.

(2) The body has an articulating facet for the head of a rib.

(3) The transverse process has an articulating facet for the tubercle of a rib.

(4) The spinous process is long and slender.

b. Lumbar vertebrae: there are five lumbar vertebrae, distinguished by four features.

(1) The body is large and bean-shaped.

(2) There are no facets for ribs.

(3) Transverse processes do not have transverse foramina.

(4) The spinous processes are square.

c. The sacrum: the sacrum is a solid, triangular mass formed from five elements.

(1) The posterior spinous processes are represented by a median crest.

(2) Fused transverse processes form a lateral mass that terminates laterally as two ear-shaped articular surfaces.

(3) The sacral promontory projects anteriorly.

(4) The sacral canal continues the vertebral canal inferiorly from the lumbar region.

(5) Four anterior and posterior pelvic foramina leave the sacral canal on either side. These transmit sacral anterior and posterior primary rami.

d. The coccyx: the coccyx is a triangular mass formed by the fusion of four segments.

(1) Pelvic component.

(a) Os coxae: the ilium, ischium, and pubic bones fuse by about age 16 to form the os coxae. The right and left os coxae form the lower hip girdle. They join with the sacrum and coccyx to form the pelvic cavity, which surrounds and protects several pelvic viscera.

(i) The ilium consists of a flared, flattened plate with a concave medial surface. It ends superiorly as the iliac crest. The iliac tubercle is a small, bony elevation on the superior-lateral aspect of the iliac crest. The anterior inferior and anterior superior iliac spines are two small elevations on the anterior surface of the iliac crest.

(ii) The inferior surface of the ischium (ischial tuberosity) supports a person when sitting.

(iii) The os pubis on each side meets in the middle at the symphysis pubis. The pubic tubercle is lateral to the symphysis. The inguinal ligament connects the pubic tubercle to the anterior superior iliac spine.

(iv) The os pubis and ischium meet and form the obturator foramen.

(v) The acetabulum serves as the receptacle for the femur.

(vi) The ischial spine projects posteriorly from the ischium. It divides the posterior aspect of the bone into the greater sciatic notch above and the lesser sciatic notch below.

(b) Pelvic cavity—is divided into an upper pelvis within the iliac crests and a lower pelvis, which is surrounded by the right and left os pubis, ischium, and sacrum. The sacrum extends into the lower pelvis as a promontory.

B. Divisions of the abdomen—the abdomen may be divided into regions according to two systems.

1. One system divides the abdomen into four quadrants, based on the median sagittal plane in the abdomen intersecting with a transverse plane.

2. The other system divides the abdomen into nine regions based on two sagittal and two transverse planes through the abdomen.

a. The sagittal planes are located by a line joining the midclavicular point to the midpoint of the inguinal ligament.

b. The transverse planes are located by a line joining the most inferior points of the costal margins and a line joining the right and left iliac tubercles on the superior aspects of the iliac crests.

C. Abdominal walls—the abdominal cavity is enclosed by four walls. They are the anterolateral wall, the posterior wall, the superior wall formed by the thoracic diaphragm, and the inferior wall formed by the pelvic diaphragm.

1. Anterolateral abdominal wall.

a. Surface features: several abdominal landmarks may be palpated, including the costal margins, xiphoid process, iliac crests, superior and inferior iliac spines, and pubic tubercles. The lateral limit of the rectus abdominis muscle is represented by linea semilunaris. Transverse bands running from the linea semilunaris and the midline represent underlying tendinous inserts of the rectus abdominis muscle. A slight crease from the anterior superior iliac spine runs toward the pubic tubercle, representing the position of the inguinal ligament.

b. Layers: the layers that comprise the anterolateral abdominal wall below the skin from superficial to deep are, in order, superficial fascia, deep fascia, muscles and aponeurosis, transversalis fascia, extraperitoneal layer, and peritoneum.

(1) Superficial fascia—also known as the *subcutaneous fatty layer*, it is usually divisible further into the more superficial Camper's fascia and the deeper Scarpa's fascia.

(2) Deep fascia—this layer is more membranous than the more superficial fascia.

(3) Muscles and aponeurosis (Table 1-27)—there are four pairs of bilateral muscles in the anterior-lateral abdominal wall. Three of the pairs are flat: the external oblique muscle, internal oblique muscle, and transverse abdominis muscle. The muscles are arranged in sheets with the fibers running in different directions for strength and meet at linea alba at the midline.

Table 1-27

Muscles of the Anterior Abdominal Wall

MUSCLE	ORIGIN	INSERTION	ACTION	NERVE
External oblique	External aspects of lower eight ribs	Iliac crest, aponeurosis of anterior abdominal wall at linea alba	Increase abdominal pressure	Segmented APR of thoracic spinal nerves
Internal oblique	Lumbodorsal fascia, iliac crest, inguinal ligament	Costal cartilages of last three ribs, linea alba of abdominal aponeurosis	Increase abdominal pressure	Segmented APR of thoracic spinal nerves
Transversus abdominis	Internal aspects of lower six costal cartilages, lumbodorsal fascia, iliac crest, inguinal ligament	Linea alba of abdominal aponeurosis	Increase abdominal pressure	Segmented APR of thoracic spinal nerves
Rectus abdominis	Pubic symphysis, pubic crest	Anterior aspect of xiphoid process, anterior aspects of costal cartilages 5, 6, and 7	Increase abdominal pressure, flex vertebral column	Segmented APR of thoracic spinal nerves

From Liebgott B: The Anatomical Basis of Dentistry, ed 2, St. Louis, Mosby, 2001, p 103.

APR, Anterior primary rami.

(a) The external oblique muscle—the outermost muscle, which courses medially from the lower ribs. When the muscles run down and approach the midline, they merge with a membranous aponeurosis. Inferior fibers attach to the iliac crest. These fibers form a border called the *inguinal ligament.*

(b) The internal oblique muscle—originates from the iliac crest. It runs upward and medially and inserts into the costal margin, the linea alba, and the os pubis, along with transverse abdominis as a conjoint tendon.

(c) The transversus abdominis muscle—originates from the lumbodorsal fascia, iliac crest, inguinal ligament, and lower costal cartilages. It runs medially, in a transverse direction, and inserts as an aponeurosis into the linea alba in the midline.

(d) The rectus abdominis muscle—runs inferiorly from the costal margin and lower thoracic cage to the pubis and is similar to a belt or strap. This muscle is enclosed in a membranous sheath formed by the aponeurosis of the three flat muscles. The muscle inserts into the anterior wall of the membranous sheath.

In lower levels of the rectus sheath, all of the aponeuroses are superficial to the muscle. The arcuate line demarcates the limit of the aponeurotic layer in the posterior wall of the rectus sheath.

(4) Transversalis fascia—a layer of deep fascia is located just deep to the anterior-lateral abdominal muscles and the rectus sheath. The fibers run in a transverse direction.

(5) Extraperitoneal layer—located between transversalis fascia and deeper peritoneum. It is a fatty layer of connective tissue. Above the umbilicus, the internal oblique aponeurosis splits to encircle the rectus abdominis muscle (Figure 1-32, *A*). Above the pubic symphysis, all of the aponeuroses are anterior to the muscle (Figure 1-32, *B*).

(6) Parietal peritoneum—is composed of organized connective tissue, in contrast to the extraperitoneal layer.

c. Blood and nerve supply.

(1) The anterior-lateral abdominal wall is supplied by the lower six intercostal nerves of the thorax. From their origin, they stream downward and medially to the abdomen. Inferiorly, the abdominal wall is supplied by two branches of the first lumbar anterior primary ramus.

These branches (iliohypogastric and ilioinguinal nerves) supply the skin and muscle of the lower portion of the anterior-lateral abdominal wall.

(2) Segmented branches of the aorta follow the spinal nerves in posterior areas. Segmented branches arise anteriorly from superior and inferior epigastric arteries in the bed of the rectus sheath.

2. Superior abdominal wall.

The thoracic and abdominal cavities are separated by the diaphragm (Figure 1-33). Because the diaphragm projects upward as a dome, abdominal contents may be found within the thoracic rib cage and yet still be part of the abdominal cavity.

a. Origins of the thoracic diaphragm—muscular slips of the diaphragm originate from three sites of attachment.

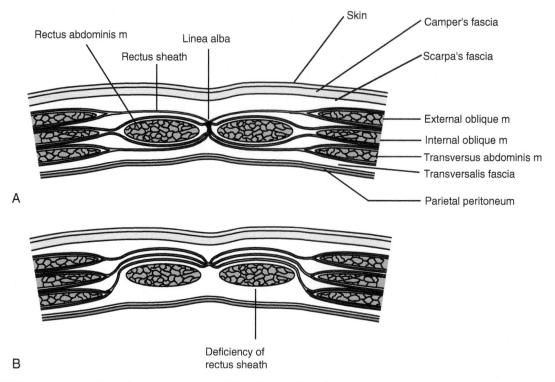

Figure 1-32 Transverse sections through anterior abdominal wall to demonstrate its layers. **A,** Above the level of the umbilicus. **B,** Above the pubic symphysis. *(From Liebgott B: The Anatomical Basis of Dentistry, ed 3, St. Louis, Mosby, 2011.)*

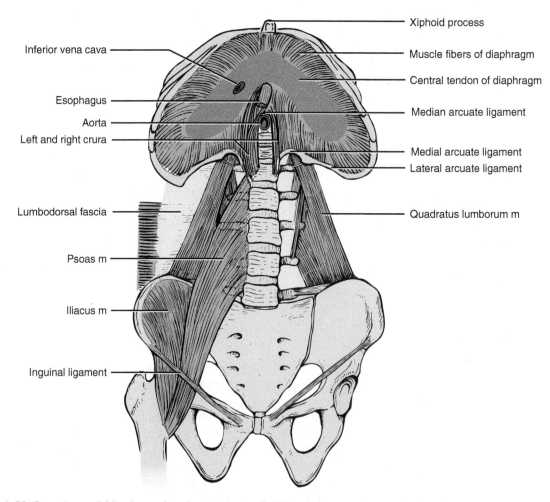

Figure 1-33 Superior wall (diaphragm) and posterior wall of the abdomen. *(From Liebgott B: The Anatomical Basis of Dentistry, ed 3, St. Louis, Mosby, 2011.)*

(1) Sternal slips originate from the posterior aspect of the xiphoid process.

(2) Costal slips originate from internal surfaces of the lower six costal cartilages and the twelfth rib.

(3) Lumbar attachments arise as a right crus from the vertebral bodies and discs of L1, L2, and L3 and a left crus arising from the two vertebral bodies and discs of L1 and L2. The two crura cross to form the median arcuate ligament, which enters the abdominal aorta. Tendons from the crura to the transverse processes of L1 form medial arcuate ligaments. Tendons from the transverse processes of L1 to the midpoints of the twelfth ribs form lateral arcuate ligaments.

b. Insertion of the diaphragm.

(1) Fibers of the diaphragm insert into the central tendon.

c. Structures passing through the diaphragm—several structures pass through the diaphragm on their way to or from the abdomen. Others pass between the diaphragm and the body wall.

(1) The aorta enters the abdomen through the median arch.

(2) The inferior vena cava passes out of the abdomen to the thorax through its own opening in the central tendon.

(3) The esophagus passes through its own opening.

(4) The thoracic duct passes through the median arch along with the aorta.

(5) The azygos vein passes through the right crus.

(6) The hemizygos vein passes through the left crus.

(7) The posterior and anterior vagal trunks pass into the abdomen, along with the esophagus, through the esophageal opening.

(8) The splanchnic nerves pass through the crura of the diaphragm.

(9) The sympathetic trunks pass behind the medial arcuate ligament to enter the abdomen.

(10) The superior epigastric arteries pass anteriorly between the sternal and costal origins of the diaphragm.

d. Functions of the diaphragm.

(1) The main function is respiration.

(2) Another function is esophageal constriction to prevent gastric regurgitation during inspiration.

e. Nerve supply to the diaphragm.

(1) The phrenic nerve is the motor and sensory supply. It arises in the neck from anterior primary rami of spinal nerves C3, C4, and C5.

(2) The phrenic nerve descends through the thoracic inlet and travels inferiorly on either side of the middle mediastinum to reach the diaphragm.

f. Blood supply of the diaphragm.

(1) From the internal thoracic artery through the pericardiophrenic and musculophrenic arteries and from aortic branches through intercostal and phrenic arteries.

3. Posterior abdominal wall—consists of skin and fascia, bone, and three muscles.

a. Lumbodorsal fascia covers the deep back muscles.

b. The inguinal ligament extends from the pubic tubercle to the anterior superior iliac spine.

c. The quadratus lumborum muscle is flat and runs from the twelfth rib and all the lumbar transverse processes down to the iliac crest.

d. Psoas major and iliacus muscles are generally considered as the iliopsoas muscle unit.

4. Inferior abdominal wall—is funnel-shaped.

a. Muscles.

(1) Levator ani muscles originate along the internal aspects of the os coxae. The fibers run medially and inferiorly toward the rectum to blend with the longitudinal smooth muscle of the rectum.

(2) The coccygeus muscle is a portion of each levator ani muscle that runs from the ischial tuberosity to the coccyx.

b. The perineum—is bound externally by the thighs and buttocks. On a deeper plane, it is bounded by the ischiopubic rami, which converge on the symphysis pubis anteriorly, and sacrotuberous ligaments converging on the coccyx posteriorly.

D. Peritoneum and peritoneal cavity.

1. Nomenclature.

a. Peritoneum is a lining tissue. Parietal peritoneum lines the inner abdominal body walls.

b. Visceral peritoneum covers viscera.

c. The peritoneal cavity is the space between the parietal and visceral layers. This space contains serous fluid, which lubricates the viscera.

d. Some abdominal organs in the peritoneal cavity are suspended by mesentery, which is a double-layered fold. Vessels and nerves pass to and from the viscera through the mesentery.

e. Retroperitoneal viscera organs lie within the extraperitoneal layer of the abdominal wall and do not possess a mesentery.

f. An omentum is a double-layered fold of peritoneum. It joins viscera.

g. Ligaments are specifically named folds of peritoneum that are parts of mesenteries or omenta.

E. Blood supply to the abdomen.

1. Arterial supply: the abdominal aorta. The descending aorta of the thorax passes through the diaphragm and becomes the abdominal aorta. At vertebral level L4, it divides into the right and left common iliac

arteries. These divide further into the right and left external iliac arteries, which descend to supply the lower limb and the right and left internal iliac arteries. The right and left internal iliac arteries supply pelvic structures.

a. Somatic branches.

(1) Inferior phrenic arteries—arise from the aorta as it passes through the diaphragm. The right and left branches ascend to supply the inferior aspect of the diaphragm.

(2) Lumbar arteries—there are five lumbar arteries. The first four pairs arise from the aorta, and the fifth pair arises from the internal iliac arteries. The internal iliac arteries turn laterally to supply the lower abdominal wall. Anteriorly, segmented lumbar arteries anastomose with collateral branches of the superior and inferior epigastric arteries.

(3) Median sacral artery—the small median sacral artery continues from the bifurcation of the aorta and supplies the anterior aspect of the sacral area.

b. Unpaired branches to the gut and associated glands—three unpaired branches arise from the abdominal aorta to supply the gut and associated glands, liver, pancreas, and spleen.

(1) Celiac trunk—arises as a short stem just below the diaphragm, at vertebral level T12 and L1, and breaks into three main branches. These branches supply the abdominal esophagus, stomach, duodenum, liver and gallbladder, part of the pancreas, and spleen.

(2) Superior mesenteric artery—arises immediately below the celiac trunk and supplies derivatives of the midgut, including the distal half of the duodenum, jejunum, ileum, cecum and appendix, ascending colon, and transverse colon.

(3) Inferior mesenteric artery—arises at vertebral level L3 and supplies derivatives of the hindgut distal to the left colic flexure.

c. Paired branches to the glands of the genitourinary system—three paired branches supply the glands of the genitourinary system; each originates from the aorta.

(1) Suprarenal arteries—arise either directly from the aorta or from the renal arteries.

(2) Renal arteries—originate from the aorta at vertebral level L1 to L2. They pass laterally to supply the right and left kidneys.

(3) Testicular or ovarian arteries—travel inferiorly to supply the gonads.

2. Venous return: inferior vena cava.

The external iliac veins, which drain the lower limbs, and the internal iliac veins, which drain the pelvis, unite within the pelvis to form the right and left common iliac veins. These veins unite at vertebral level L5 to form the inferior vena cava. The vena cava acquires several tributaries as it passes up through the diaphragm. The vena cava leaves the abdomen when it passes through the diaphragm, enters the thorax, and drains into the right atrium.

a. Somatic branches.

(1) Inferior phrenic veins—drain the inferior aspect of the diaphragm. They drain either to the superior aspect of the inferior vena cava or to the paired ascending lumbar veins.

(2) Lumbar veins—the body walls are drained by five lumbar veins. The first four drain to the inferior vena cava, and the fifth drains to the common iliac vein. Ascending lumbar veins parallel the inferior vena cava on either side. These veins arise from common iliac veins, ascend on the posterior abdominal wall, and travel through the diaphragm to the thorax. Here they become the azygos and hemiazygos veins.

(3) Median sacral vein—drains the sacral region. It joins the left common iliac vein rather than the inferior vena cava.

b. Tributaries of genitourinary glands—the renal veins receive venous blood from the right and left kidneys. The suprarenal veins receive venous blood from the right and left suprarenal glands.

c. Tributaries of the gastrointestinal tract and associated glands—veins returning from the gut join to form the portal vein. The portal vein enters the liver and ultimately ends as a bed of capillaries. The portal capillary beds are drained by hepatic veins, which enter the vena cava as several hepatic veins.

F. Nerves of the abdomen.

1. Somatic nerves.

a. The anterior rami of the lower six thoracic spinal nerves and the first lumbar nerve supply the various layers of the anterior-lateral abdominal walls. Two branches of the anterior primary rami of L1, the iliohypogastric and ilioinguinal nerves, supply the lower portion of the abdominal wall.

b. The anterior primary rami of lumbar nerves L1 to L4 unite and divide within the substance of the psoas muscle to form the lumbar plexus.

c. The anterior primary rami of L4 and L5 and S1 through S4 unite to form the sacral plexus, branches of which provide motor and sensory nerves to the perineum and the remainder of the lower limb.

2. Autonomic nerves.

a. Sympathetic nerves.

(1) Greater, lesser, and least splanchnic nerves arise bilaterally from the thoracic sympathetic trunks. Without synapsing in the sympathetic trunk, they pass inferiorly through the diaphragm to the abdomen.

(2) Lumbar splanchnic nerves arise from the sympathetic portion of the sympathetic trunk.

(3) Within the abdomen are collections of secondary neurons. The largest collection is the celiac ganglion and its plexus. The thoracic and lumbar splanchnic nerves synapse within these ganglia.

b. Parasympathetic nerves: parasympathetic innervation of abdominal viscera is shared by the vagus nerves and the pelvic splanchnic nerves.

(1) Vagus nerves—the vagal plexus within the thorax regroups as anterior and posterior vagal trunks as the vagus nerve passes through the diaphragm. The anterior trunk supplies the liver and biliary apparatus, gastric pylorus, duodenum, and pancreas. The posterior vagal trunk supplies the remainder of the stomach and then joins the celiac plexus. Vagal and celiac plexus fibers are distributed to the gut and derivatives proximal to the left colic flexure.

(2) Pelvic splanchnic nerves—within the pelvis, parasympathetic fibers from S2 through S4 join the inferior mesenteric plexus as pelvic splanchnic nerves and are distributed along with branches of the plexus. They supply the gut distal to the left colic flexure and the pelvic viscera.

Parasympathetic fibers of the abdomen travel to their sites of innervation as preganglionic fibers and synapse with secondary neurons within the substance of the organ they supply.

G. Abdominal viscera—the gut wall consists of four layers, an outer layer of visceral peritoneum, a layer of smooth muscle, a submucosal layer, and an inner lining of mucous membrane.

1. The stomach—after passing through the diaphragm, the esophagus widens to form the stomach.

a. Position: the stomach lies within the upper left quadrant. Its proximal end is immediately below the left dome of the diaphragm.

b. Features.

(1) Cardiac portion—is adjacent to the cardiac orifice. The cardiac orifice is an area of circular muscle at the entrance to the stomach. Left of the cardiac orifice is the area where the stomach bulges upward, called the *fundus*.

(2) Pylorus—toward the right, the stomach narrows, first to the pyloric antrum and then the pyloric sphincter. The pyloric sphincter controls the release of gastric contents to the duodenum.

(3) Body—the body of the stomach is located between the pylorus and cardiac portion.

(4) Curvatures—the smaller, curved right superior border of the stomach is called the *lesser curvature*, and the larger, curved left inferior border is called the *greater curvature*.

(5) Rugae—the mucosa within the stomach has a folded appearance because of the presence of rugae.

c. Stomach wall—one important function of the stomach is to break up and mix ingested food. The stomach wall is composed of a thick and strong muscular wall for that purpose.

d. Peritoneal coverings and attachments: the stomach is covered with visceral peritoneum. It is connected to other viscera by the greater and lesser omenta.

(1) Lesser omentum: connects the lesser curvature of the stomach and the proximal 3 cm of duodenum to the liver above. The common bile duct, portal vein, and hepatic artery pass through the lesser omentum in this area. The lesser omentum ends as a free edge. Immediately posterior to the free edge is the epiploic foramen, which connects the greater and lesser sacs.

(2) Greater omentum: connects the greater curvature of the stomach to three structures. The gastrocolic ligament runs down into the abdomen and curves back upward and attaches to the transverse colon, the gastrosplenic ligament runs from the curvature of the spleen, and the gastrophrenic ligament becomes continuous with the parietal peritoneum of the diaphragm.

e. Arterial supply: the blood supply to the stomach is derived from three branches of the celiac trunk.

(1) The left gastric artery passes to the left and runs superiorly to the level of the esophagus and then turns along the lesser curvature to supply the stomach.

(2) The splenic artery passes to the left behind the stomach and the lesser sac along the superior border of the pancreas. It divides into the short gastric artery and the left gastroomental artery. The short gastric artery runs superiorly along the greater curvature to the stomach. The left gastroomental artery descends along the greater curvature to supply the stomach and the greater omentum.

(3) The common hepatic artery passes to the right of the celiac trunk and divides near the duodenum into two branches, the hepatic artery and the gastroduodenal artery. The hepatic artery ascends and supplies the liver with blood. On the way to the liver, it gives off the right gastric artery, which supplies the lesser curvature of the stomach, and then anastomoses with the left gastric artery. The hepatic artery continues superiorly, sends a cystic

artery to the gallbladder, and then divides into right and left branches that supply the liver.

(4) The gastroduodenal artery passes inferiorly posterior to the duodenum and divides into two branches, the superior pancreaticoduodenal artery and the right gastroomental artery. The superior pancreaticoduodenal artery supplies part of the pancreas and duodenum. The right gastroomental artery runs to the left along the greater curvature of the stomach and anastomoses with the left gastroomental artery. It supplies portions of the stomach and greater omentum.

f. Venous return.

(1) The veins of the stomach parallel the arteries that supply the stomach. The right and left gastric veins drain directly into the portal vein. The short gastric vein and the left gastroomental vein join the splenic vein, which drains to the portal vein. The right gastroomental vein drains to the superior mesenteric vein, which joins the splenic vein to form the portal vein.

2. Duodenum—the first section of the small intestine.

a. Position: the duodenum has a semicircular shape like a "C" (Figure 1-34). It lies in front of the abdominal aorta and inferior vena cava and surrounds the head and neck of the pancreas.

b. Parts: the duodenum has four parts—a superior first part, descending second part, horizontal third part, and ascending fourth part.

c. Wall of the duodenum: the internal mucous membrane lining has many circular folds, the plicae circulares. Enzymes from the pancreas and bile

from the liver are added in the second part at the major duodenal papilla. Above the major duodenal papilla is the minor duodenal papilla. It is the entrance of the accessory pancreatic duct into the duodenum.

d. Peritoneal attachments.

(1) Most of the duodenum is retroperitoneal. As the fourth part of the duodenum ascends and curves anteriorly, the mesentery begins.

e. Arterial supply.

(1) The blood supply to the duodenum is derived from the celiac trunk and the superior mesenteric artery. The superior pancreaticoduodenal artery arises indirectly from the celiac trunk. It follows the inner curve of the duodenum and supplies the superior portion of the pancreas and duodenum.

f. Venous return.

(1) The superior and inferior pancreaticoduodenal veins transport the venous return from the duodenum to the portal vein via the superior mesenteric vein.

3. Jejunum and ileum.

a. The fourth and ascending portion of the duodenum becomes the jejunum. The jejunum and ileum together form a more mobile portion of the small intestine because they have a mesentery.

b. The jejunum and ileum are located centrally in the abdominopelvic cavity and are framed by the large intestine. The greater omentum is draped anteriorly over the small intestine.

c. Peritoneum attachments.

(1) The root of the mesentery that attaches the jejunum and ileum to the posterior body wall

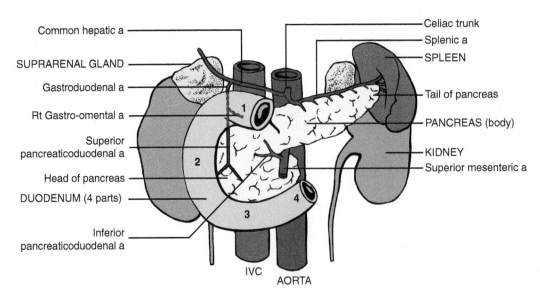

Figure 1-34 Duodenum, pancreas, spleen, and kidneys in situ. *IVC,* Inferior vena cava. *(From Liebgott B: The Anatomical Basis of Dentistry, ed 3, St. Louis, Mosby, 2011.)*

runs diagonally from the duodenal to the ileo-colic junction. Nerve and blood supply to the small intestine travels through the mesentery.

d. Small intestine wall.

(1) The mucous membrane of the surface of the small intestine has many folds covered by finger-like projections called *villi*.

e. Arterial supply.

(1) The superior mesenteric artery supplies blood to the small intestine. This artery gives off intestinal branches that travel through the mesentery. At the small intestine, the arteries join as arcades. Vasa recti arise from the arcades and supply the gut itself.

f. Venous drainage—venous return drains to small intestinal tributaries of the superior mesenteric vein. The superior mesenteric vein joins the splenic vein to form the portal vein.

4. Colon—extends from the ileocolic junction to the anus.

a. Position: the colon sits within the periphery of the abdomen, around the small intestine.

b. Features and parts: the longitudinal muscle coat has three bands, called *taeniae coli*. Contractions in taeniae coli are called *haustra*. The outer peritoneal surface of the colon has appendices epiploicae, small bags of fat-filled peritoneum hanging from its surface. The large intestine has the cecum and appendix, ascending colon, transverse colon, descending colon, sigmoid colon, rectum, and anal canal.

(1) Cecum and appendix

(a) The ileum meets the colon at the ileocecal orifice. The ileocecal valve, located at the entrance to the orifice, prevents regurgitation back into the ileum. The vermiform appendix opens into the cecum below the ileocolic orifice.

(2) Ascending colon.

(a) The ascending colon is attached to the posterior body wall. It is retroperitoneal and ascends and turns to the right as the right colic or hepatic flexure.

(3) Transverse colon.

(a) The transverse colon has a mesentery. As it approaches the left side, it ascends to the level of the spleen and turns inferiorly. The flexure is the left colic or splenic flexure.

(4) Descending colon.

(a) The descending colon is immobile. At the level of the left iliac crest, it turns medially as the sigmoid colon.

(5) Sigmoid colon.

(a) The sigmoid colon again acquires a mesentery and is mobile. It is S-shaped and, once

in the middle of the sacrum, extends inferiorly as the rectum.

(6) Rectum and anal canal.

(a) At the pelvic diaphragm, the rectum turns and becomes the anal canal. The involuntary internal sphincter ani and the voluntary external sphincter ani control the release of contents.

c. Wall of the colon.

(1) The mucous membrane lining of the large gut does not contain any villi. The surface is designed for water absorption.

d. Arterial supply: the colon is supplied by branches of superior and inferior mesenteric arteries (Figure 1-35).

(1) Superior mesenteric artery.

(a) The ileocolic artery arises from the superior mesenteric artery and travels through the mesentery toward the ileocecal junction. An ileal branch travels back to the ileum to supply the distal end of the ileum. An appendicular branch travels through the mesoappendix and supplies the appendix. Cecal branches supply the cecum, and colic branches ascend to supply the ascending colon.

(b) The right colic artery arises from the superior mesenteric artery. It supplies the superior portion of the ascending colon.

(c) The middle colic artery travels through the transverse mesocolon to supply the transverse colon.

(2) Inferior mesenteric artery.

(a) The inferior mesenteric artery arises from the abdominal aorta. It passes to the left and forms three terminal branches—left colic artery; sigmoid arteries; and rectal branches to supply the descending colon, sigmoid colon, and rectum.

e. Venous return.

(1) The cecum and ascending and transverse colon are drained by tributaries of the superior mesenteric vein. The descending colon, sigmoid colon, and rectum are drained by tributaries of the inferior mesenteric vein, which drains to the splenic vein. The superior and inferior mesenteric veins unite to form the portal vein.

H. The liver—sits under the diaphragm in the upper right quadrant. It is sheltered by the lower right ribs.

1. Surfaces and features.

a. The liver has a smooth, diaphragmatic upper surface and an inferior visceral surface. It has four lobes. The right lobe lies to the right of the inferior vena cava and the gallbladder. The left lobe lies to the left of the ligamentum teres and the ligamentum venosum. The quadrate lobe lies between the

Aorta

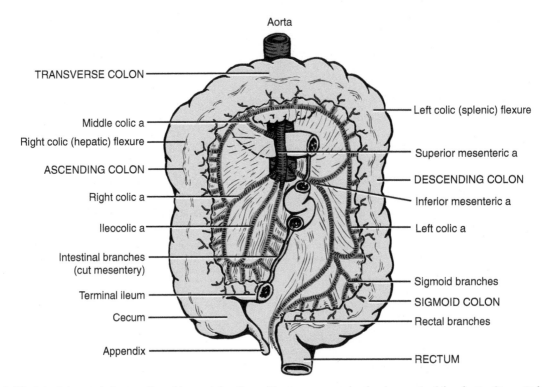

TRANSVERSE COLON

Middle colic a

Right colic (hepatic) flexure

ASCENDING COLON

Right colic a

Ileocolic a

Intestinal branches
(cut mesentery)

Terminal ileum

Cecum

Appendix

Left colic (splenic) flexure

Superior mesenteric a

DESCENDING COLON

Inferior mesenteric a

Left colic a

Sigmoid branches

SIGMOID COLON

Rectal branches

RECTUM

Figure 1-35 Arterial supply to small and large intestines. The transverse colon has been raised for clarity. *(From Liebgott B: The Anatomical Basis of Dentistry, ed 3, St. Louis, Mosby, 2011.)*

gallbladder, ligamentum teres, and porta hepatis. The caudate lobe lies between the inferior vena cava, ligamentum venosum, and porta hepatis.

2. Peritoneal attachments.

a. Coronary ligament—the visceral peritoneum that covers the liver reflects back onto the diaphragm as the diaphragmatic peritoneum. This area of reflection is called the *coronary ligament.*

b. Falciform ligament—the falciform ligament extends upward from the umbilicus to the liver. The free edge contains a thick ligament that is the remnant of the umbilical vein, called *ligamentum teres.*

c. Ligamentum venosum—the ligamentum venosum is the remnant of the ductus venosus, or umbilical vein that was the fetal bypass of the liver.

d. Lesser omentum—joins the liver to the stomach. The common bile duct, hepatic artery, and portal vein all course through the lesser omentum.

3. Blood flow to the liver—the blood flow to the liver is through the hepatic artery and portal vein.

a. Hepatic artery—arises from the common hepatic artery. It passes upward in the free edge of the lower omentum. It divides into left and right branches that supply the liver.

b. Portal vein—the inferior mesenteric vein unites with the splenic vein. The superior mesenteric vein joins the splenic vein to form the portal vein. The portal vein travels upward within the lesser

omentum and divides into right and left branches to supply the liver.

4. Venous return—blood drains from the liver via hepatic veins to the inferior vena cava.

5. Structure.

a. Liver tissue is separated into small functional units called *lobules* by fibrous septa. Each lobule consists of several sheets of epithelial cells radiating out from a central vein. Small branches of the hepatic artery, portal vein, and hepatic duct are located at the periphery of each lobule. The vessels empty their blood into spaces where exchange takes place between the epithelial cells and blood. The central vein of the lobules come together to form the hepatic vein.

6. Biliary apparatus.

a. The bile canaliculi drain bile to interlobular ducts. The interlobular ducts form right and left hepatic ducts. These ducts join to form the common hepatic duct. The gallbladder arises from the common hepatic duct. A cystic duct joins the common hepatic duct to form the common bile duct. Bile is transported to the duodenum through the common bile duct.

I. Pancreas—lies transversely in the abdomen against the posterior body wall (see Figure 1-34).

1. Features and parts.

a. The pancreas is divided into three parts. The head is surrounded by the duodenum at vertebral level

L1 to L2. The body extends to the left and ends as the tail, which touches the hilum of the spleen.

2. Peritoneum—the pancreas is retroperitoneal. It is covered by the peritoneum anteriorly and provides a base for attachment of the transverse mesocolon.

3. Structure: the pancreas contains both an exocrine and an endocrine portion.

   a. Exocrine portion.

      (1) The lobules of the pancreas are drained by ductules, which drain into a main pancreatic duct. It empties its secretions, along with the common bile duct, into the ampulla of the duodenum.

   b. Endocrine portion.

      (1) The pancreas contains clusters of cells called the islets of Langerhans, which produce insulin.

4. Arterial supply: the pancreas is supplied by branches of both the celiac trunk and the superior mesenteric artery. The splenic artery arises from the celiac trunk and supplies the pancreas.

   a. The superior pancreaticoduodenal artery arises from the gastroduodenal branch and passes inferiorly to supply both the pancreas and the duodenum.

   b. The inferior pancreaticoduodenal artery arises from the superior mesenteric artery and travels superiorly between the pancreatic head and duodenum to supply both structures.

5. Venous drainage—the splenic vein receives tributaries from the superior surface of the pancreas and courses to the left and takes part in formation of the portal vein. The superior and inferior pancreaticoduodenal veins drain directly to the portal vein.

J. Spleen—lies in the upper left quadrant of the abdomen, protected by ribs 9, 10, and 11 (see Figure 1-34).

   1. Features.

      a. The hilum of the spleen is located on the visceral surface. The tail of the pancreas contacts the hilum. Splenic vessels run to and from the hilum.

   2. Peritoneum.

      a. The spleen is attached to the stomach by the gastrosplenic ligament. The splenorenal ligament attaches the spleen to the left kidney.

   3. Structure.

      a. The spleen is divided by connective tissue septa into many compartments. Within the compartments are networks of cells surrounded by blood sinusoids.

   4. Blood supply.

      a. The spleen is supplied by the splenic artery and is drained by the splenic vein.

K. Kidneys—lie in the posterior body wall, with the medial border more anterior than the lateral border (see Figure 1-34).

   1. Features.

      a. The lateral border is rounded, and the medial border is the concave hilum of the kidney, which contains a vertical slit called the *renal sinus* through which the ureter and renal vessels pass to and from the kidney.

   2. Peritoneum.

      a. The kidneys are retroperitoneal. A layer of fibrous renal fascia anchors the kidney to the posterior body wall. The left kidney is slightly higher than the right kidney and is joined to the spleen by the splenorenal ligament.

   3. Structure.

      a. The cortex is the pale, outer layer of the kidney. The medulla is the inner layer, which appears striped because of the renal pyramids. Medullary rays are composed of medullary tissue extending into the cortex from the base of the pyramids. The apex of a medullary pyramid is called the *renal papilla*. Minor calyces receive secretions from the renal papillae. Several minor calyces join to form a major calyx. The approximately three major calyces found in the kidney unite to form the renal pelvis. The renal pelvis is drained by the ureters to the bladder.

   4. Blood supply.

      a. The renal artery arises from the abdominal aorta, passes laterally, and enters the hilum of the kidney behind the inferior vena cava. The artery gives off a branch that passes superiorly to the suprarenal gland. Within the sinus of the kidney, the renal arteries end as interlobar arteries. They course through the renal columns to reach the cortex. In the cortex, they bifurcate at right angles as arcuate arteries and anastomose with each other to form arcades.

      b. Veins leave the capillary beds and coalesce as renal veins. The right and left renal veins drain to the inferior vena cava.

L. Ureters—the ureter carries urine from the kidneys to the bladder. The ureters travel inferiorly just below the parietal peritoneum of the posterior body wall. They pass anterior to the common iliac arteries as they enter the pelvis.

   1. Blood supply.

      a. Proximally, they receive branches from the renal arteries, midportions receive branches from testicular or ovarian arteries, and the distal portion receives branches from vesicular arteries.

M. Bladder—receiving chamber for urine. The anterior border rests against the pubic bones. The superior aspect is covered with peritoneum.

   1. Entrances and exit.

      a. The right and left ureters pass to the posterior of the bladder, converge inferiorly, and then enter the bladder about 2.5 cm apart. Along with the exit of the bladder, they form the trigone of the bladder.

   2. Structure.

      a. The lumen of the bladder is lined with transitional epithelial mucosa. The walls contain smooth muscle fibers that collectively are called the *detrusor muscle*.

3. Blood supply.
   a. The superior and inferior vesical arteries arise from the internal iliac artery to supply the bladder. It is drained by veins of the same name that empty to the internal iliac vein.

N. Suprarenal glands—sit on top of the kidneys.
   1. Structure: the suprarenal glands have an outer cortex and inner medulla with distinct functions.
      a. The cortex is involved with production of steroid hormones.
      b. The medulla secretes epinephrine.

1.5 Central Nervous System and Neuroanatomy

The human nervous system maintains homeostasis by regulating the internal environment. It also interprets and reacts to external stimuli. The response to external stimuli may be unconscious or conscious.

The nervous system consists of two kinds of cells: reactive cells called *neurons* and supportive cells called *neuroglia*. The nervous system may be divided into central and peripheral components based on location, or somatic and autonomic divisions based on function.

A. Neuron—consists of cytoplasm and a nucleus surrounded by a plasma membrane. Neurons have the ability to communicate with one another at synapses through electrical impulses. Motor neurons transmit information, and sensory neurons receive information.
   1. Motor neuron.
      a. A motor neuron consists of a cell body containing a nucleus, numerous dendrites that receive information, and a single axon that transmits information.
         (1) Dendrites are short, branching cellular extensions that conduct impulses toward the body.
         (2) Axons are long, cellular extensions that conduct impulses away from the body. Near its termination, each axon branches. Each branch ends as an axon terminal or bouton. Axon terminals of motor neurons synapse with muscle cells. Several extensions arise from the cell body of motor neurons; they are termed *multipolar*.
   2. Sensory neuron.
      a. The body of a sensory neuron has only one cellular extension and is classified as unipolar. The process is short and divides into two axons. One axon, called the *peripheral process*, continues to the periphery and either functions as a sensory receptor or synapses with a sensory receptor. Some authors refer to the branching component as *dendrites*. The other axon is called the *central process*; it extends into the CNS.
   3. Synapses.
      a. Synapses are found either at the intercellular junctions of nerve processes or between nerve processes and the cells of effector organs. The presynaptic and postsynaptic cell membranes are separated by a synaptic cleft.
      b. Electrical impulses travel along the axon and cause the release of neurotransmitters from the terminus. The neurotransmitters diffuse across the synaptic cleft.
      c. The neurotransmitter may be excitatory or inhibitory. An excitatory transmitter depolarizes the postsynaptic membrane, and an inhibitory transmitter hyperpolarizes the postsynaptic membrane. Inhibitory and excitatory synapses may be mixed; one site on the target neuron may receive input from a few to 1000 synapses with other neurons.
      d. The net depolarization of the membrane determines whether the target neuron propagates the impulse.
   4. Neuroglia.
      a. Neuroglia are supportive cells. They do not transmit impulses.
         (1) Neuroglia maintain homeostasis in the extracellular environment.
         (2) They electrically insulate nerve processes from one another.
         (3) They provide nutrition for neurons.

B. Definitions and terms.
   1. Gray matter.
      a. Neuronal bodies that are grouped together are called *gray matter*. Gray matter is located in the central part of the spinal cord surrounding the central canal; on the surfaces of the cerebrum and cerebellum of the cortex of the brain; and throughout the CNS as discrete, scattered, internal patches or nuclei.
   2. White matter.
      a. Myelin speeds nerve conduction. Myelin has a shiny, white appearance, and myelinated nerves within the CNS cause nerve tissue to appear white.
   3. Peripheral nerve.
      a. A peripheral nerve is composed of a bundle of myelinated axons traveling outside the CNS.
   4. Tract.
      a. A tract is a group of myelinated axons traveling together in the CNS that share a common origin, destination, and function. Tracts run entirely within the brain and spinal cord.
   5. Nucleus.
      a. A nucleus is a group of neuronal cell bodies in the CNS that are located in the same area and share the same function.
   6. Ganglion.
      a. A ganglion is a collection of nerve cell bodies outside the CNS. Examples are dorsal root ganglia and autonomic ganglia. An exception is the basal ganglia of the cerebral hemispheres; they are nuclei by definition.

7. Afferent fibers.
   a. Afferent fibers are axons that carry nerve impulses toward the CNS or toward higher centers. They are also known as *sensory* or *ascending fibers*.
8. Efferent fibers.
   a. Efferent fibers are axons that carry impulses away from the CNS to muscles and glands. They are also known as *motor* or *descending fibers*.
C. Division based on location: the nervous system may be divided into the CNS containing the brain and spinal cord, and the peripheral nervous system consisting of the spinal and cranial nerves.
   1. CNS.
      a. Sensory component—incoming data are received at a conscious or unconscious level.
      b. Motor component—the origin of outgoing commands.
      c. Association component—connects and coordinates various CNS centers.
   2. Peripheral nervous system: peripheral nerves consist of bundles of axons that convey information to and from the CNS.
      a. 31 pairs of spinal nerves from the spinal cord.
      b. 12 pairs of cranial nerves from the brain.
D. Division based on function.
   1. Somatic nervous system.
      a. The somatic nervous system controls the body's voluntary and reflex activities through somatic sensory and somatic motor components of both the CNS and the peripheral nervous system.
   2. Autonomic nervous system.
      a. The autonomic nervous system controls involuntary smooth muscle, cardiac muscle, and glandular tissue. It is not under voluntary or conscious control. It has a motor component that controls smooth muscle contractions of viscera and blood vessels and secretions of glands. It has a sensory component to provide feedback. The autonomic nervous system is also divided into a parasympathetic division and a sympathetic division.
         (1) The parasympathetic division of the autonomic nervous system is concerned with maintenance of day-to-day activity, which is also known as *vegetative function*. Examples of vegetative function include peristalsis and digestion, slowing the heart, and stimulating glandular secretions.
         (2) The sympathetic division of the autonomic nervous system is antagonistic to the parasympathetic division and takes precedence during emergencies. It is also called the *fight-or-flight response*. During an emergency, blood is shunted to core muscles, hair stands on end, pupils dilate, the heart beats faster, respiration increases, and bronchioles dilate for more oxygenation of blood.

E. Peripheral nerves—located outside the CNS. Peripheral nerves share a common structure and function similarly; however, some have a somatic, voluntary function, and others have an autonomic function.
   1. Structure.
      a. The axon is the basic unit of a peripheral nerve. Each axon is covered by myelin-containing neurilemma, a fatty layer that acts as an insulator.
      b. The fibrous endoneurium covers each process and its coatings.
      c. The perineurium covers each bundle of processes.
      d. The epineurium is the final coating of the entire peripheral nerve.
   2. Function.
      a. Skeletal muscles form for movement and locomotion, and smooth muscle develops for peristalsis and emptying of contents.
      b. Both types of muscle have a motor (efferent) and sensory (afferent) nerve supply.
         (1) Somatic efferent to voluntary skeletal muscles.
         (2) Somatic afferent from skin and proprioception from endings in muscles, tendons, and joints.
         (3) Autonomic efferent to visceral smooth muscles and glands.
         (4) Autonomic afferent from organs and glands.
      c. Two additional modalities are found in the head, the special senses and branchial efferent nerves that supply skeletal muscles of the head and neck derived from branchial arches.
         (1) Special sensory for smell, vision, taste, hearing, and balance.
         (2) Branchial efferent for skeletal muscle in the head and neck that is derived from branchial arches.
   3. Somatic peripheral nerves (CNS origins).
      a. Voluntary motor components (efferent somatic and branchial): motor pathways comprise two groups of neurons, upper and lower.
         (1) Upper motor neurons are located in the motor cortex of the cerebrum. These axons descend in tracts that cross the midline and synapse with lower motor neurons.
         (2) Lower motor neurons give rise to motor components of peripheral nerves.
            (a) Cranial nerves.
               (i) Lower motor neurons are located in cranial nerve motor nuclei in the brainstem. The axons of these nerves leave the brainstem as motor components of cranial nerves.
               (ii) CN III, CN IV, CN VI, and CN XII carry somatic efferent fibers. These nerves innervate skeletal muscle of the head that is derived from somites.
               (iii) CN V, CN VII, CN IX, and CN X carry branchial efferent fibers that supply

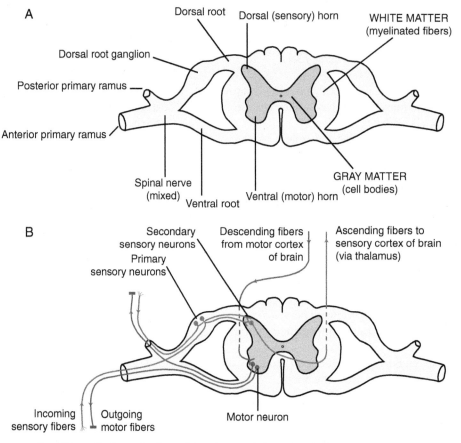

A

Dorsal root   Dorsal (sensory) horn

WHITE MATTER (myelinated fibers)

Dorsal root ganglion

Posterior primary ramus

Anterior primary ramus

Spinal nerve (mixed)   Ventral root   Ventral (motor) horn

GRAY MATTER (cell bodies)

B

Secondary sensory neurons   Descending fibers from motor cortex of brain   Ascending fibers to sensory cortex of brain (via thalamus)

Primary sensory neurons

Incoming sensory fibers   Outgoing motor fibers

Motor neuron

Figure 1-36 Cross section through the spinal cord to show origins of spinal nerves. **A,** Features seen in a typical cross section. **B,** Pathways of sensory and motor components. Note: These pathways are bilateral. Both ascending and descending pathways cross midline so that sensations and muscle movements on one side are perceived and controlled on the opposite side of the brain. *(From Liebgott B: The Anatomical Basis of Dentistry, ed 3, St. Louis, Mosby, 2011.)*

cranial muscles of branchial arch origin.

(b) Spinal nerves.

   (i) Lower motor neurons are located in the ventral horn of the spinal cord. Axons of these neurons leave the spinal cord as ventral roots that form the motor component of each of the 31 pairs of spinal nerves. These motor nerves supply all the skeletal muscles of the trunk and limbs.

b. General sensory (sensory somatic)—general sensory pathways have three sets of neurons, which synapse with neurons in the sensory cortex of the brain.

(1) Cranial nerves.

   (a) Cell bodies of the primary neurons of cranial nerves are located near the brainstem within sensory ganglia. Peripheral processes pick up stimuli from various regions of the head. The stimuli pass through the ganglia and central processes to sensory nuclei containing secondary

neurons within the brainstem. Their axons cross the midline and rise to synapse with tertiary neurons in the thalamus. These neurons send axons up to the sensory cortex.

(2) Spinal nerves.

   (a) Cell bodies of the primary neurons of spinal nerves are contained in the dorsal root ganglia adjacent to the spinal cord (Figure 1-36). Their peripheral processes transmit impulses from sensory receptors in skin or proprioceptive receptors in muscles, tendons, and joints. Central processes pass through dorsal roots into the CNS and synapse with secondary neurons within the dorsal horn. Axons cross the midline and ascend to synapse with tertiary neurons in the thalamus of the brain. These neurons send axons up to synapse with the final set of neurons located in the sensory cortex of the brain.

c. Origins of autonomic nerves in the CNS— autonomic motor. The autonomic pathway consists

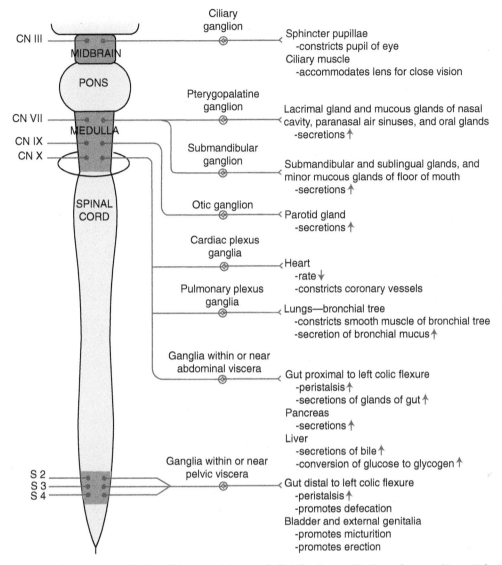

Figure 1-37 Scheme of parasympathetic division origins and distributions. *CN,* Cranial nerve. *(From Liebgott B: The Anatomical Basis of Dentistry, ed 3, St. Louis, Mosby, 2011.)*

of a two neuron chains. The first neurons are in the autonomic motor nuclei in the CNS. Axons are sent that leave the CNS and synapse with a second set within autonomic ganglia outside the CNS. The second neurons send out axons to the smooth muscle and glands of the viscera. This pathway has sympathetic and parasympathetic divisions.
(1) Parasympathetic division (Figure 1-37).
  (a) The parasympathetic division of the autonomic nervous system originates from the brain and sacral region of the spinal cord. The first neuron is found within parasympathetic motor nuclei.
    (i) Cranial preganglionic fibers arise from parasympathetic motor nuclei within the brainstem and leave as components of CN III, CN VII, CN IX, and CN X.

CN III, CN VII, and CN IX supply cranial visceral elements. CN X supplies the respiratory system, cardiac system, most of the gut, and associated glands up to the left colic flexure.
    (ii) Sacral preganglionic fibers arise from parasympathetic motor nuclei in the ventral horns of the spinal cord at levels S2, S3, and S4 and leave through the ventral roots of pelvic spinal nerves. They form pelvic splanchnic nerves that supply the distal portion of the gut and pelvic viscera.
(2) Sympathetic division.
  (a) The sympathetic division of the autonomic nervous system leaves the spinal cord at levels T1 to L2 (Figure 1-38). The first

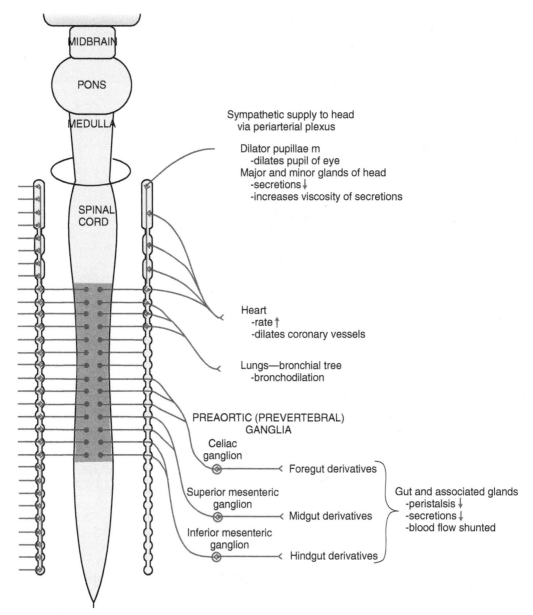

Figure 1-38 Scheme of sympathetic division origins and distributions. Note: To simplify scheme, sympathetic contributions are shown on the right side, and sympathetic innervation to the head and viscera is shown on the left side. Both sets of fibers are bilateral. *(From Liebgott B: The Anatomical Basis of Dentistry, ed 3, St. Louis, Mosby, 2011.)*

neurons are located within the intermediolateral horns, which are found only in this region of the spinal cord. Preganglionic fibers leave the spinal cord along with the anterior spinal nerve roots. The fibers leave the nerve as myelinated white communicating rami.

(b) On either side of the vertebral column are a chain of cervical ganglia. These sympathetic trunks run the entire length of the vertebral column. Each vertebral level has an associated vertebral ganglion. The ganglia at levels C1 through C4 fuse to form the superior cervical ganglion. The

ganglia at levels C5 and C6 fuse to form the middle cervical ganglion, and the ganglia at levels C7 and C8 fuse to form the inferior cervical ganglion. White communicating rami emerge from spinal levels T1 to L2 and run to the sympathetic trunk.

(c) Within the sympathetic trunk, preganglionic fibers may synapse with the neurons of the ganglion at that level, travel up or down to the sympathetic trunk to synapse in a ganglion at a higher or lower level, or leave the sympathetic trunk as splanchnic nerves. Splanchnic nerves extend into the abdomen and synapse in prevertebral ganglia. Postganglionic fibers in the first and second categories rejoin spinal nerves as unmyelinated gray communicating rami. From spinal levels T1 to L2, 14 pairs of white communicating rami arise. Leaving the sympathetic trunk to join spinal nerves are 31 pairs of gray rami.

(3) Distribution of postganglionic sympathetic fibers.

(a) Trunk and limbs.

(i) Gray rami leave the sympathetic trunk at each spinal cord level to join each pair of spinal nerves. They are distributed along with the spinal nerves to the trunk and limbs where they supply smooth muscle of blood vessels. Sympathetic fibers also pass to the skin and supply sweat glands and the arrector pili muscles that cause hair to stand on end.

(b) Head and neck.

(i) Preganglionic fibers of the sympathetic trunk rise to the superior cervical ganglion. Here, the ganglionic fibers synapse with a second set of neurons.

(ii) Postganglionic fibers leave the ganglion and join the carotid arteries as the carotid periarterial plexus. The sympathetic postganglionic fibers are distributed to visceral effector organs of the head by various branches of the external and internal carotid arteries.

(c) Thorax.

(i) Postganglionic fibers of the three cervical sympathetic ganglia stream down the thorax to form the cardiac and pulmonary plexuses. These supply the heart and smooth muscle of the bronchial tree.

(d) Abdominal and pelvic viscera.

(i) Preganglionic fibers leave the sympathetic trunk in the thorax as splanchnic nerves. These enter the abdomen and synapse in remote prevertebral ganglia.

(ii) Postganglionic fibers travel via branches of the abdominal aorta to the viscera of the abdomen. Thoracic splanchnic nerves supply derivatives of the foregut and midgut. Hindgut derivatives and urogenital pelvic viscera are supplied from lumbar splanchnic nerves from the sympathetic trunk of the lumbar region.

d. Origins of autonomic nerves in the CNS— autonomic sensory.

(1) Visceral receptors monitor smooth muscle tone in viscera and vessels, blood chemistry, blood pressure, and the content volume in hollow organs. This information is relayed back to the CNS via sensory components of autonomic nerves. Afferent impulses carrying information, such as a feeling of fullness, hunger, or nausea, travel back to the CNS along parasympathetic nerves. The pathways for visceral or autonomic sensation within the CNS are the same as the pathways for the somatic afferent nerve fibers. Feelings of pain or cramps travel back to the CNS along sympathetic nerves. The brain refers the pain to somatic sites that share the same spinal nerve innervation. The primary cell bodies are found in dorsal root ganglia of spinal nerves. Within the CNS, axons follow the same pathway as the somatic afferent fibers.

e. Nomenclature.

(1) Cranial nerves.

(a) The 12 cranial nerves originate from the brain. Each is assigned a Roman numeral. Some have one functional component, and others have more than one.

(2) Spinal nerves.

(a) Spinal nerves exit through intervertebral foramina and break into two main rami.

(i) Posterior primary rami supply mixed sensory and motor nerves to structures of the back, the back of the neck, and the back of the head.

(ii) Anterior primary rami supply mixed sensory and motor fibers to the lateral and anterior aspects of the trunk and all the upper and lower limbs.

(3) Nerve plexus.

(a) In certain areas of the spinal cord, anterior primary rami tend to join and divide in complex patterns called *nerve plexuses*.

(i) The cervical plexus is formed by the anterior primary rami of spinal nerves C1 to C4. It supplies structures in the anterior and lateral regions of the neck.

(ii) The brachial plexus is formed from the anterior primary rami of spinal nerves C5 through T1. It supplies all the structures of the upper limb.

(iii) The lumbar plexus is formed by the anterior primary rami of spinal nerves L1 through L4 and supplies the pelvis and entire lower limb.

(iv) The sacral plexus is formed by the anterior primary rami of spinal nerves L4 through S4 and supplies the perineum and lower limb.

(v) The coccygeal plexus is formed by the anterior primary rami of spinal nerves S4 to the coccygeal nerve and supplies skin of the coccygeal area.

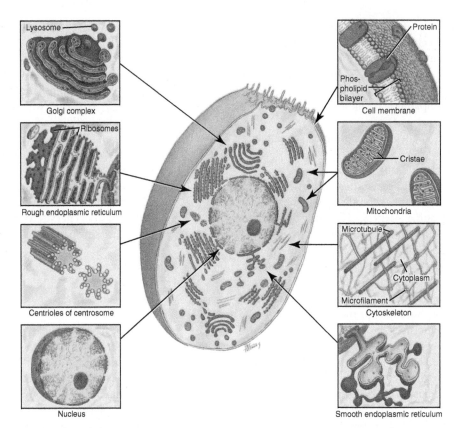

Figure 1-39 A cell with its organelles and cell membrane examined. *(From Bath-Balogh M, Fehrenbach M: Illustrated Dental Embryology, Histology, and Anatomy, ed 3, Philadelphia, Saunders, 2011.)*

f. Cutaneous distribution.
  (1) Most of the skin of the body is innervated by spinal nerves. The face and anterior scalp are innervated largely by CN V.

2.0 Histology

2.1 Ultrastructure

2.1.1 Cell

A. Cell (plasma) membrane.
  1. Consists of a phospholipid bilayer (Figure 1-39). This bilayer contains proteins that are incorporated in the membrane (integral proteins) or attached to the inner or outer surface (peripheral proteins). Some of these proteins can move freely within the phospholipids bilayer. This model of the cell membrane was first described by the fluid mosaic model.*
  2. Besides phospholipids, the membrane also contains other lipids, including cholesterols and glycolipids.
  3. The membrane proteins and lipids are held together via noncovalent interactions.

B. Cell organelles.
  1. Nucleus.
    a. Is surrounded by a nuclear envelope that consists of two (inner and outer) membranes. This envelope contains many holes, or nuclear pores, that allow for the selective passage of molecules through it (see Figure 1-39).
    b. Contains DNA and RNA.
      (1) In the nucleus, DNA appears as chromatin, which consists of a complex of DNA, histones, and proteins.
      (2) During cell division, chromatin condenses into chromosomes. Each chromosome consists of two parallel, spiral-like filaments (chromatids) that are joined together at the centromere.
        (a) Sex chromatin: the male has one Y and one X chromosome. The female has two X chromosomes.
    c. Nucleolus—a circular-shaped structure found inside the nucleus that is the site of ribosomal RNA synthesis.
    d. Barr body—in some female nuclei, during interphase, one of the X chromosomes becomes inactive and condenses to form a small, visible mass called a *Barr body.*

---

*Singer SJ: Early history of membrane biology. Annu Rev Physiol 66:1-27, 2004.

e. During apoptosis (programmed cell death), the nucleus undergoes changes.
  (1) Karyolysis—dissolution of the nucleus.
  (2) Pyknosis—the nucleus shrinks, and the chromatin condenses.
  (3) Karyorrhexis—fragmentation of the nucleus, and the chromatin disintegrates.
2. Mitochondria.
  a. The powerhouse of the cell, where adenosine triphosphate (ATP) is produced.
  b. Is surrounded by two (inner and outer) membranes. The inner membrane appears as folds that project into the inner matrix, called *cristae*.
  c. Contains circular DNA, which is similar to the genetic material found in bacteria.
3. Rough endoplasmic reticulum.
  a. Consists of a network of tubules, vesicles, and flattened sacs.
  b. Ribosomes are bound to its surface, giving the endoplasmic reticulum a rough appearance.
4. Smooth endoplasmic reticulum.
  a. Consists of a network of tubules and vesicles. No ribosomes are bound to its surface.
  b. In general, it is responsible for the synthesis of lipids. In the liver, it is involved in glycogen metabolism and detoxification of various drugs and alcohols. It also contains P450 enzymes. Cytochrome P450 enzymes are important in the detoxification process. In muscle, the smooth sarcoplasmic reticulum (equivalent to endoplasmic reticulum in other tissues) plays a major role in the storage of calcium.
5. Ribosomes.
  a. Responsible for protein synthesis.
  b. Composed of RNA subunits that are made in the nucleolus.
6. Golgi apparatus.
  a. Consists of a complex of layered, membrane-bound cisternae.
  b. Responsible for modifying and packaging proteins from the rough endoplasmic reticulum. Products are sent in vesicles to the plasma membrane, lysosomes, or secretory vesicles.
7. Lysosomes.
  a. Are small, membrane-bound vesicles that contain many hydrolytic enzymes.
  b. Play an important role in the intracellular digestion of phagocytosed particles.
8. Centrosome.
  a. Oval-shaped organelle located next to the nucleus. It plays a role in the formation of mitotic spindles during cell division (refer to Mitosis section).
  b. Contains a pair of centrioles and is composed of triplets of microtubules arranged in a cartwheel pattern.

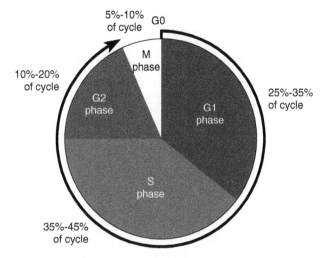

Figure 1-40 Periods of the cell cycle indicate relative time needed for each phase. *(Modified from Chiego D: Essentials of Oral Histology and Embryology: A Clinical Approach, ed 4, St. Louis, Mosby, 2014.)*

9. Cytoplasmic inclusions.
  a. Contain stored metabolites, such as fats and glycogen, pigments (melanin), or crystalline granules.
  b. May also contain residual materials such as spent lysosomes and digested materials.
10. Cilia and flagella.
  a. Are motile processes that protrude from the cell membrane.
  b. Cilia are usually shorter than flagella. They are found in multiple numbers and are organized in parallel rows. They are present on the surface of respiratory epithelium and female reproductive tracts.
  c. Flagella are typically longer than cilia and do not occur in multiple numbers.
  d. A cilium is surrounded by plasma membrane. Its central core, the axoneme, consists of a central pair or two microtubules at the center. It is surrounded by nine peripheral doublets, or pairs of microtubules. The microtubule arrangement is described as a "9 + 2 pattern." At the base of the axoneme is the basal body. The microtubule organization in the basal body consists of nine peripheral triplets.
C. Cell cycle and mitosis.
  1. The cell cycle can be divided into four phases (Figure 1-40).
  a. G_1 (first gap) phase.
    (1) Begins after mitosis and ends at the start of the S phase.
    (2) Cells grow and perform their usual functions.
    (3) This phase is typically longer than the other phases.

b. S (synthesis) phase.
  (1) DNA in the nucleus is replicated.
  (2) The sections of chromatin that appear loosely coiled and lightly colored are actively synthesizing RNA and are known as *euchromatin*. In areas of no genetic activity, the chromatin appears in clumps and stains darkly; it is called *heterochromatin*.
c. G_2 (second gap) phase.
  (1) Cells prepare for mitosis.
  (2) Includes the buildup of ATP and tubulin, which is needed for the formation of spindle fibers.
d. M—mitosis (Figure 1-41).
  (1) With the exception of sex cells, which divide via meiosis, somatic cells divide by mitotic division. Mitosis results in the production of two genetically identical daughter cells, formed from a single parent cell. Similar to the parent cell, each daughter cell carries the diploid number (46 in humans) of chromosomes.
  (2) Mitotic division can be divided into five phases.
    (a) Interphase—includes G_1, S, and G_2 phases.
    (b) Prophase—nuclear membrane and nucleolus disintegrates; chromatin condenses; centrioles in centrosomes replicate, separate, and begin migrating toward opposite poles.
    (c) Metaphase—mitotic spindles form. Chromosomes attach to mitotic spindles with their centromeres aligned with the equator of the cell.
    (d) Anaphase—centromeres (chromosomes) split. The separated chromatids are pulled by the spindles to opposite poles in the cell.
    (e) Telophase—nuclear membrane reappears. The chromosomes uncoil and lengthen to their normal form. The cytoplasm begins to divide into two daughter cells, a process known as *cytokinesis*. This process begins with the formation of a circumferential furrow, or cleavage furrow. This furrow continues to constrict the cytoplasm until it divides it into two daughter cells.
2. Cells that are nondividing or in the resting state are in G_0 phase. If stimulated, they can enter the cell cycle.
D. Meiosis.
  1. Meiosis is how sex cells divide. It differs from mitotic division in that there are two successive cycles of meiotic cell division (Figure 1-42), which results in the production of four genetically different daughter cells. Each daughter cell carries half of the diploid number (23 in humans) of chromosomes.
  2. Chiasmata formation—occurs only in meiosis, during the first meiotic division. The duplicated chromosomes cross over and exchange alleles. This rearrangement results in genetically different gametes (chromosomes).

2.2 Basic Tissues

A. Epithelium.
  1. The tissue that covers and lines all body surfaces.
  2. Classification of epithelia.
    a. Number of cell layers.
      (1) Simple epithelium—single layer of epithelial cells.
      (2) Pseudostratified epithelium—single layer of epithelial cells, where every cell contacts the basal lamina, but not all cells reach the epithelial surface. It may appear as multilayered but is actually a single layer of cells.
      (3) Stratified epithelium—more than one layer of epithelial cells.
      (4) Transitional epithelium—type of stratified epithelium. It is generally found only in the urinary tract and bladder. The epithelium appears transitional between stratified squamous (when the epithelium is stretched) and stratified cuboidal (when it is relaxed).
    b. Shape.
      (1) Squamous—flattened cells.
      (2) Cuboidal—cube-shaped (square) cells.
      (3) Columnar—rectangular cells.
    c. Epithelium also can be classified by the presence of specialized surface structures, such ciliated versus nonciliated and keratinized versus nonkeratinized epithelium.
  3. The distribution of epithelia found in the body is summarized in Table 1-28.
  4. Epithelial cell junctions.
    a. Junctional complex—consists of the zonula occludens, zonula adherens, and desmosomes.
      (1) Zonula occludens (tight junctions)—forms a seal between the plasma membrane of two adjacent cells. This seal prevents contents of the lumen from passing through.
      (2) Zonula adherens (adhering junctions)—found deep in the zonula occludens. It serves to bind the epithelial cells together and contains the glycoprotein E-cadherins.
      (3) Desmosomes (macula densa)—small, circular patches deep in the zonula adherens. It serves to bind the epithelium together and contains the glycoprotein desmogleins.
    b. Gap junctions—small pores found between adjacent cells that allow the passage of small molecules.
  5. Epithelial surfaces.
    a. Luminal surface—the surface of the lumen may contain specialized structures, such as cilia, microvilli, or stereocilia.

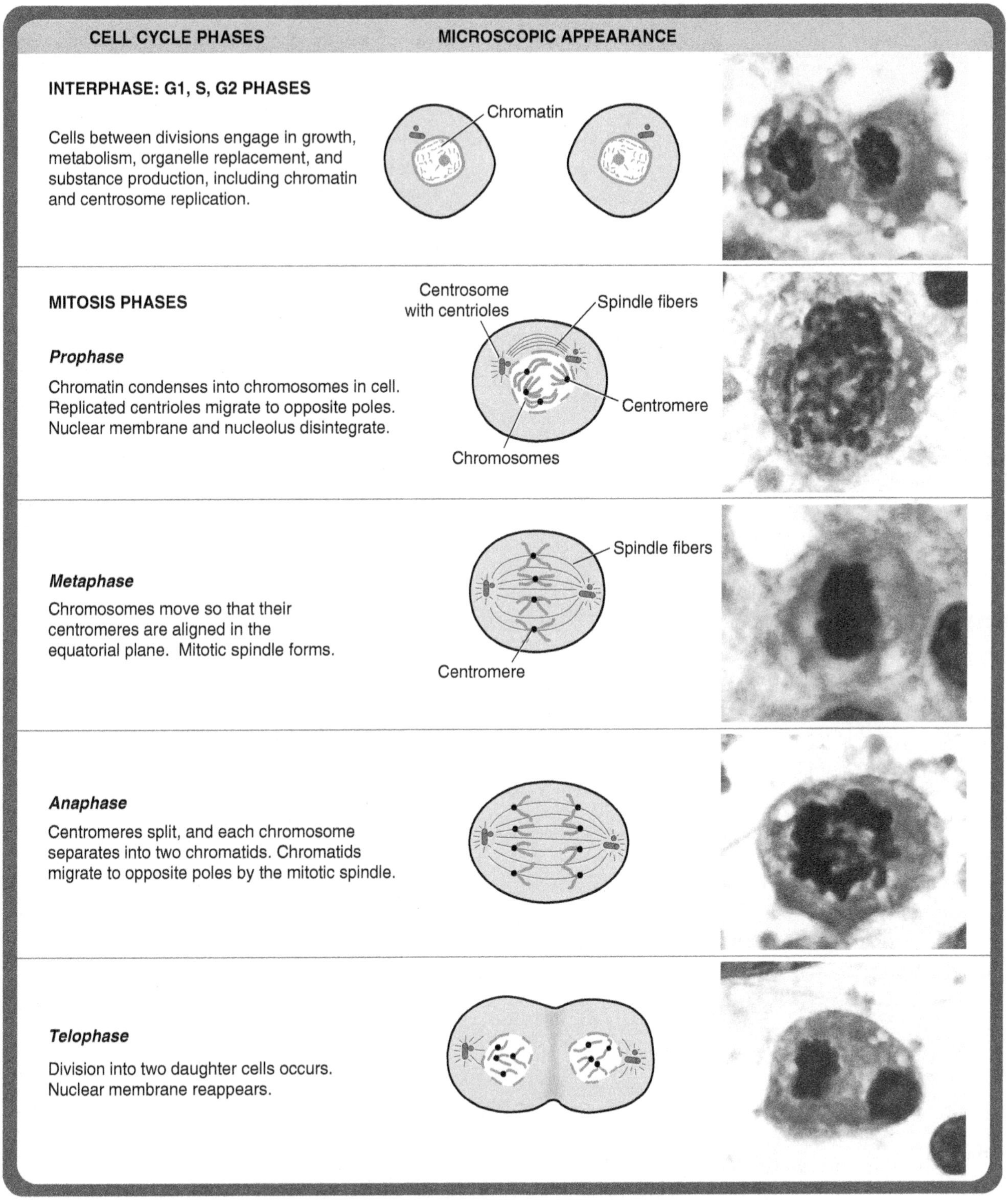
CELL CYCLE PHASES
MICROSCOPIC APPEARANCE
INTERPHASE: G1, S, G2 PHASES
Cells between divisions engage in growth, metabolism, organelle replacement, and substance production, including chromatin and centrosome replication.
Chromatin
MITOSIS PHASES
Prophase
Chromatin condenses into chromosomes in cell. Replicated centrioles migrate to opposite poles. Nuclear membrane and nucleolus disintegrate.
Centrosome with centrioles
Spindle fibers
Centromere
Chromosomes
Metaphase
Chromosomes move so that their centromeres are aligned in the equatorial plane. Mitotic spindle forms.
Spindle fibers
Centromere
Anaphase
Centromeres split, and each chromosome separates into two chromatids. Chromatids migrate to opposite poles by the mitotic spindle.
Telophase
Division into two daughter cells occurs. Nuclear membrane reappears.

Figure 1-41 Mitosis. *(From Bath-Balogh M, Fehrenbach M: Illustrated Dental Embryology, Histology, and Anatomy, ed 3, Philadelphia, Saunders, 2011.)*

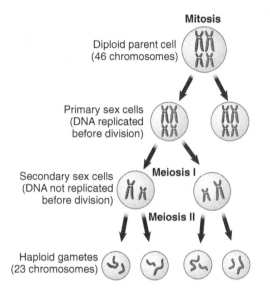

Figure 1-42 Meiosis I and II. *(From Patton KT, Thibodeau GA: Anatomy and Physiology, ed 7, St. Louis, 2010, Mosby.)*

6. Basal surface—contains hemidesmosomes, which help to anchor the epithelium to the basement membrane.

B. Basement membrane (lamina).

1. Acellular, condensed layer that forms a barrier between the epithelium and connective tissues. It is composed of type IV collagen, fibronectin, laminin, entactin, and heparan sulfate.

2. Attachment of the epithelium to the connective tissues involves a complex of hemidesmosomes and tonofilaments from the epithelium and anchoring collagen fibers from the connective tissues.

C. Connective tissue.

1. Connective tissues consist of an extracellular matrix and cells. The extracellular matrix is made up of amorphous ground substance, fibers, and glycoproteins.

a. Amorphous ground substance.

   (1) Has a semifluid, gel-like consistency that allows for the exchange of molecules and fluid between cells and the circulatory system.

Table 1-28

Three Types of Epithelia

NUMBER OF LAYERS	CELL SHAPE	FUNCTION	DISTRIBUTION
Simple	Squamous	Diffusion, filtration, and secretion	Blood vessels (endothelium) Body cavities (mesothelium) Pericardium Peritoneum Pleura
	Cuboidal	Secretion	Bronchioles Salivary glands acini Thyroid gland Ovary capsule
	Columnar	Secretion and absorption	Intestinal lining Gallbladder
Pseudostratified	Columnar—*ciliated*	Secretion	Respiratory tract (except bronchioles) Nasopharynx Paranasal sinuses Nasal cavity Eustachian tubes
	Columnar—*nonciliated*	Secretion	Salivary gland ducts Male urethra
Stratified	Squamous—*keratinized*	Protective barrier Prevent dehydration	Skin (epidermis)
	Squamous—*nonkeratinized*	Protective barrier Secretion	Oral cavity Oropharynx Laryngopharynx Esophagus Vaginal canal Anal canal
	Cuboidal	Protective barrier	Large ducts of several exocrine glands
	Transitional	Protective barrier	Bladder Urinary tract

(2) Contains proteoglycans, proteins with covalently bound glycosaminoglycan (GAG) chains.

(3) GAGs.

(a) GAGs are made of repeating sulfated disaccharide units.

(b) GAGs form hydrogen bonds with large amounts of water, forming a gel-like matrix.

(c) Ground substance stains basophilic because of the presence of GAGs contained in sulfated proteoglycans.

(d) Types of GAGs.

(i) Chondroitin sulfate (chondroitin 4-sulfate, chondroitin 6-sulfate)—the most abundant GAG. It is found in cartilage.

(ii) Keratan sulfate—found in cartilage and the cornea.

(iii) Heparan sulfate—found in cell membranes and basement membranes.

(iv) Dermatan sulfate—found in skin, blood vessels, and heart valves.

(v) Hyaluronic acid.

(e) Known as the "cement substance of tissue."

(f) Found in bone, cartilage, tendons, synovial fluid, and vitreous humor of the eye.

b. Fibers.

(1) Collagen.

(a) Most abundant protein in the body, about 30% dry weight.

(b) Is secreted as tropocollagen (a triple helix containing hydroxylysine and hydroxyproline), which polymerizes in the extracellular matrix to form collagen.

(c) Type I collagen—most abundant type of collagen. Found in connective tissues, tendons, ligaments, bone, teeth, and dermis of the skin.

(d) Type II collagen—found in hyaline cartilage.

(e) Type III collagen—constitutes reticulin fibers. These fibers play a role in the structural component in the liver, bone marrow, and lymphoid organs.

(f) Type IV collagen—found in basement membranes. Does not form fibers or fibrils.

(2) Elastin—a flexible protein that is arranged into elastic fibers. These fibers also contain fibrillin.

c. Glycoproteins.

(1) Glycoproteins are found in the extracellular matrix.

(2) Types of glycoproteins.

(a) Fibrillin—plays a role in the deposition of elastic fibers.

(b) Fibronectin—plays a role in the deposition of collagen fibers. It also aids in the attachment of cells to collagen.

(c) Laminin—found in basement membranes.

(d) Entactin—binds laminin to type IV collagen in basement membranes.

(e) Tenascin—plays a role in the embryologic development of nerve cells.

2. Miscellaneous cells.

a. Fibroblasts—produce collagenous, reticular, and elastic fibers.

b. Immune cells—includes macrophages, mast cells, plasma cells, and lymphocytes.

c. Adipocytes—fat cells that store and metabolize fat. Collectively, they form adipose tissue.

D. Muscle.

1. There are three types of muscle: smooth, skeletal, and cardiac. Their histologic characteristics are summarized in Table 1-29.

a. Smooth (visceral) muscle.

(1) Smooth muscle is under autonomic or hormonal control, or involuntary control.

(2) Cells are capable of mitosis.

(3) Smooth muscle is found in the walls of blood vessels, organs, and visceral structures, including the gastrointestinal tract, the uterus, and the urinary bladder.

b. Skeletal muscle.

(1) Skeletal muscle is under conscious or voluntary control.

(2) Cells are incapable of mitosis.

(3) Anatomic organization (Figure 1-43).

(a) Skeletal muscle is covered by a dense collagenous tissue called the *epimysium.*

(b) Muscle fibers are grouped into bundles (muscle fasciculi). The connective tissues covering the muscle fibers and fasciculi are known as *endomysium* and *perimysium,* respectively.

Table 1-29	
Three Types of Muscle	
	HISTOLOGIC CHARACTERISTICS
Smooth muscle	Nonstriated muscle Spindle-shaped (fusiform) cells Gap junctions (nexi) Nucleus centered in *widest* part of cell
Skeletal muscle	Striated muscle Prominent A bands and I bands Multiple nuclei found at the cell periphery
Cardiac muscle	Striated muscle Specialized gap junctions (intercalated discs) and desmosomes Nucleus centered in cells

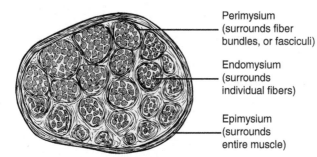

Perimysium (surrounds fiber bundles, or fasciculi)

Endomysium (surrounds individual fibers)

Epimysium (surrounds entire muscle)

Figure 1-43 Cross section of skeletal muscle. (*From Liebgott B: The Anatomical Basis of Dentistry, ed 3, St. Louis, Mosby, 2011.*)

(c) Histologic staining (hematoxylin-eosin staining) of a muscle fiber reveals A bands and I bands.
  (i) A band—dark band with a light band (H band) in the center.
  (ii) I band—light band with a thin band (Z line) bisecting it.
  (iii) The contractile unit of skeletal muscle, or sarcomere, is the area between two Z lines.
  (iv) Sarcomeres contain two types of filaments, thick and thin. Thick filaments consist mostly of myosin, and thin filaments consist mostly of actin.
c. Cardiac muscle.
  (1) Is incapable of mitosis.
  (2) Histologic organization.
    (a) Consists of rows of myocardial cells connected in a series.
    (b) Myocardial cells are separated by intercalated discs, which consist of gap junctions and desmosomes.
      (i) Gap junctions—areas of communication between the cells that allow electrical currents to travel through them.
      (ii) Desmosomes ("spot welds")—attach cells together.
  (3) Histologic appearance compared with skeletal muscle.
    (a) Similarities.
      (i) Both are striated muscle.
      (ii) The contractile unit for both is sarcomere consisting of thin and thick filaments.
    (b) Differences.
      (i) Cardiac muscles have larger T tubules and more mitochondria.
      (ii) Nuclei are centered in cells.
      (iii) Presence of intercalated discs between cells.

E. Nervous tissue.
  1. Neurons consist of a cell body, a single axon, and dendrite(s).
    a. Cell body—contains the nucleus and cell organelles.
    b. Dendrites.
      (1) Receive and transmit information toward the cell body.
      (2) Are usually short and highly branched.
    c. Axon.
      (1) Transmits impulses away from the cell body.
      (2) A long, uniform process that is usually surrounded by a myelin sheath. The myelin sheath consists of Schwann cells that are separated by spaces called *nodes of Ranvier*.
  2. There are three types of neurons.
    a. Multipolar neurons—have dendrites extending directly from the cell body. Example: motor neurons (Figure 1-44, *A*).
    b. Bipolar neurons—have a single dendrite that extends from the cell body. Example: neurons that function in the senses of smell and sight or that coordinate balance.
    c. Pseudounipolar—have a single dendrite. The dendrite and the axon are joined. Example: most primary sensory neurons (Figure 1-44, *B*).
  3. Glial cells.
    a. Function as support cells to neurons and include Schwann cells and oligodendrocytes.
    b. Schwann cells—make up the myelin sheath around myelinated axons in the parasympathetic nervous system.
    c. Oligodendrocytes—make up the myelin sheath around myelinated axons in the CNS.
  4. Synapse.
    a. The site at which a nerve impulse (action potential) passes from one nerve to another (i.e., nerve impulses are sent from one nerve's axon to the receiving nerve's dendrites) (see Figure 1-44).
    b. Synaptic transmission: refer to Biochemistry and Physiology Review.

2.3 Bone, Cartilage, and Joints

2.3.1 Bone

A. General characteristics.
  1. Bone plays many roles, including providing support against mechanical stresses, hematopoiesis, and calcium homeostasis (i.e., calcium storage).
  2. Bone consists of the following components.
    a. A calcified (mineralized) matrix—contains inorganic substances consisting mostly of calcium hydroxyapatite. Osteogenin, a glycoprotein that binds calcium and collagen, is also present.
    b. Extracellular matrix—contains organic substances including type I collagen and GAGs (i.e., ground substance).

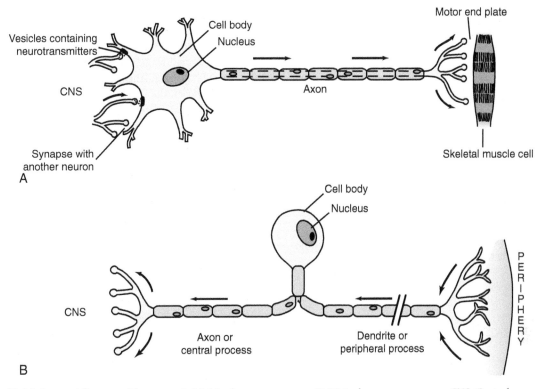

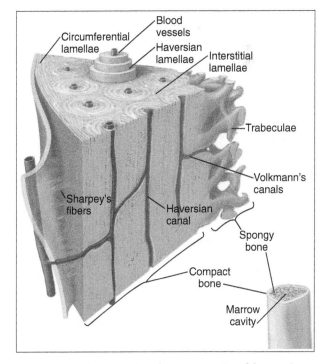

Figure 1-44 Motor and Sensory Neurons. **A,** Multipolar motor neuron. **B,** Unipolar sensory neuron. *CNS,* Central nervous system. *(From Liebgott B: The Anatomical Basis of Dentistry, ed 3, St. Louis, Mosby, 2011.)*

c. Cells, including osteoblasts, osteoclasts, and osteocytes.

d. Note: during the calcification (mineralization) of bone, its inorganic content increases, and its water content decreases. The amount of collagen does not change.

e. Osteoid—bone that has not yet been calcified (i.e., contains no mineralized matrix).

B. Two types of bone.

1. Cortical (compact) bone (Figure 1-45).

   a. 70% of bone in the body.

   b. Dense bone that consists of parallel cylinders tightly stacked together, called *haversian systems* or *osteons.*

   c. A haversian system consists of layers of bone (lamellae) that are concentrically arranged, with the oldest layer near the periphery. The lamellae circumscribe a neurovascular canal (haversian canal), which contains nerves, lymphatics, and blood vessels.

   d. Haversian canals are interconnected by Volkmann's canals.

   e. As bone is laid down, osteocytes get trapped in spaces called *lacunae.* Lacunae have minicanals known as *canaliculi,* which connect them with the central canal.

   f. Cortical bone is covered by a thick, connective tissue called the *periosteum.* The periosteum

Figure 1-45 Organizational components of bone. *(From Pollard TD, Earnshaw WC: Cell Biology, Philadelphia, Saunders, 2002.)*

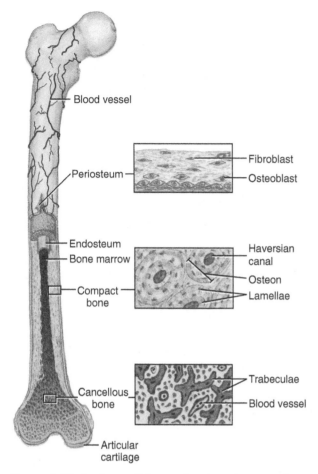

Figure 1-46 Anatomy of bone showing close-up views of its periosteum and compact or cancellous bone. Note the endosteum and bone marrow. *(From Bath-Balogh M, Fehrenbach M: Illustrated Dental Embryology, Histology, and Anatomy, ed 3, Philadelphia, Saunders, 2011.)*

attaches to the bone by Sharpey's fibers. Note: Sharpey's fibers also attach the periodontal ligament (PDL) to alveolar bone. Endosteum lines the medullary cavity of bone on the inside of cortical cancellous bone.

   g. During bone apposition, resting lines appear between the old and newly formed cortical bone.

  2. Cancellous (trabecular, spongy) bone (Figure 1-46).

   a. Protected by an outer shell of cortical bone.

   b. The major site for bone remodeling and metabolic activity.

   c. Consists of a spongelike structure with a network of bony plates (trabeculae) that are filled with pockets of bone marrow.

   d. It is not arranged in concentric layers.

C. Anatomy of long bones.

  1. Long bones can be divided into three zones (see Figure 1-46).

   a. Diaphysis—the shaft (midportion) of the bone.

   b. Epiphysis—the ends of the bone. If the epiphysis articulates with another bone, it will likely be surrounded by articular cartilage.

   c. Metaphysis—the area where the bone narrows between the epiphysis and diaphysis.

  2. Epiphyseal plate (physis)—found between the epiphysis and metaphysis in children who are still growing.

D. Osteogenesis (bone development).

  1. Cellular players.

   a. Osteoblasts (see Figure 1-46).

    (1) Secrete (create) bone. They also play a role in bone remodeling.

    (2) Appear as cuboidal cells with a polarized nucleus on the side of the cell opposite from the bony surface.

    (3) Synthesize alkaline phosphatase. Note: alkaline phosphatase is also produced in the kidney and liver. Increased serum alkaline phosphatase is often indicative of bone disease.

   b. Osteocytes—osteoblasts that become trapped in bone (i.e., develop from osteoblasts).

   c. Osteoclasts.

    (1) Resorb (destroy) bone.

    (2) Appear as multinucleated, giant cells.

    (3) Derived from the fusion of bloodborne monocytes.

    (4) Bone resorption creates depressions called *Howship's lacunae.*

  2. Osteogenesis—two processes.

   a. Endochondral ossification.

    (1) Associated with the growth of long bones.

    (2) Increases the length of bones via interstitial growth at the epiphyseal plates.

    (3) Includes most skeletal bones (i.e., tibia, fibia, femur) and a few bones in the skull (ethmoid, sphenoid, temporal, occipital bones, and the base of the skull).

    (4) Process of bone development.

     (a) Chondrocytes differentiate from mesenchymal cells present in connective tissue.

     (b) Chondrocytes secrete a cartilage (hyaline) matrix, which is covered by perichondrium. The matrix then calcifies.

     (c) Chondrocytes die, leaving spaces that become filled with vascular tissue.

     (d) Osteoblasts differentiate from mesenchymal cells in adjacent tissues and secrete bone onto the preformed cartilage scaffold.

   b. Intramembranous ossification (appositional growth).

    (1) Associated with increasing the diameter or width of flat bones (i.e., bones grow "out").

    (2) Includes flat bones of the skull, part of the mandible, and a portion of the clavicle.

Table 1-30

Three Types of Cartilage

	GENERAL CHARACTERISTICS	DISTRIBUTION
Hyaline (articular) cartilage	Fibrous matrix of type II collagen Slightly elastic Covered by perichondrium	Ends of bones (articular joints) Costal cartilage (ribs) Respiratory cartilage (nasal septum, larynx, trachea, bronchial walls) Auditory cartilage (external auditory meatus, pharyngotympanic tube) Synchondroses Cartilage matrix for endochondral ossification Embryonic skeleton formation
Elastic cartilage	Like hyaline cartilage with type II collagen, but less dense Elastic Covered by perichondrium	Ear—external ear, pinna, auditory tube Epiglottis
Fibrocartilage	Dense, fibrous matrix of type I collagen Not elastic No perichondrium	Articular discs—TMJ, knee meniscus Intervertebral discs Pubic symphysis Insertions of tendons or ligaments

TMJ, Temporomandibular joint.

(3) Process of bone development.
  (a) Osteoblasts differentiate from mesenchymal cells present in connective tissue.
  (b) Osteoblasts secrete bone directly into connective tissues, forming trabeculae (long strands of bone) matrix. This initial type of bony matrix is known as *woven bone*.
  (c) Osteoblasts that become trapped in the matrix, in spaces known as *lacunae*, are called *osteocytes*. They continue to lay down bone, forming compact bone. The bone mineralizes.
 c. Bone remodeling—bone is constantly being remodeled. This process includes both osteoclasts removing bone and osteoblasts reforming bone in the resorbed area.

2.3.2 Cartilage

A. Cartilage is a tissue that consists of the following components.
  1. Water.
  2. Type II collagen.
  3. Sulfated proteoglycans, which results in basophilic staining of cartilage.
  4. Chondrocytes.
B. Perichondrium.
  1. Fibrous connective tissue that lines the surfaces of cartilage except articulate surfaces (i.e., nonarticulate surfaces).
  2. Is the vascular supply for cartilage.
  3. Cannot be viewed on radiographs because of lack of calcium salts.
  4. Contains chondroblasts.

C. Growth of cartilage.
  1. Interstitial growth—growth by cell division of chondrocytes. Note: bones do not grow interstitially (from within) except at the epiphyseal plates. This is one of the ways cartilage growth differs from bone development.
  2. Appositional growth—growth by layering (i.e., deposition of a cartilage matrix by chondroblasts).
D. There are three types of cartilage: hyaline (articular) cartilage, elastic cartilage, and fibrocartilage. Their general characteristics and distribution are summarized in Table 1-30.

2.3.3 Joints

A. Classification of joints.
  1. Synarthroses—joints with little or no movement.
    a. Syndesmoses.
      (1) Bones joined by dense fibrous tissue. No cartilage is present.
      (2) Example: cranial sutures in children.
      (3) Gomphosis—a type of syndesmosis joint that is described as a cone-shaped process placed in a socket.
      (4) Example: tooth in alveolar bone.
    b. Synchondroses.
      (1) Bones joined by cartilage. No synovial cavity is present.
      (2) Example: ribs, sternum.
    c. Synostoses.
      (1) Bones joined by bone.
      (2) In many circumstances can be considered a pathologic condition (i.e., ankylosis).
      (3) Example: cranial sutures in adults.

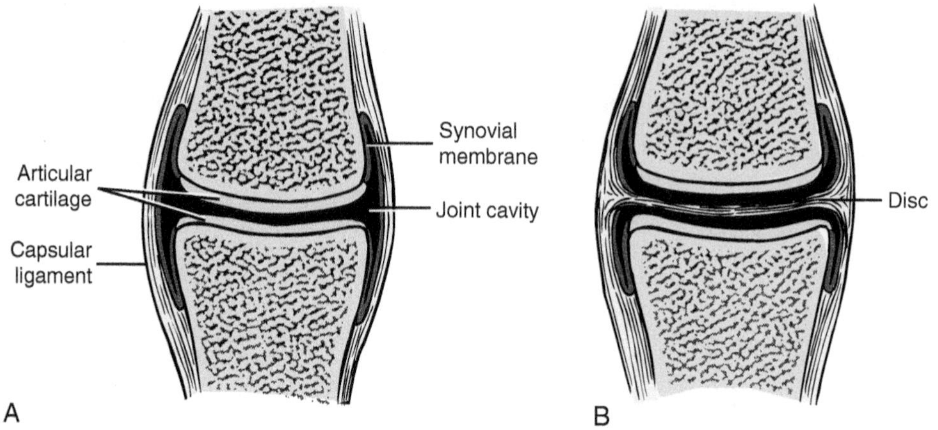

Figure 1-47 Synovial joint. **A,** Typical view of synovial joint. **B,** Synovial joint with articular disc. *(From Liebgott B: The Anatomical Basis of Dentistry, ed 3, St. Louis, Mosby, 2011.)*

d. Symphyses
  (1) Bones joined by fibrocartilage and ligaments.
  (2) May be classified as an amphiarthrosis (slightly movable) joint.
  (3) Example: pubic symphysis, intervertebral discs.
2. Synovial (diarthrodial or diarthroses) joints—freely movable joints.
  a. Consists of two bone ends articulating in an enclosed capsule (Figure 1-47).
  b. Articular cartilage (see Figure 1-46).
    (1) Consists of hyaline cartilage that covers the ends of the two opposing bones.
    (2) Has no vascular or nerve supply.
    (3) Synovial fluid provides its nourishment.
  c. Articular capsule.
    (1) Consists of dense, fibrous connective tissue that encloses the joint space.
    (2) Continuous with the periosteum and synovium.
3. Synovial cavity (joint space).
  a. Synovial fluid.
    (1) Fluid that fills the joint space.
    (2) It is responsible for providing lubrication for frictionless movement and nourishment of the articular cartilage.
    (3) Consists of hyaluronic acid, glycoproteins including lubricin, and lysosomal enzymes that are secreted by macrophages.
  b. Synovial membrane (synovium).
    (1) Lines the synovial cavity.
    (2) Secretes synovial fluid.
    (3) Lined with macrophages and fibroblasts.

2.3.4 Blood

In general, circulating blood constitutes 5% to 7% of body weight. Blood is a tissue that consists of cells and molecules in a fluid medium known as *plasma*.

A. Composition of blood.
  1. Plasma—55% of blood volume.
    a. Components.
      (1) Water.
      (2) Proteins—three types.
        (a) Carrier proteins—include albumin and lipoproteins. Albumin makes up two thirds of plasma proteins; it is the major source of colloid osmotic pressure in plasma.
        (b) Immunoproteins—includes immunoglobulins (antibodies) and complement.
        (c) Coagulation proteins—includes fibrinogen, prothrombin, and proteins of the coagulation cascade.
      (3) Other substances, including electrolytes, glucose, and hormones.
    b. Serum—supernatant that separates from blood after it has clotted (i.e., plasma without the fibrinogen).
  2. Formed elements (cells)—45% of blood volume.
    a. Erythrocytes (red blood cells [RBCs])
      (1) Shaped as biconcave discs. Do not contain a nucleus or mitochondria.
      (2) Have a life span of 120 days.
      (3) Function to carry oxygen to tissue and carbon dioxide from tissues.
      (4) Hemoglobin—the protein in RBCs that is responsible for binding oxygen and carbon dioxide.
    b. Platelets (thrombocytes).
      (1) Disc-shaped fragments. Do not contain a nucleus.
      (2) Play a role, along with coagulation proteins, in blood coagulation.
    c. Leukocytes (white blood cells [WBCs]).
      (1) Contain a nucleus.
      (2) Are capable of locomotion within tissues.
      (3) Play a role in immune defense.

CELLS	MICROSCOPIC APPEARANCE	DESCRIPTION	FUNCTIONS
Polymorphonuclear leukocyte (PMN) (neutrophile)	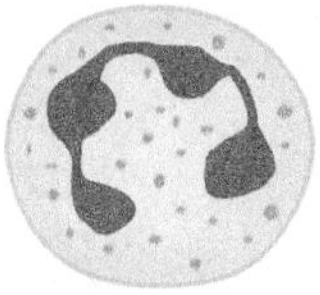	Multilobed nucleus with granules	Inflammatory response: phagocytosis
Lymphocyte	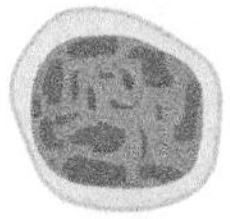	Eccentric round nucleus without granules; B, T, and NK cells	B and T cell: immune response humoral and cell-mediated NK; defense against tumor and virally infected cells
Plasma cell	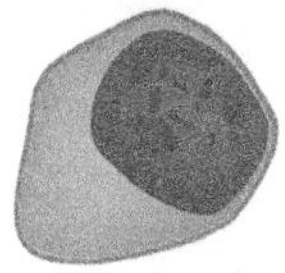	Round cartwheel nucleus derived from B-cell lymphocytes	Humoral immune response: produces immunoglobulins (antibodies)
Monocyte (blood)/ **macrophage** (tissue)	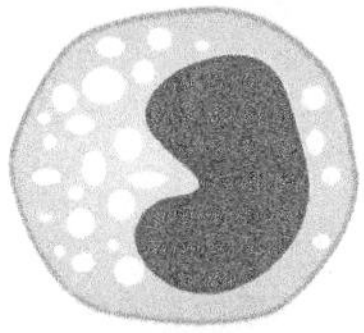	Bean-shaped nucleus with poorly staining granules	Inflammatory and immune response: phagocytosis, as well as process and present immunogens (antigens)
Eosinophil	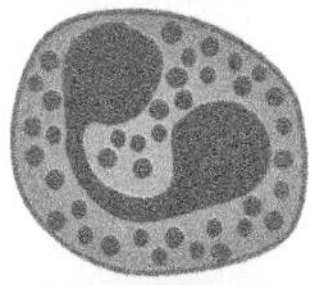	Bilobed nucleus with granules	Hypersensitivity response
Basophil	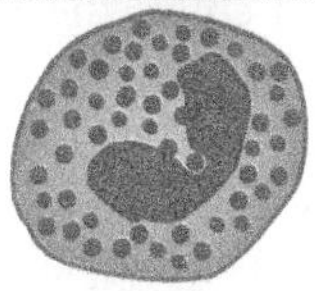	Irregularly shaped bilobed/trilobed nucleus with granules	Hypersensitivity response
Mast cell (tissue)	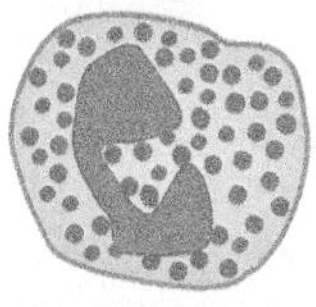	Irregularly shaped bilobed nucleus with granules	Hypersensitivity response

Figure 1-48 Blood cells and related tissue cells. *(From Bath-Balogh M, Fehrenbach M: Illustrated Dental Embryology, Histology, and Anatomy, ed 3, Philadelphia, Saunders, 2011.)*

(4) Cell types (Figure 1-48).
    (a) Granulocytes—WBCs that are observed with particular nuclear shapes and granules; includes neutrophils (polymorphonuclear leukocytes), eosinophils, and basophils.
    (b) Lymphocytes (B and T cells)—the smallest leukocyte; they contain a large nucleus with a relatively small amount of cytoplasm.
    (c) Monocytes—contain a kidney-shaped nucleus. They mature into macrophages when they enter tissues.
    (d) Plasma cells.

B. Hematopoiesis (hemopoiesis).
    1. All blood cells develop from a common source of undifferentiated cells (pluripotent hematopoietic stem cells). This process of blood cell differentiation and proliferation is known as *hematopoiesis* (Figure 1-49).
    2. Hematopoiesis occurs in the fetus and adults.
        a. Fetus—bone marrow, liver, and spleen.
        b. Adult—bone marrow.
    3. Bone marrow.
        a. Two types.
            (1) Red bone marrow—site of hematopoiesis.
            (2) Yellow bone marrow—consists mainly of fat.

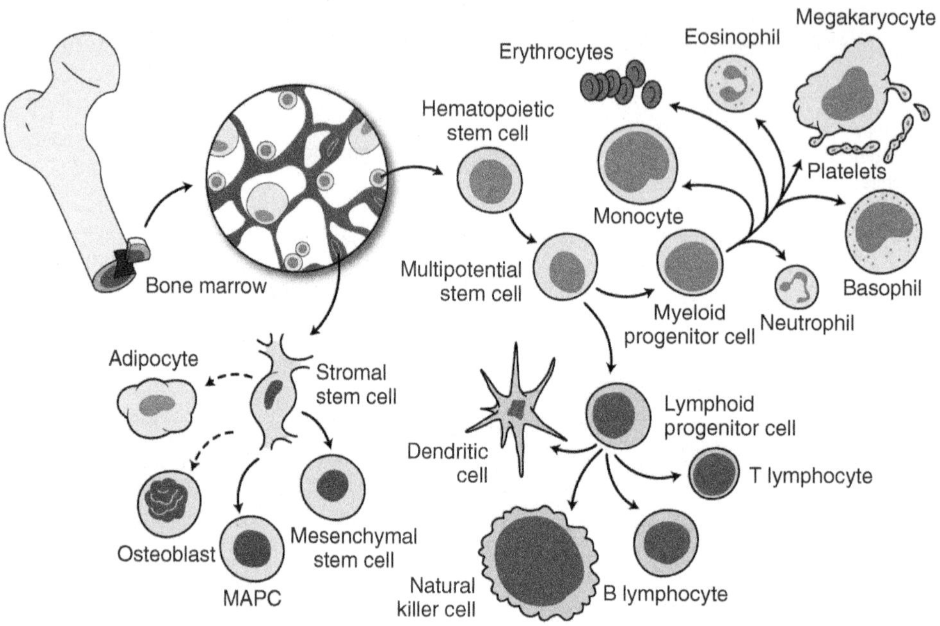

Figure 1-49 Stem cells in the bone marrow (hematopoietic) have been studied extensively. These cells can differentiate into blood and immune cell lines. Other stem cells in the bone marrow are stromal stem cells, and they have been reported to be able to differentiate into fat and bone cell precursors. Other stem cells have been discovered in the brain, eyes, skin, muscle, dental pulp, blood vessels, and gastrointestinal tract. *MAPC, Multipotent adult progenitor cell. (Modified from Chiego D, Essentials of Oral Histology and Embryology: A Clinical Approach, ed 4, St. Louis, Mosby, 2014.)*

b. In a growing child, most of the bone marrow is devoted to hematopoiesis (red). As people age, fat (yellow) largely replaces red bone marrow.

2.4 Lymphatic and Circulatory Systems

2.4.1 Circulatory System

A. Heart.
   1. The heart and its vessels are enclosed by an outer fibrous sac known as the *pericardium*. It consists of inner (visceral pericardium) and outer (parietal pericardium) sacs that are separated by a layer of pericardial fluid.
   2. The heart wall consists of three layers (listed in order from outer to inner).
      a. Epicardium—the outermost layer of the heart that is equivalent to the visceral pericardium.
      b. Myocardium
         (1) Is the thickest layer of the heart that contains cardiac muscle cells. Cardiac myocytes are incapable of mitosis.
         (2) Includes the papillary muscles and chordae tendineae.
      c. Endocardium—the innermost layer of the heart that consists of endothelial cells lining the inner chambers and heart valves.
B. Blood vessels.
   1. Arteries.
      a. Arteries transfer blood from the heart to capillary beds throughout the body.

   b. As blood enters the arterial system, it forces arterial walls to expand. The subsequent elastic recoil of these walls aids in the maintenance of blood pressure between ventricular heartbeats.
   c. Blood flow to various organs and tissues can be controlled by varying the diameter of small arteries or arterioles (i.e., via vasoconstriction and vasodilatation). This is accomplished by the presence of smooth muscle in the vessel walls, which is primarily controlled by the sympathetic nervous system and hormones from the adrenal medulla.
   d. Three main types of arteries.
      (1) Elastic arteries—the largest arteries including the aorta and common carotid, subclavian, and pulmonary arteries.
      (2) Muscular arteries—main distribution arterial branches that provide vascular supply to different organs and tissues. These include the radial, femoral, coronary, and cerebral arteries.
      (3) Arterioles—terminal branches of the arterial tree that provide and control the blood supply to the capillary beds.
   2. Veins
      a. Veins function under a low-pressure system and return blood from the capillary beds back to the heart. More than 70% of total blood volume is in this portion.

b. Because the pressure in the veins remains low, veins contain valves to help prevent the backflow of blood.

c. Veins can be categorized as small, medium, or large. Smaller veins are also known as *venules*.

3. The walls of blood vessels are composed of three basic layers:

a. Tunica intima—the innermost layer, which consists of a single layer of endothelial cells and a subendothelial layer of supporting connective tissue.

b. Tunica media—the middle layer, which consists of varying amounts of smooth muscle fibers and elastin. Of the three layers in arterial walls, it is the broadest layer.

c. Tunica adventitia—the outermost layer, which consists of connective tissue containing collagen and elastin. In some large vessels, it also contains the vasa vasorum. The vasa vasorum consists of small arteries that provide nutrients to the outer tissues. Of the three layers in the walls of veins, it is the broadest layer. The adventitia frequently contains longitudinal bundles of smooth muscles.

d. Arterial walls—in general, the amount of elastic tissue decreases and the amount of smooth muscle increases as the vessels decrease in size. For example, the tunica media of the aorta is extremely elastic with few smooth muscle fibers. In contrast, the tunica media of arterioles consists mostly of smooth muscle with very few elastic fibers.

e. Venous walls—the walls of veins usually contain little elastin and are thinner than arterial walls. Their tunica media is thin, and the diameter of their lumen is large compared with arteries. In general, the thickness of the tunica adventitia increases as the size of the vein increases.

4. Capillaries.

a. Capillaries consist of a thin layer of endothelial cells with an average diameter of 8 μm.

b. The interchange of gases, fluids, nutrients, and metabolic waste products between the blood and tissues occurs in the capillaries.

c. Blood enters the capillary beds through arterioles. Blood flow is controlled by smooth muscle sphincters, called *precapillary sphincters*, at the arteriole-capillary junctions. Blood from the capillaries drains into venules.

d. There are three types of capillaries.

(1) Continuous capillaries—the endothelia contain no pores. They are the most common type of capillary.

(2) Fenestrated capillaries—the endothelia contain a large number of pores.

(3) Discontinuous capillaries (sinusoids)—consist of a large lumen and with discontinuous endothelia. They are found in the liver.

2.4.2 Lymphatic System

A. Lymphatic circulation.

1. Excess fluid from the circulation (lymph) is drained into the lymphatic circulation. Lymph is first drained into lymphatic capillaries and then transported by a series of progressively larger lymphatic vessels. It is filtered in lymph nodes along the way and ultimately drains into the venous system via the left or the right thoracic duct.

2. Similar to veins, lymphatic vessels also contain valves, but their lumens are larger and their walls are thinner. They also do not contain any RBCs.

3. Lymphoid organs.

a. Primary lymphoid organs—site where lymphocyte precursors mature and are programmed to recognize a specific antigen; include the bone marrow (B cell) and thymus (T cell).

b. Secondary lymphoid organs—areas where collected antigens are used to stimulate clonal expansion of mature T and B cells. Examples are lymph nodes, tonsils, and the spleen.

B. Lymph nodes.

1. Lymph is filtered as it enters the lymph node through an afferent lymphatic vessel. It exits the gland at the hilum via an efferent lymphatic vessel (Figure 1-50).

2. A secondary lymphoid organ is where antigen-stimulated activation and clonal expansion of T and B cells occur.

3. Lymph nodes are encapsulated by a layer of dense connective tissue. The capsule is pierced by many afferent lymphatic vessels and has inward trabecular projections that partially compartmentalize the cortex.

4. Consists of a cortex and medulla.

a. Cortex.

(1) Outer cortex—consists of B cells, organized in lymphatic nodules or follicles. Germinal centers (the central, lighter staining areas) may be observed in the follicles.

(2) Paracortex—consists of T cells and is found between the outer cortex and medulla.

b. Medulla.

(1) Located centrally in the lymph node.

(2) Is less cellular than the cortex.

(3) Contain the medullary sinuses.

C. Tonsils.

1. Partially encapsulated or nonencapsulated masses of lymphoid tissue that are found near the airway and food passages. In contrast to lymph nodes, they are not located along lymphatic vessels.

2. Located in the lamina propria of oral mucosa. Their epithelial lining consists of stratified squamous epithelium that is continuous with the surrounding oral mucosa.

3. Palatine tonsils.

a. Located bilaterally at the opening of the pharynx, between the anterior and posterior faucial pillars.

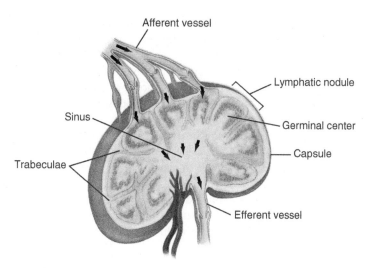

Figure 1-50 **Lymph node and its features.** Diagram showing entering of lymph by the afferent vessels and exiting of the efferent vessel *(arrows).* *(From Fehrenbach MJ, Herring SW: Illustrated Anatomy of the Head and Neck, ed 3, Philadelphia, Saunders, 2007.)*

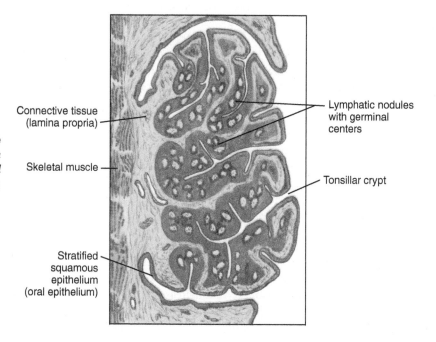

Figure 1-51 Histologic features of the palatine tonsillar tissue. *(Modified from Bath-Balogh M, Fehrenbach M: Illustrated Dental Embryology, Histology, and Anatomy, ed 3, Philadelphia, Saunders, 2011.)*

b. Histologically consists of lymphatic nodules with germinal centers. There are also numerous epithelial invaginations, which form tonsillar crypts (Figure 1-51).

4. Pharyngeal tonsil.
   a. A single tonsil that lies in the superior-posterior wall of the nasopharynx.
   b. It has no crypts, has a thinner capsule, and is composed of mucosa overlying diffuse lymphoid tissue and nodules.

5. Lingual tonsil.
   a. Located at the base of the tongue.
   b. Histologically consists of lymphatic nodules with germinal centers and one associated tonsillar crypt.

6. Together, the palatine, lingual, and pharyngeal tonsils form a tonsillar ring, known as *Waldeyer's ring.*

D. Spleen.
   1. A secondary lymph organ, the functions of which include the following.
      a. The filtration of blood. This includes removing pathogens from the circulation and destroying defective or old RBCs.
      b. Antigen-stimulated activation of lymphocytes, which is similar to the function of a lymph node.
      c. In the fetus, it also plays a role in hematopoiesis (forming RBCs).
   2. Can be divided into two parts, the red and white pulps.
      a. White pulp.
         (1) Site of activation and clonal expansion lymphocytes.

(2) T cells congregate around central arteries of the white pulp, forming the periarterial lymphatic sheath. B cells are found in follicles, adjacent to the arterioles.
  b. Marginal zone.
    (1) The sinusoidal interface between the red and white pulp.
    (2) Area where antigen-presenting cells interact and activate T helper cells, which activate B cells.
  c. Red pulp.
    (1) Site of blood filtration.
    (2) Consists of cords (Billroth's cords) containing numerous macrophages that lie between the venous sinusoids.
E. Thymus.
  1. Primary lymph organ that is the site of T-cell maturation. Because it is not involved in filtering lymph, it contains no afferent lymphatic vessels. It does contain efferent lymphatic vessels.
  2. Is located in the anterior mediastinum.
  3. Is active at birth and increases in size until puberty, after which it gradually atrophies and is replaced by fatty tissue.
  4. Can be divided into two parts separated by connective tissue capsules.
    a. Cortex—outer zone.
      (1) The darker staining, outer zone consists of T cells and epithelial reticular cells.
      (2) Is the site of T-cell maturation, where T cells are programmed to recognize specific antigens.
    b. Medulla—central zone.
      (1) The lighter staining (less dense) central area, where mature T cells leave the medulla.
      (2) Contains Hassall's corpuscles, which consist of epithelial cells with keratohyaline granules.

2.5 Endocrine System
2.5.1 Pituitary Gland (Hypophysis)

The pituitary gland is found in the hypophyseal fossa, protected in the sella turcica of the sphenoid bone. The two components of the pituitary gland are functionally different and are of separate embryologic origins: the oral (Rathke's pouch) and neural ectoderm. The two regions of the pituitary gland are divided into an anterior and posterior lobe.
A. Anterior pituitary (adenohypophysis, anterior lobe).
  1. Hormones.
    a. Anterior pituitary hormones: growth hormone (somatotropin), prolactin, adrenocorticotropic hormone (ACTH), thyroid-stimulating hormone (TSH), and gonadotropic hormones, follicle-stimulating hormone (FSH) and luteinizing hormone (LH).
    b. Hypothalamic control.
      (1) The control of hormone secretion from the anterior pituitary is mediated by specific releasing and inhibitory hormones from the hypothalamus (e.g., growth hormone–releasing hormone), with the exception of prolactin, which is under the inhibitory control of dopamine.
      (2) Hypothalamohypophyseal portal veins—the axons of hypothalamic neurosecretory cells terminate in the median eminence. The hypothalamic hormones are transferred to the anterior pituitary via a system of portal veins and capillary beds (Figure 1-52).
  2. Can be divided into three parts.
    a. Pars distalis—contains endocrine cells. It serves as the primary source of hormones of the anterior pituitary.

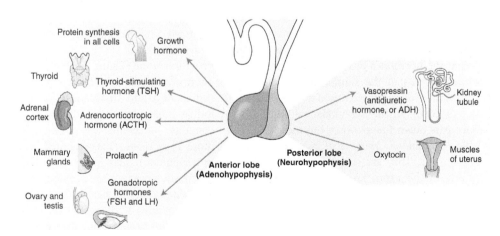

Figure 1-52 Pituitary hormones. Some of the major organs of the anterior and posterior lobes and their principal target organs. *FSH,* Follicle-stimulating hormone; *LH,* luteinizing hormone. (*Adapted from McKenry LM, Tessier E, Hogan MA: Mosby's pharmacology in nursing, ed 22, St. Louis, Mosby, 2006. IN Lilley L, Collins S, Snyder J: Pharmacology and the nursing process, ed 7, Mosby, St. Louis, 2014.*)

b. Pars tuberalis—surrounds the infundibulum and carries portal veins of the hypophyseal portal system; contains endocrine cells but plays only a minor role in hormone release.

c. Pars intermedia.

    (1) A thin layer of tissue found between the anterior and posterior lobes.

    (2) Is rudimentary in humans but may play a role in the synthesis and secretion of melanocyte-stimulating hormone.

    (3) A vestigial cleft consisting of cystlike spaces (Rathke's cysts) may be found between the pars intermedia and anterior lobe. It represents the vestigial lumen of Rathke's pouch.

3. Consists of two groups of cells.

    a. Chromophils—secrete hormones. There are two cell types that are divided according to their histologic staining.

        (1) Acidophils—stain a pinkish or orange color and include the following cells.

            (a) Somatotrophs—secrete growth hormone.

            (b) Mammotrophs (lactotrophs)—secrete prolactin.

        (2) Basophils—stain a bluish color and include the following cells.

            (a) Corticotrophs—secrete ACTH.

            (b) Thyrotrophs—secrete TSH.

            (c) Gonadotrophs—secrete FSH and LH.

    b. Chromophobes—have no secretory function. They likely represent degranulated chromophils.

B. Posterior pituitary (neurohypophysis, pars nervosa, posterior lobe).

1. Hormones.

    a. Posterior pituitary hormones: vasopressin (antidiuretic hormone [ADH]) and oxytocin.

    b. Hypothalamic control and synthesis.

        (1) The control of hormone secretion from the posterior pituitary is via nerve impulses from the hypothalamus, a regulation process known as *neurosecretion*.

        (2) Hypothalamohypophyseal (hypothalamopituitary) tract: the hormones are synthesized by neurosecretory cells of the supraoptic nuclei (produce ADH) and paraventricular nuclei (produce oxytocin) of the hypothalamus. The hormones pass down the axons of these cells, called the *hypothalamohypophyseal tract*, into the pars nervosa. They are stored in the terminal parts of the axon, known as *Herring bodies*.

2. The posterior lobe is divided into two parts.

    a. Pars nervosa—consists of the following components.

        (1) The nonmyelinated axons of neurosecretory cells, whose cell bodies remain in the hypothalamus.

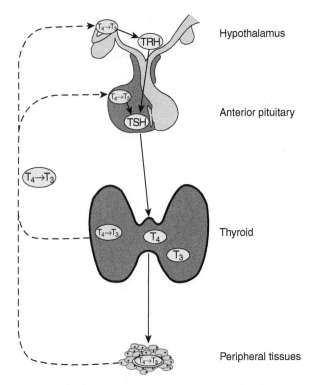

Figure 1-53 Hypothalamic-pituitary-thyroid axis. *T_3,* Triiodothyronine; *T_4,* thyroxine; *TRH,* thyrotropin-releasing hormone; *TSH,* thyroid-stimulating hormone. *(Redrawn from DeGroot LJ, Jameson JL: Endocrinology, ed 5, vol 2, Philadelphia, Saunders, 2006.)*

        (2) Pituicytes, which are similar neuroglial cells of the CNS and act as supporting cells for the axons of neurosecretory cells.

    b. Infundibulum—connects the pars nervosa to the hypothalamus. It also carries axons of neurosecretory cells.

2.5.2 Thyroid

The thyroid is the largest endocrine gland. It consists of a right and left lobe that are connected by an isthmus. It is located anterior to the trachea, around the level of the cricoid cartilage.

A. Thyroid hormone (Figure 1-53).

1. There are two forms of thyroid hormone: triiodothyronine (T_3) and thyroxine (T_4). T_3 contains three iodine molecules and is the more potent form; T_4 contains four iodine molecules. Although there is more T_4 secreted, T_4 is converted (deiodinated) to T_3 in peripheral tissues.

2. Synthesis, storage, and secretion of T_3 and T_4.

    a. Synthesis and storage: thyroglobulin synthesis from amino acids occurs on rough endoplasmic reticulum within follicular cells; thyroglobulin is released into the colloid in the follicle, where iodination (catalyzed by thyroid peroxidase) of thyroglobulin occurs. This results in the formation of T_3 and T_4 on tyrosine residues of thyroglobulin.

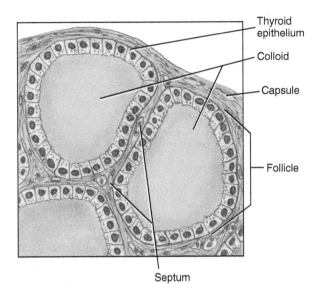

Figure labels: Thyroid epithelium, Colloid, Capsule, Follicle, Septum

Figure 1-54 Histology of the thyroid gland. *(Modified from Bath-Balogh M, Fehrenbach M: Illustrated Dental Embryology, Histology, and Anatomy, ed 3, Philadelphia, Saunders, 2011.)*

b. Secretion of hormone: TSH from the anterior pituitary stimulates the release of thyroid hormone. Endocytosis of colloid (containing iodinated thyroglobulin) occurs. A lysosome fuses with the endocytosed vacuole, allowing for lysosomal enzymes to cleave the hormone from thyroglobulin; T_3 and T_4 are secreted into the bloodstream.

B. Thyroid follicles.
  1. Site of synthesis, storage, and release of thyroid hormone.
  2. Thyroid follicles are spherical structures that make up the thyroid gland. They consist of follicular cells surrounding a lumen filled with colloid (Figure 1-54).
  3. Follicular cells.
    a. Derived from the endoderm of the thyroglossal duct.
    b. Histologically, during the synthesis of thyroglobulin, the morphology of the cell appears as low cuboidal cells. During the secretion of thyroid hormone, their morphology changes to resemble taller cuboidal cells.
    c. Their apical membranes (facing the colloid) contain thyroid peroxidase, an enzyme that iodinates tyrosine residues of thyroglobulin.
  4. Colloid.
    a. Fills the lumen of the thyroid follicle.
    b. Consists of a viscous gel that primarily contains iodinated thyroglobulin (i.e., it also serves as a storage reserve for thyroid hormone).

C. Parafollicular cells (clear cells).
  1. Derived from the endoderm of the ultimobranchial body, a diverticulum of the fifth pharyngeal pouch.
  2. Are located at the periphery of thyroid follicles.

3. Histologically, compared with follicular cells, their cytoplasm appears paler in color.
4. Secrete calcitonin, a hormone that plays an important role in the regulation of calcium and phosphates. It suppresses bone resorption by decreasing calcium and phosphate release.

2.5.3 Parathyroid Gland

There are usually four parathyroid glands in humans. The glands are located just posterior to the thyroid gland. Parathyroid hormone (PTH) plays an important role in the metabolism of calcium.

A. PTH.
  1. Is synthesized and secreted by the parathyroid gland.
  2. Is secreted when calcium levels fall.
  3. Overall effects of PTH.
    a. Increased serum calcium.
    b. Decreased serum phosphate.
  4. Actions of PTH.
    a. Bone: increased resorption by stimulating osteoblasts to release osteoclast-activating factor.
    b. Kidney: increased calcium reabsorption (i.e., decreased calcium excretion), decreased phosphate reabsorption.
    c. Digestive tract: indirectly increases absorption of dietary calcium by stimulating vitamin D activity.
    d. Activation of vitamin D in the kidney.

B. Parathyroid gland.
  1. Usually there are two pairs of glands.
  2. Chief (principal) cells.
    a. Secrete PTH.
    b. Histologically, active cells have dark cytoplasm (basophilic) with numerous granules. Inactive cells have light cytoplasm (acidophilic) with fewer granules.

2.5.4 Adrenal (Suprarenal) Glands

The adrenal glands are located superior and medial to the upper pole of each kidney. The gland consists of two components that function independently and have different embryologic origins. The two regions are the adrenal cortex and medulla.

A. Adrenal cortex.
  1. Derived from the mesodermal epithelium from the root of the dorsal mesentery.
  2. Divided into three zones (Figure 1-55).
    a. Zona glomerulosa.
      (1) Secretes mineralocorticoids (mainly aldosterone), which are important in the regulation of electrolyte and water balance.
      (2) Secretory cells are arranged in irregular, ovoid clumps.
    b. Zona fasciculata.
      (1) Secretes glucocorticoids (mainly cortisol), which play a role in the regulation of general metabolism.

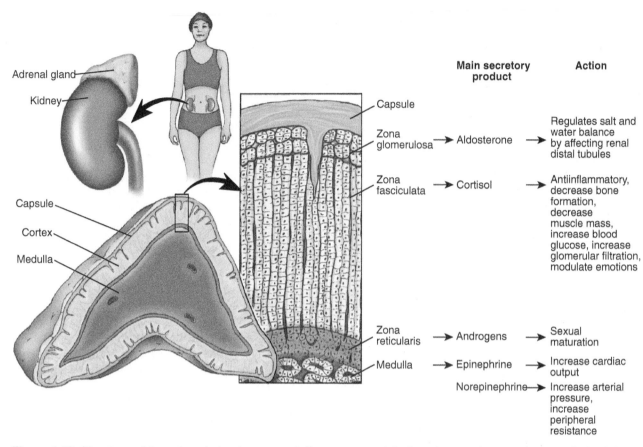

Figure 1-55 Structure of the adrenal gland, representative zones, and their main secretory products and physiologic actions. (*Adapted from Thibodeau GA, Patton KT: Anatomy and Physiology, ed 7, St. Louis, Mosby, 2010.*)

(2) Secretory cells are arranged in narrow cords.

c. Zona reticularis.

(1) Secretes androgens. The androgens produced are considered weak, but they can be converted in peripheral tissues to testosterone or the estrone estrogen.

(2) Secretory cells are arranged in an irregular network of anastomosing cords and clumps.

B. Adrenal medulla.

1. Derived from neuroectoderm (neural crest cells).

2. Consists of chromaffin cells.

a. Are modified postganglionic sympathetic neurons that synthesize, store, and secrete catecholamines.

b. There are two types of chromaffin cells: one produces epinephrine (75%) and the other produces norepinephrine (25%).

3. Secretion of catecholamines is stimulated by the release of acetylcholine from preganglionic-type sympathetic axons that form junctions on chromaffin cells.

2.5.5 Endocrine Pancreas

The pancreas functions as both an exocrine and an endocrine gland. The exocrine portion comprises more than 95% of the pancreatic mass and consists of a network of ducts and pancreatic cells, including acinar and centroacinar cells. The endocrine tissue (islets of Langerhans) can be found scattered throughout the exocrine pancreas.

A. Islets of Langerhans.

1. Are most numerous in the tail of the pancreas.

2. Cell types.

a. Alpha (A) cells—secrete glucagon, which, in response to low levels of blood glucose, raises blood glucose levels.

b. Beta (B) cells—secrete insulin, which, in response to high levels of blood glucose, lowers blood glucose levels.

c. Delta (D) cells—secrete somatostatin, an inhibitory hormone that inhibits the release of numerous hormones, including glucagon, insulin, and growth hormone.

d. F cells—secrete pancreatic polypeptide.

2.5.6 Pineal Gland (Epiphysis Cerebri)

The pineal gland is a very small gland located along the roof of the third ventricle. It is contained within the pia mater and is largest in early childhood. It secretes the hormone melatonin.

A. Melatonin.
1. Is produced from serotonin.
2. Circadian fluctuations—blood melatonin levels are three times higher at night than during the day.
3. Antigonadotropic effect.
   a. Has an inhibitory effect on hypothalamic gonadotropin-releasing hormones.
   b. Because the pineal gland involutes rapidly near the time of puberty, it plays a role in the onset of puberty (i.e., early destruction of the pineal gland causes precocious puberty).
   c. Administration of melatonin to a child delays the onset of puberty.
B. Cell types.
1. Pinealocytes—produce serotonin and melatonin.
2. Neuroglial cells—act as support cells to the pinealocytes.

2.6 Respiratory System

The respiratory system consists of progressively smaller passageways that lead to the alveoli where exchange of gases occurs. The system is characterized by respiratory epithelium throughout the conducting portion and the respiratory portion itself.
A. Respiratory epithelium—composed of pseudostratified ciliated columnar epithelium, which lines all or part of the larger conducting areas.
1. Cell types located in respiratory epithelium.
   a. Goblet cells—contain mucin granules. The mucus they secrete traps inhaled particles such as bacteria and dust.
   b. Ciliated columnar cells—move mucus upward toward the oropharynx to remove particles so they may be swallowed or expectorated.
   c. Nonciliated columnar cells—have microvilli on their apical surface; however, they do not possess cilia.
   d. Basal cells—stem cells that differentiate into goblet cells or columnar cells.
   e. Small granule cells—synthesize and release catecholamines.
2. Lamina propria deep to respiratory epithelium—is formed of loose areolar connective tissue. It contains seromucous and mucous glands and diffuse lymphatic tissue, including plasma cells, lymphocytes, and macrophages.
B. Conducting portion.
   Air is warmed, moistened, and cleaned as it passes through the conducting portion. The order of passage is from the nasal cavity to nasopharynx and oropharynx, larynx, trachea, bronchi, bronchioles, and terminal bronchioles.
1. Nasal cavity and nasopharynx.
   a. Oral epithelium composed of a nonkeratinized stratified squamous epithelium that covers some of the areas of the nasopharynx inspired air first crosses.
   b. Blood vessels in the lamina propria help warm air, and watery secretions moisten it.
   c. Olfactory mucosa extending from the third cranial nerve is present in the superior aspect of the nasal cavity.
2. Larynx—hyaline and elastic cartilage helps support the walls of the larynx.
   a. Epiglottis—the anterior-superior extension of the larynx. It protects the airway during swallowing.
      (1) Elastic cartilage surrounded by lamina propria is at the core of the epiglottis.
      (2) The digestive part of the epiglottis is covered by oral epithelium.
      (3) The respiratory part of the epiglottis is covered by respiratory epithelium.
3. Vocal apparatus—consists of two pairs of folds of the laryngeal mucosa that span the laryngeal space.
   a. False vocal cords are the superior pair of folds. They are covered by respiratory epithelium and contain seromucous glands in the lamina propria.
   b. True vocal cords are the inferior pair of folds. They produce sound when air passes over them. They are covered by oral epithelium and do not have seromucous glands in the lamina propria.
4. Trachea (Figure 1-56).
   a. The mucosa of the trachea is covered with respiratory epithelium.
   b. The submucosa is separated from the mucosa by elastic fibers. The submucosa contains seromucous glands.
   c. Hyaline cartilage rings lie deep to the submucosa.
      (1) The cartilage is covered by a perichondrium, surrounded by an adventitia of loose connective tissue that is shared with the esophagus.
      (2) The hyaline cartilage is shaped like a "C"; the open end of the ring faces toward the posterior.
      (3) Smooth muscle extends across the open end of each cartilage.
   d. Extrapulmonary bronchi arise by division of the trachea outside the lungs and are histologically similar to trachea.
5. Intrapulmonary bronchi—divide many times within the lungs.
   a. Hyaline cartilage provides structure. The pieces are variably shaped and break up into small blocks in the walls of intrapulmonary bronchi.
   b. The layers of the wall become thinner as the bronchi penetrate farther into the lung.
6. Conducting bronchioles—are characterized by an absence of cartilage and smooth muscle in the walls.
   a. The diameter of the bronchioles is controlled by contraction of smooth muscle under sympathetic control of the autonomic nervous system. Epinephrine causes relaxation of these muscles.

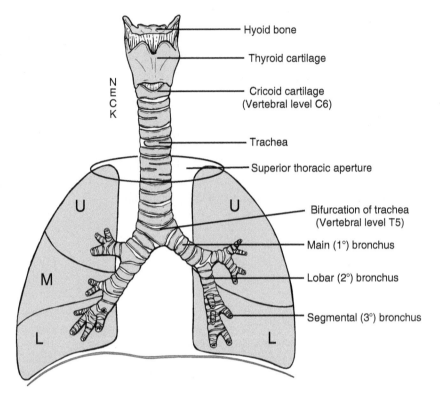

Figure 1-56 Trachea. *(From Liebgott B: The Anatomical Basis of Dentistry, ed 3, St. Louis, Mosby, 2011.)*

Labels on figure:
- Hyoid bone
- Thyroid cartilage
- Cricoid cartilage (Vertebral level C6)
- Trachea
- Superior thoracic aperture
- Bifurcation of trachea (Vertebral level T5)
- Main (1°) bronchus
- Lobar (2°) bronchus
- Segmental (3°) bronchus
- NECK

b. The epithelium changes from respiratory to ciliated columnar, ciliated cuboidal, and nonciliated cuboidal as the bronchioles become smaller in diameter.

c. In contrast to the trachea, there are no seromucous glands in the conducting bronchioles.

d. Goblet cells are found only in the larger bronchioles.

7. Terminal bronchioles.

   a. The most distal part of the conducting tree.

   b. No goblet cells, so no mucus is produced.

   c. Contains ciliated cuboidal cells.

C. Respiratory portion.

1. Pulmonary lobules—the lung is composed of lobules, distal to terminal bronchioles.

   a. Each lobule contains a central respiratory bronchiole, leading to alveolar ducts.

   b. The alveolar ducts terminate in alveolar sacs.

   c. Pulmonary veins drain oxygenated blood from the periphery of each lobule.

2. Alveoli—the sites of gaseous exchange in the lungs.

   a. Adjacent alveoli are separated by connective tissue partitions called *interalveolar septa*, which contain pulmonary capillaries.

   b. Alveoli share air through pores of Kohn in interalveolar septa.

   c. Alveolar walls are lined by an epithelium with two kinds of pneumocytes.

     (1) Type I pneumocytes—cover most of the alveolar surface. They are connected by tight junctions, and the basal lamina of these cells may be fused with the basal lamina of nearby capillary endothelial cells.

     (2) Type II pneumocytes—may also be called *greater alveolar cells*. They bulge into the alveolar lumen and function as cells that repair the alveoli by dividing and replacing type I pneumocytes, which do not divide.

   d. Pulmonary surfactant is a phospholipid-protein mixture secreted by type II pneumocytes that spreads over alveolar walls.

     (1) The surfactant reduces surface tension in the alveoli, allowing them to expand easily during inspiration and contract without collapsing during expiration.

3. Gaseous exchange.

   a. Oxygen diffuses from the alveolar airspace into RBCs, where it binds to heme groups in hemoglobin. Carbon dioxide diffuses back to the alveolar airspace.

   b. The respiratory membrane is about 0.2 μm thick.

   c. The respiratory membrane contains the following elements, in order from lung surface: surfactant, type I pneumocyte, basal lamina of type I pneumocyte, basal lamina of capillary endothelial cell, endothelial cell, blood plasma, plasmalemma of RBC.

4. Alveolar macrophages—called *dust cells*, are derived from monocytes. They migrate from capillaries in the interalveolar septa and ingest bacteria and other inhaled substances on the alveolar surface.

E. Visceral and parietal pleurae.
  1. Serous membranes—the pleural cavity contains serous membranes composed of surface mesothelium and an underlying lamina propria.
    a. Visceral pleura invests the lungs, and parietal pleura lines the thoracic cavity.
    b. Visceral and parietal pleura slide over one another to permit movement of the lungs within the thoracic cavity.

2.7 Gastrointestinal System

The gastrointestinal system consists of a hollow tube, also known as the *alimentary canal*, extending from the lips to the anus. The digestive system also includes several extramural glands such as the salivary glands, liver, and gallbladder. The secretions of these glands are delivered to the gastrointestinal system.

A. Major layers—the wall of the gastrointestinal system consists of four major layers.
  1. Mucosa—lines the lumen of the gastrointestinal tract. It has three distinct sublayers.
    a. A nonkeratinized stratified, squamous epithelium with secretory, absorptive, and protective functions.
    b. A lamina propria of loose areolar connective tissue deep to the epithelium. The lamina propria contains glands and gut-associated lymphoid tissue (GALT).
    c. A muscularis mucosae with one to three layers of fine smooth muscle.
  2. Submucosa—is composed of dense, irregular connective tissue.
    a. The submucosa contains (Meissner's) autonomic plexuses or ganglia.
  3. Muscularis externa—contains an inner circular and an outer longitudinal layer of smooth muscle.
    a. The muscularis externa contains Auerbach's myenteric autonomic plexus or ganglia between the layers of muscle.
  4. Serosa or fibrosa (adventitia).
    a. The serosa consists of a mesothelial lining and a layer of submesothelial connective tissue.
      (1) It forms the visceral peritoneum, a reflection of the parietal peritoneum that forms the serosal lining of the abdominal wall.
      (2) It covers the intraperitoneal portions of the alimentary canal, surface of the gallbladder exposed to the peritoneal cavity, and surface of the colon facing the peritoneal cavity.
    b. Fibrosa—consists of dense, irregular connective tissue containing adipose.
      (1) It blends with connective tissue around adjacent organs.
      (2) It covers retroperitoneal portions of the alimentary canal, surface of gallbladder embedded in the liver, and surface of the colon facing the posterior body wall.

B. Innervation.
   Peristalsis of the gastrointestinal tract depends on innervation to the smooth muscle.
  1. Postganglionic sympathetic fibers from the sympathetic chain pass through the gut wall to glands and smooth muscle.
  2. Preganglionic parasympathetic fibers arrive on cell bodies of parasympathetic postganglionic neurons in ganglia in the gut wall.
  3. Postganglionic parasympathetic fibers pass to glands and smooth muscle.

C. GALT.
   Lining epithelium is coated with secretory immunoglobulin A (IgA) produced by Peyer's patches and other GALT.
  1. Lymph follicles.
    a. Specialized squamous epithelial cells called *M cells*, located in the luminal epithelium, acquire antigens from the lumen and transport them to lymph follicles in the underlying lamina propria.
    b. Antigen-stimulating B cells within follicles differentiate into IgA-secreting plasma cells.
  2. Diffuse lymphatic tissue of the lamina propria, including lymphocytes, macrophages, and IgA-secreting plasma cells.
  3. Aggregated lymph follicles.
    a. Waldeyer's ring of tonsillar tissue in the oropharynx.
    b. Peyer's patches in the submucosa of the ileum.

D. Oral cavity—extends from the lips to the pharynx (Figure 1-57).
  1. Lips.
    a. The lips have a core of skeletal muscle, the orbicularis oris.
    b. The anterior surface is covered with dermis and epidermis.
    c. The posterior surface is covered by a nonkeratinized, stratified squamous epithelium (oral epithelium) and a lamina propria.
  2. Teeth.
    a. Cementum covers the external surface of the tooth root. It is similar to bone in composition. Sharpey's fibers extend from the surface of the cementum into the bony tooth socket.
    b. Enamel covers the external surface of the tooth crown. It is highly mineralized, contains 98% hydroxyapatite by weight, and is the hardest substance in the body.
    c. Dentin is found around the pulp in both the crown and the root of the tooth. It forms the bulk of the tooth.
    d. Pulp contains fibroblasts, odontoblasts, nerves, and blood vessels.

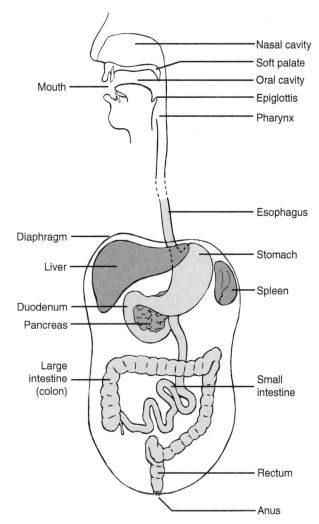

Nasal cavity
Soft palate
Oral cavity
Mouth
Epiglottis
Pharynx
Esophagus
Diaphragm
Liver
Stomach
Duodenum
Spleen
Pancreas
Large intestine (colon)
Small intestine
Rectum
Anus

Figure 1-57 Scheme of gastrointestinal system. *(From Liebgott B: The Anatomical Basis of Dentistry, ed 3, St. Louis, Mosby, 2011.)*

3. Tongue—a strong, muscular organ with specialized mucosa for taste.
   a. The skeletal muscle fibers of the tongue run in three different directions.
   b. The mucosa of the tongue lacks a muscularis mucosa on the dorsal surface and an underlying submucosa on the dorsal surface.
      (1) The ventral surface is covered by oral epithelium, a nonkeratinized, stratified squamous epithelium.
      (2) The dorsal surface is covered by a parakeratinized, stratified squamous epithelium.
   c. Lingual papillae project from the dorsal surface of the anterior two thirds of the tongue.
      (1) Filiform papillae do not have taste buds.
      (2) Fungiform and circumvallate papillae have taste buds.
      (3) Glands of von Ebner rise out the trenches surrounding circumvallate papillae with a serous secretion.

4. Hard palate.
   a. The mucosa of the hard palate is firmly attached to the bone.
   b. Nasal mucosa is lined with a pseudostratified, ciliated, columnar epithelium, called *respiratory epithelium*, containing seromucous glands.
   c. Lingual mucosa is lined with parakeratinized, stratified, squamous epithelium containing mucous glands.
5. Soft palate.
   a. The mucosa is similar to the lingual mucosa of the hard palate.
   b. The uvula is surfaced by oral epithelium.
6. Pharynx—is continuous with the nasal and oral cavities and with the lumen of the esophagus.
   a. Pharyngeal mucosa contains respiratory epithelium where air transits and oral epithelium where food passes.
   b. Pharyngeal constrictor muscles are found beneath the mucosa.
E. Alimentary canal.
   1. Esophagus.
      a. Mucosa—has surface mucosal folds when food is not present.
         (1) The mucosa is surfaced by oral epithelium, a nonkeratinized, stratified, squamous epithelium.
      b. Muscularis externa.
         (1) The upper third of the esophagus contains skeletal muscle.
         (2) The middle third of the esophagus contains both skeletal and smooth muscle.
         (3) The lower third of the esophagus contains smooth muscle.
      c. Mucous glands.
         (1) The submucosa contains esophageal glands.
         (2) The lamina propria contains esophageal cardiac glands.
   2. Stomach.
      a. The gastric mucosa is surfaced by a simple epithelium of mucous columnar cells.
      b. The muscularis externa has a third layer, an inner oblique layer of smooth muscle.
      c. Gastric glands are simple, branched tubular glands. These glands consist of an isthmus opening into the bottom of a gastric pit, a neck, and a base or fundus that traverses the lamina propria.
         (1) Mucous neck cells secrete mucus.
         (2) Stem cells proliferate and differentiate to replace the other cells of the gland, pit, and surface epithelium.
         (3) Chief cells secrete pepsinogen.
         (4) Parietal cells located primarily in the body and fundus of the stomach secrete intrinsic factor needed for absorption of vitamin B_{12} and manufacture hydrogen chloride.

(5) Enteroendocrine cells secrete hormones toward capillaries in the lamina propria.

3. Small intestine—has numerous specializations that increase the surface area for absorption, including microvilli, villi, and plicae circulares.

  a. Glands with secretions that enter the intestinal lumen.

    (1) Brunner's glands are submucosal glands in the duodenum that secrete an alkaline mucus.

    (2) Goblet cells within the epithelium of the lumen.

    (3) Crypts of Lieberkühn open between adjacent villi and extend to muscularis mucosae.

  b. Cells of the intestinal lining.

    (1) Enterocytes are the primary cell type of surface epithelium.

      (a) They are tall, columnar cells containing closely packed microvilli forming a brush border.

    (2) Goblet cells containing mucigen granules.

    (3) Enteroendocrine cells producing hormones.

    (4) Paneth's cells containing eosinophilic granules. These cells secrete digestive enzymes and lysosome and phagocytize some microorganisms.

    (5) Stem cells replace cells of the intestinal lining.

4. Large intestine—the primary function of the large intestine is to absorb water and electrolytes and lubricate feces with mucus.

  a. From cecum to the anal canal, enterocytes decrease.

  b. Goblet cells increase in number.

  c. The outer longitudinal layer of muscularis externa forms three strong, flat strips.

  d. Myenteric (Auerbach's) ganglia are located between taeniae coli and the subjacent circular layer of smooth muscle.

5. Anal canal.

  a. The upper portion is continuous with the rectum.

  b. The lower portion is surfaced by nonkeratinized, stratified, squamous epithelium.

F. Extramural glands of the digestive system—exocrine secretions enter the oral cavity from the salivary glands and the small intestine from the liver, gallbladder, and pancreas.

1. Major salivary glands.

  a. Components of saliva.

    (1) Water and salivary glycoproteins clean and lubricate the oral cavity.

    (2) IgA, lysozyme, and lactoferrin defend against pathogens.

    (3) Amylase begins the digestion of carbohydrates.

  b. Liver.

    (1) Hepatic sinusoids arise near the periphery of the lobule and course between cords of hepatocytes to drain toward the central vein. The sinusoids are lined by sinusoidal endothelial cells and Kupffer's cells, which are phagocytic.

    (2) The space of Disse between sinusoid endothelium and adjacent hepatocytes contains reticular fibers, which are lipocytes (Ito cells) that store vitamin A, and blood plasma minus formed elements.

    (3) Hepatocytes exchange material with contents of the space of Disse.

      (a) Microvilli are present on surfaces facing space of Disse.

      (b) Bile canaliculi occur as tiny grooves between abutting surfaces of adjacent hepatocytes.

      (c) Basophilic cytoplasmic regions contain rough endoplasmic reticulum and free polysomes.

      (d) Acidophilic cytoplasmic regions contain mitochondria and peroxisomes.

      (e) Unstained cytoplasmic regions contain multiple Golgi bodies, glycogen inclusions, and droplets of lipid.

  c. Gallbladder—releases bile in response to the presence of fat in the duodenum. Cholecystokinin released by enteroendocrine cells in the duodenum stimulates release of bile.

    (1) The mucosa is composed of simple, columnar epithelium with microvilli and junctional complexes and a richly vascularized lamina propria.

    (2) The muscularis externa is thin, with three indistinct layers.

    (3) The external surface has serosa facing the peritoneal cavity and fibrosa facing the liver.

  d. Exocrine pancreas.

    (1) Pancreatic acinar cells contain basally located nuclei and rough endoplasmic reticulum, prominent Golgi apparatus, and apically located secretory granules.

    (2) Centroacinar cells within the acini form the beginning of the duct system.

2.8 Genitourinary System

2.8.1 Male Reproductive System

A. Structure.

1. The testes produce male gametes (spermatozoa).

  a. The tunica albuginea is a connective tissue capsule surrounding each testis.

    (1) The thickened, posterior region of each capsule contains incomplete connective tissue septa. The septa divide each testis into numerous lobules.

    (2) Each lobule contains two to four highly convoluted seminiferous tubules.

      (a) Seminiferous epithelium lining the tubules is a specialized, glandlike epithelium where spermatogenesis occurs.

(3) Intratesticular ducts conveying spermatozoa to the surface of the testis include tubuli recti and rete testis.

    (a) Tubuli recti are straight, terminal portions of the seminiferous tubules lined by simple columnar epithelium. They drain into the rete testis.

    (b) Rete testis is an anastomosing network of channels located at the mediastinum and lined by simple cuboidal epithelium.

2. Extratesticular ducts conduct spermatozoa outside the body.

3. Specialized glands produce and release secretions that provide nutritive and lubricative elements to semen.

  a. Seminal vesicles.

  b. Prostate gland.

  c. Bulbourethral (Cowper's) glands.

4. Glandular function of the testes.

  a. Exocrine function.

    (1) Production of a holocrine cytogenic secretion containing spermatozoa occurs within the seminiferous epithelium.

  b. Endocrine function.

    (1) Synthesis and secretion of hormones is carried out by Leydig cells within the interstitium and by Sertoli cells within the seminiferous epithelium.

B. Spermatogenesis.

1. Composition of seminiferous epithelium.

  a. Spermatogenic cells.

    (1) Present in a gradient from undifferentiated cells to differentiated spermatids that are ready to be released into the lumen.

  b. Sertoli cells.

    (1) Tall, columnar cells extending from the basement membrane to the lumen.

    (2) Support and protect germ cells within the seminiferous epithelium.

    (3) Secrete inhibin and androgen-binding protein.

    (4) Are nondividing cells and remain in the senescent gonad after degeneration of germ cells.

C. Hormonal control of male reproductive system.

1. Pituitary hormones—release of pituitary hormones that promote testicular hormone production is stimulated by gonadotropin-releasing hormone from the hypothalamus.

  a. LH stimulates Leydig cells to release testosterone.

  b. FSH stimulates Sertoli cells to secrete inhibin and androgen-binding protein.

2. Effects of testicular hormones.

  a. Testosterone.

    (1) Promotes development of secondary sex characteristics.

    (2) Stimulates spermatogenesis.

    (3) Maintains the function of ducts and accessory glands.

    (4) Acts on the hypothalamus to reduce release of gonadotropin-releasing hormone, exhibiting negative feedback on LH and FSH secretion.

  b. Androgen-binding protein.

    (1) Binds testosterone and helps transport it across seminiferous epithelium to tubular lumen.

    (2) Helps maintain high local concentration of testosterone.

    (3) Inhibin acts on the anterior pituitary to decrease FSH secretion.

2.8.2 Female Reproductive System

A. Structure—organs of the female reproductive system.

1. Ovaries.

  a. Features.

    (1) A simple, squamous to cuboidal epithelium covers the surface.

    (2) The tunica albuginea of fibrous connective tissue lies under the surface epithelium.

    (3) The cortex contains ovarian follicles in various stages of maturation.

    (4) The medulla is not well-defined.

2. Oviducts.

  a. Regions.

    (1) The infundibulum is a funnel-shaped free end with finger-like projections called *fimbria*.

    (2) The ampulla is a dilated region proximal to the infundibulum where fertilization usually occurs.

    (3) The isthmus is a nondilated region proximal to the ampulla.

    (4) Pars intramuralis is the part passing through the uterine wall.

  b. Oviduct wall.

    (1) The mucosa is a simple, columnar epithelium containing ciliated cells and secretory cells.

    (2) The lamina propria is edematous during the premenstrual phase.

    (3) Contractions of the muscularis stimulates movement of the zygote toward the uterus.

3. Uterus.

  a. Uterine wall.

    (1) The perimetrium is an external uterine covering that is serosa or adventitia, depending on the peritoneal reflection.

    (2) The myometrium is the vascularized smooth muscle tunic of the uterus.

    (3) The endometrium is the mucosal lining of the uterus. It is composed of a simple, columnar epithelium, highly vascular lamina propria, and endometrial glands.

4. Breasts.

  a. Lobes.

    (1) Each gland has 15 to 25 lobes that are separated by a dense connective tissue septa.

(2) Each lobe has compound tubuloalveolar glands that drain into intralobular ducts, interlobular ducts, lactiferous sinus, lactiferous duct, and finally the nipple.

b. Lactiferous ducts.

(1) Stratified cuboidal and columnar epithelium lines the largest ducts, and simple cuboidal epithelium lines the smallest ducts.

(2) The epithelium is surrounded by loose areolar connective tissue, outside of which is dense irregular connective tissue with adipose cells.

c. Alveoli.

(1) Dilated ends of intralobular ducts are lined by simple cuboidal epithelium and surrounded by a discontinuous layer of stellate myoepithelial cells.

B. Oogenesis.

1. Formation of primordial follicles.

a. Primordial germ cells migrate from yolk sac endoderm into the ovaries early in the embryonic period.

b. Oogonia proliferate until 20 to 28 weeks of gestation, yielding 3 million oogonia per ovary.

(1) After ceasing mitosis, oogonia are arrested in prophase I of meiosis.

(2) Additional oocytes are not formed later in life.

c. The primordial follicle consists of one primary oocyte surrounded by a single layer of squamous epithelial cells and a basal lamina.

(1) The number of primordial follicles is reduced to approximately 200,000 per ovary at menarche.

2. Maturation of ovarian follicles—characterized by progressive morphologic changes in the oocyte, surrounding follicular cells, and adjacent stroma.

a. Unilaminar primary follicle.

(1) Simple, squamous epithelium changes to a single layer of cuboidal follicular cells.

(2) Differentiation of primary oocyte begins, marked by increases in size and number of mitochondria, Golgi apparatus, rough endoplasmic reticulum, and polysomes, which augment the synthetic capacity of the oocyte.

(3) Zona pellucida, synthesized by both the oocyte and the follicular cells, begins to form around the oocyte.

b. Multilaminar primary follicle.

(1) Stratification of cuboidal follicular cells occurs, forming a granulosa layer.

(2) Stromal cells begin to form the thecal layer around the follicle.

c. Secondary (antral) follicle.

(1) Spaces filled with fluid appear between granulosa cells. They eventually coalesce into a single large antrum.

(2) A mound of granular cells called the *cumulus oophorus* attaches the oocyte to the follicular wall.

(3) The theca interna secretes a 17-ketosteroid, which is known as *androstenedione.*

(a) Androstenedione is enzymatically converted to testosterone.

(b) FSH stimulates enzymatic conversion of these androgens to estrogen in granulosa cells.

d. Graafian follicle.

(1) The primary oocyte completes its first meiotic division within the mature follicle shortly before ovulation, forming a large secondary oocyte and small polar body.

(2) The secondary oocyte enters the second meiotic division but is halted in metaphase II at the time of ovulation.

3. Ovulation and the fate of secondary oocyte.

a. A surge of LH, induced by an increasing level of estrogen, triggers the release of a secondary oocyte surrounded by its corona radiata from a graafian follicle.

b. The ovulated secondary oocyte normally is caught in the fimbria of the oviduct.

2.8.3 Urinary System

The urinary system consists of the paired kidneys and ureters and the unpaired bladder and urethra.

A. Structure.

1. The uriniferous tubule is a continuous tubular structure with regional specializations that constitute the functional unit of the kidney.

a. Each uriniferous tubule consists of a nephron and the collecting tubules into which it drains.

(1) The nephron includes a renal corpuscle, a proximal convoluted tubule, the loop of Henle, and a distal convoluted tubule.

(2) Collecting tubules extend from arched collecting tubules to the papillary duct.

B. Uriniferous tubules and urine production (Figure 1-58).

1. Renal (malpighian) corpuscle—consists of the glomerulus and Bowman's capsule.

a. Glomerulus.

(1) Blood flows from the afferent arteriole through the glomerular capillary network to the efferent arteriole.

(2) Mesangial cells are located around glomerular capillaries. These cells are phagocytic and help support capillary loops.

b. Bowman's capsule.

(1) The visceral layer is formed of podocytes, which are responsible for synthesis of the glomerular basement membrane.

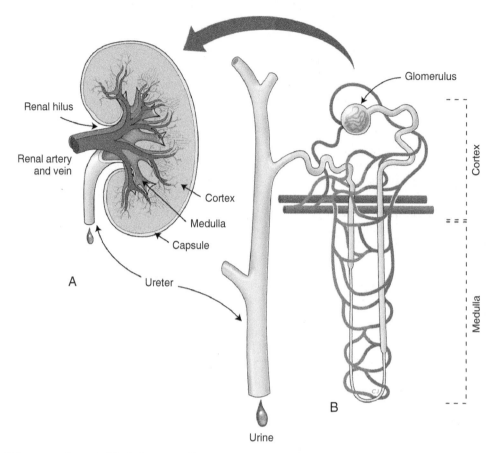

Figure 1-58 **Urinary system. A,** The kidneys are filters, removing toxins but conserving water, proteins, glucose, salts, and other essential substances. The kidneys also help regulate blood pressure and acid-base balance. The kidneys deliver urine to the urinary bladder. **B,** Uriniferous tubules. All fluids pass through the tubule system as they carry fluid to the glomeruli and urine to the medullary area of the kidney. These highly cellular structures remove important elements and allow the urine to collect for passage to the urinary bladder. The glomeruli are important in recirculating and in toxin removal and retaining water, protein, sugars, and other important elements. *(From Chiego D: Essentials of Oral Histology and Embryology: A Clinical Approach, ed 4, St. Louis, Mosby, 2014.)*

(2) Bowman's urinary space is the narrow cavity between the visceral and parietal layers into which the glomerular filtrate drains.

(3) The parietal layer is composed of simple, squamous epithelium and forms the outer wall of Bowman's capsule.

2. Renal tubule.
  a. Proximal convoluted tubule.
    (1) The wall is composed of large, cuboidal epithelial cells and numerous structures.
      (a) Abundant microvilli called a *brush border.*
      (b) Apical tubular invaginations called *canaliculi, vesicles,* and *granules.*
      (c) Infoldings of basal plasmalemma.
      (d) Numerous mitochondria.
  b. Thin segment of the loop of Henle.
    (1) The wall is composed of squamous epithelial cells.
    (2) Apical surfaces possess sparse microvilli.

  c. Thick ascending segment of the loop of Henle.
    (1) The wall is composed of cuboidal epithelial cells.
  d. Distal convoluted tubule.
    (1) The wall is similar to the thick ascending segment of the loop of Henle; it also is impermeable to water.
  e. Collecting tubules and ducts.
    (1) The arched collecting tubule is lined by simple cuboidal epithelium, which connects the distal convoluted tubule of a nephron and the collecting tubule into which it drains.
    (2) The collecting duct is a straight tubule formed by the convergence of arched tubules from multiple nephrons.
      (a) The upper, cortical portion has cuboidal epithelium and lies within a medullary ray.
      (b) The lower, medullary portion has columnar epithelium and lies within a medullary pyramid.

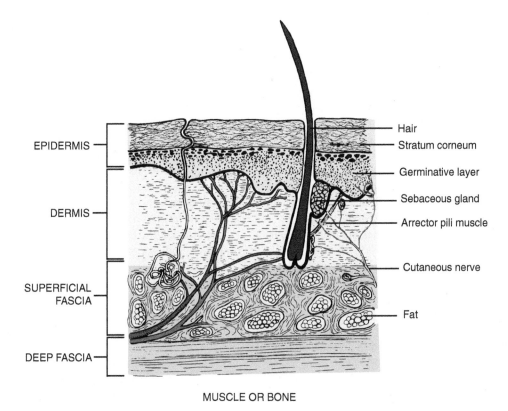

Figure 1-59 Skin and fascia. *(From Liebgott B: The Anatomical Basis of Dentistry, ed 3, St. Louis, Mosby, 2011.)*

(3) Papillary ducts of Bellini are large collecting tubules with simple columnar epithelium.

C. Juxtaglomerular apparatus—functions in the regulation of blood pressure.

   1. Components.

      a. Macula densa are specialized cells of the distal convoluted tubule where it contacts the afferent arteriole.

      b. Juxtaglomerular cells are myoepithelial cells derived from smooth muscle in the tunica media of the afferent arteriole.

   2. Renin-angiotensin-aldosterone system

      a. Renin is secreted by juxtaglomerular cells in response to a decrease in blood pressure.

      b. Renin converts angiotensin I to angiotensin II in circulation.

      c. Angiotensin-converting enzyme is located in endothelial cells of blood vessels and hydrolyzes angiotensin I to angiotensin II.

      d. Angiotensin II increases blood pressure.

         (1) Directly by stimulating vasoconstriction.

         (2) Indirectly by stimulating aldosterone secretion.

2.9 Integument

The integument consists of the skin and its appendages, including hair follicles, nails, sweat glands, and sebaceous glands.

A. Components (Figure 1-59).

   1. Epidermis—superficial layer of stratified, squamous, keratinized epithelium.

   2. Dermis—dense, fibrous, irregular connective tissue layer beneath the epidermis.

   3. Hypodermis—layer of loose connective tissue underlying the dermis.

      a. The hypodermis binds skin to adjacent tissue.

B. Epidermis.

   1. Keratinocytes—form a stratified, squamous, keratinized epithelium containing five strata.

      a. Stratum basale—the deepest layer of epidermis; it is a single layer of cuboidal to columnar keratinocytes.

         (1) These keratinocytes are mitotically active.

         (2) The keratinocytes are attached to the basement membrane by hemidesmosomes.

         (3) The keratinocytes produce low-molecular-weight keratins.

         (4) Basal cells give rise to additional nondifferentiating stem cells, which remain in this layer, as well as to differentiating keratinocytes, which migrate into the stratum spinosum.

      b. Stratum spinosum—contains several layers of polyhedral-shaped keratinocytes (prickle cells) that proliferate and differentiate.

         (1) High-molecular-weight keratins are produced and assembled into intermediate filaments

(tonofibrils) that terminate in numerous desmosomes.

(2) Lamellar bodies containing lipid, carbohydrate, and hydrolytic enzymes become evident.

(3) The stratum germinativum consists of the stratum basale and stratum spinosum.

c. Stratum granulosum—consists of three to five layers of flattened keratinocytes.

(1) Disulfide bonds begin to cross-link keratin filaments.

(2) Glycolipid and sterols secreted from lamellar bodies into the intercellular space form an impermeable, waterproof barrier.

(3) Lysosomal activity degrades organelles as cells move superficially.

d. Stratum lucidum—a clear, homogeneous layer composed of flat keratinocytes lacking nuclei and organelles.

(1) The cytoplasm consists almost entirely of keratin filaments.

(2) The layer is well-defined only in thick skin.

e. Stratum corneum—the most superficial layer, composed of 5 to 50 layers of flattened, keratinized dead cells.

(1) The cells, called *squames*, are filled with cross-linked keratin filaments.

(2) Squames are continuously shed from the surface and are replaced with differentiating cells from the basal layer.

2. Nonkeratinocytes include melanocytes, Langerhans' cells, and Merkel cells.

a. Melanocytes—synthesize melanin, which absorbs ultraviolet (UV) radiation and protects cells in the skin from UV-induced damage.

(1) Melanocytes are located in the stratum basale, the papillary layer of the dermis, and hair follicles.

(2) Synthesis of melanin occurs in melanosomes, granules containing tyrosinase, and other enzymes that participate in the metabolic pathway whereby tyrosine is converted to melanin.

(3) Chromatophores are cells in the dermis that take up melanin by phagocytosis.

b. Langerhans' cells.

(1) Langerhans' cells are located primarily in the stratum spinosum.

(2) They are derived from precursor cells in bone marrow.

c. Merkel cells.

(1) Contain small granules filled with catecholamines.

(2) May act as sensory mechanoreceptors or as diffuse neuroendocrine cells.

C. Dermis—composed of dense, fibrous, irregular connective tissue.

1. Layers—both the papillary and the reticular layers of dermis contain an elastic fiber network continuous throughout the bundles of collagen.

a. Papillary layer.

(1) The papillary layer is composed of moderately dense connective tissue arranged in fine, interlacing-bands of thin, collagenous bundles.

b. Reticular layer.

(1) The reticular layer is composed of dense connective tissue arranged in thick, interlacing collagenous bands.

D. Appendages.

Hair follicles and glands extend into the dermis and occasionally the hypodermis.

1. Hair and hair follicles.

a. Structure: the hair shaft is located in a multilayered follicle.

(1) Ducts of sebaceous glands and apocrine sweat glands empty into hair follicles.

(2) A dermal sheath surrounds each follicle and extends a protrusion through the follicular layers into the base of the shaft.

(3) The arrector pili muscle originates on the dermal sheath of the hair follicle and inserts into the papillary layer of the dermis.

2. Glands of the skin (Table 1-31).

a. Glands in the skin include sebaceous, eccrine sweat, and apocrine sweat glands.

3. Nails.

a. The proximal root is embedded in epidermis.

(1) The eponychium (cuticle) is the stratum corneum of the nail fold that overlies the proximal root.

(2) The nail matrix is the area of epidermal cells covered by eponychium where nail synthesis takes place.

(3) The lunula is an extension of the nail matrix beyond the eponychium. It is visible as a white crescent.

b. The distal free edge is underlaid by hyponychium, a thickened stratum corneum.

E. Vasculature of the skin—the epidermis does not have a blood supply; the deeper layers and all skin appendages have a network of small vessels.

1. Arterial plexuses.

a. Rete cutaneum at the border of the dermis and hypodermis.

b. Rete subpapillare at the border of papillary and reticular layers of the dermis.

(1) Arterioles from this plexus give rise to a single capillary loop around each dermal papilla.

2. Venous plexuses.

a. Located in the middle of the dermis, between papillary and reticular layers of the dermis, and at the border of the dermis and hypodermis.

Table 1-31

Glands of the Skin

PROPERTY	TYPE OF GLAND		
	SEBACEOUS	ECCRINE SWEAT	APOCRINE SWEAT
Location within skin	Dermis	Dermis	Dermis and hypodermis
Body distribution	Throughout body except for palms and soles	Throughout body	Axilla, mons pubis, areola of nipple, perianal region
General structure	Branched acinar gland with short duct	Simple, tubular gland	Large, complex gland
Myoepithelial cells	Absent	Present	Present
Type of secretion	Thick, lipid-containing substance (sebum)	Clear, watery secretion	Viscous substance rich in protein and cellular debris
Secretion mechanism	Holocrine	Merocrine	Mixed
Duct opening	Hair follicle (usually)	Surface of skin (sweat pore)	Hair follicle
Period of activity	Inactive until puberty	Active throughout life	Inactive until puberty
Other features	Excess androgen-mediated secretion can plug hair follicles, predisposing to acne	Secretion stimulated by high temperature and stress	Activity is linked to menstrual cycle in girls and women

From Burns ER, Cave MD: Histology and Cell Biology, St. Louis, Mosby, 2002.

3. Arteriovenous anastomoses.
   a. Direct connections between arterioles and venules (arteriovenous shunts). They occur in deeper skin and are important in thermoregulation.
   b. Blood flow through arteriovenous shunts is regulated by autonomic nerve fibers and certain hormones.
F. Nerves of the skin.
   1. Motor nerves are postganglionic fibers from sympathetic ganglia of the paravertebral chain.
      a. Autonomic nerve supply functions primarily in thermoregulation.
   2. Sensory nerve endings.
      a. Free nerve endings are located at epidermal openings, and the root sheaths of hair follicles function as mechanoreceptors.
      b. Encapsulated sensory receptors, located in the skin and associated mucous membranes, include the pacinian corpuscle, the Meissner corpuscle, and the Krause end-bulb.

3.0 Oral Histology

3.1 Tooth and Supporting Structures

A. Enamel.
   1. Composition.
      a. Inorganic (96%)—calcium hydroxyapatite crystals.
      b. Organic (4%)—water and proteins, including amelogenins and enamelins.
   2. Structural characteristics and microscopic features.
      a. Enamel rods or prisms.
         (1) Basic structural unit of enamel.
         (2) Consists of tightly packed hydroxyapatite crystals. Hydroxyapatite crystals in enamel are four times larger and more tightly packed than hydroxyapatite found in other calcified tissues (i.e., it is harder than bone).
         (3) Each rod extends the entire thickness of enamel and is perpendicular to the dentinoenamel junction (DEJ).
      b. Aprismatic enamel.
         (1) The thin outer layer of enamel found on the surface of newly erupted teeth.
         (2) Consists of enamel crystals that are aligned perpendicular to the surface.
         (3) It is aprismatic (i.e., prismless) and is more mineralized than the enamel beneath it.
         (4) It results from the absence of Tomes' processes on the ameloblasts during the final stages of enamel deposition.
      c. Lines of Retzius (enamel striae).
         (1) Microscopic features.
            (a) In longitudinal sections, they are observed as brown lines that extend from the DEJ to the tooth surface.
            (b) In transverse sections, they appear as dark, concentric rings similar to growth rings in a tree.
         (2) The lines appear weekly during the formation of enamel.

(3) Although the cause of striae formation is unknown, the lines may represent appositional or incremental growth of enamel. They may also result from metabolic disturbances of ameloblasts.

(4) Neonatal line.

(a) An accentuated, dark line of Retzius that results from the effect of physiologic changes on ameloblasts at birth.

(b) Found in all primary teeth and some cusps of permanent first molars.

d. Perikymata.

(1) Lines of Retzius terminate on the tooth surface in shallow grooves known a *perikymata*.

(2) These grooves are usually lost through wear but may be observed on the surfaces of developing teeth or nonmasticatory surfaces of formed teeth.

e. Hunter-Schreger bands.

(1) Enamel rods run in different directions. In longitudinal sections, these changes in direction result in a banding pattern known as *Hunter-Schreger bands*.

(2) These bands represent an optical phenomenon of enamel and consist of a series of alternating dark and light lines when the section is viewed with reflected or polarized light.

f. Enamel tufts.

(1) Consist of hypomineralized groups of enamel rods.

(2) They are observed as short, dark projections found near or at the DEJ.

(3) They have no known clinical significance.

g. Enamel lamellae.

(1) Small, sheetlike cracks found on the surface of enamel that extend its entire thickness.

(2) Consist of hypocalcified enamel.

(3) The open crack may be filled with organic material from leftover enamel organ components, connective tissues of the developing tooth, or debris from the oral cavity.

(4) Both enamel tufts and lamellae may be likened to geologic faults in mature enamel.

h. Enamel spindle (Figure 1-60).

(1) Remnants of odontoblastic processes that become trapped after crossing the DEJ during the differentiation of ameloblasts.

(2) Spindles are more pronounced beneath the cusps or incisal edges of teeth (i.e., areas where occlusal stresses are the greatest).

i. Note: to evaluate enamel microscopically, slides cannot be decalcified because of the low content of organic matrix in enamel. Only ground sections can be used.

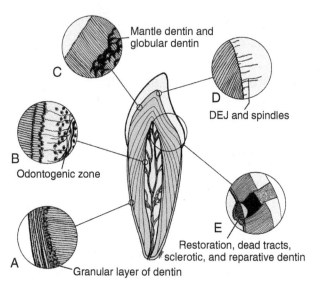

Figure 1-60 Various structures in dentin. **A,** Granular layer of dentin and adjacent cementum. **B,** Odontogenic zone and predentin. **C,** Mantle dentin and interglobular or globular dentin. **D,** Dentinoenamel junction (DEJ) and spindles. **E,** Restoration, dead tracts, sclerotic dentin, and reparative dentin. *(From Chiego D: Essentials of Oral Histology and Embryology: A Clinical Approach, ed 4, St. Louis, Mosby, 2014.)*

B. Dentin.

1. Composition.

a. Inorganic (70%)—calcium hydroxyapatite crystals.

b. Organic (30%)—water and type I collagen.

2. Types of dentin (see Figure 1-60).

a. Primary dentin.

(1) Dentin formed during tooth development, before completion of root formation. It constitutes most dentin found in a tooth.

(2) Consists of normal organization of dentinal tubules.

(3) Circumpulpal dentin.

(a) The layer of primary dentin that surrounds the pulp chamber. It is formed after the mantle dentin.

(b) Its collagen fibers are parallel to the DEJ.

b. Secondary dentin.

(1) Dentin formed after root formation is complete.

(2) Is deposited unevenly around the pulp chamber, forming along the layer of dentin closest to the pulp. It contributes to the decrease in the size of the pulp chamber as one ages.

(3) It consists of a normal, or slightly less regular, organization of dentinal tubules. However, compared with primary dentin, it is deposited at a slower rate.

(4) Although the dentinal tubules in secondary dentin can be continuous with dentinal tubules in primary dentin, there is usually a tubular angle change between the two layers.

c. Tertiary (reparative, reactive) dentin.

   (1) Dentin that is formed in localized areas in response to trauma or other stimuli such as caries, tooth wear, or dental work.

   (2) Its consistency and organization vary. It has no defined dentinal tubule pattern (see Figure 1-60).

d. Mantle dentin.

   (1) The outermost layer of dentin (see Figure 1-60).

   (2) Is the first layer of dentin laid down by odontoblasts adjacent to the DEJ.

   (3) Is slightly less mineralized than primary dentin.

   (4) Has collagen fibers that are perpendicular to the DEJ.

   (5) Dentinal tubules branch abundantly in this area.

e. Sclerotic (transparent) dentin.

   (1) Describes dentinal tubules that have become occluded with calcified material (see Figure 1-60).

   (2) Occurs when the odontoblastic processes retreat, filling the dentinal tubule with calcium phosphate crystals.

   (3) Occurs with aging.

f. Dead tracts.

   (1) When odontoblasts die, they leave behind empty dentinal tubules, or dead tracts (see Figure 1-60).

   (2) Occurs with aging or trauma.

   (3) Empty tubules are potential paths for bacterial invasion.

3. Structural characteristics and microscopic features.

a. Dentinal tubules (Figure 1-61).

   (1) Tubules extend from the DEJ to the pulp chamber.

   (2) The tubules taper peripherally (i.e., their diameters are wider as they get closer to the pulp). Because the tubules are distanced farther apart at the periphery, the density of tubules is greater closer to the pulp.

   (3) Each tubule contains an odontoblastic process or Tomes' fiber. Odontoblastic processes are characterized by the presence of a network of microtubules, with occasional mitochondria and vesicles present. Note: the odontoblast's cell body remains in the pulp chamber.

   (4) Coronal tubules follow an S-shaped path, which may result from the crowding of odontoblasts as they migrate toward the pulp during dentin formation.

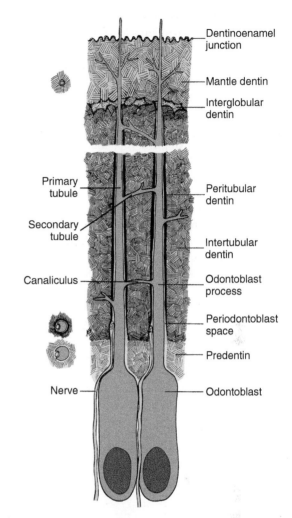

Figure 1-61 Odontoblast process in the dentinal tubule and extending from the dentinoenamel junction above to the pulp below. *(From Bhaskar SN, editor: Orban's Oral Histology and Embryology, ed 11, St. Louis, Mosby, 1991.)*

b. Peritubular dentin (intratubular dentin).

   (1) Is deposited on the walls of the dentinal tubule, which affects (i.e., narrows) the diameter of the tubule.

   (2) It differs from intertubular dentin by lacking a collagenous fibrous matrix. It is also more mineralized than intertubular dentin.

c. Intertubular dentin.

   (1) The main part of dentin, which fills the space between dentinal tubules.

   (2) Is mineralized and contains a collagenous matrix.

d. Interglobular dentin.

   (1) Areas of hypomineralized or unmineralized dentin caused by the failure of globules or calcospherites to fuse uniformly with mature dentin.

(2) Dentinal tubules are left undisturbed as they pass through interglobular dentin; however, no peritubular dentin is present.

(3) Interglobular dentin is found in the crown and root.

(a) Crown—just beneath the mantle dentin.

(b) Root—beneath the dentinocemental junction, giving the root the appearance of a granular layer (of Tomes).

e. Incremental lines.

(1) Dentin is deposited at a daily rate of approximately 4 μm.

(2) As dentin is laid down, small differences in collagen fiber orientation result in the formation of incremental lines.

(3) Called *imbrication lines of von Ebner.*

(a) Every 5 days, or about every 20 μm, the changes in collagen fiber orientation appear more accentuated. This results in a darker staining line, known as the *imbrication line of von Ebner.*

(b) These lines are similar to the lines of Retzius seen in enamel.

f. Contour lines of Owen.

(1) An optical phenomenon that occurs when the secondary curvatures of adjacent dentinal tubules coincide, resulting in the appearance of lines known as *contour lines of Owen.*

(2) Contour lines of Owen may also refer to lines that appear similar to those just described; however, these lines result from disturbances in mineralization.

g. Granular layer of Tomes (see Figure 1-60).

(1) A granular or spotty-appearing band that can be observed on the root surface adjacent to the dentinocemental junction, just beneath the cementum.

(2) The cause is unknown.

C. Pulp.

1. Four zones—listed from dentin inward (Figure 1-62).

a. Odontoblastic layer.

(1) Contains the cell bodies of odontoblasts. Note: their processes remain in dentinal tubules.

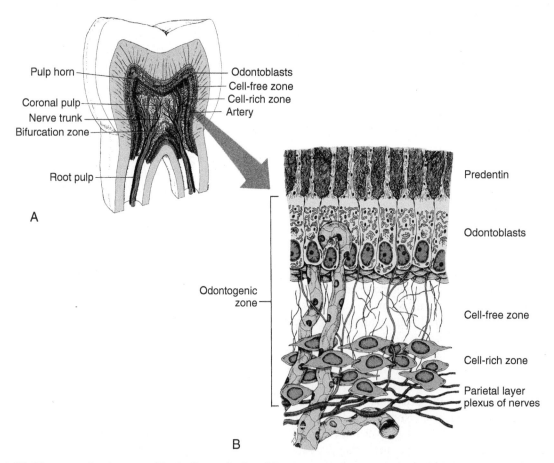

Figure 1-62 Diagram of pulp organ illustrating pulpal architecture. **A,** There appears to be high organization of the peripheral pulp and appearance of centrally located nerve trunks (dark) and blood vessels (light). **B,** Odontogenic zone of pulp. *Top to bottom:* Predentin, odontoblasts, cell-free and cell-rich zones, and parietal layer of nerves. *(From Bhaskar SN, editor: Orban's Oral Histology and Embryology, ed 11, St. Louis, Mosby, 1991.)*

(2) Capillaries, nerve fibers, and dendritic cells may also be present.

b. Cell-free or cell-poor zone (zone of Weil).

(1) Contains capillaries and unmyelinated nerve fibers.

c. Cell-rich zone.

(1) Consists mainly of fibroblasts. Macrophages, lymphocytes, and dendritic cells may also be present.

d. Pulp (pulp proper, central zone).

(1) The central mass of the pulp.

(2) Consists of loose connective tissue, larger vessels, and nerves. Also contains fibroblasts and pulpal cells.

2. Pulpal innervation.

a. When pulpal nerves are stimulated, they can transmit only one signal—pain.

b. There are no proprioceptors in the pulp.

c. Types of nerves.

(1) A-delta fibers.

(a) Myelinated sensory nerve fibers.

(b) Stimulation results in the sensation of fast, sharp pain.

(c) Found in the coronal (odontoblastic) area of the pulp.

(2) C fibers.

(a) Unmyelinated sensory nerve fibers.

(b) Transmits information of noxious stimuli centrally.

(c) Stimulation results in pain that is slower, duller, and more diffuse in nature.

(d) Found in the central region of the pulp.

(3) Sympathetic fibers.

(a) Found deeper within the pulp.

(b) Sympathetic stimulation results in vasoconstriction of vessels.

3.1.1 Periodontium

The periodontium consists of tissues supporting and investing the tooth and includes cementum, the PDL, and alveolar bone. Parts of the gingiva adjacent to the tooth also give minor support, although the gingiva is not considered to be part of the periodontium in many texts. For our purposes here, the groups of gingival fibers related to tooth investment are discussed in this section.

A. Cementum.

1. Composition.

a. Inorganic (50%)—calcium hydroxyapatite crystals.

b. Organic (50%)—water, proteins, and type I collagen.

c. Note: compared with other dental tissues, the composition of cementum is most similar to bone; however, in contrast to bone, cementum is avascular (i.e., no haversian systems or other vessels are present).

2. The main function of cementum is to attach PDL fibers to the root surface.

3. Cementum is generally thickest at the root apex and in interradicular areas of multirooted teeth. It is thinnest in the cervical area.

4. Types of cementum.

a. Acellular (primary) cementum.

(1) A thin layer of cementum that surrounds the root, adjacent to the dentin.

(2) May be covered by a layer of cellular cementum, which most often occurs in the middle and apical root.

(3) It does not contain any cells.

b. Cellular (secondary) cementum.

(1) A thicker, less mineralized layer of cementum that is most prevalent along the apical root and in interradicular (furcal) areas of multirooted teeth.

(2) Contains cementocytes.

(3) Lacunae and canaliculi.

(a) Cementocytes (cementoblasts that become trapped in the extracellular matrix during cementogenesis) are observed in their entrapped spaces, known as *lacunae*.

(b) The processes of cementocytes extend through narrow channels called *canaliculi*.

(4) Microscopically, the best way to differentiate between acellular and cellular cementum is the presence of lacunae in cellular cementum.

c. Differences between acellular and cellular cementum are listed in Table 1-32.

B. PDL

1. Composition.

a. Consists mostly of collagenous (alveolodental) fibers. Note: the portions of the fibers embedded in cementum and the alveolar bone proper are known as *Sharpey's fibers*.

Table 1-32

Differences between Acellular and Cellular Cementum

	ACELLULAR CEMENTUM	CELLULAR CEMENTUM
Presence of cells	None	Cementocytes
Dentin border	Not clearly demarcated	Clearly demarcated
Rate of development	Slow	Fast
Incremental lines	Close together	Relatively wide apart
Precementum layer	Largely absent	Present
Function	Anchorage	Adaptation and repair

b. Oxytalan fibers (a type of elastic fiber) are also present. Although their function is unknown, they may play a role in the regulation of vascular flow.

c. Contains mostly type I collagen, although smaller amounts of type III and XII collagen are also present.

d. Has a rich vascular and nerve supply. Both sensory and autonomic nerves are present.
   (1) The sensory nerves in the PDL differ from pulpal nerves in that PDL nerve endings can detect both proprioception (via mechanoreceptors) and pain (via nociceptors).
   (2) The autonomic nerve fibers are associated with the regulation of periodontal vascular flow.
   (3) Nerve fibers may be myelinated (sensory) or unmyelinated (sensory or autonomic).

2. Cells
   a. Cells present in the PDL include fibroblasts; epithelial cells; cementoblasts and cementoclasts; osteoblasts and osteoclasts; and immune cells such as macrophages, mast cells, or eosinophils.
   b. These cells play a role in forming or destroying cementum, alveolar bone, or PDL.
   c. Epithelial cells often appear in clusters, known as *rests of Malassez.*

3. Types of alveolodental fibers (Figure 1-63).
   a. Alveolar crest fibers—radiate downward from cementum, just below the cementoenamel junction (CEJ), to the crest of alveolar bone.
   b. Horizontal fibers—radiate perpendicular to the tooth surface from cementum to alveolar bone, just below the alveolar crest.

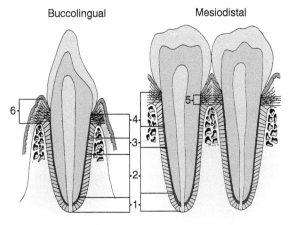

Buccolingual   Mesiodistal

1. Apical
2. Oblique
3. Horizontal
4. Alveolar crest
5. Transseptal
6. Gingival group

Figure 1-63 Principal fiber groups of the periodontal ligament. *(Modified from Chiego D: Essentials of Oral Histology and Embryology: A Clinical Approach, ed 4, St. Louis, Mosby, 2014.)*

c. Oblique fibers.
   (1) Radiate downward from the alveolar bone to cementum.
   (2) The most numerous type of PDL fiber.
   (3) Resist occlusal forces that occur along the long axis of the tooth.

d. Apical fibers.
   (1) Radiate from the cementum at the apex of the tooth into the alveolar bone.
   (2) Resist forces that pull the tooth in an occlusal direction (i.e., forces that try to pull the tooth from its socket).

e. Interradicular fibers.
   (1) Found only in the furcal area of multirooted teeth.
   (2) Resist forces that pull the tooth in an occlusal direction.

4. Gingival fibers.
   a. The fibers of the gingival ligament are not strictly part of the PDL, but they play a role in the maintenance of the periodontium.
   b. Gingival fibers are packed in groups and are found in the lamina propria of gingiva (see Figure 1-63).
   c. Gingival fiber groups.
      (1) Transseptal (interdental) fibers.
         (a) Extend from the cementum of one tooth (just apical to the junctional epithelium), over the alveolar crest, to the corresponding area of the cementum of the adjacent tooth.
         (b) Collectively, these fibers form the interdental ligament, which functions to resist rotational forces and retain adjacent teeth in interproximal contact.
         (c) These fibers have been implicated as a major cause of postretention relapse of teeth that have undergone orthodontic treatment.
      (2) Circular (circumferential) fibers.
         (a) Extend around tooth near the CEJ.
         (b) Function in binding free gingiva to the tooth and resisting rotational forces.
      (3) Alveologingival fibers—extend from the alveolar crest to lamina propria of free and attached gingiva.
      (4) Dentogingival fibers—extend from cervical cementum to the lamina propria of free and attached gingiva.
      (5) Dentoperiosteal fibers—extend from cervical cementum, over the alveolar crest, to the periosteum of the alveolar bone.

C. Alveolar bone (process).
   1. The bone in the jaws that contains the teeth alveoli (sockets).
   2. Three types of bone.
      a. Cribriform plate (alveolar bone proper).
         (1) Directly lines and forms the tooth socket. It is compact bone that contains many holes,

allowing for the passage of blood vessels. It has no periosteum.

   (2) Serves as the attachment site for PDL (Sharpey's) fibers.

   (3) The tooth socket is constantly being remodeled in response to occlusal forces. The bone laid down on the cribriform plate, which also provides attachment for PDL fibers, is known as *bundle bone*.

   (4) It is radiographically known as the *lamina dura*.

   b. Cortical (compact) bone.

   (1) Lines the buccal and lingual surfaces of the mandible and maxilla.

   (2) Is typical compact bone with a periosteum and contains haversian systems.

   (3) Is generally thinner in the maxilla and thicker in the mandible, especially around the buccal area of the mandibular premolar and molar.

   c. Trabecular (cancellous, spongy) bone.

   (1) Is typical cancellous bone containing haversian systems.

   (2) Is absent in the maxillary anterior teeth region.

3. Alveolar crest (septa).

   a. The height of the alveolar crest is usually 1.5 to 2 mm below the CEJ junction.

   b. The width is determined by the shape of adjacent teeth.

   (1) Narrow crests—found between teeth with relatively flat surfaces.

   (2) Widened crests—found between teeth with convex surfaces or teeth spaced apart.

3.2 Soft Oral Tissues

3.2.1 Oral Mucosa

The oral mucosa consists mainly of two types of tissues: the oral epithelium, which consists of stratified, squamous epithelium, and the underlying connective tissue layer, known as the *lamina propria* (Figure 1-64). There are three variations of oral mucosa.

A. Oral epithelium.

   1. Consists of stratified, squamous epithelium.

   2. Four layers. Note: cells mature as they progress from the deepest (basal) layer to the most superficial (cornified) layer.

   a. Basal layer (stratum germinativum or basale).

   (1) A single layer of cuboidal or columnar cells overlying the lamina propria.

   (2) Contains progenitor cells and provides cells to the epithelial layers above.

   (3) Site of cell division (mitosis).

   b. Prickle cell layer (stratum spinosum).

   (1) Consists of several layers of larger, ovoid-shaped cells.

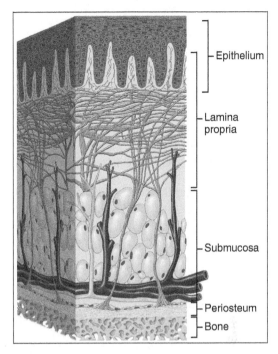

Figure 1-64 Main tissue components of the oral mucosa. *(From Nanci A: Ten Cate's Oral Histology, St. Louis, Mosby, 2013.)*

   c. Granular layer (stratum granulosum).

   (1) Cells appear larger and flattened.

   (2) Granules (known as *keratohyaline granules*) are present in the cells.

   (3) This layer is absent in nonkeratinized epithelium.

   d. Cornified layer (stratum corneum, keratin, or horny layer).

   (1) In keratinized epithelium.

   (a) Orthokeratinized epithelium—the squamous cells on the surface appear flat and contain keratin. They have no nuclei present.

   (b) Parakeratinized epithelium—the squamous cells appear flat and contain keratin; nuclei are present within the cells.

   (2) In parakeratinized epithelium, both squamous cells without nuclei and cells with shriveled (pyknotic) nuclei are present.

   (3) In nonkeratinized epithelium, the cells appear slightly flattened and contain nuclei.

B. Lamina propria.

   1. Consists of type I and III collagen, elastic fibers, and ground substance. It also contains many cell types, including fibroblasts, endothelial cells, immune cells, and a rich vascular and nerve supply.

   2. Two layers.

   a. Superficial, papillary layer.

   (1) Located around and between the epithelial ridges.

   (2) Collagen fibers are thin and loosely arranged.

b. Reticular layer.
    (1) Located beneath the papillary layer.
    (2) Collagen fibers are organized in thick, parallel bundles.
C. Types of oral mucosa (Table 1-33).
  1. Masticatory mucosa.
    a. Found in areas that have to withstand compressive and shear forces.
    b. Clinically, it has a rubbery, firm texture.
    c. Regions: gingiva, hard palate.
  2. Lining mucosa.
    a. Found in areas that are exposed to high levels of friction, but must also be mobile and distensible.

b. Clinically, it has a softer, more elastic texture.
c. Regions: alveolar mucosa, buccal mucosa, lips, floor of the mouth, ventral side of the tongue, and soft palate.
  3. Specialized mucosa.
    a. Similar to masticatory mucosa, specialized mucosa is able to tolerate high compressive and shear forces; however, it is unique in that it forms lingual papillae.
    b. Region: dorsum of the tongue.
D. Submucosa.
  1. Submucosa is the connective tissue found beneath the mucosa (see Figure 1-64) that contains blood vessels and nerves and may contain fatty tissue and minor salivary glands.
  2. Submucosa is not present in all regions of the oral cavity, such as attached gingiva, the tongue, and hard palate. Its presence tends to increase the mobility of the tissue overlying it.
E. Gingiva.
  1. The portion of oral mucosa that attaches to the teeth and alveolar bone.
  2. There are two types of gingiva: attached and free gingiva. The boundary at which they meet is known as the *free gingival groove* (Figure 1-65).
    a. Attached gingiva.
      (1) Directly binds to the alveolar bone and tooth.
      (2) It extends from the free gingival groove to the mucogingival junction.
    b. Free gingiva.
      (1) Coronal to the attached gingiva, it is not bound to any hard tissue.
      (2) It extends from the gingival margin to the free gingival groove.

Table 1-33

Three Types of Oral Mucosa

	MUCOSA	REGIONS
Masticatory mucosa	Thick epithelium Keratinized Numerous rete ridges Long papilla	Gingiva (free, attached) Hard palate
Lining mucosa	Thin epithelium* Nonkeratinized Few rete ridges Short papilla	Alveolar mucosa Labial and buccal mucosa Lips Floor of mouth Ventral side of tongue Soft palate
Specialized mucosa	Nonkeratinized Forms lingual papillae	Dorsum of tongue

*An exception is the epithelium of labial and buccal mucosa—it is thick.

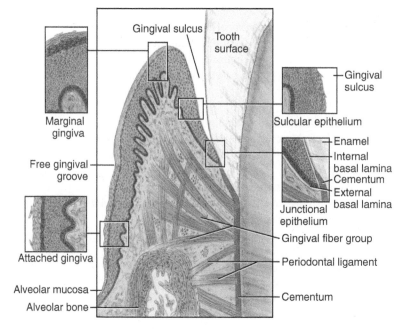

Figure 1-65 Gingival and dentogingival junctional tissue: marginal gingiva, sulcular epithelium, and junctional epithelium. *(From Bath-Balogh M, Fehrenbach M: Illustrated Dental Embryology, Histology, and Anatomy, ed 3, Philadelphia, Saunders, 2011.)*

c. Together, the free and attached gingiva form the interdental papilla (described subsequently).

F. Alveolar mucosa.

1. The tissue just apical to the attached gingiva.

2. The alveolar mucosa and attached gingiva meet at the mucogingival junction (see Figure 1-65).

3. Histologic differences in mucosal structure between gingiva and alveolar mucosa are summarized in Table 1-34.

G. Junctional epithelium.

1. Area where the oral mucosa attaches to the tooth, forming the principal seal between the oral cavity and underlying tissues.

2. Is unique in that it consists of two basal lamina, an internal and external (Figure 1-66). The internal basal lamina, along with hemidesmosomes, constitutes the attachment apparatus (the epithelial attachment). This serves to attach the epithelium directly to the tooth.

3. Histologically, it remains as immature, poorly differentiated tissue. This allows it to maintain its ability to develop hemidesmosomal attachments.

4. Has the highest rate of cell turnover of any oral mucosal tissue.

H. Interdental papilla (interdental gingiva).

1. Occupies the interproximal space between two teeth. It is formed by free and attached gingiva.

2. Functions to prevent food from entering the (interproximal) area beneath the contact point of two adjacent teeth. It plays an important role in maintaining the health of the gingiva.

3. Col.

a. If the interdental papilla is cross-sectioned in a buccolingual plane, it shows two peaks (buccal and lingual) with a dip between them, known as the *col* or *interdental col*. This depression occurs around the contact point of the two adjacent teeth.

b. Histologically, col epithelium is the same as junctional epithelium.

3.3 Temporomandibular Joint

A. Description.

1. The TMJ features two types of movements: rotary and translatory (gliding). It is described as a synovial sliding-ginglymoid joint. It may also be referred to as a *hinge* and *sliding joint*.

2. The TMJ is different from other diarthrodial joints in that its articulating surfaces are covered with fibrocartilage rather than hyaline cartilage.

3. The TMJ is different from compound (complex) joints, which consist of three bones. The TMJ consists of two bones and a disc.

B. Structure and anatomy.

1. Bones.

a. The TMJ is formed from two bones: temporal bone (mandibular fossa) and mandible (condyle).

Table 1-34		
Gingiva and Alveolar Mucosa: Differences in Mucosal Structure		
	GINGIVA	**ALVEOLAR MUCOSA**
Oral mucosa type	Lining mucosa	Masticatory mucosa
Epithelium	Thick, keratinized stratified squamous	Thin, nonkeratinized stratified squamous
Lamina propria	Long papillae	Short, poorly developed papillae
	Very vascular	Less vascular
Submucosa	No distinct layer	Extensive layer

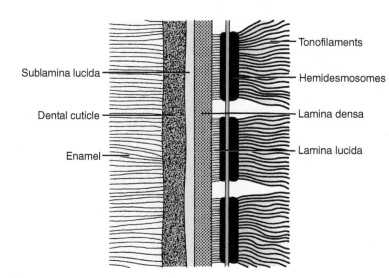

Sublamina lucida

Dental cuticle

Enamel

Tonofilaments

Hemidesmosomes

Lamina densa

Lamina lucida

Figure 1-66 The means of gingival attachment with the tooth surface. *(Modified from Chiego D: Essentials of Oral Histology and Embryology: A Clinical Approach, ed 4, St. Louis, Mosby, 2014.)*

b. Mandibular (articular) fossa.
  (1) Part of the squamous portion of the temporal bone (see Figure 1-12).
  (2) Anterior to the mandibular fossa is the articular eminence. Posterior to it lies the postglenoid process.
c. The articulating surfaces of the TMJ are covered with fibrocartilage, directly overlying periosteum. The nonarticulating surfaces are covered with periosteum.
2. Articular (joint) capsule.
  a. Thick, fibrous capsule that encloses the joint space (Figure 1-67).
  b. Attachments.
    (1) Superiorly, the capsule attaches to the margin of the articular eminence (anteriorly) and fossa and extends posteriorly to the squamotympanic fissure of the temporal bone.
    (2) Inferiorly, it attaches to the neck of the condyle.
  c. Consists of two layers.
    (1) Outer layer—thick, fibrous tissue that is supported laterally by the temporomandibular ligament.
    (2) Inner layer—consists of synovial membrane, which secretes synovial fluid to help lubricate and nourish the joint.
  d. Note: the superior head of the lateral pterygoid muscle attaches to the anterior portion of the articular capsule (see Figure 1-67). When chewing food, the contraction of the superior head helps to stabilize the TMJ on the nonchewing side.

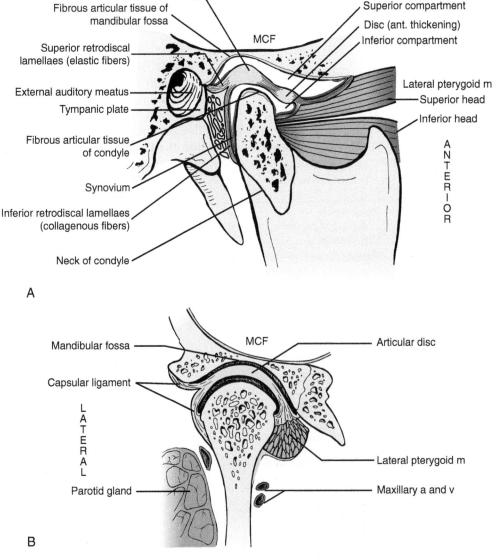

Figure 1-67 Internal features of the temporomandibular joint. **A,** Sagittal section. **B,** Coronal section. *MCF,* Middle cranial fossa. *(From Liebgott B: The Anatomical Basis of Dentistry, ed 3, St. Louis, Mosby, 2011.)*

3. Articular disc (meniscus).
   a. Consists of dense, fibrous tissue.
   b. Divides the TMJ into two compartments: the upper and lower synovial cavities. These two cavities are involved in translational and rotational TMJ movements, respectively (refer to TMJ movements, later).
   c. Disc thickness.
      (1) Lateral aspect (from widest to narrowest): posterior → anterior → middle.
      (2) Coronal aspect: medial side is wider than lateral side (see Figure 1-67, *B*).
   d. Attachments.
      (1) The anterior end of the disc fuses with the articular capsule.
      (2) The posterior end is divided into two sections: the upper portion attaches to the postglenoid process of the temporal bone; the lower portion attaches to the neck of the condyle.
      (3) Fibers of the superior head of the lateral pterygoid muscle attach to the anterior end of the disc. This helps to balance and stabilize the disc during closure.
   e. The central part of the disc is void of any blood vessels or nerves. The posterior portion of the disc (specifically, the retrodiscal space between the upper and lower posterior portions) contains vascular and nerve tissue.
4. Upper elastic lamina (superior retrodiscal lamina).
   a. Attachments: extends from the tympanic plate of the temporal bone to the upper portion of the posterior disc (see Figure 1-67, *A*).
   b. Contains elastic fibers.
   c. Produces a posterior pull on the disc.
      (1) During mouth opening, the condyles rotate forward. The disc, attached to the poles of the condyle, has a tendency to move forward with it. However, the elastic lamina pulls the disc back, allowing the disc and condyle to rotate on one another.
      (2) During retrusion (i.e., as the mandible returns to centric relation), the superior head of the lateral pterygoid relaxes. This relaxation balances the posterior pull of the elastic lamina.
5. Lower collagenous lamina.
   a. Attachments: extends from the posterior condylar neck to the lower portion of the posterior disc.
   b. Prevents anterior displacement of the disc and upper elastic lamina.
6. Functional ligaments.
   a. Collateral (discal) ligaments.
      (1) Attach to the medial and lateral sides of the disc (see Figure 1-67).
      (2) The lateral side is shorter than the medial side.

(3) These ligaments help to restrict medial and lateral rotation of the disc.
   b. Capsular ligament.
      (1) Wraps around the entire ligament.
      (2) Helps to keep the disc together.
   c. Temporomandibular (lateral) ligament.
      (1) Prevents posterior, inferior, and some lateral displacement of the mandible.
      (2) Provides lateral reinforcement to the articular capsule.
      (3) Consists of two ligaments (running in different directions), which function as a single unit.
         (a) Oblique—outer ligament.
            (i) Extends from the articular eminence posteriorly and inferiorly to the outer surface of the neck of the condyle.
            (ii) Prevents lateral and inferior displacement of the mandible.
         (b) Horizontal—inner ligament.
            (i) Extends from the articular eminence posteriorly to the lateral pole of the condyle.
            (ii) Prevents posterior displacement of the mandible.
7. Accessory ligaments.
   a. Sphenomandibular ligament.
      (1) Extends from the spine of the sphenoid bone to the lingula of the mandibular foramen.
      (2) Local anesthesia considerations—the IAN courses between the sphenomandibular ligament and the ramus of the mandible before entering the mandibular foramen. The sphenomandibular ligament may be damaged during the administration of an IAN block.
   b. Stylomandibular ligament.
      (1) Extends from the styloid process of the temporal bone to the angle of the mandible.
      (2) Restricts anterior (protrusive) movement of the mandible.
C. Nerve and vascular supply.
   1. Innervation—provided by branches of the trigeminal nerve, mandibular division (CN V_3).
      a. Auriculotemporal nerve.
      b. Sensory fibers from the masseteric and posterior temporal nerve.
   2. Blood supply—provided by branches of the external carotid artery.
      a. Superficial temporal artery.
      b. Branches from the deep auricular, anterior tympanic, ascending pharyngeal, and maxillary arteries may also be involved.
D. TMJ movement.
   1. Two motions.
      a. Rotational.
         (1) A hingelike motion, which occurs around a horizontal axis.

(2) Isolated rotation is possible only when the mandible is retruded, in the centric relation position.

(3) Involves the disc and condyle in the lower synovial cavity (i.e., during rotation, the shape of the lower synovial cavity would be more affected).

(4) Terminal hinge movement—rotation that occurs when the discs are positioned superiorly in the articular fossa, with the condyles directly underneath them.

b. Translational, sliding motion.

(1) Translation occurs as the disc slides along the slope of the articular eminence.

(2) Isolated translation occurs during protrusion (i.e., when the jaw moves forward).

(3) Involves the disc and anterior eminence in the upper synovial cavity.

2. Mouth opening—when the mouth opens, both rotational and translational movements occur. The condyles initially rotate and then translate forward. Note: rotational movement continues during translation.

4.0 Developmental Biology

4.1 Osteogenesis

A. Intramembranous ossification.

The process of intramembranous ossification involves differentiation of mesenchyme directly into bone without formation of an intervening cartilage. Flat bones of the skull and subperiosteal lamellar bone are formed by intramembranous ossification.

1. Steps in intramembranous ossification.

a. Stellate mesenchymal cells differentiate into osteoblasts and form spicules of aggregated cells.

b. Osteoblasts commence producing osteoid.

(1) Osteoid traps some of the osteoblasts, which form osteocytes in the interior of spicules.

c. Mineralization of the developing spicule occurs gradually.

(1) The basophilic core is composed of mineralized, older osteoid.

(2) The thin, eosinophilic peripheral zone is composed of nonmineralized, younger osteoid.

d. Spicules anastomose with one another to produce immature woven bone.

(1) Woven bone does not contain lamellae.

(2) It has loosely packed, randomly arranged collagen fibers.

(3) It has a greater cell density than mature bone.

e. Anastomosing spicules eventually enclose mesenchymal areas, which contain blood vessels and nerves.

f. Deposition of osteoid is greatest on the side of the spicule nearest the vessels.

2. Remodeling of immature bone creates mature compact bone.

B. Endochondral ossification (Figure 1-68).

This process of bone formation begins with differentiation of mesenchyme into a hyaline cartilage model. It is then reworked into adult compact bone. Long bones of the limbs, vertebral column, shoulder and pelvic girdles, and ribs are formed by endochondral ossification.

1. Formation of diaphyseal (primary) center of ossification.

a. Based on the hyaline cartilage model.

(1) Structure is formed from fetal mesenchyme containing chondroblasts and chondrocytes. It is surrounded by perichondrium except at the ends.

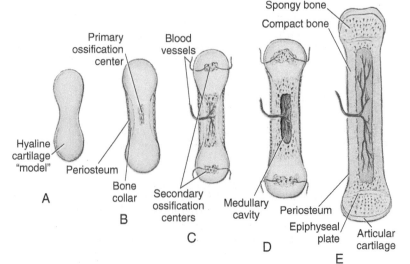

Figure 1-68 Endochondral ossification over time. **A-E,** The formation of osteoid within a cartilage model that subsequently becomes mineralized and dies. *(From Applegate EJ: The Anatomy and Physiology Learning System, ed 4, WB Saunders, St. Louis, 2011.)*

(2) Interstitial growth increases the length of the model.

(3) Appositional growth increases the width.

b. Vascularization of the perichondrium induces differentiation of osteoblasts from regional mesenchyme.

(1) The outer layer is transformed into periosteum.

c. The periosteal collar of bone is produced by intramembranous ossification of the periosteum.

d. Hypertrophy and death of chondrocytes at the center of the cartilage leaves spicules of calcified cartilage and lacunae.

(1) These form the primitive marrow cavity.

(2) Enlargement of the cavity occurs by addition of bone on the outside of the diaphyseal collar and removal of bone from its endosteal surface.

e. The periosteal bud, containing blood vessels, osteoprogenitor cells, and mesenchymal cells, extends from the diaphyseal periosteum into the center of the degenerating cartilage.

f. Osteoprogenitor cells of the periosteal bud attach to spicules of calcified cartilage and become osteoblasts.

(1) This establishes the primary center of ossification.

g. Osteoblasts begin elaborating matrix, which become mineralized to form a spicule.

(1) Spicules have calcified cartilage in the center surrounded by mineralized bone matrix.

(2) The mineralized bone matrix is covered with a thin zone of unmineralized bone matrix, which is under the peripheral layer of osteoblasts.

h. The formation of bone proceeds toward both epiphyseal ends.

i. The marrow cavity is enlarged by osteoclastic removal of the oldest spicules of endochondral ossification.

2. Formation of epiphyseal centers of ossification.

a. Following birth, a center of ossification develops in each epiphysis.

(1) This occurs by the same process used in formation of the diaphyseal center.

b. Epiphyseal and diaphyseal centers of ossification are separated by epiphyseal plates composed of hyaline cartilage.

c. Addition of new hyaline cartilage at the epiphyseal ends of long bones and its replacement by bone at the diaphyseal ends cause migration of the epiphyseal plates outward, leading to lengthening of long bones.

d. Cartilage is enlarged by interstitial growth of hyaline cartilage in the articular region and its ossification.

e. Epiphyseal surfaces remain covered by hyaline cartilage and have no periosteum.

C. Epiphyseal plates.

Bone formation at the epiphyseal plates is stimulated by pituitary growth hormone.

1. Zones in epiphyseal plates can be distinguished histologically.

2. The zones occur in the following order from epiphyseal to diaphyseal side.

a. Zone of resting cartilage composed of small, randomly arranged chondrocytes.

b. Zone of proliferation composed of rows of isogenous cell groups owing to interstitial growth of chondrocytes.

c. Zone of hypertrophy composed of enlarged chondrocytes that release alkaline phosphatase.

d. Zone of calcified cartilage containing dead or dying chondrocytes and calcified cartilage spicules.

e. Zone of ossification with a continuous secretion of osteoid by osteoblasts attached to spicules of calcified cartilage and subsequent mineralization of older osteoid.

3. Closure of epiphyses occurs within epiphyseal plates and makes them nonfunctional.

a. Closure occurs in young adults at 20 to 30 years of age.

b. Epiphyseal closure marks the end of growth in length of long bones.

D. Remodeling of bone.

1. Bone remodeling results from combined activity of osteoclasts and osteoblasts.

2. Adult bone turns over completely in about 7 to 10 years.

4.2 Tooth Development, Eruption, and Movement

A. Tooth development.

1. Dental lamina.

a. Neural crest cells migrate down the sides of the head and induce oral epithelial cells to form the dental lamina.

b. The first sign of a dental structure is a narrow band of thickened oral epithelium.

c. The lamina forms the oral epithelium that subsequently develops into the inner enamel epithelium and induces the formation of dentin from mesenchymal cells.

d. After forming, the lamina wraps around the perimeter of the jaws, and 20 tooth buds appear.

e. The buds may be called the *enamel organ*.

f. The enamel organ consists of knobs of tissue that periodically arise from the dental lamina.

g. The lamina develops 32 permanent tooth buds lingual to the primary buds.

(1) If the permanent tooth follows a primary tooth, it develops from successional lamina.

(2) If there was no primary tooth, it develops as did the primary teeth from general lamina.

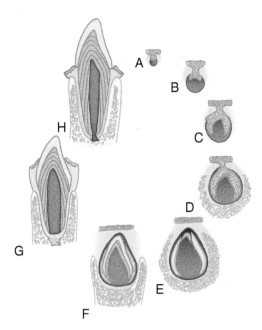

Figure 1-69 Stages of tooth development. A, Bud. **B,** Cap.
C, Bell. **D** and **E,** Dentinogenesis and amelogenesis. **F,** Crown
formation. **G,** Root formation and eruption. **H,** Function. *(From
Chiego D: Essentials of Oral Histology and Embryology: A Clinical
Approach, ed 4, St. Louis, Mosby, 2014.)*

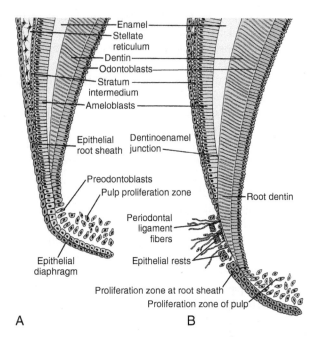

Figure 1-70 Root formation, showing the root sheath
and epithelial diaphragm. A, Time of epithelial root sheath
formation showing fusion of the outer and inner enamel epithelium to form the epithelial root sheath, which includes the vertical
epithelial root trunk and inward bending epithelial diaphragm.
B, Later stages of root sheath development. *(Modified from Chiego
D: Essentials of Oral Histology and Embryology: A Clinical
Approach, ed 4, St. Louis, Mosby, 2014.)*

B. Stages of tooth development (Figure 1-69).
  1. Bud.
    a. A localized growth of epithelial cells that develops
       from the dental lamina to create an enamel organ.
  2. Cap.
    a. The cells acquire a concave lower surface.
    b. The epithelial cells now become the enamel organ
       and remain attached to the lamina.
    c. Mesenchymal cells form the dental papilla, which
       becomes the pulp.
    d. The tissue surrounding these structures is the
       dental follicle.
  3. Bell.
    a. The enamel organ has developed into an outer and
       inner enamel epithelium.
    b. The inner enamel epithelium differentiates into
       ameloblasts that create enamel.
    c. The ameloblasts induce cells in the dental papillae
       to differentiate into odontoblasts that start to lay
       down dentin before the ameloblasts start laying
       down enamel.
    d. Between the inner and outer enamel epithelium
       are stellate reticulum cells.
    e. Another layer adjacent to the inner enamel epithe-
       lium in the enamel organ is called the *stratum
       intermedium.*
C. Dental papilla.
  1. Densely packed fibroblasts are seen in the dental
     papilla.

  2. These cells are thought to be significant in furthering
     the formation of the enamel organ in the bud and cap
     stages.
  3. Blood vessels and nerves may also be seen, initially
     in the central region.
D. Dentinogenesis.
  1. Odontoblasts move toward the pulp, forming incre-
     ments of dentin.
  2. First, the dentin matrix is a matrix of collagen fibers,
     but it becomes calcified within 24 hours.
  3. Dentinogenesis takes place in two phases.
    a. Initial collagen matrix formation.
    b. Deposition of calcium phosphate crystals
       (hydroxyapatite).
      (1) The crystals grow, spread, and coalesce until
          the matrix is mineralized.
E. Amelogenesis.
  1. Ameloblasts begin to deposit enamel shortly after
     dentin deposition has begun.
  2. The enamel matrix is formed within the cell and
     migrates in vesicles to the apical end of the cell, where
     it is deposited.
F. Root sheath (Figure 1-70).
  1. Inner and outer enamel epithelial cells lengthen after
     crown completion.

2. The double layer of cells is called the *epithelial root sheath (Hertwig's sheath)*.
   a. At the apex, it bends inward at a 45-degree angle (epithelial diaphragm).
3. The inner cell layer induces odontoblasts to form root dentin.
4. The outer cell layer deposits a cuticular membrane (enameloid) on the root surface.
5. Mesenchymal cells appear in the pulp in what is known as the *pulp proliferative zone*.
6. These cells create new odontoblasts for dentin and fibroblasts for pulp.
7. The dentin tapers to the apical foramen.

G. Single root formation.
   1. After deposition of enameloid, the root sheath breaks up, creating epithelial rests (rests of Malassez).
   2. Mesenchymal cells move in to contact the root surface and become cementoblasts.
   3. Cementoblasts secrete cementoid, which mineralizes to form cementum.
   4. Near the CEJ, cementum is thinner and acellular.
   5. Cementum nearer the apex is thicker and cellular.
   6. It contains cementocytes and is formed after tooth eruption.

H. Multiple root formation.
   1. The shape of roots depends on the interaction of the inner and outer enamel epithelial cells and adjacent pulp mesenchymal cells.
   2. Extensions of the epithelial diaphragm grow at an increased rate until they fuse.
   3. Each extension forms the same as a single-rooted tooth.

I. Supporting structures.
   1. The PDL connects cementum and alveolar bone.
   2. The PDL and alveolar bone form from mesenchymal cells in the dental follicle.
   3. Fibroblasts develop from mesenchyme and appear on cementum in the cervical area of the tooth.
   4. Fibroblasts produce the collagen that forms connective tissue.
   5. The alveolar process develops as a bony trench around the teeth.
   6. Septa appear between teeth to create crypts.
   7. The collagen formed by fibroblasts attaches to cementum on one end and alveolar bone on the other to create the PDL.

J. Prefunctional eruptive phase.
   1. The prefunctional eruptive phase continues until the clinical crown contacts the opposing crown.
   2. Macrophages appear in soft tissue and release enzymes along the eruptive path, causing bone resorption.
   3. For permanent teeth replacing primary teeth, the resorptive process is similar to bony resorption in primary teeth.
   4. Monocytes form osteoclasts that resorb bone and primary roots.
   5. The alveolus grows in size as the tooth root grows.
   6. Occasionally, trauma may cause primary or permanent teeth to fuse to bone (ankylosis).
   7. Compensating alveolar process development continues while teeth are in function.
   8. It may take 2 to 3 years for completion of root formation after teeth are in function.
   9. Teeth may erupt slightly even later in life to compensate for wear.

K. Physiologic tooth movement.
   1. The arches grow in a vertical, facial, and buccal direction.
   2. The alveolar process must compensate for growth of the roots of permanent incisors and changes in position.
   3. Children pass through a mixed dentition stage as teeth erupt.
   4. Anterior force on teeth causes them to drift forward toward the midline (mesial drift).
   5. The teeth are also wearing occlusally and proximally.
   6. Mesial drift may create anterior crowding that is accentuated as a person ages.
   7. Crowding may create oral hygiene difficulties and periodontal problems.

L. Orthodontic movement of teeth.
   1. Bone is more easily remodeled than cementum.
   2. Remodeled bone shows arrest and reversal lines.
   3. It is easier to tilt teeth rather than move them bodily and extrude rather than intrude teeth.

4.3 Facial and Branchial Arch Development

A. Development of the oropharynx.
   The face begins forming in the fourth week; at that time, the body is about $\frac{1}{16}$ inch long.
   1. The neural plate bends ventrally, pushing the heart ventrally.
      a. An oral pocket develops between the forebrain and the heart, which eventually becomes the oral cavity.

B. Branchial (pharyngeal) arches (Figure 1-71).
   1. Externally, they appear as swellings; internally, they form pharyngeal pouches.
      a. Resemble gill slits.
   2. Externally, they disappear by the end of the fifth week as the second grows down to contact the fifth branchial arch (Figure 1-72).
      a. There are five or six branchial arches.
      b. They are separated by branchial clefts or grooves.

C. Branchial grooves and pharyngeal pouches.
   1. Clefts seen between the arches.
      a. The first branchial groove deepens to become the external auditory canal leading to the middle ear.
      b. The membrane at the depth of the first branchial groove becomes the tympanic membrane.

c. The middle ear and eustachian tube develop from the corresponding first pharyngeal pouch.

d. The second pharyngeal pouch becomes the palatine tonsils.

  (1) Tonsils function in the development of lymphocytes.

e. The third pharyngeal pouch becomes the inferior parathyroids and thymus.

f. The fourth pharyngeal pouch becomes the superior parathyroid.

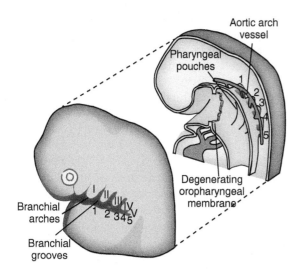

Figure 1-71 Sagittal view of pharyngeal arches with corresponding groove between each arch. *(Modified from Chiego D: Essentials of Oral Histology and Embryology: A Clinical Approach, ed 4, St. Louis, Mosby, 2014.)*

g. The fifth pharyngeal pouch becomes the ultimobranchial body.

  (1) Ultimobranchial function is unknown.

D. Vascular development.

  Each of the branchial arches has a right and left aortic arch vessel that leads from the heart through the arches to the face, brain, and posterior of the body.

1. The first and second branchial arches begin to develop in the fourth week and disappear in the fifth week.

2. The third arch vessels become prominent, taking over the facial area from the first two.

3. As the fourth and fifth arch vessels arise, the fourth becomes prominent, and the fifth disappears.

4. Finally, the sixth arch vessels arise and become dominant, along with the third and fourth.

5. The third arch vessels become the common carotid arteries, which supply the neck, face, and brain.

6. The fourth arch vessels become the dorsal aorta, which supplies the rest of the body.

7. The sixth arch vessels supply the lungs.

E. Muscular and neural development.

  Muscle cells become apparent in the first arch in the fifth week.

1. They spread within the mandibular arch into each muscle's site of origin in the sixth and seventh weeks.

2. The muscles of the first arch become the muscles of mastication.

3. By the 10th week, the muscles of the second arch have formed a thin sheet extending over the face and posterior to the ear.

4. The muscles of the fourth arch form the pharyngeal constrictor muscles.

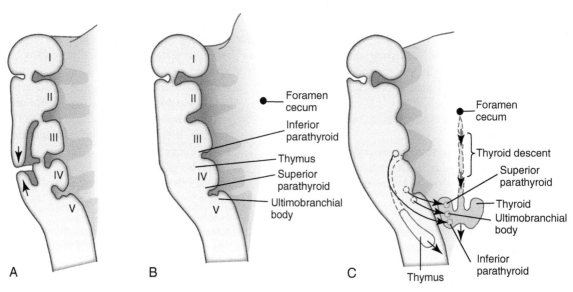

Figure 1-72 Cross section of the pharyngeal arches. **A,** Tissues of pharyngeal arches II and V overgrow together, which results in disappearance of arches II to V and external smoothing of the neck. **B,** Resulting external appearance follows overgrowth. **C,** Contribution of the pharyngeal pouches. *(From Chiego D: Essentials of Oral Histology and Embryology: A Clinical Approach, ed 4, St. Louis, Mosby, 2014.)*

5. By the end of the seventh week, CN V (first arch) and CN VII (second arch) have interdigitated with their respective muscle groups.

6. CN IX interdigitates with the third arch.

7. CN X interdigitates with the fourth arch.

F. Cartilaginous skeletal development (Figure 1-73).

  1. Meckel's cartilages appear bilaterally in the first arch.

    a. These structures are later absorbed into the forming jaw.

    b. Their posterior hinge becomes the malleus of the ear.

  2. Reichert's cartilage appears in the second arch.

    a. The stapes, styloid process, lesser horn, and upper body of the hyoid arise from this arch.

  3. The third arch forms the greater horn and lower part of the hyoid.

  4. The fourth arch forms hyoid cartilage.

  5. The fifth arch has no adult cartilage derivative.

  6. The sixth arch forms the laryngeal cartilage.

G. Cartilages of the face.

  The cartilaginous nasal capsule (ethmoid), the sphenoid, the auditory capsules, and the basioccipital cartilages are the first skeletal structures seen in the craniofacial area.

  1. They are called the *cranial base.*

  2. Later, these separate to form individual bones by endochondral bone formation.

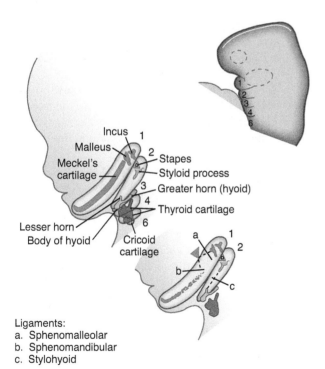

Ligaments:
a. Sphenomalleolar
b. Sphenomandibular
c. Stylohyoid

Figure 1-73 Cartilages derived from the pharyngeal arches. *(Modified from Chiego D: Essentials of Oral Histology and Embryology: A Clinical Approach, ed 4, St. Louis, Mosby, 2014.)*

H. Bones of the face.

  1. The protective bones of the face do not form from cartilage.

    a. These include the frontal, parietal, and squamous portions of the temporal and interoccipital bones.

  2. Facial bones also do not form from cartilage.

    a. They include the premaxillary, maxillary, zygomatic, and petrous portions of the temporal bone.

  3. Maxillary bones also grow medially into the palate to support the palatine shelf tissue.

  4. Mandibular bones grow laterally to the first arch cartilage and posteriorly to meet the bony body of the cartilaginous condyle.

  5. Together these replace Meckel's cartilage.

  6. The mandible forms from several units.

    a. Condylar.

      (1) Forms the articulation.

    b. Body.

      (1) Center of all growth.

    c. Angular process.

      (1) Responds to lateral pterygoid and masseter muscles.

    d. Coronoid process.

      (1) Responds to temporalis muscle development.

    e. Alveolar process.

      (1) Responds to development of the teeth.

I. Sutures of the face.

  Sutures are fibrous joints (articulations) in which opposing surfaces are closely joined.

  1. Sutures are named for the bones they join.

    a. The articulations may consist of a band of connective tissue.

  2. External face.

    a. All sutures have a central zone or proliferating connective tissue cells along peripheral bony fronts.

    b. All are surrounded by fibrous connective tissue.

    c. There are three types of sutures of the face.

      (1) Simple.

      (2) Serrated.

        (a) Interdigitating type of suture.

      (3) Squamosal.

        (a) Beveled or overlapping.

  3. Internal face.

    a. Synchondrosis—all have an interposing band of cartilage.

    b. Grow by forming new cartilage in the center of the suture.

J. Structures derived from branchial arches (Figure 1-74).

K. Formation of structures.

  1. Week by week.

    a. Between the fourth and eighth weeks, all structures are formed and are recognizable. From that point on, they add mass.

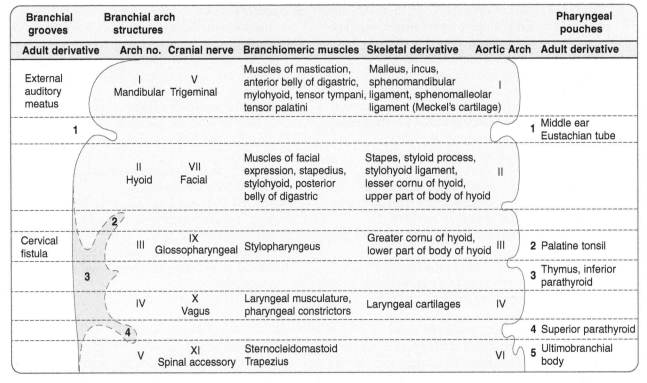

Branchial grooves	Branchial arch structures						Pharyngeal pouches
Adult derivative	Arch no.	Cranial nerve	Branchiomeric muscles	Skeletal derivative	Aortic Arch	Adult derivative	
External auditory meatus	I Mandibular	V Trigeminal	Muscles of mastication, anterior belly of digastric, mylohyoid, tensor tympani, tensor palatini	Malleus, incus, sphenomandibular ligament, sphenomalleolar ligament (Meckel's cartilage)	I		
1						1 Middle ear Eustachian tube	
	II Hyoid	VII Facial	Muscles of facial expression, stapedius, stylohyoid, posterior belly of digastric	Stapes, styloid process, stylohyoid ligament, lesser cornu of hyoid, upper part of body of hyoid	II		
Cervical fistula	2 III	IX Glossopharyngeal	Stylopharyngeus	Greater cornu of hyoid, lower part of body of hyoid	III	2 Palatine tonsil	
3						3 Thymus, inferior parathyroid	
	IV	X Vagus	Laryngeal musculature, pharyngeal constrictors	Laryngeal cartilages	IV		
	4					4 Superior parathyroid	
	V	XI Spinal accessory	Sternocleidomastoid Trapezius		VI	5 Ultimobranchial body	

Figure 1-74 Summary of structures that develop from pharyngeal arches, pharyngeal grooves, and pharyngeal pouches. *(From Chiego D: Essentials of Oral Histology and Embryology: A Clinical Approach, ed 4, St. Louis, Mosby, 2014.)*

2. Week 4.
  a. By the end of the third week, branchial arch I (called the *mandibular arch*) has divided into left and right maxillary and mandibular processes.
  b. By the beginning of the fourth week, the primitive mouth (stomodeum) has formed.
  c. The buccopharyngeal membrane separates the stomodeum and foregut and is located in the area of the palatine tonsils.
3. Week 5.
  a. The embryo is ¼ inch long.
  b. Depressions called *nasal pits* appear in the frontal process.
  c. Nasal pits divide the frontal process.
    (1) Medial nasal processes.
    (2) Lateral nasal processes.
  d. Oropharyngeal membrane ruptures.
  e. Eyes form on side of the head.
4. Week 6.
  a. Globular processes appear on the medial nasal process.
    (1) Form the philtrum of the lip.
  b. The primary palate forms, later known as the *premaxilla*.
  c. The globular processes begin to fuse with the lateral nasal processes and the maxillary processes.
    (1) Takes about 2 weeks.

5. Week 7.
  a. The face has a more human appearance.
  b. Lateral growth of the brain moves eyes to the front of the face.
  c. Upper lip has fused, creating the medially located philtrum.
  d. The hillocks have fused to form the ears.
L. Development of vascular blood supply to the face.
  1. Aortic arch formation and changes.
  2. A dorsal aortic arch forms corresponding to each branchial arch.
    a. The first and second aortic arch shrivel.
    b. The third aortic arch becomes the common carotid.
    c. The fourth aortic arch becomes the dorsal aorta.
    d. The dorsal aorta becomes the internal carotid, which develops a stapedial artery.
    e. The sixth aortic arch forms the pulmonary circulation.
    f. The ventral aorta becomes the ventral pharyngeal artery.
  3. Shift from internal to external carotid artery (Figure 1-75).
    a. The stapedial artery dwindles, and vessels arising from it become attached to the external carotid artery and will supply the face.
    b. The internal carotid subsequently supplies the brain.

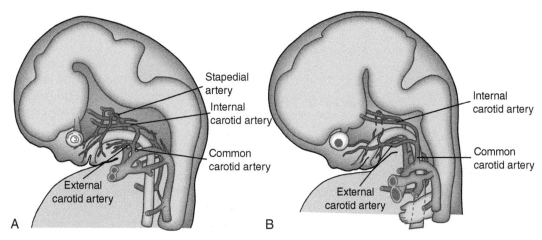

Figure 1-75 Shift in vascular supply of the face. **A,** The face and brain are first supplied by the internal carotid artery. **B,** The facial vessels at 7 weeks of gestation detach from the internal carotid artery and attach to the external carotid artery. *(From Chiego D: Essentials of Oral Histology and Embryology: A Clinical Approach, ed 4, St. Louis, Mosby, 2014.)*

M. Medial and lateral palatal processes.

The palate develops from an anterior, wedge-shaped medial part and two lateral palatine processes.

1. Medial palate.
   a. Also called the *primary palate*.
   b. Develops from the globular processes near the end of the sixth week.
   c. Is a floor to the nasal pits.
2. Lateral palatine processes.
   a. Appear at the eighth week.
   b. Arise as left and right palatine processes coming off the left and right maxillary processes.
   c. Form the posterior portion of the hard palate and the soft palate.

N. Palatal elevation.

1. Occurs rapidly as the palatine processes flip up over the descending tongue.
2. Fusion of the hard palate begins in the ninth week, following palatal elevation.
3. Contact between segments is initially made behind the medial palatine segment.
   a. Continues in an anterior and posterior direction until the entire palate is complete by the end of the 12th week.

4.3.1 Internal Facial Development

A. Muscle development.

1. Muscle cells become apparent during the fifth week and spread during the sixth and seventh weeks.
   a. They grow over the face and attach to developing bones.

B. Neural development.

1. The CNS begins forming during the third week.
2. Cranial nerves grow from the area of the developing brain to innervate the muscles of the head.

   a. CN V—innervates muscles of mastication.
   b. CN VII—innervates stylohyoid and stapedius muscles and posterior belly of the digastric muscle.
   c. CN IX—innervates stylopharyngeal and upper pharyngeal constrictor muscles.
   d. CN X—innervates inferior constrictor and laryngeal muscles.

C. Cartilaginous skeletal development.

1. First branchial arch.
   a. Meckel's cartilage.
      (1) Originally articulates with the malleus, which becomes a hearing bone of the middle ear.
   b. Eventually the TMJ becomes functional, and Meckel's cartilage is incorporated into the mandible.
2. Second branchial arch.
   a. Reichert's cartilage.
      (1) Forms the stapes, styloid process, and the lesser horn and upper part of the body of the hyoid.
3. Third branchial arch.
   a. Forms the greater horn and lower part of the hyoid body.
4. Fourth branchial arch.
   a. Forms the thyroid cartilage.
5. Sixth branchial arch.
   a. Forms the laryngeal cartilage.

D. Tongue (Figure 1-76).

1. Muscles of the head (including the tongue) arise from blocks of mesoderm (myotomes).
2. Nerves.
   a. CN V—sensory nerve to anterior tongue.
   b. CN VII—special sensory nerve to anterior two thirds (body) of tongue.
   c. CN IX—sensory nerve to posterior third (base) of tongue.
   d. CN X—also innervates the base of the tongue.

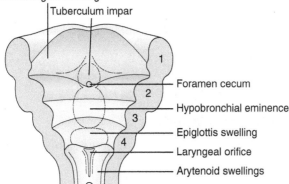

Figure 1-76 Early tongue development. *(From Coburne MT, DiBiase AT: Handbook of Orthodontics, St. Louis, Mosby, 2010.)*

3. Body.
   a. The anterior, more movable, part of the tongue develops from the first branchial arch during the fourth week.
   b. Extends from the tip to a V-shaped groove called the *terminal sulcus* behind the circumvallate papillae.
4. Root.
   a. The posterior, less movable, part of the tongue develops from the second and third branchial arches.
5. Development.
   a. Arises from two mounds of tissue called *lateral lingual swellings* and the *tuberculum impar*.
   b. The lateral parts rapidly enlarge and merge.
   c. A U-shaped sulcus develops around the anterior part of the tongue.
E. Thyroid gland.
   At the point of the V-shaped groove (called the *terminal sulcus*) is a depression known as *foramen cecum*.
   1. This location is the embryologic beginning point of the thyroid gland.
   2. During development, the epithelium in this area begins to migrate into the neck.
   3. The path is called the *thyroglossal duct*.
   4. The glandular tissue that forms the thyroid is carried into the neck with the epithelium.
   5. The pathway usually disappears eventually.
   6. A remnant can persist, and aberrant thyroid tissue that can cause a cyst may be found anywhere along the path.
F. Facial clefts.
   1. May be unilateral, bilateral, or medial.
   2. May be complete with no joining of tissue.
   3. May be incomplete with joining of soft tissue but not bone.
   4. Normally, philtrum ridges are the line of fusion.

G. Palatal clefts.
   1. Most cleft palates occur in combination with cleft lips.
   2. They may also occur as isolated defects.
   3. Palatal clefts must extend around the medial palatal segment before they reach the midline.
H. Other defects—are involved with defects in fusion and merging.
   1. Fusion.
      a. Epithelial adhesion followed by reorganization of the deep tissues to mesenchyme.
      b. After the ectoderm has fused, it is replaced by mesenchyme.
      c. Sometimes globules of ectoderm persist and become epithelial rests, which may become cysts.
   2. Merging.
      a. Filling in of a cleft.
      b. If failure occurs at the junction of the lateral nasal and maxillary processes, it causes an oblique facial cleft.
      c. If failure occurs at the globular processes, it causes a midsagittal cleft in the upper lip.

4.4 General Embryology

The study of embryology allows us to see how a single cell can develop to form an entire person. The journey begins with fertilization of the egg. After fertilization, the egg (now called a *zygote*) begins a trip along the fallopian tube toward the uterus. As it travels, it starts to divide, first into two cells, then four, then eight, and so on. Eventually, it forms a solid ball called a *morula* (for mulberry). The morula continues to grow, and as it does, the interior becomes hollow. At this stage, the aggregation of cells is called a *blastocyst*. Along the interior of one side of the blastocyst, a mass of cells begins forming; it arches into the cavity of the blastocyst until there is a second, smaller cavity under the group of cells. The organism itself forms from this small group of cells, with most of the blastocyst forming the yolk sac and the yolk that will be consumed by the developing organism.

The small mass of cells is called the *embryonic disk*. At first, it is only one cell layer thick; however, it soon divides into three layers. These primordial layers are significant because each forms distinct structural parts of the body.

The layer facing the smaller cavity is called *ectoderm*. Ectoderm forms nervous tissue; sensory epithelia of the eye, ear, and nose; epidermis, hair, and nails; mammary and cutaneous glands; epithelia of sinuses; oral and nasal cavities; intraoral glands; and tooth enamel.

The middle layer is called *mesoderm*. Mesoderm forms muscles, connective tissue, bone, cartilage, blood, dentin, cementum, pulp, and the PDL.

The layer facing the larger cavity forms *endoderm*. Endoderm forms the gastrointestinal tract epithelium.

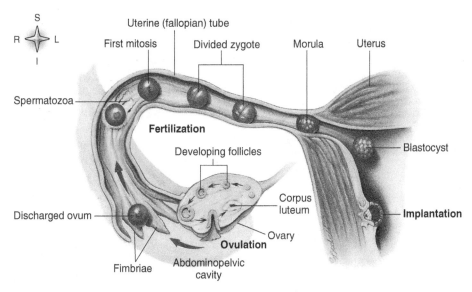

Figure 1-77 Implantation of a fertilized ovum (zygote) in the wall of the uterus. *(From Sanders MJ: Mosby's Paramedic Textbook, ed 4, St. Louis, Mosby, 2012.)*

A. Definition of basic terms.
 1. Embryology.
  a. The study of the development of the individual during the first 8 weeks after conception.
   (1) Formation of the organs occurs in this period.
  b. Histology.
   (1) Microscopic anatomy.
   (2) Portion of anatomy dealing with the minute structure, composition, and function of tissues.
  c. Cytology.
   (1) The study of individual cells and their parts.
B. Embryo.
 1. Periods of prenatal development.
  a. 0 to 2 weeks—proliferative.
   (1) Includes fertilization, implantation, and formation of the embryonic disc.
  b. 2 to 8 weeks—embryonic.
   (1) Tissues develop to create organ systems.
  c. 8 weeks to 9 months—fetal.
   (1) Increase in body weight and size.
 2. Fertilization—the egg is fertilized in the distal portion of the uterine tube, which is called the *ampulla of the oviduct* (Figure 1-77).
  a. The fertilized egg is first called a *zygote*.
  b. As it travels toward the uterus, the number of cells begins to increase, but the size does not increase at first.
   (1) At this point, the many-celled ball is called a *morula*.
  c. After 5 to 6 days, it has 16 to 32 cells and reaches the uterus, where the endometrium has developed to receive it.
   (1) The morula becomes a blastocyst as it increases in size and becomes hollow.

3. Implantation—usually occurs 6 to 10 days after conception.
  a. Soon after entering the uterine cavity, the blastocyst sticks to the uterine lining.
  b. The lining deteriorates at the site of adhesion, and the blastocyst becomes embedded in the wall of the endometrium.
4. Blastocyst—a hollow mass of cells that forms as cells pull away from the center of the morula.
  a. The peripheral cells are called the *trophoblast*, with the blastocele being the cavity.
  b. This hollow ball of cells develops an inner cell mass against one wall.
  c. The small mass enlarges to form an area separating two small cavities.
   (1) This layer is called the *embryonic disc*.
  d. Cells facing the smaller cavity form the primordial ectodermal layer, and cells facing the larger one form the primordial endodermal layer.
5. Yolk sac—implantation of the blastocyst causes breakdown of endometrial tissue.
  a. This provides food and materials for the embryo for a few weeks.
  b. The embryo sends out branches of umbilical arteries and veins.
  c. The yolk supplies nutrition to the embryo through the vitelline arteries.
  d. At the same time, the placenta and its blood supply are forming.
  e. When the yolk sac becomes depleted, the placenta takes over supplying nutrients and removing waste.
  f. The umbilical and placental system is in place 5 weeks after implantation.
  g. Nutrients and wastes cross, but maternal and fetal blood do not mix.

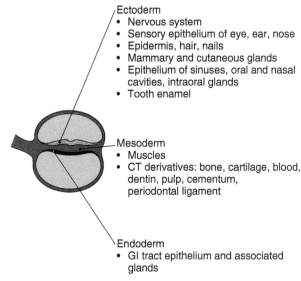

Ectoderm
- Nervous system
- Sensory epithelium of eye, ear, nose
- Epidermis, hair, nails
- Mammary and cutaneous glands
- Epithelium of sinuses, oral and nasal cavities, intraoral glands
- Tooth enamel

Mesoderm
- Muscles
- CT derivatives: bone, cartilage, blood, dentin, pulp, cementum, periodontal ligament

Endoderm
- GI tract epithelium and associated glands

Figure 1-78 Derivatives of ectoderm, mesoderm, and endoderm germ layers. *CT,* connective tissue; *GI,* gastrointestinal. *(From Chiego D: Essentials of Oral Histology and Embryology: A Clinical Approach, ed 4, St. Louis, Mosby, 2014.)*

6. Extraembryonic coelom—at 9 or 10 days, the trophoblast portion of the blastocyst produces mesoblasts, which begin to fill the blastocyst cavity.
   a. The blastocyst grows faster than these cells can fill the space, so they end up lining the cavity around the actual embryo.
   b. These cells form the amnion, vitelline sac, and chorion.
C. Primordial layers (Figure 1-78).
D. Development of human tissues.
   1. Epithelial structures and derivatives.
      a. Mesoderm.
         (1) Forms the dermis of the epithelium and the visceral mesoderm that covers the yolk sac and subsequently becomes the gastrointestinal tract.
      b. Ectoderm.
         (1) Initially, the embryo is covered by a single layer of ectodermal cells.
         (2) By 11 to 12 weeks, this thickens into four layers.
         (3) Later melanocytes invade and pigment the skin.
   2. Nervous system.
      a. Folds arise in the neural plate in the third week.
         (1) The fold facing the smaller cavity shows three areas that form the forebrain, midbrain, and hindbrain.
      b. The forebrain curls down toward the chest as the cranial nerves develop.
   3. Connective tissue.
      a. Develops from somites as fibroblasts migrating from either side of the neural tube.

4. Cartilage and bone—cartilage cells arise from the sclerotome and migrate to surround the notochord and spinal cord.
   a. The skeleton forms in a segmental pattern.
   b. Cartilage grows both by apposition and by interstitial growth.
   c. Bone replaces cartilage through a process called *endochondral bone development* or by intramembranous bone formation.
5. Muscle—by the 10th prenatal week, myoblasts migrate from the myotome.
6. Cardiovascular system—originates from angioblasts, which arise from mesoderm in the walls of the yolk sac.
   a. For the first few weeks, nutrition is provided through the vitelline vascular system.
   b. The heart starts pumping in the fourth week.

Acknowledgments

The section editor acknowledges Dr. Jean Yang for her contributions as author and editor of Section 1, Edition 1.

Sample Questions

1. The lateral pterygoid muscle attaches to which of the following?
   A. Lateral surface of the lateral pterygoid plate
   B. Medial surface of the lateral pterygoid plate
   C. Lateral surface of the medial pterygoid plate
   D. Medial surface of the medial pterygoid plate
   E. Pyramidal process of palatine bone
2. Which of the following muscles is responsible for the formation of the posterior tonsillar pillar?
   A. Stylopharyngeus
   B. Tensor veli palatini
   C. Palatoglossus
   D. Palatopharyngeus
   E. Levator veli palatini
3. The superior and inferior ophthalmic veins drain into the _____.
   A. Internal jugular vein
   B. Pterygoid plexus
   C. Frontal vein
   D. Infraorbital vein
   E. Facial vein
4. The masseter originates from the _____.
   A. Condyle of the mandible
   B. Infratemporal crest of the sphenoid bone
   C. Inferior border of the zygomatic arch
   D. Pyramidal process of the palatine bone
   E. Mastoid process of temporal bone
5. Which of the following muscles adducts the vocal cords?

A. Lateral cricoarytenoid
B. Posterior cricoarytenoid
C. Cricothyroid
D. Vocalis
E. Tensor veli palatini

6. Which of the following strata of oral epithelium is engaged in mitosis?
   A. Basale
   B. Granulosum
   C. Corneum
   D. Spinosum

7. The auriculotemporal nerve encircles which of the following vessels?
   A. Maxillary artery
   B. Superficial temporal artery
   C. Deep auricular artery
   D. Middle meningeal artery
   E. Anterior tympanic artery

8. The muscle that is found in the walls of the heart is characterized by _____.
   A. A peripherally placed nucleus
   B. Multiple nuclei
   C. Intercalated discs
   D. Fibers with spindle-shaped cells

9. All of the following are found in the posterior triangle of the neck *except* one. Which one is the *exception*?
   A. External jugular vein
   B. Subclavian vein
   C. Hypoglossal nerve
   D. Phrenic nerve
   E. Brachial plexus

10. Deoxygenated blood from the transverse sinus drains into the _____.
    A. Inferior sagittal sinus
    B. Confluence of sinuses
    C. Sigmoid sinus
    D. Straight sinus
    E. Internal jugular vein

11. The vestigial cleft of Rathke's pouch in the hypophysis is located between the _____.
    A. Anterior and posterior lobes
    B. Anterior lobe and hypothalamus
    C. Posterior lobe and hypothalamus
    D. Median eminence and optic chiasm

12. Involution of the thymus would occur following which year in a healthy individual?
    A. 0 years (at birth)
    B. 12th year
    C. 20th year
    D. 60th year

13. Blood from the internal carotid artery reaches the posterior cerebral artery by the _____.
    A. Anterior cerebral artery
    B. Anterior communicating artery
    C. Posterior communicating artery

D. Posterior superior cerebellar artery
E. Basilar artery

14. The infraorbital nerve is a branch of the _____.
    A. Optic nerve
    B. Oculomotor nerve
    C. Ophthalmic nerve
    D. Maxillary nerve
    E. Mandibular nerve

15. Which of the following cells are capable of mitosis?
    A. Smooth muscle
    B. Skeletal muscle
    C. Cardiac muscle
    D. Type I pneumocytes
    E. Neurons

16. Which of the following types of epithelium lines acinar units of salivary glands?
    A. Simple squamous
    B. Stratified squamous
    C. Simple cuboidal
    D. Simple columnar
    E. Pseudostratified columnar

17. To which of the following bones is the tensor tympani attached?
    A. Incus
    B. Malleus
    C. Stapes
    D. Hyoid
    E. Mandible

18. In mature dentin, the ratio of inorganic to organic matter is approximately _____.
    A. 94:6
    B. 50:50
    C. 70:30
    D. 80:20
    E. 60:40

19. Which of the following cells forms the myelin sheath around myelinated nerves in the CNS?
    A. Schwann cells
    B. Astrocytes
    C. Microglia
    D. Oligodendrocytes
    E. Amphicytes

20. Which of the following nerves supplies taste sensation to the anterior two thirds of the tongue?
    A. Hypoglossal
    B. Glossopharyngeal
    C. Lingual
    D. Facial
    E. Mental

Test items 21-26 refer to the following scenario.
A 24-year-old man presents to your office for an emergency visit after being hit on the left side of his face with a soccer ball. He complains that his "tooth got knocked out" and that his jaw feels "out of place." He has no other medical conditions.

21. During the intraoral examination, you find that the patient's lower second premolar is missing. Which type of alveolodental fibers was *least* involved in resisting the force that pulled this patient's tooth out of its socket?
    A. Apical
    B. Oblique
    C. Alveolar crest
    D. Interradicular

22. You also notice that a cusp of his mandibular second molar has fractured off and that dentin is exposed. If this patient were to drink something cold, what would he sense?
    A. Pain
    B. Pressure
    C. Vibration
    D. Temperature

23. You decide to take a radiograph of the fractured tooth. On the first film, you miss the apex of the tooth, so you decide to take another radiograph. Relaxation of which of the patient's muscles would help you in taking the second film?
    A. Geniohyoid
    B. Stylohyoid
    C. Mylohyoid
    D. Levator veli palatini
    E. Palatopharyngeus

24. On further examination, you determine that the articular disc of the patient's TMJ has been displaced. If the patient contracts his lateral pterygoid muscle, the disc will move _____.
    A. Posteriorly and medially
    B. Anteriorly and medially
    C. Posteriorly and laterally
    D. Anteriorly and laterally

25. During the examination, the patient observes that he cannot feel it when you touch part of his cheek and his upper lip. Which of the following nerves was probably damaged during the accident?
    A. Lingual
    B. Maxillary
    C. Long buccal
    D. Superior alveolar
    E. Inferior alveolar

26. You decide to restore the missing cusp on the patient's molar. During the administration of the IAN block, which of the following ligaments is *most* likely damaged?
    A. Sphenomandibular
    B. Stylomandibular
    C. Temporomandibular
    D. Interdental

27. The lateral thoracic wall of the axilla is covered by which of the following muscles?
    A. Pectoralis major
    B. Pectoralis minor
    C. Serratus anterior
    D. Subscapularis
    E. Latissimus dorsi

28. The trochlea of the humerus bone articulates with the _____.
    A. Ulna of the forearm
    B. Radius of the forearm
    C. Coronoid process of the ulna of the forearm
    D. Olecranon of the ulna of the forearm
    E. Medial epicondyle

29. Which of the following muscles of the back is supplied by CN XI?
    A. Levator scapulae
    B. Latissimus dorsi
    C. Trapezius
    D. Major rhomboid
    E. Minor rhomboid

30. There are _____ pairs of true ribs.
    A. 4
    B. 5
    C. 7
    D. 11
    E. 12

31. _____ vertebrae are characterized by a heart-shaped body.
    A. Cervical
    B. Thoracic
    C. Lumbar
    D. Sacral
    E. Coccygeal

32. The sternal angle between the manubrium and the sternum marks the position of the _____ rib.
    A. First
    B. Second
    C. Third
    D. Fourth
    E. Fifth

33. Which muscle of the anterolateral abdominal wall is described as being beltlike or straplike?
    A. External oblique muscle
    B. Internal oblique muscle
    C. Transversus abdominis muscle
    D. Rectus abdominis muscle
    E. Quadratus lumborum muscle

34. In addition to the esophagus itself, which of the following structures also passes through the diaphragm through the esophageal opening?
    A. Aorta
    B. Inferior vena cava
    C. Azygos vein
    D. Posterior and anterior vagal trunks
    E. Splanchnic nerves

35. The inferior aspect of the diaphragm is supplied with blood by which of the following arteries?
    A. Median sacral artery
    B. Lumbar arteries

C. Inferior phrenic arteries
D. Celiac trunk
E. Superior mesenteric artery

36. Oral epithelium is composed of _____ epithelium.
    A. Keratinized simple squamous
    B. Keratinized stratified squamous
    C. Nonkeratinized simple squamous
    D. Nonkeratinized stratified squamous
    E. Nonkeratinized stratified columnar

37. Which of the following statements is *true* of the histology of the trachea?
    A. The mucosa is covered with oral epithelium.
    B. Elastic cartilage rings lie deep to the submucosa.
    C. The cartilage is ring-shaped; the open end of the ring faces anterior.
    D. The cartilage is covered by a perichondrium.
    E. Skeletal muscle extends across the open end of each cartilage.

38. Terminal bronchioles are characterized by _____ cells.
    A. Goblet
    B. Ciliated cuboidal
    C. Nonciliated cuboidal
    D. Ciliated squamous
    E. Nonciliated squamous

39. The most superficial layer of the epidermis is the stratum _____.
    A. Spinosum
    B. Basale
    C. Granulosum
    D. Lucidum
    E. Corneum

40. Langerhans' cells are located primarily in stratum _____.
    A. Corneum
    B. Lucidum
    C. Granulosum
    D. Spinosum
    E. Basale

41. Arteriovenous anastomoses in deeper skin are important in _____.
    A. Immunity
    B. Thermoregulation
    C. Controlling the arrector (erector) pili muscle
    D. Pigmentation
    E. Pain sensation

42. Which of the following bones is formed by intramembranous ossification?
    A. Humerus
    B. Lumbar vertebrae
    C. Frontal bone of the skull
    D. Ribs
    E. Clavicle

43. Osteocytes are found in _____ in mature bone.
    A. Trabeculae
    B. Lacunae
    C. The central canal

D. Canaliculi
E. Spicules

44. _____ marks the end of growth in length of long bones.
    A. Diaphyseal closure
    B. Epiphyseal closure
    C. Ossification
    D. Formation of periosteum
    E. Cessation of bone remodeling

45. The branchial arches disappear when the _____ branchial arch grows down to contact the _____.
    A. Second; third branchial arch
    B. Second; fifth branchial arch
    C. Third; fifth branchial arch
    D. First; first branchial groove
    E. First; sixth branchial groove

46. Facial nerves are derived from the _____ branchial arch.
    A. First
    B. Second
    C. Third
    D. Fourth
    E. Fifth and sixth

47. Cytochrome P450 enzymes may be found in which of the following cellular organelles?
    A. Mitochondria
    B. Golgi apparatus
    C. Lysosome
    D. Ribosome
    E. Endoplasmic reticulum

48. What type of collagen is found in cementum?
    A. Type I collagen
    B. Type II collagen
    C. Type III collagen
    D. Type IV collagen
    E. Type V collagen

49. Calcium binds to which of the following for contraction in smooth muscle?
    A. Troponin C
    B. Calmodulin
    C. Myosin
    D. Actin
    E. Desmosomes

50. Lymph from the mandibular incisors drains chiefly into _____.
    A. Submandibular nodes
    B. Submental nodes
    C. Superficial parotid nodes
    D. Deep cervical nodes
    E. Occipital nodes

51. Which of the following muscles attaches to the anterior end of the articular disc of the TMJ?
    A. Superficial head of the medial pterygoid muscle
    B. Deep head of the medial pterygoid muscle
    C. Superior head of the lateral pterygoid muscle
    D. Inferior head of the lateral pterygoid muscle

52. All of the following arteries are branches of the mandibular division of the maxillary artery *except* one. Which one is the *exception*?
    A. Incisive artery
    B. Submental artery
    C. Middle meningeal artery
    D. Mylohyoid artery
    E. Deep auricular artery

53. The maxillary nerve passes through which of the following?
    A. Superior orbital fissure
    B. Internal acoustic meatus
    C. Foramen ovale
    D. Foramen rotundum
    E. Foramen spinosum

54. Injury to which of the following nerves would affect abduction of the eyeball?
    A. Optic nerve
    B. Oculomotor
    C. Trochlear
    D. Trigeminal
    E. Abducens

55. Nucleus ambiguus contains the cell bodies of which of the following cranial nerves?
    A. CN III, CN IV, and CN V
    B. CN VII, CN IX, and CN X
    C. CN VII, CN IX, and CN XI
    D. CN IX, CN X, and CN XI
    E. CN IX, CN X, and CN XII

56. The articulating surfaces of the TMJ are covered with _____.
    A. Fibrocartilage
    B. Hyaline cartilage
    C. Articular cartilage
    D. Elastic cartilage
    E. Perichondrium

57. The primary sensory neurons' nucleus of termination involved in the jaw jerk reflex is the _____.
    A. Facial nucleus
    B. Trochlear nucleus
    C. Mesencephalic nucleus
    D. Spinal trigeminal nucleus
    E. Nucleus of solitary tract

58. Red pulp in the spleen consists of _____.
    A. Fibroblasts
    B. T lymphocytes
    C. B lymphocytes
    D. Macrophages
    E. Chromaffin cells

59. The vertebral artery meets with the basilar artery at the lower border of the _____.
    A. Midbrain
    B. Pons
    C. Medulla
    D. Temporal lobe
    E. C1

60. Where are the cells that produce calcitonin located?
    A. Red marrow
    B. Adrenal gland
    C. Parathyroid gland
    D. Thyroid gland
    E. Spleen

61. Chromosomes line up at a cell's equator during which phase of mitosis?
    A. Telophase
    B. Metaphase
    C. Interphase
    D. Anaphase
    E. Prophase

62. Which of the following types of epithelium lines the oropharynx?
    A. Simple squamous
    B. Stratified squamous
    C. Simple cuboidal
    D. Simple columnar
    E. Pseudostratified columnar

63. Which of the following organelles is surrounded by a double membrane?
    A. Ribosome
    B. Golgi apparatus
    C. Lysosome
    D. Cytoplasmic inclusion
    E. Mitochondria

64. Hassall's corpuscles are found in the medulla of which of the following glands?
    A. Thymus
    B. Thyroid
    C. Parathyroid
    D. Pineal
    E. Suprarenal

65. Which of the following are the *most* abundant in the fovea centralis of the eyeball?
    A. Rod cells
    B. Cone cells
    C. Rod and cone cells
    D. Amacrine cells
    E. Ganglion cells

66. Which of the following bones is part of the superior wall (roof) of the orbit?
    A. Zygomatic
    B. Lacrimal
    C. Sphenoid
    D. Maxilla
    E. Ethmoid

Test items 67-70 refer to the following scenario.

A 30-year-old woman comes to your office for a dental examination. She has not been to the dentist in 2 years. The patient has type 1 diabetes, which requires her to take insulin. She is otherwise in good health. On intraoral examination, you notice that the dorsum of her tongue has a thick, matted appearance and diagnose hairy tongue. You also find that the patient has deep caries in her upper second maxillary molar.

67. Which type of papillae is affected that causes the hair-like appearance of her tongue?
    A. Foliate
    B. Circumvallate
    C. Fungiform
    D. Filiform

68. On the patient's radiograph, you notice that the pulp chamber in the carious molar appears smaller than the surrounding teeth. This is *most* likely due to the deposition of which type of dentin?
    A. Secondary
    B. Tertiary
    C. Mantle
    D. Sclerotic

69. You decide to remove the caries and prepare the patient for anesthesia. Which nerve must you anesthetize to ensure adequate anesthesia for the patient?
    A. Nasopalatine nerve
    B. Greater palatine nerve
    C. Anterior superior alveolar nerve
    D. Middle superior alveolar nerve
    E. Posterior superior alveolar nerve

70. After administering the anesthetic, the patient complains that her "heart feels like it's racing." You explain to her that it may be from the epinephrine in the anesthesia. Which of the following glands could *most* likely cause the same symptoms in the patient?
    A. Hypophysis
    B. Thyroid
    C. Pineal
    D. Suprarenal

71. All of the following are rotator cuff muscles *except* one. Which one is the *exception*?
    A. Supraspinatous muscle
    B. Infraspinatous muscle
    C. Teres minor muscle
    D. Teres major muscle
    E. Subscapularis muscle

72. The brachial plexus of nerves arises from which of the following roots of the anterior primary rami of spinal nerves?
    A. All cervical roots (C1–C8)
    B. All thoracic roots (T1–T12)
    C. C8 and T1.
    D. C5 through C8 and T1
    E. C5 through C8 and T1 through T4

73. The right subclavian artery arises from the _____, and the left subclavian artery arises from the _____.
    A. Axillary artery; aortic arch
    B. Brachiocephalic artery; aortic arch
    C. Aortic arch; brachiocephalic artery
    D. Brachiocephalic artery; axillary artery
    E. Axillary artery; brachial artery

74. The pulmonary vein of the lung carries:
    A. Unoxygenated blood from the lungs to the heart
    B. Oxygenated blood from the lungs to the heart
    C. Unoxygenated blood to the lungs from the heart
    D. Oxygenated blood to the lungs from the heart
    E. Oxygenated blood from the heart to the lungs

75. The _____ of the heart is also known as the mitral valve.
    A. Right atrioventricular valve
    B. Left atrioventricular valve
    C. Pulmonary valve
    D. Aortic valve
    E. Tricuspid valve

76. The cricopharyngeus muscle of the esophagus _____.
    A. Is a parasympathetic stimulator of peristalsis
    B. Is a sympathetic inhibitor of peristalsis
    C. Prevents swallowing air at the pharyngeal end
    D. Prevents regurgitation of stomach contents at the abdominal end
    E. Controls the gag reflex

77. The pancreas is enveloped at its head by the _____.
    A. First part of the duodenum
    B. Second part of the duodenum
    C. Third part of the duodenum
    D. Fourth part of the duodenum
    E. First part of the jejunum

78. The gallbladder arises from the _____.
    A. Common hepatic duct
    B. Common bile duct
    C. Left hepatic duct
    D. Cystic duct
    E. Bile canaliculi

79. The apex of a medullary pyramid in the kidney is called the _____.
    A. Cortex
    B. Medulla
    C. Renal papilla
    D. Major calyx
    E. Minor calyx

80. Ureters travel inferiorly just _____ the parietal peritoneum of the posterior body wall. They pass _____ to the common iliac arteries as they enter the pelvis.
    A. Above; posterior
    B. Above; anterior
    C. Below; posterior
    D. Below; anterior
    E. Above; superior

81. The lumen of the gastrointestinal tract is lined with _____.
    A. Mucosa
    B. Submucosa
    C. Muscularis externa
    D. Fibrosa
    E. Adventitia

82. GALT produces secretory _____.
    A. IgA
    B. IgD
    C. IgE
    D. IgG
    E. IgM

83. The muscularis externa has a third layer in the _____.
    A. Esophagus
    B. Stomach
    C. Liver
    D. Small intestine
    E. Large intestine

84. Which portion of uriniferous tubules contains squamous epithelial cells?
    A. Proximal convoluted tubule
    B. Thick descending limb of Henle's loop
    C. Thin segment of Henle's loop
    D. Thick ascending segment of Henle's loop
    E. Distal convoluted tubule

85. The _____ is a component of the juxtaglomerular apparatus that functions in regulation of blood pressure.
    A. Proximal convoluted tubule
    B. Distal convoluted tubule
    C. Bowman's capsule
    D. Glomerulus
    E. Macula densa

86. Urinary filtrate is most hypotonic in the _____.
    A. Proximal convoluted tubule
    B. Descending limb of Henle's loop
    C. Thin segment of Henle's loop
    D. Thick ascending segment of Henle's loop
    E. Distal convoluted tubule

87. The _____ differentiates into ameloblasts.
    A. Stellate reticulum
    B. Inner enamel epithelium in the cap stage
    C. Inner enamel epithelium in the bell stage
    D. Outer enamel epithelium in the cap stage
    E. Outer enamel epithelium in the bell stage

88. The dental lamina arises from _____.
    A. Somites
    B. Neural crest cells
    C. The first branchial arch
    D. The second branchial arch
    E. The buccopharyngeal membrane

89. The correct order of tooth formation is _____.
    A. Ameloblasts form, odontoblasts form, ameloblasts start to form enamel, odontoblasts start to form dentin
    B. Ameloblasts form, odontoblasts form, odontoblasts start to form dentin, ameloblasts start to form enamel
    C. Odontoblasts form, odontoblasts start to form dentin, ameloblasts form, ameloblasts start to form enamel
    D. Ameloblasts form, ameloblasts start to form enamel, odontoblasts form, odontoblasts start to form dentin
    E. Odontoblasts form, ameloblasts form, odontoblasts start to form dentin, ameloblasts start to form enamel

90. The auricular hillocks are derived from the _____.
    A. First branchial arch
    B. Second branchial arch
    C. First and second branchial arches
    D. Lateral nasal process
    E. Medial nasal process

91. Reduction division occurs during the _____.
    A. First stage of mitosis
    B. Second stage of mitosis
    C. First stage of meiosis
    D. Second stage of meiosis
    E. Third stage of meiosis

92. The embryo develops specifically from the _____.
    A. The entire blastocyst
    B. The entire trophoblast
    C. The embryonic disc
    D. The extraembryonic coelom
    E. The morula

93. Tooth enamel is derived from _____.
    A. Endoderm
    B. Mesoderm
    C. Ectoderm
    D. Endoderm and mesoderm
    E. Ectoderm and mesoderm

94. The olecranon fossa is located on the _____ surface of the _____.
    A. Superior; radius
    B. Anterior; humerus
    C. Posterior; humerus
    D. Anterior; radius

95. The latissimus dorsi muscle is supplied by the _____ nerve.
    A. Medial pectoral
    B. CN XI
    C. Dorsal scapular
    D. Thoracodorsal

96. The middle trunk of the brachial plexus of nerves arises from:
    A. C5
    B. C6
    C. C7
    D. C8

97. Which of the following ribs cannot be palpated?
    A. First
    B. Second
    C. Third
    D. A and B

98. An infection in a mandibular incisor with an apex below the mylohyoid muscle drains into which of the following spaces?

A. Sublingual space
B. Submental space
C. Submandibular space
D. Parapharyngeal space

99. The spread of an odontogenic infection to which of the following spaces would *most* likely be considered life-threatening?
    A. Submandibular space
    B. Sublingual space
    C. Parapharyngeal space
    D. Retropharyngeal space
    E. Pterygomandibular space

100. The median pharyngeal raphe serves as the attachment site for which of the following muscles?
    A. Lateral pterygoid
    B. Palatopharyngeus
    C. Levator veli palatini
    D. Salpingopharyngeus
    E. Superior constrictor

101. The right subclavian artery arises:
    A. Directly from the arch of the aorta.
    B. From the brachiocephalic trunk.
    C. From the common carotid artery.
    D. From the external carotid artery.
    E. From the internal carotid artery.

102. Cerebrospinal fluid is drained by reabsorption into which of the following vessels?
    A. Cisterna chyli
    B. Thoracic duct
    C. Superior sagittal sinus
    D. Inferior sagittal sinus
    E. Falx cerebri

103. Which of the following lymph nodes is located most inferiorly?
    A. Mastoid node
    B. Jugulodigastric node
    C. Juguloomohyoid node
    D. Parotid node
    E. Deep cervical node

104. The _____ nerve joins the lingual nerve before it meets the submandibular gland.
    A. Greater petrosal
    B. Inferior alveolar
    C. Tensor veli palatini
    D. Chorda tympani
    E. Auriculotemporal

105. Which of the following spaces is the site for the IAN block?
    A. Sublingual space
    B. Pterygomandibular space
    C. Infratemporal space
    D. Submasseteric space
    E. Temporal space

106. Which of the following sutures joins the parietal and temporal bones?

A. Coronal suture
B. Squamosal suture
C. Temporozygomatic suture
D. Lambdoidal suture
E. Sagittal suture

107. Which of the following structures forms the posterior border of the posterior triangle of the neck?
    A. Posterior border of SCM muscle
    B. Clavicle
    C. Levator scapulae muscle
    D. Anterior border of trapezius muscle
    E. Posterior border of trapezius muscle

108. Which of the following cranial nerves supplies motor innervation for all intrinsic and extrinsic muscles of the tongue?
    A. CN V
    B. CN VII
    C. CN IX
    D. CN XI
    E. CN XII

109. Which of the following nerves of the brachial plexus is sensory to the shoulder joint?
    A. Suprascapular nerve
    B. Medial pectoral nerve
    C. Lateral pectoral nerve
    D. Dorsal scapular nerve
    E. Long thoracic nerve

110. Which of the following veins of the arm is the preferred site for venipuncture?
    A. Cephalic vein
    B. Median antebrachial vein
    C. Median cubital vein
    D. Basilic vein
    E. Dorsal venous arch

111. Occlusion of which of the following arteries would result in "heart block"?
    A. Right coronary artery
    B. Left coronary artery
    C. Anterior interventricular artery
    D. Posterior interventricular artery
    E. Circumflex artery

112. At which of the following vertebral levels does the descending aorta become the abdominal aorta?
    A. T4
    B. T8
    C. T12
    D. L2
    E. S1

113. Which of the following nerves provides motor and sensory supply to the diaphragm?
    A. Vagus nerve
    B. Intercostal nerve
    C. Greater splanchnic nerve
    D. Least splanchnic nerve
    E. Phrenic nerve

114. Which lobe of the liver lies between the gallbladder, the ligamentum teres, and the porta hepatis?
    A. Right lobe
    B. Left lobe
    C. Quadrate lobe
    D. Caudate lobe

115. Type II collagen is found in which of the following tissues?
    A. Teeth
    B. Hyaline cartilage
    C. Basement membrane
    D. Tendons and ligaments
    E. Reticulin fibers

116. Osteocytes are found in spaces in bone known as
    _____.
    A. Lamellae
    B. Lacunae
    C. Osteons
    D. Central canals
    E. GAGs

117. Which is the most common type of granular leukocyte?
    A. Plasma cell
    B. Monocyte
    C. Polymorphonuclear leukocyte
    D. Lymphocyte
    E. Basophil

118. Which of the following are extensions of dentinal tubules that pass through the DEJ into enamel?
    A. Enamel lamellae
    B. Enamel tufts
    C. Enamel spindles
    D. Perikymata
    E. Incremental lines

119. Which of the following is a gingival rather than alveolodental fiber of the PDL?
    A. Oblique fibers
    B. Interradicular fibers
    C. Transseptal fibers
    D. Alveolar crest fibers
    E. Horizontal fibers

120. Which of the following muscles attaches to the anterior end of the articular disc of the TMJ?
    A. Superior head of the lateral pterygoid muscle
    B. Inferior head of the lateral pterygoid muscle
    C. Medial pterygoid muscle
    D. Masseter muscle
    E. Stylopharyngeus muscle

Biochemistry and Physiology

KATHERINE M. HOWARD

OUTLINE

1.0 Biologic Compounds

Biologic systems depend on molecules that serve various functions. They may serve as structural components, regulatory agents, energy sources, enzymatic agents, osmotic regulators, transport agents, and agents of hereditary information. Each of these compounds has unique characteristics that enable them to perform their function in both the intracellular and the extracellular environments. This section focuses on these biochemical agents and relates their function to biologic systems in which they participate.

1.1 Sugars and Carbohydrates

A. Carbohydrate nomenclature and structure.
  1. Empiric formula $(CH_2O)_n$.
  2. Simple carbohydrate (sugar)—polyhydroxylated aldehyde or ketone (up to seven carbon atoms). Examples are shown in Figure 2-1.
    a. Classified based on the number of carbons.
      (1) Trioses (three).
      (2) Tetroses (four).
      (3) Pentoses (five).
      (4) Hexoses (six).
    b. Aldose—contains an aldehyde as the most oxidized functional group.
      (1) Glyceraldehydes (aldotriose).
      (2) Glucose (aldohexose).
    c. Ketose—contains a keto group as the most oxidized functional group. Fructose is a ketohexose.
    d. Sugar derivatives—OH group is replaced by a $-NH_2$ or an acetylated $-NH_2$ (glucosamine and acetylglucosamine).
  3. Isomers—the chemical formula is the same, but the structure is different.
  4. Epimers—configuration around one carbon differs.
B. Carbohydrate classification—carbohydrates are classified based on the number of simple sugar units they contain. Sugar units are joined by glycosidic bonds.
  1. Monosaccharides (glyceraldehydes, ribose, xylose, glucose, mannose, galactose, fructose).
  2. Disaccharides (lactose, maltose, sucrose).
  3. Oligosaccharides—three to six monosaccharides (often found in glycoprotein).
  4. Polysaccharides—more than six monosaccharides.
    a. Amylose—unbranched glucose chain of α-1,4-glycosidic bonds.
    b. Amylopectin—α-1,4-linked glucose chains with branches of α-1,6-glycosidic bonds.
    c. Glycogen—α-1,4-linked glucose chains with highly branched α-1,6-glycosidic bonds, the principal carbohydrate storage molecule in vertebrates and are found predominately in liver and skeletal muscle.
    d. Cellulose—unbranched glucose polymer linked by β-1,4-glycosidic bonds; major structural polysaccharide in plants. Mammals cannot digest this type of glycosidic bond.
    e. Mucopolysaccharide (glycosaminoglycan)—long, unbranched polysaccharide consisting of alternating residues of uronic acid and either glucosamine or galactosamine. Mucopolysaccharidoses are hereditary disorders that produce a deficiency of

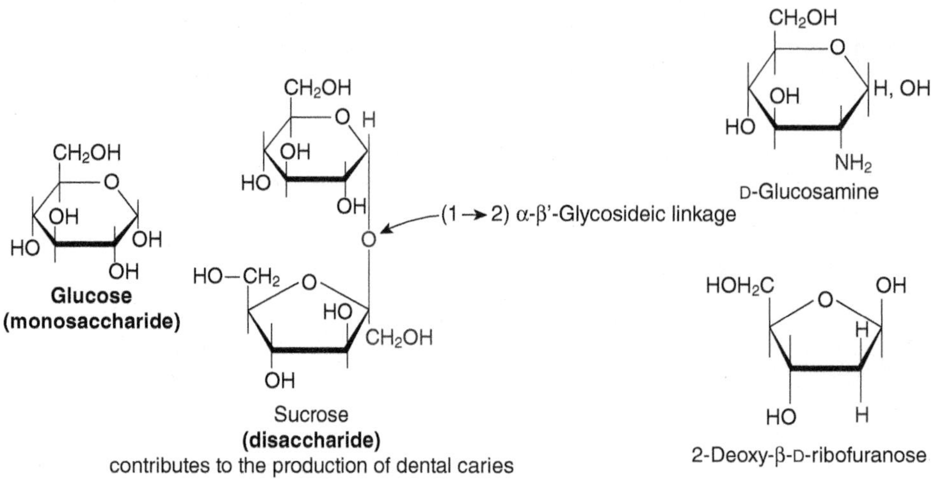

CH2OH
OH
HO
OH
OH
Glucose
(monosaccharide)
CH2OH
O H
OH
HO
OH
O
HO—CH2
HO
CH2OH
OH
Sucrose
(disaccharide)
contributes to the production of dental caries
(1→2) α-β'-Glycosideic linkage
CH2OH
OH
H, OH
HO
NH2
D-Glucosamine
HOH2C
OH
H
HO
H
2-Deoxy-β-D-ribofuranose

Figure 2-1 Chemical structure of several simple carbohydrates.

lysosomal hydrolases (degrade heparan sulfate or dermatan sulfate) resulting in the accumulation of glycosaminoglycans in tissues.

C. Function of carbohydrates.
   1. Important source of energy and energy stores.
   2. Metabolic intermediates.
   3. Component of ribonucleic acid (RNA) and deoxyribonucleic acid (DNA).
   4. Structural component of plants and animals.

D. Nutritional implications of carbohydrates.
   1. See Section 4.4 and 4.5, Metabolism, for discussion of regulation of blood glucose and glycogen metabolism.
   2. See Section 12, Digestion, for discussion of digestion and absorption of carbohydrates.

1.2 Amino Acids and Proteins

A. Amino acids.
   1. Building blocks of proteins consisting of a carboxyl group, an amino group, and a distinctive side chain (R) attached to a central carbon (α carbon) (Figure 2-2).
   2. There are 20 common amino acids grouped according to characteristics derived from the chemical nature of the side chain.
      a. Nonpolar side chains (glycine, alanine, valine, leucine, isoleucine, phenylalanine, tryptophan, methionine, and proline). These promote hydrophobic interactions.
      b. Uncharged polar side chains (asparagine, cysteine, glutamine, tyrosine, threonine, and serine). These have no charge at neutral pH but may participate in hydrogen bond formation with other compounds and are more hydrophilic.
      c. Acidic side chains (aspartic acid and glutamic acid). These have negative charges at neutral pH owing to the charge on the carboxyl group.

H3N+ — C — COO- + H3N+ — C — COO-
R1
R2
Amino acid 1
Amino acid 2
Energy
Peptide Bond
H3N+ — C — C — N — C — COO- + H2O
Dipeptide

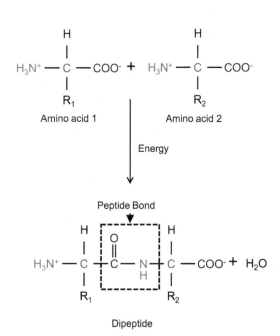

Figure 2-2 General structure of an amino acid and the formation of a peptide bond.

      d. Basic side chains (arginine, lysine, and histidine). These have positive charges at neutral pH owing to the ability to accept protons.
   3. Modified amino acids.
      a. Hydroxyproline and hydroxylysine—present in collagen and require vitamin C for formation.
      b. γ-Carboxyglutamate—present in blood-clotting protein prothrombin and requires vitamin K as a cofactor for formation.
   4. Amino acids are amphoteric—having both basic and acid side chains. Charge on protein from amino acids depends on pH of the solution.

5. Characteristics of weak acids and weak bases. The Henderson-Hasselbalch equation describes the relationship between pK_a and pH. This equation can be used to determine the dissociation constant of ionizable groups at a given pH.
   a. pH = −log [H^+].
   b. pK_a of an acid is defined as the pH at which the acid is half-dissociated: pK_a = −log(K_a).

B. Proteins.
   1. Peptide bond—amide bond that is formed between the free amino end of the peptide or amino acid and the free carboxyl end of the peptide or amino acid. Formation requires energy and releases water (see Figure 2-2).
   2. Structure.
      a. Primary structure—sequence of amino acids.
      b. Secondary structure—folding of the polypeptide chain owing to hydrogen bonds formed through interactions of the carbonyl oxygens and amide hydrogens.
         (1) α helix—coiled polypeptide core with amino acid side chains extending outward to avoid steric interference. Keratins and myoglobin are examples.
         (2) β sheets—characterized by hydrogen bonds between two or more polypeptide chains.
      c. Tertiary structure—three-dimensional structure owing to side chain interactions resulting from hydrophobic or hydrophilic interactions, hydrogen bonding, disulfide bonds, or ionic interactions.
      d. Quaternary structure—two or more polypeptides arranged in aggregates to form functional protein.
      e. Misfolding of proteins—associated with many diseases (amyloidoses), including Alzheimer's disease and bovine spongiform encephalopathy.
      f. Hemoglobinopathies—disorder produced by abnormal hemoglobin molecules or insufficient amount of the globular protein. Examples include sickle cell anemia (abnormal β-chain) and thalassemia (imbalance of α and β chains).
   3. Classification.
      a. Fibrous—structural proteins.
         (1) Collagen.
         (2) Elastin.
         (3) Keratin.
         (4) Fibrin.
      b. Globular—functional proteins.
         (1) Hydrophilic amino acids found on surface of proteins.
         (2) Hydrophobic amino acids found in interior of proteins.
   4. Functions—structural support, catalysts, signaling molecules, transport and storage of molecules, movement, regulatory molecules, transmission of nerve impulses, and control of growth and differentiation.

1.3 Lipids

A. Classification of lipids.
   1. Fatty acids—straight-chained hydrocarbon compounds that possess a terminal carboxyl group that provides polarity and establishes an amphipathic (contain both hydrophilic and hydrophobic moieties) character to the molecule.
      a. Saturated fatty acid—contains no double bonds.
      b. Unsaturated fatty acid—contains double bonds that are identified with δ or ω terminology. May be either monounsaturated or polyunsaturated.
      c. Essential fatty acids cannot be synthesized in the body.
         (1) Linoleic acid.
         (2) Linolenic acid.
         (3) Arachidonic acid if linoleic acid is missing from the diet.
      d. Functions as metabolic fuel.
   2. Triacylglycerols (triglyceride)—esters of glycerol and three fatty acids (Figure 2-3). Triacylglycerols are most abundant lipid class and the principal fat storage molecule; they are acted on by lipases to release the fatty acids.
   3. Phospholipids—composed of glycerol or sphingosine, one or two fatty acids attached via an ester linkage, and a polar head group attached via an ester linkage to the phosphate group forming a phosphodiester bond. Phospholipids have hydrophobic (fatty acid) and hydrophilic (polar head group) domains, which, in an aqueous environment, form bimolecular layers, which are the biologic basis of membranes.
      a. Phosphoglycerides—glycerol backbone, two fatty acids, and polar head group.
         (1) Phosphatidic acid (PA)—parent compound of other phosphoglycerides (see Figure 2-3).
         (2) PA and serine = phosphatidylserine—important component of membranes.
         (3) PA and ethanolamine = phosphatidylethanolamine (cephalin)—important for mitochondrial activity.

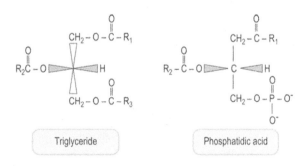

Figure 2-3 General structure of triglyceride and phosphatidic acid. *(From Baynes JW, Dominiczak MH: Medical Biochemistry, New York, Mosby, 2005.)*

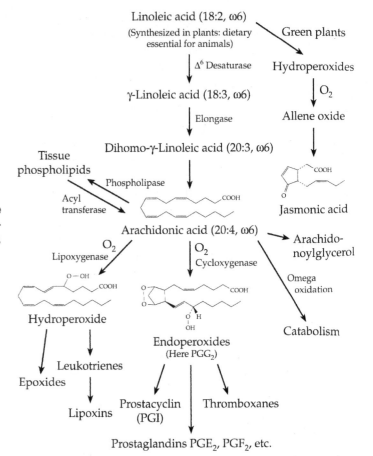

Figure 2-4 Arachidonic acid is a precursor of the eicosanoids, which function as hormonelike molecules in most tissues. *(From Metzler DE: Biochemistry, ed 2, San Diego, Academic Press, 2003.)*

(4) PA and choline = phosphatidylcholine (lecithin)—major constituent of surfactant. Lack of surfactant (dipalmitoyl lecithin) results in respiratory distress syndrome.

(5) PA and inositol = phosphatidylinositol—precursor of second messengers diacylglycerol and inositol triphosphate (IP$_3$).

(6) PA and glycerol = phosphatidylglycerol.

4. Glycolipids—composed of glycerol or sphingosine, with one or two fatty acids and one or more carbohydrates.

5. Sphingolipids—either a phospholipid or glycolipid. Sphingosine and fatty acid = ceramide (structural parent of all sphingolipids).

   a. Phosphosphingolipids—derivative of phosphorylated ceramide (PC). PC and choline = sphingomyelin—an important constituent of myelin.

   b. Glycosphingolipids—composed of ceramide and one or more carbohydrates; often found on plasma membrane surfaces, especially in nervous tissue. One sugar unit = cerebrosides; oligosaccharides and sialic acid = gangliosides, which are determinants for O, A, and B human blood group types.

6. Sterols—steroid nucleus consisting of four fused rings. Cholesterol is the major sterol in animal tissue consisting of the sterol ring, hydrocarbon tail (hydrophobic), and hydroxyl (polar) group on the steroid nucleus.

7. Eicosanoids—20-carbon fatty acid derivatives of arachidonic acid that function as hormonelike molecules in most tissues (Figure 2-4). Prostaglandins, thromboxanes, and leukotrienes are examples of these molecules. If linoleic acid is missing from the diet, arachidonic acid becomes essential.

B. Function of lipids.

1. Component of biologic membranes (phospholipids and sphingolipids).

2. Facilitate the interactions between membrane proteins and hydrophobic environments in the membrane (e.g., covalent modification of the protein with myristic and palmitic acids).

3. Source of energy (triacylglycerol).

4. Provides insulation and protection (triacylglycerol).

5. Precursor of hormones and intracellular messengers (fatty acids).

6. Precursor of steroid hormones, vitamin D, bile acids and salts, and membranes (cholesterol).

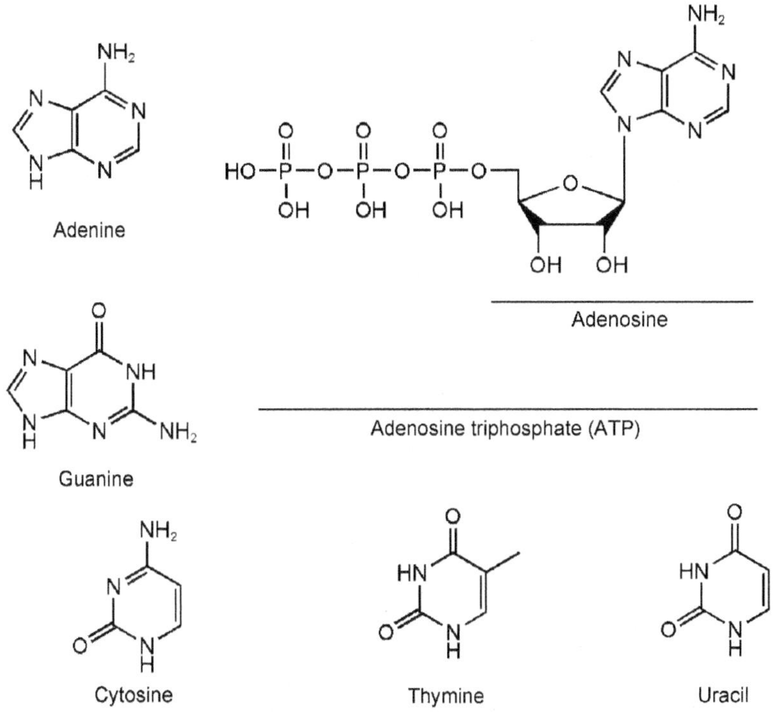

Figure 2-5 Chemical structures of the purines, adenine and guanine, and pyrimidines, cytosine, thymine, and uracil. The structures of the nucleoside, adenosine, and the nucleotide, adenosine triphosphate (ATP), are also shown.

1.4 Nucleotides and Nucleic Acids

A. Nucleotides
   1. Composition—nitrogenous base, pentose, and phosphate (Figure 2-5).
      a. Nitrogenous base.
         (1) Purines (adenine and guanine).
         (2) Pyrimidines (cytosine, thymine, and uracil).
      b. Nucleoside—purine or pyrimidine base linked via a glycosidic bond to pentose sugar (no phosphate).
      c. Nucleotide—nucleoside and phosphate.
         (1) Adenine + ribose + phosphate = adenosine monophosphate.
         (2) Cytosine + deoxyribose + phosphate = deoxycytidine monophosphate.
   2. Functions.
      a. Component of DNA and RNA.
      b. Component of cofactors (e.g., reduced nicotinamide adenine dinucleotide [NADH], reduced nicotinamide adenine dinucleotide phosphate [NADPH]).
      c. Energy currency (adenosine triphoshate [ATP] and guanosine triphosphate [GTP]).
      d. Second messengers (cyclic adenosine monophosphate [cAMP] and cyclic guanosine monophosphate [cGMP]).
B. Nucleic acids—polynucleotide chain formed by removing a molecule of water between the phosphate group of one nucleotide and the sugar group of the other (phosphodiester bond). The chains formed are either

polyribonucleotides (RNA) or polydeoxyribonucleotides (DNA).
   1. DNA.
      a. Composed of four bases linked to deoxyribose (2′ position lacks the hydroxyl group) and phosphate.
         (1) Adenine.
         (2) Guanine.
         (3) Cytosine.
         (4) Thymine.
      b. Consists of two strands of nucleotides in the form of a double helix.
      c. Double helix is held together by hydrogen bonds.
      d. Only adenine and thymine and guanine and cytosine are paired. The two strands are said to be complementary.
   2. RNA.
      a. Composed of four bases linked to ribose and phosphate.
         (1) Adenine.
         (2) Guanine.
         (3) Cytosine.
         (4) Uracil.
      b. Types of RNA.
         (1) Ribosomal RNA (rRNA)—integral component of ribosomes, the site of protein synthesis.
         (2) Messenger RNA (mRNA)—carries the genetic information of DNA and directs protein synthesis.
         (3) Transfer RNA (tRNA)—delivers amino acids to ribosome. Cloverleaf structure contains an

Table 2-1

Fat-Soluble and Water-Soluble Vitamins

VITAMIN	FUNCTION	DEFICIENCY DEFECTS
Fat-Soluble		
A	Vision, differentiation	Night blindness
D	Calcium and phosphate metabolism	Rickets, osteomalacia
E	Lipid antioxidant	Lipid peroxidation
K	Blood coagulation enzymes	Bleeding
Water-Soluble		
Thiamine (B_1)	Oxidative decarboxylation, transketolation Coenzyme: Thiamine pyrophosphate	Impaired carbohydrate metabolism and lipid biosynthesis, beriberi
Riboflavin (B_2)	Oxidation-reduction reactions in respiratory chain Coenzyme: Flavin mononucleotide (FMN) and flavin adenine dinucleotide (FAD)	Angular cheilosis and glossitis, dermatitis
Pantothenic acid	Acyl-group transfer in metabolism Coenzyme: Coenzyme A	
Niacin	Oxidation-reduction reactions Coenzyme: Nicotinamide adenine dinucleotide (NAD) and nicotinamide adenine dinucleotide phosphate (NADPH)	Pellagra
Pyridoxine (B_6)	Transamination reactions in amino acid metabolism Coenzyme: Pyridoxal phosphate	Seborrheic dermatitis, cheilosis, glossitis, and stomatitis
Biotin	Carboxylation and carboxyl-group transfer	Dermatitis, alopecia
Folic acid	Transfer of one-carbon units for purine and pyrimidine synthesis and the formation of heme Coenzyme: Tetrahydrofolate	Anemia, neural tube defects
Cobalamin (B_{12})	Transfer of methyl groups Intrinsic factor required for absorption Coenzyme: Adenosylcobalamin	Pernicious anemia, neurologic degeneration
Ascorbic acid (C)	Antioxidant, collagen formation	Scurvy

Adapted from Montgomery R: Biochemistry: A Case-Oriented Approach,, 6th ed. St. Louis, Mosby, 1996.

anticodon triplet of bases to base pair with mRNA.

C. Function of nucleic acids.
1. DNA is responsible for transmitting genetic information from generation to generation. The process of transcription makes RNA from DNA.
2. RNA transmits the genetic information stored in DNA for the synthesis of proteins. The process of translation makes polypeptides from mRNA.

1.5 Micronutrients

A. Vitamins—traditionally divided into fat-soluble and water-soluble vitamins. Vitamins A, D, K, and E are fat-soluble, and the remaining nine vitamins are water-soluble. Fat-soluble vitamins can be retained in lipid throughout the body; the potential for toxicity is generally greater than that of water-soluble vitamins.

Table 2-1 lists the vitamins and their corresponding functions and deficiency defects.

B. Minerals—in biologic systems, minerals are often associated with enzymes, and they function as cofactors. Following are examples of cofactors (minerals) and the enzymes with which they are associated.
1. Fe^{2+} or Fe^{3+}—cytochrome oxidase, catalase, and peroxidase.
2. Cu^{2+}—cytochrome oxidase.
3. Zn^{2+}—DNA polymerase, carbonic anhydrase, and alcohol dehydrogenase.
4. Mg^{2+}—hexokinase and glucose-6-phosphatase.
5. Mn^{2+}—arginase.
6. K^{2+}—pyruvate kinase.
7. Ni^{2+}—urease.
8. Mo—nitrate reductase.
9. Se—glutathione peroxidase.

2.0 Cellular and Molecular Biology

2.1 Cellular Organization

A. Cell (plasma) membrane.
  1. Phospholipid bilayer and proteins.
  2. Selectively permeable to small nonpolar molecules and polar molecules.
  3. Establishes transport systems and regulates cell-cell interactions (see Section 3, Membranes).
B. Cytoplasm—all of the cell outside of the nucleus.
C. Cytosol.
  1. Aqueous area between the plasma membrane and membrane-bound organelles in the cytoplasm.
  2. Contains a solution of water, proteins, electrolytes, small molecules, and carbohydrates.
  3. Site of important biochemical functions: glycolysis, translation, cell signaling.
D. Nucleus.
  1. Control center for cell division and cell activities; surrounded by nuclear membrane bilayer.
  2. Contains: DNA (and proteins such as histones to form chromosomes) and nucleolus (rRNA synthesis).
E. Nucleolus.
  1. Non–membrane-bound structure composed of proteins and nucleic acids.
  2. Transcribes and assembles rRNA.
F. Mitochondria.
  1. Powerhouse of the cell.
  2. Bilayered: outer membrane is permeable to small solutes.
  3. Site of aerobic respiration in the cell: generates ATP via oxidative phosphorylation.
G. Ribosome.
  1. Assembled in cytoplasm.
  2. Synthesizes proteins; located in cytoplasm and outer membrane of endoplasmic reticulum (rough endoplasmic reticulum).
H. Endoplasmic reticulum.
  1. Tubular and vascular structure that is continuous with the nuclear envelope.
  2. Transports material throughout cell.
  3. Two regions.
    a. Rough endoplasmic reticulum—contains ribosomes; synthesizes proteins.
    b. Smooth endoplasmic reticulum—lacks ribosomes; synthesizes lipids, phospholipids, and steroids. It also assists in carbohydrate metabolism, drug detoxification, and calcium storage.
I. Golgi apparatus.
  1. Contains stacked, flattened membranous sacs called cisternae that have polarity.
  2. Posttranslational modification: modifies, concentrates, and packages rough endoplasmic reticulum products for exocytosis.
J. Lysosomes—formed by Golgi apparatus; contains hydrolytic enzymes that break down ingested cell material.
K. Centrioles—microtubules used for spindle organization in cell division.
L. Cytoskeleton.
  1. Structural framework of the cell, made up of microtubules, actin filaments, intermediate filaments, and thick filaments.
  2. Enables transport of materials by adapting shape to maintain support, shape, and function of cell.

2.2 DNA Replication

A. DNA replication—DNA → DNA: produces a new DNA strand synthesized from 5′ → 3′.
  1. Complementary base pairing as parent strand is template for daughter strand.
  2. Replication is semiconservative—contains original parent strand plus new strand.
  3. Chromatin—double-stranded helical structure of DNA.
    a. Histones are complexed with DNA to form nucleosomes, which fold and form extended loops. These loops are compressed and folded to form a long (250 nm) fiber, which tightly coils to become the chromatid of a chromosome (1400 nm).
    b. DNA → DNA (Figure 2-6).
      (1) DNA double helix is unwound by helicases, exposing single strands to serve as templates for reproduction. RNA primer is laid down by primase on leading strand.
      (2) DNA polymerase III binds leading strand of DNA from 5′ → 3′. This is referred to as *chain elongation.*
      (3) DNA polymerase I replaces regions of RNA primers with DNA, which simultaneously replicates the complementary strand.
      (4) Lagging (complementary) strand: RNA primase attaches RNA primer.
      (5) Polymerase III synthesizes complementary strand DNA in pieces (Okazaki fragments) between the RNA primers.
      (6) DNA polymerase I replaces RNA primers with DNA.
      (7) DNA ligase forms links via phosphodiester bonds between 5′ P and 3′ OH group of Okazaki fragments.

2.3 RNA Synthesis

A. Transcription—DNA → RNA: new RNA is synthesized from 5′ → 3′.
  1. Process occurs in nucleus.
  2. Base DNA transcribed into mRNA strands, which leave the nucleus to go into cytoplasm.

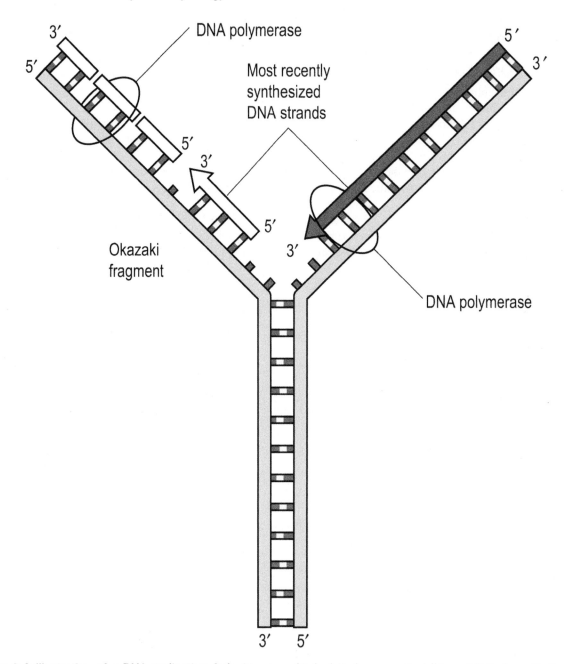

Figure 2-6 Illustration of a DNA replication fork. *(Courtesy of Baback Roshanravan, In Adkinson NF, Bochner BS, Busse WW: Middleton's Allergy: Principles and Practice, ed 7, St. Louis, Mosby, 2009.)*

3. DNA → RNA: only one DNA strand ("template strand") used for RNA copy because it provides the template for RNA nucleotide sequence. Other strand is "coding strand" because its sequence is identical to the new RNA sequence (except T → U).
4. RNA polymerase reads DNA template strand from 3′ → 5′ so that RNA polymerase can make new strand from 5′ → 3′.
5. RNA polymerase binds to 3′ end of gene ("promotor") and moves to 5′ end. Primase is not needed, *but* a promotor (i.e., TATA sequence) is needed:

transcription factors bind → RNA polymerase binds → initiation starts.
6. Transcription is terminated by Rho protein.

2.4 Protein Synthesis

A. Translation—RNA → protein = mRNA is read from 5′ → 3′. Process occurs in the cytoplasm such that mRNA codons are translated into an amino acid sequence.
1. tRNA.
   a. Brings amino acids to ribosomes; recognizes amino acid and mRNA codon via its three-dimensional

structure, which contains an anticodon (complement to mRNA codon) and an amino acid attachment site.

  b. Each amino acid has aminoacyl-tRNA synthetase, whose active site binds to its amino acid and corresponding tRNA forming an aminoacyl-tRNA complex.

2. Ribosomes.
   a. Contain two subunits: protein and rRNA.
   b. Offers three binding sites: one for mRNA and two for tRNA (P and A site).
      (1) P site—binds tRNA to the polypeptide chain.
      (2) A site—binds to the incoming aminoacyl-tRNA complex.

3. Polypeptide synthesis (three phases).
   a. Initiation.
      (1) Ribosome binds to mRNA near 5′ end and finds start codon (AUG).
      (2) Met-tRNA (with anticodon UAC) and aminoacyl-tRNA complex bind to mRNA P site.
      (3) Initiation complex is stabilized by GTP hydrolyzation.

  b. Elongation.
      (1) Hydrogen bonding occurs between mRNA and incoming aminoacyl-tRNA on A site.
      (2) Amino acids on P and A site attach together via peptide bond.
      (3) Translocation—ribosome moves three nucleotides over on mRNA in 5′ → 3′ direction, causing tRNA to dissociate from P site. This allows tRNA on A site to become the new P site to open a new A site for the process to continue.
      (4) Elongation continues to termination.
   c. Termination.
      (1) Stop codon release factors (UAA, UAG, or UGA) bind to the ribosome A site.
      (2) Protein is released, and ribosome complex dissociates into subunits (polyribosome).
      (3) mRNA is released, terminating translation.

2.5 Cell Cycle for Growth and Division

A. Cell cycle (Figure 2-7)—interphase (G_1, S, and G_2 phase).
   1. Cell spends 90% of time here. Chromosomes are copied to give two identical sister chromatids held by a centromere (S phase).

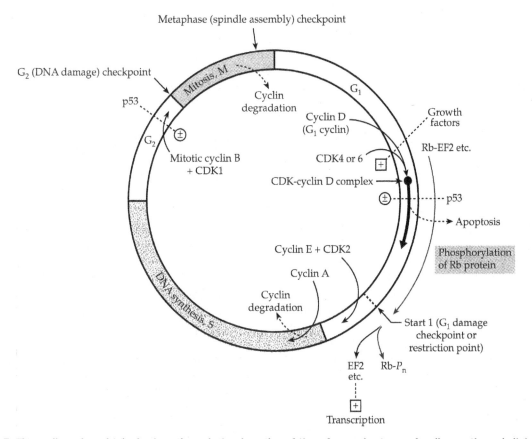

Figure 2-7 The cell cycle, which depicts the relative lengths of time for each stage of cell growth and division. After mitosis (M), the cell grows during the G_1 (gap) period. At the G_1 checkpoint, the cell prepares to divide, with DNA synthesis occurring during the S phase. After a second gap (G_2), mitosis occurs to complete the cycle. (*From Metzler DE: Biochemistry, ed 2, San Diego, Academic Press, 2003.*)

B. Mitosis.
  1. Division of DNA to make two daughter cells with copies of original genome—diploid (2n) *via* karyokinesis then cytokinesis (division of nucleus then cytoplasm).
  2. Five phases.
    a. Prophase—chromosomes condense, centrioles move to opposite poles, and spindles form.
    b. Metaphase—spindle fibers align chromosomes along midline of cell to form metaphase plate.
    c. Anaphase—spindle fibers shorten to separate chromatids, pulling them to either end of cell.
    d. Telophase—formation of a new nuclear membrane containing diploid (2n) chromosomes. Chromosomes uncoil resembling interphase.
    e. Cytokinesis—cytoplasm divides, and cleavage furrow separates along cell midline to create two daughter cells.
C. Meiosis.
  1. Production of haploid (1n) sex cells (gametes).
  2. Two divisions—four haploids formed.
  3. Interphase—same as mitosis to give two daughter cells.
    a. First meiotic division.
      (1) Prophase I—spindle forms pulling homologous chromosomes together (synapse). Homologous chromosomes and sister chromosomes make a tetrad where crossing over may occur via chiasmata in homologous/nonidentical chromosomes.
      (2) Metaphase I—homologous pairs align at midline.
      (3) Anaphase I—pairs undergo disjunction leading to random distribution of parent chromosomes.
      (4) Telophase I—nuclear membrane forms.
    b. Second meiotic division—not preceded by chromosomal replication.
      (1) Metaphase II—chromosomes meet at equator.
      (2) Anaphase II—chromosomes separate to 1n and move to poles.
      (3) Telophase II—nuclear membrane forms.
      (4) New cells have haploid (1n) number of chromosomes—four 1n gametes.
        Note: in females the process of oogenesis produces only one daughter cell (oocyte, 1n) and 3 non-functional polar bodies. In males, the process of spermatogenesis produces four functional gametes (sperm, 1n).

2.6 Genetic Engineering

A. Restriction endonucleases.
  1. Bacterial enzymes that hydrolyze double-stranded DNA at specific sites.
  2. Resultant DNA fragments can be incorporated into a different DNA molecule using DNA ligase.

B. Complementary DNA (cDNA) libraries.
  1. cDNA is synthesized using reverse transcriptase, which uses mRNA as a template.
  2. Multiple copies of cDNA can be made using DNA polymerase (polymerase chain reaction [PCR]).
  3. All expressed genes of the cell can be cloned when this library is made.
C. PCR
  1. A sample of DNA is added to a mixture of DNA primer, deoxyribonucleoside triphosphates (dNTPs), and a thermophilic DNA polymerase.
  2. The mixture is heated to separate the strands of DNA, which permits the primers to bind.
  3. The mixture is cooled, and polymerase synthesizes cDNA.
  4. The mixture is heated again, and strands separate, permitting primers to bind to DNA.
  5. The mixture is cooled, permitting another synthesis of cDNA.
  6. The process continues through many cycles, resulting in many copies.
D. Genetic transfer (genetic engineering).
  1. Cloned cDNA is incorporated into a vector (bacterial plasmids, bacterial virus), which introduces cDNA into a host DNA.
  2. The host DNA is able to express the cDNA product.
E. Terminology.
  1. Southern blots analyze DNA.
  2. Northern blots analyze RNA.
  3. Western blots analyze protein.
  4. Enzyme-linked immunosorbent assays analyze protein.

3.0 Membranes

3.1 Structure

A. Lipid bilayer—formation of two layers of lipids oriented with the polar head groups toward the aqueous environments and the hydrophobic tails inward. It creates an inner and outer leaflet (Figure 2-8).
B. Lipid composition.
  1. Phospholipids (see Section 1.3, Lipids).
  2. Cholesterol—stabilizes the membrane, maintains fluidity.
  3. Glycolipids—have several functions.
    a. Surface markers to regulate tissue growth.
    b. Important for cell recognition.
C. Protein composition (see Figure 2-8).
  1. Intrinsic or integral proteins.
    a. Mostly composed of hydrophobic amino acids.
    b. Difficult to remove from the membrane.
    c. Often span the membrane (transmembrane), may pass through membrane multiple times.

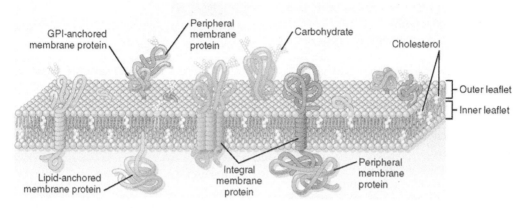

Figure 2-8 Schematic diagram of the cell plasma membrane. *(From Koeppen BM, Stanton BA, Berne RM: Berne & Levy Physiology, ed 6, Philadelphia, Saunders, 2010.)*

d. Examples.
   (1) Regulated channels that selectively permit ions to move across the membrane.
   (2) Carrier molecules unique to certain tissues.
   (3) Receptor proteins—specific surface molecules that initiate membrane and cellular events (may require second messenger systems).
2. Lipid anchored proteins—proteins covalently attached to lipid molecules, which are embedded in one leaflet of the bilayer.
   a. Outer leaflet—glycosylphosphatidylinositol anchors.
   b. Inner leaflet.
      (1) N-terminus of protein via fatty acids myristate or palmitate.
      (2) C-terminus of protein via prenyl anchors (farnesyl or geranylgeranyl).
3. Extrinsic or peripheral proteins.
   a. Composed of both hydrophobic and hydrophilic amino acids.
   b. Found near the surface of the membrane mostly on the cytoplasmic face.
   c. Function as enzymes or in a structural capacity.

3.2 Functions

Membranes provide a means for the selective permeability of molecules into and out of the cell or organelle and in doing so create distinct compartments and give organization to the cell. Membranes function in several capacities.
A. Provide structural integrity.
B. Control movement of substances.
C. Establish transport systems.
D. Regulate cell-cell interactions.
E. Establish membrane potentials by separating ionic charges.
F. Facilitate cell adhesion and specialized cell junctions.

3.3 Membrane Transport

A. Passive transport (diffusion)—movement across a membrane using energy from normal kinetic motion of molecules. Movement continues until gradient is eliminated. It may be either simple diffusion or facilitated diffusion.
   1. Simple diffusion—down a concentration gradient without the need for carrier proteins. Osmosis and bulk flow are associated with simple diffusion. Hydrophobic molecules and very small molecules (e.g., O_2 and CO_2) diffuse through the interstices of the lipid bilayer. Charged molecules (ions) use transmembrane watery protein channels. Protein channels can be gated as a way to control permeability.
      a. Voltage-gated—responds to electrical potential across the membrane.
      b. Ligand-gated—opens by the binding of another molecule (ion channels, neurotransmitter-gated, nucleotide-gated).
   2. Facilitated diffusion—uses intrinsic carrier proteins to transport large, lipid-insoluble molecules (amino acids, glucose). It also moves down a concentration gradient. Intrinsic proteins undergo conformational changes to facilitate diffusion (saturable and specific). Energy is from normal kinetic motion of molecules. Facilitated diffusion shows Michaelis-Menten kinetics (glucose transport). Carrier proteins can be uniport, symport, or antiport.
      a. Uniport—single molecule moving one way.
      b. Symport (coupled)—two molecules moving one way.
      c. Antiport (coupled)—two molecules moving opposite ways.
   3. Osmosis—diffusion of water from lower solute concentration (number of particles/unit volume) to higher solute concentration. Extracellular fluid (ECF)

and intracellular fluid (ICF) have the same osmolarity (approximately 300 mOsm).

    a. Isotonic extracellular solution—no cell volume change.

    b. Hypertonic extracellular solution—cells shrink.

    c. Hypotonic extracellular solution—cells swell.

B. Active transport—movement across a membrane against an electrochemical gradient. It involves carrier proteins and demonstrates Michaelis-Menten kinetics. Energy (ATP) is required.

  1. Primary active transport—energy derived from ATP. Specific carriers are used, which are saturable.

    a. Ca^{2+}—ATPase pumps are important active transports in sarcoplasmic reticulum (SR) membranes.

    b. Na^+-K^+-ATPase pump is present in all plasma membranes.

      (1) Establishes and maintains Na^+ and K^+ gradient by transporting Na^+ out and K^+ into the cell.

      (2) Na^+ concentration gradient is the force for secondary active transport mechanisms.

  2. Secondary active transport—ATP establishes an ionic gradient, which is the driving force (secondary transport).

    a. Na^+ gradient established by membrane pumps drives this system.

    b. Protein carriers bind both substance transported and Na^+.

    c. Cotransport systems—Na^+ and substance transported move in the same direction.

      (1) Glucose and galactose across gastrointestinal (GI) mucosa and reabsorption in renal tubule.

      (2) Amino acid transport in GI mucosa and renal tubules.

    d. Countertransport—Na^+ and transported substance move in opposite directions.

      (1) Na^+/H^+ exchange—H^+ out and Na^+ into cells.

      (2) Na^+/Ca^{2+} exchange—Ca^{2+} out and Na^+ into cells.

D. Transport of large molecules across the membrane.

  1. Endocytosis—vacuole formation using plasma membrane and released inside the cell; may result in degradation. If vacuole is fused with lysozymes, degradation results.

    a. Pinocytosis—internalization of interstitial fluid.

    b. Phagocytosis—internalization of material and subsequent lysosomal digestion.

    c. Receptor-mediated endocytosis—selective internalization of receptor/ligand complex. Receptor complex may return to surface.

  2. Exocytosis—secretory vesicle membrane from within the cell fuses with the plasma membrane, and the contents of the vesicle are released outside the cell.

3.4 Membrane and Action Potentials

A. Membrane potentials—measured electrical potential difference across all cell membranes in millivolts

Table 2-2

Approximate Compositions of Extracellular and Intracellular Fluids

SUBSTANCE AND UNITS	EXTRACELLULAR FLUID	INTRACELLULAR FLUID*
Na^+ (mEq/L)	140	14
K^+ (mEq/L)	4	120
Ca^{2+}, ionized (mEq/L)	2.5[†]	1×10^{-4}
Cl^- (mEq/L)	105	10
HCO_3^- (mEq/L)	24	10
pH[‡]	7.4	7.1
Osmolarity (mOsm/L)	290	290

From Costanzo LS: Physiology, ed 3, Philadelphia, Saunders, 2004.

*The major anions of intracellular fluid are proteins and organic phosphates.

[†]The corresponding total [Ca^{2+}] in extracellular fluid is 5 mEq/L or 10 mg/dL.

[‡]pH is $-\log_{10}$ of the [H^+]; pH 7.4 corresponds to [H^+] of 40×10^{-9} Eq/L.

(measured charge is inside cell). This results from concentration differences of permeable ions. Nerve and muscle cells are excitable and capable of self-generating electrochemical impulses.

  1. The separation of charges (ions) results in a slight excess of negative charges inside and more positive charges outside.

  2. An electrochemical gradient is established secondary to the ion and chemical concentration differences. The electrochemical gradient determines the diffusion of ions.

  3. Resting membrane potential is determined by the diffusion potentials of the ions and membrane.

    a. At rest, K^+ is far more permeable than Na^+.

    b. Table 2-2 shows the composition of ECF and ICF.

    c. As a result of the diffusion of K^+ out of the cell, the resting membrane potential is negative and near the equilibrium potential of K^+.

    d. The resting membrane potential is maintained by the Na^+-K^+-ATPase pump (−40 to −90 mV). For every two K^+ ions pumped into the cell, three Na^+ ions are pumped out of the cell.

    e. Hyperkalemia reduces the concentration gradient for potassium out of the cell, making the inside less negative.

B. Graded membrane potentials—local changes in membrane potentials that result in gradations of membrane potentials and sensitivity to stimulation.

  1. Postsynaptic potentials in synapses.

  2. Sensory receptor potentials.

  3. Skeletal muscle end-plate potential.

  4. Pacemaker potential in cardiac and smooth muscle.

C. Action potentials—rapid changes in membrane potentials results in change from normal resting negative potential to positive potential and back to negative potential; this occurs only when a threshold potential has been reached.

1. Resting stage—resting slightly negative membrane potential.

2. Depolarization stage—sudden permeability to Na^+ ions usually caused by opening of voltage-gated sodium channels resulting in a large and rapid influx of sodium diffusing into the cell (inward current).

3. Repolarization stage—sodium channels close, and voltage-gated potassium channels open further to allow K^+ to flow to the exterior.

4. Refractory period—period during which another normal action potential cannot be elicited.

   a. Relative refractory period—action potential can be elicited if a greater than usual depolarization is applied.

   b. Absolute refractory period—another action potential cannot be elicited.

5. Propagation of action potential—occurs by local currents depolarizing adjacent areas of membrane. Propagation velocity can be increased by the following factors.

   a. Increasing fiber size.

   b. Increasing stimulation intensity.

   c. Myelination, which results in action potentials jumping from node to node (saltatory conduction).

4.0 Metabolism

Metabolism refers to the sum of all the physical and chemical processes by which a living organized substance is produced and maintained as well as the transformation by which energy is made available for use by the organism.

4.1 Bioenergetics

A. Study of the energy transductions that occur in living cells and the chemical processes underlying these transductions.

B. Terminology.

1. Entropy (δS)—degree of randomness in a system.

2. Enthalpy (δH)—heat change during a chemical reaction owing to differences in bond energy.

3. Exergonic—the free energy (δG) of the products is lower than the dG of the reactants ($\delta G < 0$). (Net energy is released as a result of the reaction.)

4. Endergonic—the δG of the products is higher than the dG of the reactants ($\delta G > 0$). (Net energy is consumed as a result of the reaction.)

5. Equilibrium constant (K_{eq})—ratio of the concentration of products to reactants when the reaction reaches equilibrium. The larger the K_{eq}, the more favorable the reaction.

6. Free energy (δG)—the energy that can drive a chemical reaction.

   a. Negative δG—the reaction proceeds in the direction written.

   b. Positive δG—the reaction goes in the opposite direction.

   c. δG is 0—the reaction is at equilibrium.

7. Free energy of activation—energy required to reach the transition state.

8. Transition state—highest energy arrangement of the atoms that occurs between the reactants and the products.

9. Thermodynamics—the energy state of a system and the direction in which the reaction will proceed.

10. Kinetics—the rate of the reaction and the factors that affect the rate. The rate of the reaction can be increased in two ways.

    a. Increase the temperature to activate more molecules to reach the transition state.

    b. Lower the activation of energy of the transition state by using a catalyst.

4.2 Enzymology

Enzymes are biologic compounds that catalyze chemical reactions. Enzymes can alter the rates of reactions by providing a reaction mechanism that has a lower energy of activation. Enzymes *do not* alter the equilibrium of the reaction and are not consumed in the reaction. Most enzymes are highly specific because they associate with substrates through specific sites in the catalytic center of the enzyme. The rate of an enzyme catalyzed reaction depends on the temperature, pH, and concentrations of the enzyme and substrate.

A. Classification of enzymes.

1. Oxidoreductases—one substrate is oxidized, while the other is reduced.

2. Transferases—transfer functional groups between two substrates.

3. Hydrolases—catalyze the hydrolysis of proteins and carbohydrates.

4. Lyases—remove two groups from a substrate, leaving a double bond.

5. Isomerases—interconvert isomers.

6. Ligases—catalyze the formation of covalent bonds, using the hydrolysis of ATP or some other high-energy compound.

B. Michaelis-Menten equation—examines the kinetics of enzyme catalyzed reactions.

1. At constant substrate concentration, increasing the concentration of enzyme increases the rate of the reaction.

2. At low substrate concentrations, increasing the substrate concentration increases the reaction rate. However, at high substrate concentrations, the rate of

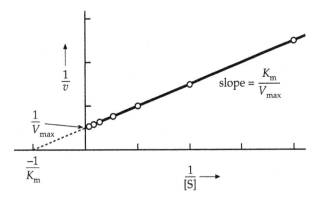

Figure 2-9 Double-reciprocal or Lineweaver-Burk plot of 1/v versus 1/[S]. The intercept on the vertical axis gives $1/V_{max}$, and the slope gives K_m/V_{max}. The intercept on the horizontal axis equals $-1/K_m$. *(From Metzler DE: Biochemistry, ed 2, San Diego, Academic Press, 2003.)*

the reaction is independent of substrate concentration and reaches a maximal velocity. This is because the substrate has saturated the enzyme active site, and the reaction cannot proceed any faster.

C. Enzyme kinetics plot (velocity versus substrate) (Figure 2-9).
   1. V_{max}—maximum velocity of the reaction.
   2. K_m—the substrate concentration at which the velocity is 50% of the maximum velocity.

D. Enzyme inhibition—numerous substances (including drugs and metabolites) can interfere with enzyme activity. This inhibition may be reversible or irreversible. Three types of reversible inhibitory mechanisms can be identified by enzyme kinetic plots.
   1. Competitive inhibition.
      a. Substances are similar to the substrate and compete for binding at the active site.
      b. K_m is increased, but there is no change in V_{max}.
   2. Uncompetitive inhibition.
      a. The inhibitor binds only to the substrate-enzyme complex.
      b. Both V_{max} and K_m are reduced.
   3. Noncompetitive inhibition.
      a. The inhibitor can bind to the substrate-enzyme complex or free enzyme.
      b. V_{max} is decreased, but K_m is unaffected.

E. Enzyme regulation can occur by the following mechanisms.
   1. Increased synthesis of the enzyme.
   2. Activation or inactivation by proteolytic enzymes.
   3. Activation or inactivation by covalent modification (phosphorylation).
   4. Allosteric modification.
   5. Degradation of enzymes by proteases.

F. Measurement of enzymes is useful in the diagnosis of disease. Examples are alanine aminotransferase (liver

damage), creatine kinase, troponin T, and lactate dehydrogenase (myocardial infarction).

4.3 Basic Concepts of Metabolism

A. Catabolism—degradation of large, complex molecules into smaller, simpler products: releases energy.
B. Anabolism—conversion of small, simple molecules or precursors into larger, more complex molecules: requires energy.
C. Catabolic and anabolic pathways are distinct and usually located in different cellular compartments.
D. Highly integrated network of chemical reactions (Figure 2-10).
E. Highly regulated chemical reactions that are regulated by the synthesis and degradation rates of enzymes; the control of enzymatic activity via allosteric control, reversible covalent modifications, and inhibitors; and the accessibility and amount of substrate via compartmentation and control of substrate flux.
F. Thermodynamically unfavorable reactions are driven by coupling to thermodynamically favorable reactions.
G. ATP—the universal energy carrier.
   1. Conserves energy in high-energy phosphoanhydride bond.
   2. ATP–adenosine diphosphate (ADP) cycle is the fundamental mode of energy exchange.
      a. ATP acts as phosphate donor.
      b. ADP acts as phosphate acceptor.
H. Electron carrier molecules.
   1. NAD^+—accepts one hydrogen and two electrons. Electron acceptor in the oxidation of fuels.
   2. Flavin adenine dinucleotide (FAD)—accepts two hydrogens and two electrons. Electron acceptor in the oxidation of fuels.
   3. $NADP^+$—P at 2′ position of adenosine moiety. Also accepts one hydrogen and two electrons. NADPH is the electron donor for reductive biosyntheses.
I. Coenzyme A (CoA)—universal carrier of acyl groups.

4.4 Catabolism

A. Degradation of large, complex molecules into smaller, simpler products.
B. Carbohydrate catabolism.
   1. Glycolysis (Figure 2-11)—series of reactions that convert one 6-carbon glucose to two 3-carbon pyruvate or lactate molecules; also produce intermediates for other pathways of metabolism.
      a. The process is located in the cytosol.
      b. Under aerobic conditions, two pyruvate, two NADH, and two ATP are produced.
      c. Under anaerobic conditions, lactate and ATP are produced by using NADH.
      d. Important enzymes.
         (1) Hexokinase (most cells)—irreversible reaction trapping glucose in cell.

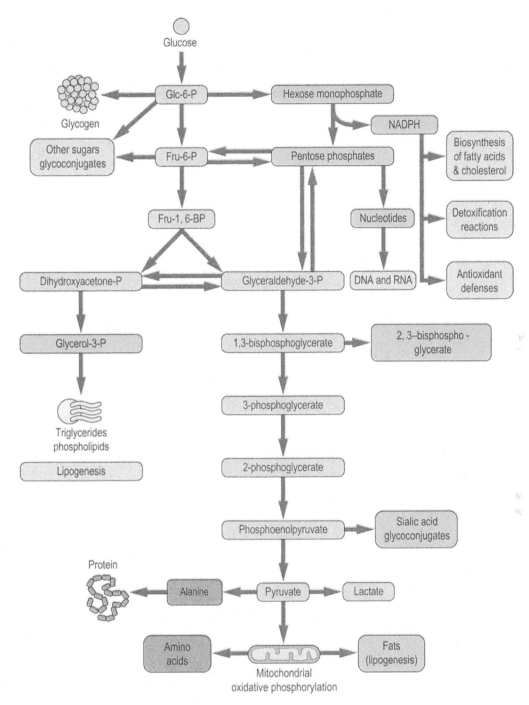

Figure 2-10 Interactions between glycolysis and other metabolic pathways. *(From Baynes JW, Dominiczak MH: Medical Biochemistry, ed 3, New York, Mosby, 2009.)*

(2) Glucokinase—found in liver; has high K_m and V_{max}.

(3) Phosphofructokinase—irreversible reaction forming fructose-1,6-bisphosphate; the principal rate-limiting step in the pathway.

(4) Pyruvate kinase—catalyzes formation of ATP and production of pyruvate.

e. Regulators.

(1) Hexokinase—inhibited by glucose 6-phosphate (feedback inhibition).

(2) Glucokinase—via glucokinase regulatory protein.

(a) Inhibited by fructose 6-phosphate.

(b) Stimulated by glucose.

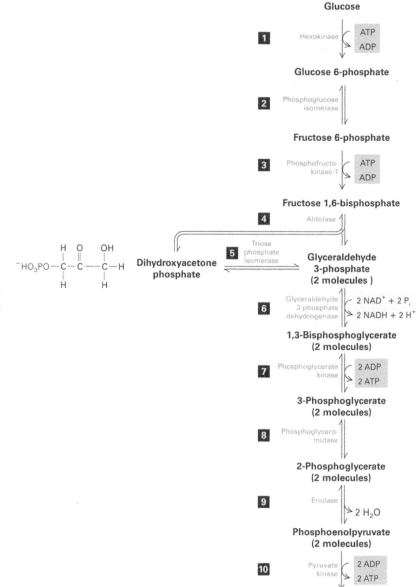

Figure 2-11 The glycolytic pathway.
(From Lodish HF: Molecular Cell Biology, ed 7, New York, WH Freeman & Co, 2013.)

(3) Phosphofructokinase—inhibited by ATP and citrate, stimulated by AMP and fructose-2,6-bisphosphate.

(4) Pyruvate kinase—in muscle, activated by fructose-1,6-bisphosphate and inhibited by ATP; in the liver, inhibited by ATP and alanine.

(5) Lactic acidosis occurs when pyruvate metabolism is blocked.

f. Endocrine regulation of glycolysis.

(1) Insulin stimulates.

(2) Glucagon inhibits.

(3) Epinephrine stimulates in muscle and inhibits in liver.

2. Pentose phosphate pathway (hexose monophosphate shunt).

a. Source of pentoses for nucleotide synthesis.

b. Major source of NADPH for synthesis of fatty acids, cholesterol, and steroids.

c. Overall reaction (glucose 6-phosphate + 2 NADP → ribulose—5 + CO_2 and 2 NADPH).

d. Transketolase and transaldolase catalyze reversible reactions in the pathway.

e. Does not consume or produce ATP.

3. Tricarboxylic acid (TCA) cycle (Krebs cycle, citric acid cycle) (Figure 2-12).

a. Complete oxidation of acetyl CoA to CO_2.

b. Process located in mitochondria.

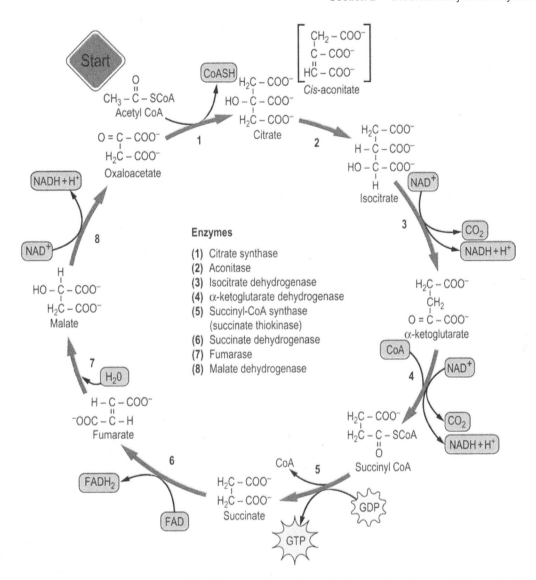

Figure 2-12 Intermediates and enzymes of the tricarboxylic acid cycle. (*Adapted from Baynes JW, Dominiczak MH: Medical Biochemistry, ed 3, New York, Mosby, 2009.*)

c. Consists of eight reactions that require five coenzymes.
   (1) FAD.
   (2) Thiamine pyrophosphate.
   (3) Lipoic acid.
   (4) CoA.
   (5) NAD$^+$.
d. Provides substrates for biosynthetic processes.
   (1) Citrate used for fatty acid synthesis.
   (2) Succinyl CoA for heme synthesis.
   (3) Oxaloacetate for glucose synthesis.
   (4) α-Ketoglutarate for nonessential amino acid synthesis.
e. Important irreversible regulatory enzymes.
   (1) Citrate synthase—pace setting enzyme of TCA cycle. Rate controlled by availability of oxaloacetate and acetyl CoA, inhibited by high citrate levels.
   (2) Isocitrate dehydrogenase—inhibited by ATP and NADH and stimulated by ADP.
   (3) α-Ketoglutarate dehydrogenase—inhibited by NADH, ATP, and succinyl CoA.
f. Overall reaction.
   (1) Acetyl CoA + 3 NAD + FAD + GDP + P_i = 2 CO_2 + 3 NADH + reduced form of flavin adenine dinucleotide ($FADH_2$) + GTP.
      (a) Three NADH oxidized to produce 7.5 moles of ATP.
      (b) $FADH_2$ produces 1.5 moles of ATP.
      (c) GTP converted to ATP by nucleoside diphosphate kinase.
      (d) One cycle of TCA produces 10 moles of ATP.

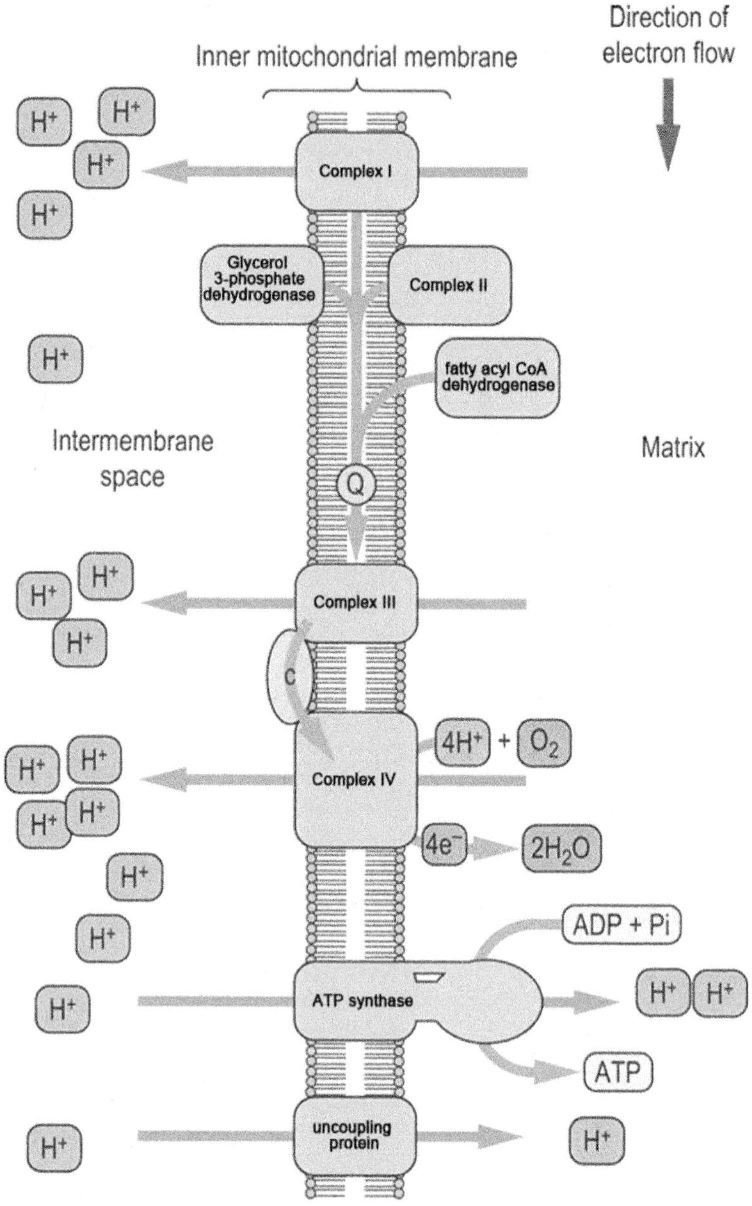

Figure 2-13 Schematic diagram of the electron transport chain and oxidative phosphorylation. *(Adapted from Baynes JW, Dominiczak MH: Medical Biochemistry, ed 3, New York, Mosby, 2009.)*

4. Electron transport chain and oxidative phosphorylation (Figure 2-13): series of electron carriers that pass electrons from NADH and $FADH_2$ to O_2 to form water; the liberated free energy is used to synthesize ATP from ADP.
   a. Associated with inner mitochondrial membrane.
   b. Transport chain composed of four multisubunit protein complexes with prosthetic groups for electron transport.
      (1) NADH–coenzyme Q (CoQ) reductase (complex I): prosthetic groups flavin mononucleotide (FMN), Fe-S, and nonheme iron clusters.
      (2) Succinyl–CoQ reductase (complex II): prosthetic groups FAD, Fe-S, and nonheme iron clusters.
      (3) Cytochrome-*c* reductase (complex III): prosthetic groups hemes, Fe-S, and nonheme iron clusters.
      (4) Cytochrome-*c* oxidase (complex IV): prosthetic groups hemes, Cu_A, and Cu_B (inhibited by cyanide, carbon monoxide, and azide).
   c. NADH $\rightarrow$ complex I $\rightarrow$ CoQ $\rightarrow$ complex III $\rightarrow$ cytochrome-*c* $\rightarrow$ complex IV.
   d. $FADH_2$ $\rightarrow$ complex II $\rightarrow$ CoQ $\rightarrow$ complex III $\rightarrow$ cytochrome-*c* $\rightarrow$ complex IV.
   e. Transfer of electrons results in the pumping of protons from the matrix to the intermembrane space, which establishes a membrane potential.
   f. Energy in membrane potential is conserved by pumping protons across the inner mitochondrial

membrane via ATP synthase to generate ATP from $ADP + P_i$.

5. Glycogenolysis—the breakdown of glycogen to form glucose. Degradation occurs at the nonreducing end of glycogen.
   a. Important enzymes.
      (1) Glycogen phosphorylase—phosphorylates the α-1,4 bonds of glycogen, resulting in the release of glucose 1-phosphate. Phosphorylase stops four residues short of branch points in glycogen. Enzyme requires pyridoxal phosphate, a derivative of vitamin B_6.
      (2) Transferase enzyme and α-1,6-glucosidase (debranching enzyme)—responsible for cleaving α-1,6 bonds in a two-step process to release free glucose.
   b. Regulation.
      (1) Glucagons and epinephrine through cAMP activate protein kinases A, which phosphorylates the phosphorylase enzyme, converting it to the active form of the enzyme.
      (2) Insulin dephosphorylates the phosphorylase enzyme, inactivating it.
      (3) Allosteric inhibitors of phosphorylase include ATP, creatine phosphate, and glucose-6-phosphate.
      (4) Allosteric stimulators include AMP and glucose (in liver).
6. Glycogen storage disease comprises numerous diseases that result from defects in enzymes required for glycogen synthesis or glycogen degradation (e.g., von Gierke disease results from deficiencies of glucose-6-phosphatase).

C. Lipid catabolism.
   1. β oxidation of fatty acids—fatty acids constitute a major source of energy. The fatty acids are oxidized to acetyl CoA, and ultimately the acetyl CoA is oxidized to CO_2 in the TCA cycle, producing NADH and $FADH_2$ for the electron transport chain.
      a. The process is located in the mitochondria.
      b. Fatty acids are activated to acyl CoA by acyl CoA synthetase in the outer mitochondrial membrane. Fatty acids are delivered into the mitochondria by the carnitine shuttle.
         (1) Two enzymes are involved in transporting large fatty acids into mitochondria.
            (a) Carnitine acyltransferase-1—associates carnitine with the fatty acid to form acyl carnitine (releases CoA).
            (b) Carnitine acyltransferase-2—reassociates the fatty acid with CoA. This enzyme is inhibited by malonyl CoA.
      c. Important enzymes for β oxidation: each round of β oxidation shortens the acyl CoA by two carbons and produces one $FADH_2$, one NADH, and one acetyl CoA (for the TCA cycle).
         (1) Fatty acyl CoA dehydrogenases—specific for fatty acids of different chain lengths. Ultimately, a β ketoacyl CoA and NADH are produced.
         (2) Thiolase—adds a CoA, which results in the release of acetyl CoA.
      d. Regulators: act primarily through activation or inhibition of hormone-sensitive lipase (degrades triglycerides into fatty acids and glycerol in adipocytes). Free fatty acids readily enter the cell and become fatty acid acyl CoA.
         (1) Glucagons, epinephrine, and ACTH stimulate hormone-sensitive lipase.
         (2) Insulin inhibits hormone-sensitive lipase.
   2. Ketone metabolism—under conditions of reduced intake of carbohydrate and increased β oxidation of fatty acids, ketone bodies are formed. Because most of the oxaloacetate is being used for gluconeogenesis, acetyl CoA resulting from β oxidation cannot be condensed and metabolized further in the TCA cycle. Acetyl CoA is conserved by converting it to acetoacetate and β-hydroxybutyrate in the liver mitochondria.
      a. Ketone bodies may serve as a source of energy for extrahepatic tissues.
         (1) Heart.
         (2) Skeletal muscle.
         (3) Kidney.
         (4) Brain.
      b. Accumulation of ketone bodies results in ketoacidosis.
      c. Ketoacidosis occurs with excessive fatty acid oxidation associated with a lack of insulin.
   3. Hyperlipidemia results from defects in lipoprotein metabolism.
      a. Type I results from the accumulation of triglycerides.
      b. Type II results from the accumulation of cholesterol.
      c. Type III results from the accumulation of both triglyceride and cholesterol.
   4. Cholesterol catabolism.
      a. Most cholesterol is eliminated from the body via the feces after conversion to bile salt in the liver.
         (1) Cholic acid and chenodeoxycholic acid are the major bile acids.
         (2) Bile salts are produced by the addition of an amino acid to the bile acid.
            (a) Glycocholate (cholic acid and glycine).
            (b) Glycochenodeoxycholic acid (chenodeoxycholic acid and glycine).
            (c) Taurine may also be added to bile acids to produce comparable bile salts.
      b. Enterohepatic circulation accounts for reabsorption of most of the bile acids secreted from the liver.

D. Protein catabolism.
1. Two major enzyme systems are responsible for protein degradation.
    a. Ubiquitin-proteosome mechanism—proteins tagged with molecules of ubiquitin are recognized by the proteolytic molecule proteasome, which degrades the protein to amino acids.
    b. Lysosomes—primarily responsible for digesting extracellular enzymes to amino acids.
2. The liver is the main site for amino acid catabolism, where amino groups are removed, converted to urea, and excreted. The remaining carbon skeleton is then metabolized.
3. Pyridoxal phosphate (vitamin B_6) is an important coenzyme in transamination reactions using a class of enzymes known as *aminotransferases*. The products of this reaction (α-keto acids and glutamate) can be used as amino group donors for the synthesis of essential amino acids (glutamate) or enter metabolic pathways for energy metabolism (α-keto acids).
4. Every amino acid has a corresponding α-keto acid that can be metabolized for energy.
    a. α-Ketoglutarate (glutamate).
    b. Oxaloacetate (aspartate).
    c. Pyruvate (alanine).
5. The carbon groups are further metabolized to pyruvate, acetyl CoA, acetoacetyl CoA, α-ketoglutarate, succinyl CoA, fumarate, or oxaloacetate.
6. Peripheral amino acids can be transported to the liver as part of alanine (alanine aminotransferase), glutamate (glutamate aminotransferase), or glutamine.
7. Phenylketonuria, caused by a deficiency of phenylalanine hydroxylase, results in the inability to metabolize phenylalanine. Aspartame contains phenylalanine and is contraindicated in individuals with this deficiency.
8. Maple syrup urine disease is caused by a deficiency in branched-chain α-keto acid dehydrogenase.
9. Albinism is caused by a defect in tyrosine metabolism and subsequent inability to produce melanin.
10. Because these enzymes are normally intracellular enzymes, elevated plasma levels of aminotransferases indicate damage to tissues containing cells rich in these enzymes (i.e., the liver).
11. Only the liver makes urea because it is the only tissue that has arginase. Four ATPs are needed for each cycle.
12. Urea cycle (Figure 2-14).

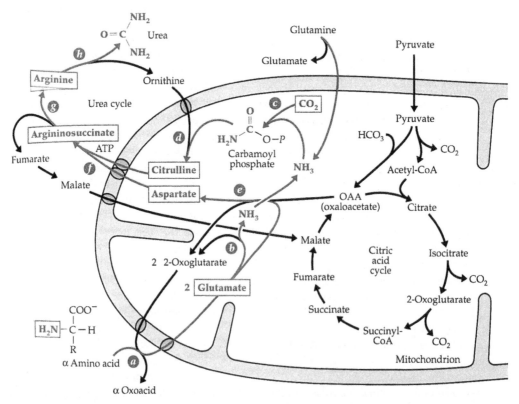

Figure 2-14 Integration of the urea cycle with mitochondrial metabolism. Thinner lines trace the flow of nitrogen into urea on deamination of amino acids or on removal of nitrogen from the side chain of glutamine. *(From Metzler DE: Biochemistry, ed 2, San Diego, Academic Press, 2003.)*

E. Nucleotide catabolism.
1. Purine nucleotides—degraded to uric acid through a series of reactions catalyzed by enzymes.
   a. Adenosine deaminase—removes the amino group.
   b. 5′-Nucleotidase—converts the nucleotide to nucleoside.
   c. Purine nucleoside phosphorylase—releases the bases (guanine and hypoxanthine).
   d. Guanine is deaminated and hypoxanthine oxidized to xanthine.
   e. Xanthine is oxidized to uric acid.
   f. Gout—caused by the overproduction or underexcretion of uric acid.
2. Pyrimidine nucleotides—pyrimidine ring is opened and degraded to β-alanine and β-aminoisobutyrate, which can be further metabolized in the citric acid cycle.

4.5 Anabolism

A. Process by which small, simple compounds are used to synthesize larger, more complex molecules, including carbohydrates, lipids, proteins, and nucleic acids.
B. Carbohydrate anabolism.
1. Glycogenesis—process by which glucose is stored as a polymer consisting of α-1,4 and α-1,6 glycosidic bonds.
2. Process occurs in the liver and muscle.
3. Important enzymes for glycogen synthesis.
   a. Glycogen is synthesized from a series of reactions that use glucose-6-phosphate trapped within the cell by either glucokinase (liver) or hexokinase (muscle).
   b. Glucose-6-phosphate is converted to glucose-1-phosphate, which reacts with uridine triphosphate, producing uridine diphosphate (UDP) glucose the activated carrier of glycosyl units (irreversible step).
   c. UDP-glucose transfers the glycosyl unit to the nonreducing ends of glycogen in a reaction catalyzed by glycogen synthase (UDP-glycosyltransferase).
   d. When the chain contains 6 to 11 residues, a branching enzyme transfers the oligosaccharide to an interior site of the glycogen molecule, creating an α-1,6 glycosidic bond.
4. Regulation of glycogen synthesis is by insulin that activates protein phosphatase 1, which, by removing phosphate groups from glycogen synthase, activates the enzyme. Epinephrine (muscle) and glucagon (liver) via cAMP and protein kinase A inactivate glycogen synthase via phosphorylation.
C. Lipid anabolism—occurs when energy sources (acetyl CoA, citrate) are high.
1. Synthesis of fatty acids occurs in the cytoplasm by sequential addition of two carbon units (acetyl CoA) to the carboxyl end.

2. Acetyl CoA carboxylase (biotin serving as a coenzyme) catalyzes the rate-limiting step in the production of malonyl CoA, which is the committed step in the synthesis of fatty acids. The enzyme is regulated by two mechanisms.
   a. Allosteric control.
      (1) Citrate activates.
      (2) Malonyl CoA and AMP inhibit.
   b. Covalent modulation (phosphorylation and dephosphorylation).
      (1) Insulin activates.
      (2) Epinephrine and glucagons inactivate.
3. Fatty acid synthase—a multienzyme complex that synthesizes palmitic acid.
   a. Uses NADPH as reducing source.
   b. Located in cytosol.
   c. Net reaction: 8 acetyl CoA + 7 ATP + 14 NADPH + H^+ → palmitate + 14 NADP + 8 CoA + 6 H_2O + 7 ADP + 7 P_i.
4. Synthesis of triacylglycerides (triglycerides).
   a. Glycerol phosphate serves as the initial acceptor of the fatty acid. Glycerol phosphate can be synthesized by glycolysis in liver and adipose cells or from glycerol in liver.
   b. The fatty acids are activated by thiokinases (CoA attachment).
   c. Final synthetic pathway involves the addition of the fatty acids and phosphate removal.
D. Cholesterol anabolism.
1. Synthesized through a series of reactions from carbon atoms provided by acetyl CoA.
2. Rate-limiting step and control of synthesis is exerted through regulation of 3-hydroxy-3-methylglutaryl (HMG) CoA reductase.
   a. Inhibitors of HMG CoA reductase—cholesterol, glucagons, glucocorticoids, bile acids, and medications (statin drugs).
   b. Stimulators of HMG CoA reductase—insulin, thyroxine, and fat ingestion.
3. Familial hypercholesterolemia is caused by a defect in the low-density lipoprotein (LDL) receptor.
E. Protein anabolism.
1. Protein synthesis involves transcription and translation of DNA and RNA (see Section 2.2 and 2.3, Cellular and Molecular Biology).
2. Essential amino acids (isoleucine, leucine, lysine, methionine, phenylalanine, valine, tryptophan, threonine) must be obtained in the diet because humans cannot synthesize them in sufficient quantities.
3. Nonessential amino acids—can be synthesized in humans.
   a. Alanine—transamination from pyruvate.
   b. Aspartate—transamination from oxaloacetate.
   c. Asparginine—addition of ammonia to aspartate.
   d. Cysteine—skeleton from serine and sulfur from methionine.

e. Glutamate—transamination from α-ketoglutarate.
f. Glutamine—addition of ammonia to glutamate.
g. Glycine—removal of hydroxymethyl from serine, de novo synthesis by action of glycine synthetase or oxidation of choline.
h. Proline—from α-ketoglutarate.
i. Serine—from 3-phosphoglycerate and transamination.
j. Tyrosine—from phenylalanine.

4. Products and utilization of individual amino acids.
   a. Precursor of γ-aminobutyric acid (GABA)—important intermediate in transamination reactions.
   b. Alanine—important in gluconeogenesis.
   c. Glycine—precursor for purine and porphyrin synthesis.
   d. Aspartate—involved in purine synthesis, urea structure, and gluconeogenesis.
   e. Serine—source of one-carbon fragments for folic acid coenzymes.
   f. Proline—major collagen amino acid. Converted to hydroxyproline.
   g. Glutamine—major role in NH_4^+ metabolism and transfer of amino groups to sugars, pyrimidines, and purines.
   h. Histidine—precursor of histamine.
   i. Tyrosine—precursor of thyroxine, melanin, and catecholamines.
   j. Arginine—precursor of urea and creatine.
   k. Phenylalanine—precursor of tyrosine.
   l. Tryptophan—precursor of serotonin.
   m. Cysteine—precursor of taurine and source of sulfur.
   n. Methionine—precursor of cysteine, adenosylmethionine (transmethylation reactions), and source of sulfur.
   o. Nitric oxide (NO)—mediator of numerous physiologic activities, including smooth muscle relaxation, macrophage stimulation, and inhibition of platelet aggregation. Its synthesis requires NO synthase. In the reaction, arginine, O_2, and NADPH are converted to NO and citrulline.

F. Nucleotide anabolism.
   1. Purine biosynthesis.
      a. Addition of amino group from glutamine to phosphoribosyl-1-pyrophosphate (amidophosphoribosyltransferase catalyzes this committed step). This addition is inhibited by purines.
      b. Closure of rings by addition of single carbons using tetrahydrofolate, biotin, and cobalamine.
      c. Purines also can be synthesized from intact bases obtained from dietary sources or nucleotide degradation.
   2. Pyrimidine biosynthesis.
      a. Orotate is synthesized from carbamoyl phosphate in cytosol.

b. Ribose phosphate is added followed by subsequent reductase reactions to form uridine monophosphate, uridine triphosphate, and cytidine triphosphate.

5.0 Connective Tissue and Bone

A. Connective tissue—biologic tissue that supports, connects, or separates epithelial, muscle, and nervous tissue. It consists of three components: cells, fibers, and ground substance.
   1. Cells.
      a. Fixed cells—fibroblasts, myofibroblasts, pericytes, adipose cells, mast cells, and macrophages.
      b. Transient cells—plasma cells and leukocytes (neutrophils, eosinophils, and lymphocytes).
   2. Fibers.
      a. Collagen.
         (1) Most abundant protein in humans, characterized by its high rigidity and tensile strength.
         (2) Approximately one third of collagen is glycine (every third position), and 10% is proline.
         (3) Hydroxyproline and hydroxylysine are formed from proline and lysine, respectively, after translation (posttranslational modification). This requires ascorbate, Fe^{2+}, and O_2.
         (4) The tertiary structure is a triple helix (tropocollagen) formed by hydrogen bonds and modified by glycosylation of hydroxylysine.
         (5) Tropocollagen spontaneously aggregates, and cross-links form between lysine and hydroxylysine.
         (6) Several types of collagen exist.
            (a) Type I—skin, tendon, bone, and dentin.
            (b) Type II—cartilage.
            (c) Type III—aorta and fetal skin.
            (d) Type IV—basement membrane.
            (e) Type V—placenta and skin.
         (7) Collagen is degraded by mammalian enzymes, which cleave tropocollagen. Cleavage of tropocollagen permits further digestion by proteases.
         (8) Osteogenesis imperfecta is an inherited disease that is due to an amino acid substitution in collagen that interferes with the normal folding of the protein into a triple helix conformation.
      b. Elastic—provides elasticity to connective tissue.
         (1) Rich in proline and other nonpolar side chains. Approximately one third of elastin amino acids are glycines.
         (2) Does not have a stable tertiary structure, but cross-links are derived from lysine condensation.
         (3) Because of its elastic properties, it is found in arterial walls, lung pleura, and parenchyma.

(4) Elastin is degraded by elastases by inflammatory cells or cells involved in tissue remodeling.

c. Keratin.

(1) Fibrous, insoluble proteins derived from epidermis.

(2) Forms a helical structure stabilized by hydrogen bonds.

(3) Overall properties depend on the degree of disulfide cross-linking.

(a) Low level of cross-linking—more flexibility (e.g., hair, skin).

(b) High level of cross-linking—less flexibility (e.g., nails).

3. Ground substance—ground substance and fibers constitute the extracellular matrix (ECM).

a. Glycosaminoglycans—long, inflexible, unbranched polysaccharides, sulfated (keratin sulfate, heparan sulfate, heparin, chondroitin sulfate, dermatan sulfate) and nonsulfated (hyaluronic acid).

b. Proteoglycans—core protein and glycosaminoglycans.

c. Adhesive glycoproteins: integrins, fibronectin, laminin, tenascin, chondronectin, and osteonectin.

B. Cartilage—specialized connective tissue composed of chondrocytes and a specialized ECM.

1. Hyaline—homogeneous amorphous matrix (glycosaminoglycans, hyaluronic acid, chondroitin sulfate, and keratan sulfate).

2. Elastic—elastic fibers and lamellae; elastin in matrix.

3. Fibrocartilage—large bundles of type I collagen.

C. Bone—connective tissue characterized by a mineralized ECM.

1. Hydroxyapatite.

a. $Ca_{10}(PO_4)_6(OH)_2$.

b. Hydroxyapatite can vary in ion content. Most substituted ions increase the solubility of the crystal. Fluoride *decreases* the solubility.

(1) Ca^{2+} may be substituted by Mg^{2+}, Sr^{2+}, and Pb^{2+}.

(2) PO_4^{3-} may be substituted by HPO_4^- and citrate.

(3) OH^- may be substituted by Cl^-, F^-, and HCO_3^-.

2. Mineralization.

a. Supersaturated solutions of calcium and P_i (1.5 mM of each) may exist without hydroxyapatite formation (crystals of hydroxyapatite promote precipitation).

b. Increasing the concentration of calcium and P_i more than 3 mM of each results in the formation of amorphous calcium phosphate $CaHPO_4\text{-}2H_2O$ (brushite).

c. Mineralization process.

(1) Initiation—ions become aligned on the surface of the initiator protein (phosphoryns).

(a) Contain phosphorylated side chains for binding Ca^{2+}.

(b) Cationic side chains attract PO_4^{3+} and OH^-.

Table 2-3

Composition of Calcified Tissue

TISSUE	% INORGANIC	% ORGANIC	% H$_2$O
Enamel	95	1	4
Dentin	70	20	10
Bone	60	25	15
Calculus	84	10	6

(2) Crystal growth.

(a) Osteoblasts (and odontoblasts) secrete phosphoryns between collagen matrix.

(b) Growth of crystals facilitated by concentrating calcium and P_i in matrix vesicles.

(i) Phospholipid membrane vesicles produced by budding from osteoblasts.

(ii) Calcium pump driven by ATP hydrolysis.

(c) Composition of mineralized tissues (Table 2-3).

6.0 Nervous System

6.1 General Properties

A. The central nervous system (CNS) consists of highly integrated neurons (spinal cord and brain) surrounded by cerebrospinal fluid.

B. The peripheral nervous system is an interface between the CNS and the environment.

1. Autonomic neurons.

a. Parasympathetic.

b. Sympathetic.

c. Enteric.

2. Sensory receptors and afferent neurons (vision, hearing, chemical, and touch).

3. Somatic motoneurons (muscle, endocrine, and exocrine gland secretion).

6.2 Central Nervous System

A. Spinal cord—contains sensory (afferent or ascending pathways) and motor (efferent or descending pathways) nerves.

B. Brainstem.

1. Medulla—responsible for regulation or coordination.

a. Blood pressure.

b. Breathing.

c. Swallowing.

d. Coughing.

e. Vomiting.

2. Pons—participates in respiratory regulation and the relay of information from cerebral hemispheres to the cerebellum.

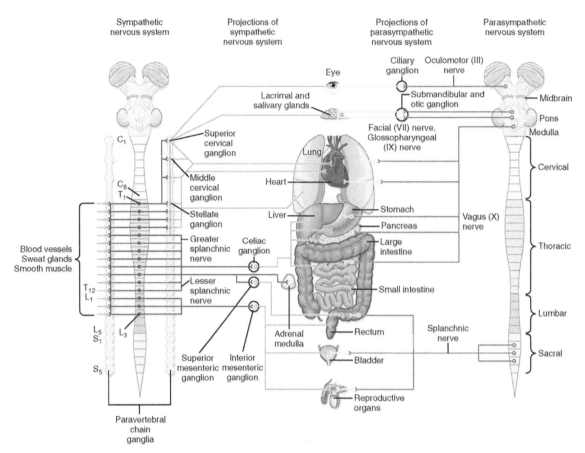

Sympathetic
nervous system

Projections of
sympathetic
nervous system

Projections of
parasympathetic
nervous system

Parasympathetic
nervous system

Figure 2-15 Parasympathetic and sympathetic nervous system. *(From Koeppen BM, Stanton BA, Berne RM: Berne & Levy Physiology, ed 6. Philadelphia, Saunders, 2010.)*

3. Midbrain—participates in coordination of visual and auditory systems.

C. Cerebellum—responsible for posture and coordination of movement.

D. Thalamus—processes sensory information going to and motor information coming from the cerebral cortex.

E. Hypothalamus—essentially an endocrine gland that is involved with the regulation of body temperature, water balance, and food intake (see Section 13.1, Endocrine System).

F. Cerebral cortex—receives and processes sensory information and integrates motor function in response to peripheral input.

G. Basal ganglia—involved with movement control; modulates information from the thalamus to the motor cortex in the execution of movement. GABA is an important neurotransmitter for many inhibitory synaptic connections.

H. Hippocampus and amygdala—involved with emotions and the autonomic responses mediated through the hypothalamus (e.g., pupil size, heart rate, hypothalamic hormone secretion).

6.3 Autonomic Nervous System

A. Involuntary regulation of visceral organs. The autonomic nervous system (ANS) is highly integrated in the hypothalamus, but reflexes often involve only the medulla or spinal cord. Most tissues are tonically innervated by both sympathetic and parasympathetic systems, resulting in dual control (inhibitory and stimulatory). An exception is the salivary gland, where both systems are stimulatory.

B. Parasympathetic system (Figure 2-15).
   1. Preganglionic neurons have cell bodies in brainstem or sacral region of spinal cord (S1–S4) (long fibers).
   2. Postganglionic cell bodies are found in ganglia located near target tissues (short fibers).
   3. Both preganglionic and postganglionic neurons are cholinergic (acetylcholine is synthesized, stored, and used as a neurotransmitter in nerve terminal).
   4. Two types of cholinergic receptors (cholinoreceptors) exist (Table 2-4).
      a. Nicotinic receptors.
         (1) Found in autonomic ganglion, neuromuscular junction of skeletal muscle, and chromaffin cells of the adrenal medulla.

Table 2-4

Location and Mechanism of Action of Autonomic Receptors

RECEPTOR	TARGET TISSUE	SIGNALING MECHANISM
Adrenoceptors		
α_1	Vascular smooth muscle, skin, renal, and splanchnic GI tract, sphincters Bladder, sphincter Radial muscle, iris	IP_3, ↑ intracellular (Ca^{2+})
α_2	GI tract, wall Presynaptic adrenergic neurons	Inhibition of adenylyl cyclase, ↓ cAMP
β_1	Heart Salivary glands Adipose tissue Kidney	Stimulation of adenylyl cyclase, ↑ cAMP
β_2	Vascular smooth muscle of skeletal muscle GI tract, wall Bladder, wall Bronchioles	Stimulation of adenylyl cyclase, ↑ cAMP
Cholinergic Receptors		
Nicotinic	Skeletal muscle, motor end plate Postganglionic neurons, SNS and PNS Adrenal medulla	Opening Na^+ and K^+ channels → depolarization
Muscarinic	All effector organs, PNS Sweat glands, SNS	IP_3, ↑ intracellular (Ca^{2+})

From Costanzo LS: Physiology, ed 3, Philadelphia, Saunders, 2004.

cAMP, Cyclic adenosine monophosphate; *GI*, gastrointestinal; *PNS*, parasympathetic nervous system; *SNS*, sympathetic nervous system.

(2) Agonists include acetylcholine, nicotine, and carbachol.

(3) Antagonists include curare (skeletal neuromuscular junction–selective) and hexamethonium (ganglion-selective).

(4) Activation of the receptor by the agonist results in the opening of Na^+/K^+ ion channels, resulting in excitation.

b. Muscarinic receptors.

(1) Found in all effector organs of the parasympathetic nervous system (smooth muscle, cardiac muscle, and most glands) and in sweat glands (innervated by the sympathetic nervous system).

(2) Activation results in G protein–mediated activation of phospholipase C and generation of IP_3 and diacylglycerol with subsequent release of Ca^{2+} to produce tissue-specific physiologic actions (similar to α_1-adrenoreceptors).

(3) Other muscarinic receptors use G proteins to act directly on ion channels (e.g., K^+ channels in cardiac tissue).

5. Acetylcholine activity is terminated through the activity of acetylcholinesterase, which degrades acetylcholine.

C. Sympathetic system (see Figure 2-15).

1. Preganglionic neurons have cell bodies in the thoracolumbar spinal cord segments (T1–L3).

2. Postganglionic cell bodies are located in the vertebral ganglia or paravertebral ganglia (e.g., mesenteric or celiac).

3. Preganglionic neurons are cholinergic; release acetylcholine to interact with nicotinic receptors.

4. Postganglionic neurons are adrenergic; synthesize, store, and release norepinephrine to interact with adrenoceptors. (Postganglionic neurons to sweat glands are cholinergic.)

5. The adrenal medulla is a specialized endocrine organ, which, on stimulation from sympathetic neurons, secretes catecholamines (80% epinephrine and 20% norepinephrine).

6. Several classes of adrenergic receptors exist (see Table 2-4).

7. Norepinephrine is removed from the terminal by neuronal reuptake and reused or metabolized by monoamine oxidase (MAO).

D. Enteric system—intrinsic neuronal system of the GI tract. Neurons and neuromodulators are contained totally in the tissues but are influenced by input from the sympathetic and parasympathetic nervous system.

Table 2-5					

Classification of Nerve Fibers

CLASSIFICATION	TYPE OF NERVE FIBER	EXAMPLE	RELATIVE DIAMETER	RELATIVE CONDUCTION VELOCITY	MYELINATION
Sensory and motor	Aα	α motoneurons	Largest	Fastest	Yes
	Aβ	Touch, pressure	Medium	Medium	Yes
	Aγ	γ motoneurons to muscle spindles (intrafusal fibers)	Medium	Medium	Yes
	Aδ	Touch, pressure, temperature, pain	Small	Medium	Yes
	B	Preganglionic autonomic nerves	Small	Medium	Yes
	C	Slow pain; postganglionic autonomic nerves; olfaction	Smallest	Slowest	No
Sensory only*	Ia (Aα)	Muscle spindle afferents	Largest	Fastest	Yes
	Ib (Aα)	Golgi tendon organ afferents	Largest	Fastest	Yes
	II (Aβ)	Secondary afferents of muscle spindles; touch, pressure	Medium	Medium	Yes
	III (Aδ)	Touch, pressure, fast pain, temperature	Small	Medium	Yes
	IV (C)	Pain, temperature; olfaction	Smallest	Slowest	No

From Costanzo LS: Physiology, ed 3, Philadelphia, Saunders, 2004.

*The numerical system is an alternative way to classify sensory nerves.

6.4 Sensory Systems

A. Consist of nerve fibers, which are responsible for transmitting sensory information from receptors to the CNS (afferent input).
B. Nerve fibers (pathways)—classified according to their conduction velocity, which depends on their size and degree of myelination (Table 2-5).
C. Sensory receptors—classified according to their specificity.
   1. Mechanoreceptors—activated by pressure or change in pressure.
      a. Hair cells in the organ of Corti.
      b. Pacinian corpuscles.
      c. Meissner's corpuscles.
      d. Baroreceptors in carotid sinus and carotid arch.
      e. Golgi tendon organs.
   2. Photoreceptors—activated by light (rods and cones in retina).
   3. Chemoreceptors—activated by chemicals (olfactory, gustation, osmoreceptors, pH, O_2 receptors, and CO_2 receptors).
   4. Thermoreceptors—activated by temperature change.
   5. Nociceptors—activated by extremes in pressure, temperature, or noxious chemicals.
   6. Receptors for pain are free nerve endings. Fast pain is carried by group Aδ fibers, and slow pain is carried by group C fibers. Among the neurotransmitters is substance P (release inhibited by opioids).

D. Sensory transduction—the process by which sensory information is transformed into nerve impulses.
   1. Stimulus reacts with receptor.
   2. Ion channels open, producing depolarization or hyperpolarization.
   3. Change in membrane potential (receptor potential) increases or decreases the likelihood that an action potential will be generated. The type, magnitude, and duration determine the number and frequency of the generated action potential.
      a. Depolarizing—moves toward threshold, increasing likelihood of generating an action potential.
      b. Hyperpolarizing—moves away from threshold, decreasing likelihood of generating action potential.
E. Sensory adaptation—the fall in action potential frequency with time despite continuous stimulation.
   1. Phasic receptors—detect onset and offset of a stimulus by generating action potentials. Reduced response follows until stimulus is terminated. These receptors adapt rapidly.
   2. Tonic receptors—respond to the onset of the stimulus and remain depolarized for the duration of the stimulus. These receptors adapt slowly.
F. Somatosensory pathways.
   1. Dorsal column system—responsible for transmitting information about discriminative touch, pressure, vibration, and proprioception.

2. Anterolateral system—responsible for transmitting information about pain, temperature, and light touch.
3. General patterns of transmission.
   a. First-order neuron (primary afferent neuron)—signal transmitted to CNS by the primary afferent neuron. The nerve cell body is located in the dorsal root.
   b. Second-order neuron—signal is transmitted from first-order neurons, and information is then transmitted to the thalamus; located in spinal cord or brainstem.
   c. Third-order neuron—located in the somatosensory nuclei of thalamus; projects information to cerebral cortex.
   d. Fourth-order neuron—located in the somatosensory cortex; responsible for conscious perception of the stimulus.

6.5 Neurotransmission

A. Synaptic transmission—transfer of information from one cell to another.
   1. Electrical synapse—current moves from one cell to another through areas of low resistance (gap junctions). Examples include muscle in cardiac, uterine, and bladder tissue.
   2. Chemical synapse—information transferred through the synaptic cleft by the release of neurotransmitters (e.g., acetylcholine, norepinephrine, dopamine).
      a. Presynaptic neuron.
         (1) Action potential causes Ca^{2+} channels to open, which causes neurotransmitters stored in vesicles to be released.
         (2) Neurotransmitters diffuse across cleft to interact with postsynaptic receptors.
      b. Postsynaptic neuron.
         (1) Neurotransmitter interacts with receptor to open ion channels, which can be either excitatory (cause depolarization by opening sodium ion channels) or inhibitory (cause hyperpolarization by opening chloride ion channels).
         (2) Postsynaptic neurons receive input from many presynaptic terminals, which, when integrated, result in overall stimulation (excitatory postsynaptic potential) or overall inhibition (inhibitory postsynaptic potential). These potentials are graded so that the magnitude determines the frequency of the action potential transmitted down the postsynaptic neuron.
            (a) Spatial summation—occurs when multiple neurons arrive at the postsynaptic neuron simultaneously.
            (b) Temporal summation—occurs when multiple presynaptic inputs arrive in rapid succession, permitting the inputs to overlap in time.

B. Neurotransmitters.
   1. Acetylcholine.
      a. Neuromuscular transmission.
      b. Neurotransmitter in all parasympathetic preganglionic and postganglionic neurons.
      c. Neurotransmitter from all sympathetic preganglionic neurons and from most sympathetic postganglionic neurons to sweat glands.
      d. Activity is terminated through the action of acetylcholinesterase.
      e. Myasthenia gravis is an autoimmune disease that interferes with the acetylcholine receptors on the motor end-plates.
   2. Catecholamines (epinephrine, norepinephrine, and dopamine).
      a. Synthesized from tyrosine.
      b. Activity is terminated by catechol O-methyltransferase (in tissues) or MAO (in nerve).
   3. Serotonin—synthesized from tryptophan.
   4. Histamine—synthesized from histidine.
   5. Glutamate—excitatory neurotransmitter in CNS.
   6. Glycine.
      a. Inhibitory neurotransmitter in CNS.
      b. Causes hyperpolarization by increasing chloride ion conductance.
   7. GABA.
      a. Synthesized from glutamic acid.
      b. Causes hyperpolarization by increasing chloride conductance (GABA$_A$) or potassium conductance (GABA$_B$) in postsynaptic cell.
      c. GABA$_A$ is the receptor site for the action of benzodiazepines and barbiturates.

6.6 Somatic Nervous System (Motoneurons)

A. Motor unit—the single neuron and the muscle fibers it innervates.
   1. Fine movements—single motoneurons innervating a small number of muscle fibers.
   2. Forceful movements—single motoneurons innervating many fibers.
B. Muscle reflexes—automatic response produced through the stimulation of receptors (sensors) in muscle.
   1. Knee-jerk reflex—due to stretching of muscle spindles (intrafusal fibers arranged in parallel with the larger, force-generating extrafusal fibers).
      a. Mechanical stretch of muscle spindle increases afferent fiber firing.
      b. Afferent fibers synapse (monosynaptic reflex) with a motoneuron in spinal cord.
      c. α motoneuron stimulates muscle contraction, returning muscle length to normal.
      d. Muscle spindles are responsible for maintenance of posture and resting muscle length.
      e. Knee-jerk reflex is used to test function of CNS.

2. Withdrawal reflex—response to noxious stimulus (polysynaptic reflex).
3. Golgi tendon reflex—responds to too much tension and results in inhibition of α motoneurons.

7.0 Muscle

7.1 Skeletal Muscle

A. General considerations.
   1. Location—attached to bone, skin deep fascia.
   2. Appearance—striated, peripherally located multinuclei in each fiber (cell), unbranched.
   3. Nervous control—voluntary; controlled by somatic nerves.
   4. Function.
      a. Movement of skeletal system.
      b. Maintain posture.
      c. Movement of diaphragm to change intrathoracic volume.
B. Structural considerations.
   1. Functional unit—each muscle fiber (covered by sarcolemma membranes) is innervated by a motoneuron and contains bundles of myofibrils arranged in repeating structures called *sarcomeres*. Sarcomeres contain repeating units of contractile myofilaments (Figure 2-16).
   2. Thick filaments—composed primarily of myosin myofilaments (200 to 300 myosin molecules).
      a. Present in the A band.
      b. Myosin molecule contains two myosin heads that bind ATP and are responsible for cross-bridging to actin.
   3. Thin filaments—composed of actin, tropomyosin, and troponin.

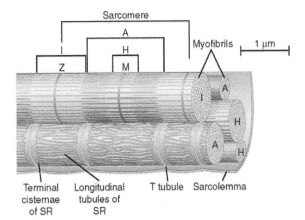

Figure 2-16 Thick and thin filament organization in the sarcomere of myofibrils. *(From Koeppen BM, Stanton BA, Berne RM: Berne & Levy Physiology, ed 6. Philadelphia, Saunders, 2010.)*

   a. Actin is a globular (spherical) protein that forms F-actin and contains binding sites for myosin, tropomyosin, and troponin.
   b. Tropomyosin—elongated protein that covers the cross-bridge binding sites on actin when the muscle is resting.
   c. Troponin—regulator protein that permits cross-bridging when it binds calcium.
   d. Transverse tubules (T-tubules)—sarcolemma membrane that invaginates into the muscle fiber at the A-to-I junction.
C. Excitation-contraction coupling (Figure 2-17).
   1. Action potential—depolarization initiated at the neuromuscular junction owing to the release of acetylcholine and graded end-plate potential (see Section 6.6, Somatic Nervous System [Motoneurons]).
   2. Depolarization of T-tubules—produces a conformational change in the dihydropyridine receptor, an L-type voltage-gated Ca^{2+} channel. The conformational change results in the opening of ryanodine receptors in the terminal cisternae of SR to release Ca^{2+}. This is called *electromechanical coupling*.
D. Skeletal muscle contraction.
   1. In the relaxed state, ATP is hydrolyzed, and the cross-bridge is in a cocked position (Figure 2-18, *A*).
   2. Ca^{2+} released from the SR binds to troponin C, producing a conformational change on the thin filament, which causes tropomyosin to be moved exposing the myosin binding site on actin.
   3. Cross-bridges form between actin and myosin (Figure 2-18, *B*).
   4. A conformational change in myosin, the "ratchet action," pulls the actin filament toward the center of the sarcomere (Figure 2-18, *C*). ADP and P_i are released in the process.
   5. ATP binding to myosin produces a conformational change, decreasing its affinity for actin and causing a displacement of myosin (Figure 2-18, *D*). Without ATP, myosin remains tightly bound, resulting in rigor.
   6. ATP is hydrolyzed to ADP and P_i but not released, recocking the myosin head to the resting position.
   7. The cross-bridging continues as long as Ca^{2+} is bound to troponin. When Ca^{2+} is sequestered again by the SR, calcium is released from troponin, and tropomyosin returns to its resting position, blocking the myosin-binding site on actin.
E. Skeletal muscle mechanics.
   1. Spatial summation—more motor units (fibers) recruited, resulting in greater tension and stronger contraction.
   2. Temporal summation—increased frequency of stimulation to each motor unit, resulting in a summation of twitches.
   3. Tetanus—maximum, sustained muscle contraction with rapid stimulation.

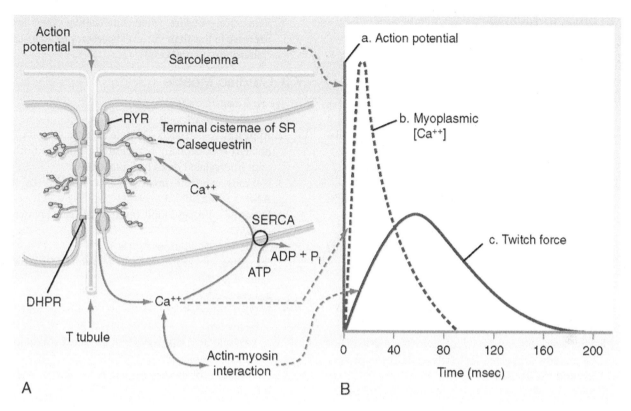

Figure 2-17 A and **B,** Excitation-contraction coupling in skeletal muscle. *(From Bers DM: Cardiac excitation: contraction coupling, nature 415:198-205, 2002.)*

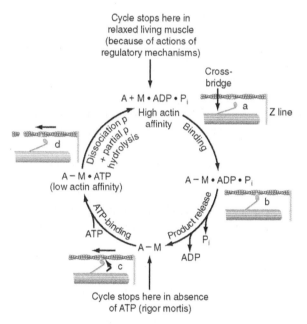

Figure 2-18 A-D, Cross-bridge cycle during skeletal muscle contraction. *(From Koeppen BM, Stanton BA, Berne RM: Berne & Levy Physiology, ed 6. Philadelphia, Saunders, 2010.)*

F. Length-tension relationship.
1. Isometric—tension develops, but muscle does not shorten; load is too great to permit shortening.
2. Isotonic—muscle tension remains constant, and muscle shortens.

G. Energy sources for muscle contraction.
1. ATP—necessary for muscle contraction but limited amounts are available. ATP can be generated by different metabolic pathways.
2. Creatine phosphate—serves as a storage pool of high-energy phosphate. It is an important supply for short bursts of high-intensity activity.
3. Glycolysis.
   a. Aerobic—supply ATP at very high rates (two ATP produced when pyruvate is formed from glucose).
   b. Anaerobic—in the absence of O_2, ATP is produced, and lactic acid is formed from pyruvate.
4. Oxidative phosphorylation—a slow process that uses O_2 and substrates to generate ATP.

H. Fiber types—based on ATP production and consumption rates.
1. Type I (oxidative metabolism)—slow speed, weak contractions, resistant to fatigue.
2. Type IIB (glycolytic metabolism)—fast speed, strong contraction, fatigable.
3. Type IIA (oxidative metabolism)—fast speed, intermediate strength of contraction, resistant to fatigue.

7.2 Smooth Muscle

A. General considerations.
   1. Location.
      a. Walls of hollow organs.
      b. Blood vessels.
      c. Iris and ciliary muscles of eye.
      d. Erector pili (hair).
   2. Appearance—no striations, single nucleus, spindle-shaped fibers, no T-tubules.
   3. Nervous control—involuntary control of ANS.
   4. Function.
      a. Mixes and propels luminal contents through GI tract.
      b. Regulates blood flow in cardiovascular system.
      c. Contracts urinary bladder, gallbladder, and spleen.
      d. Modulates tone in sphincter muscles.
      e. Regulates pupil diameter and lens shape.
      f. Causes hair to stand up (erector pili muscles).
B. Structural considerations.
   1. Multiunit—little or no coupling between cells; must be directly stimulated for contraction (examples are iris and vas deferens).
   2. Unitary (single unit)—have gap junctions that permit fast spread of electrical activity and coordinated contraction (examples are GI tract, bladder, uterus, and ureter); characterized as having pacemaker (slow wave) activity.
   3. Myofilaments.
      a. Thin filament—actin and tropomyosin; no troponin; connected to dense bodies analogous to Z-disc.
      b. Thick filament—myosin but a different isoform than skeletal muscle.
   4. Have caveolae (small invaginations of sarcolemma) that are analogous to T-tubules.
C. Excitation-contraction coupling.
   1. Action potential—depolarization opens voltage-gated Ca^{2+} channels in the sarcolemmal membrane, producing an increase in intracellular Ca^{2+} concentration.
   2. Hormones and neurotransmitters—may produce additional increase in intracellular Ca^{2+} via ligand-gated Ca^{2+} channels or IP_3-gated Ca^{2+} release channels (pharmacomechanical coupling).
   3. Calmodulin binding—increased Ca^{2+} binds to calmodulin, which activates myosin-light-chain kinase.
   4. Myosin-light-chain kinase phosphorylates myosin (uses ATP), which permits it to bind actin to form cross-bridges and produce a contraction. Cross-bridge cycle is identical to that for skeletal muscle.
   5. Myosin dephosphorylation—due to reduced intracellular Ca^{2+}, which activates myosin phosphatase. Myosin and actin remain attached but not by cross-bridges.
   6. Relaxation—occurs when intercellular Ca^{2+} levels decrease to less than the level necessary to form Ca^{2+}-calmodulin complexes.

7.3 Cardiac Muscle

A. General considerations.
   1. Location—heart.
   2. Appearance—striated, single centrally located nucleus (occasionally binucleated), branched, fibers with intercalated discs (cell junctions).
   3. Nervous control—involuntary, controlled by the ANS.
   4. Function—propel blood through the cardiovascular system.
B. Structural considerations.
   1. Structure of cardiac muscle is similar to striated muscle.
      a. Less SR.
      b. Diad instead of triad for T-tubule and SR formation.
      c. T-tubule at Z-disc rather than A-to-I junction in skeletal muscle.
   2. Contraction of cardiac muscle is similar to skeletal muscle.
C. Excitation-contraction coupling (Figure 2-19).
   1. Action potential—initiated in the myocardial cell membrane and spreads to the interior of the cell by way of the T-tubules. This causes an influx of Ca^{2+} through a voltage-gated L-type Ca^{2+} channel (one subunit is the dihydropyridine receptor seen in skeletal muscle). The increase in Ca^{2+} triggers the Ca^{2+}-gated Ca^{2+} channel ryanodine receptors to release more Ca^{2+} from the SR; this is called *electrochemical coupling.*
   2. The resulting increase in Ca^{2+} causes cross-bridge formation and contraction identical to that described for skeletal muscle.
   3. The magnitude of tension developed by myocardial cells is proportional to the intracellular Ca^{2+} concentration.
   4. When Ca^{2+} is sequestered by the SR by the action of Ca^{2+} ATPase, relaxation occurs. In addition, Ca^{2+} is extruded from the cell in exchange for Na^+ in the sarcolemmal membrane.
   5. Cardiac glycosides produce a positive inotropic effect by inhibiting Na^+/K^+ ATPase. This results in an increased intracellular sodium concentration and reduced Na/Ca exchange. The increased intracellular calcium results in an increased contraction.

8.0 Circulation

A. Homeostasis—maintenance of constant conditions in the internal environment of the body. Homeostasis is accomplished through the coordinated efforts of organ

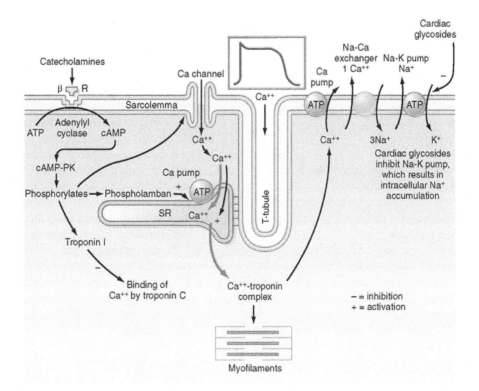

Figure 2-19 Schematic diagram of the movement of calcium in excitation-contraction coupling in cardiac muscle. *(From Koeppen BM, Stanton BA, Berne RM: Berne & Levy Physiology, ed 6. Philadelphia, Saunders, 2010.)*

systems in the body, which are integrated through neuronal and endocrine communication.

1. Internal environment (of a 70-kg adult human)—maintained by organ systems.
   a. ECF (20% of total body weight, 14 L), which includes the following.
      (1) Interstitial fluid (11 L).
         (a) High in sodium and chloride.
         (b) Low in potassium, magnesium, and phosphate.
      (2) Plasma (3 L).
         (a) Similar ionic composition to interstitial fluid.
         (b) Higher concentration of protein compared with interstitial fluid.
   b. ICF (28 L), separated from ECF by the cell membrane, which is highly permeable to water but not to many of the electrolytes and proteins.
      (1) High in phosphate and potassium.
      (2) Low in calcium ions.
2. Factors that must be maintained within very narrow limits and the organs responsible for regulating the concentrations of each include the following.
   a. Electrolytes—GI and renal systems.
   b. Water—GI, circulatory, and renal systems.
   c. pH—renal and respiratory systems.
   d. Temperature—cardiovascular, respiratory, musculatory, and integumentary systems.

e. Nutrients—cardiovascular, renal, and GI systems.
f. O_2, CO_2—respiratory and renal systems.
g. Wastes—circulatory, renal, and GI systems.

3. Control mechanisms for homeostasis.
   a. Intrinsic control—within an organ.
   b. Extrinsic control—neuronal and endocrine systems.
4. Types of control.
   a. Negative feedback—effector decreases or terminates the original stimulus (blood pressure, blood glucose, blood gases, and pH).
   b. Positive feedback—effector results in continued enhancement of original stimulus (e.g., blood-clotting cascade).

B. Anatomic considerations.
   1. Arteries.
      a. Large vessels containing numerous layers of elastin (stretch) and collagen (tensile strength).
      b. Offer little resistance to flow owing to their large radius.
      c. Capable of elastic recoil; serve as a pressure reservoir.
   2. Arterioles.
      a. Less elastic and more muscular.
      b. Provide the greatest resistance to blood flow.
   3. Capillaries.
      a. Heavily branched, thin-walled vessels (one cell thick).

b. Location of the exchange of fluid and substances between blood and interstitial fluid.

c. Precapillary sphincter muscles regulate local blood flow.

4. Veins.

a. Have large radii and low resistance to flow.

b. Valves ensure one-way flow.

c. Serve as a blood reservoir.

5. Lymphatics.

a. One-way vessels that return interstitial fluid and contents to venous circulation.

b. One-way valves and skeletal muscle contraction ensure proper flow.

C. Pressure, resistance, and flow.

1. Relationship of pressure, flow, and resistance.

a. Pressure gradient (δP)—difference in pressure between the beginning and end of a vessel. This is the driving force for blood flow. Blood flows from high to low pressure.

b. Resistance (R)—impediment to blood flow.

c. Flow rate (Q)—volume of blood through a vessel per unit of time.

d. Ohm's law: $Q = \delta P/R$.

2. Blood flow is characterized as two types.

a. Laminar flow.

(1) Velocity is greatest in the center of the vessel.

(2) Fluid passes more readily through a large vessel than through a small vessel because a given volume of blood comes into contact with more surface area in the small vessel.

b. Turbulent flow.

(1) Blood flows crosswise.

(2) Caused by obstructions to flow and rough surfaces in the vessel.

3. Resistance.

a. Caused by friction between the moving blood and the vessel wall.

b. As the blood flows through the vessel, the pressure decreases secondary to frictional losses.

(1) As resistance increases, flow decreases.

(2) To maintain the same flow with increased resistance, pressure must increase.

c. Resistance to blood flow depends on three factors.

(1) Viscosity of blood.

(2) Vessel length (usually remains the same).

(3) Vessel radius (most important factor because this can change).

d. Poiseuille's law—effect of vessel diameter (or radius [r]) on resistance and flow.

(1) Flow is proportional to r^4, or resistance is inversely proportional to r^4. Fluid passes more readily through a large vessel because a given volume of blood comes into contact with more surface area in a small vessel.

(2) Resistance is proportional to $1/r^4$, and because radius can be regulated, this is the most

important factor in controlling overall resistance to blood flow.

e. Viscosity and blood flow.

(1) Viscosity increases as hematocrit (percent of cells in blood) increases.

(2) The greater the hematocrit, the less the flow owing to increased resistance.

D. Blood pressure and vascular compliance.

1. Blood pressure—depends on the volume of blood contained within the vessel and the compliance or distensibility of the vessel wall.

a. Systolic pressure—the pressure at the height of each pulse; measured when the ventricle ejects the stroke volume (normal average = 120 mm Hg).

b. Diastolic pressure—the lowest point pressure (normal average = 80 mm Hg).

c. Pulse pressure (systolic pressure − diastolic pressure)—depends on two factors.

(1) Stroke volume output.

(2) Compliance (total dispensability) of arterial tree.

d. Mean arterial pressure (MAP)—the average of all pressures measured at any time point.

E. Arteriole resistance—very important to the understanding of blood pressure.

1. The radii of the arterioles are responsible for regulation of blood pressure and distribution of cardiac output (CO).

2. Vascular tone—normal state of partial vascular constriction secondary to inherent contractile activity and ongoing sympathetic stimulation.

3. Arteriole smooth muscle is responsible for adjustments in arteriole resistance. This may result in either vasoconstriction or vasodilation. Factors that produce these changes are intrinsic (local) or extrinsic (neuronal or hormonal).

a. Local factors producing vasodilation.

(1) Increased CO_2.

(2) Decreased O_2.

(3) Histamine.

(4) Heat.

(5) Decreased myogenic activity.

(a) In response to increased metabolism (reactive hyperemia).

(b) In response to reduced blood flow (pressure autoregulation).

(6) Decreased pH (carbonic and lactic acids).

(7) Increased K^+.

(8) Increased osmolarity.

(9) Adenosine (cardiac vessels).

(10) Prostaglandins (prostaglandin E and prostaglandin I_2).

(11) Nitric oxide.

b. Local factors producing vasoconstriction.

(1) Decreased CO_2.

(2) Increased O_2.

(3) Cold.

(4) Increased myogenic activity in response to decreased metabolism or increased blood flow and pressure.

c. Extrinsic factors producing vasodilation are primarily via decreased sympathetic activity.

d. Extrinsic factors producing vasoconstriction.

(1) Epinephrine and norepinephrine from adrenal medulla.

(2) Vasopressin.

(3) Angiotensin II.

e. Regulatory factors in special tissues.

(1) Coronary circulation—hypoxia and adenosine.

(2) Cerebral circulation—CO_2 or H^+.

(3) Pulmonary circulation—CO_2 causes vasoconstriction.

(4) Renal circulation—autoregulation.

(5) Skeletal muscle—sympathetic innervation at rest, local metabolites (lactate, adenosine, and K^+) during exercise.

(6) Skin—sympathetic innervation and vasoactive substances (histamine).

F. Capillary exchange.

1. Types of exchange.

a. Passive diffusion—key factor in the exchange of gases, substrates, and waste products between capillaries and tissue cells. This exchange occurs readily owing to the following reasons.

(1) Distance is small.

(2) Capillary walls are composed of single cells with pores.

(a) Responsible for passage of water-soluble substances (e.g., ions, amino acids).

(b) Pore size varies (liver has large pores, brain has no pores).

(c) Pore size is increased by histamine.

(3) There are a large number of capillaries.

(4) Flow in capillaries is slow.

(5) Lipid-soluble substances and gases pass directly through the capillary membrane.

(6) Proteins not exchanged by vesicular transport are retained in the capillary.

b. Bulk flow—volume of protein-free plasma that passes in and out of the capillary. Bulk flow determines the distribution of ECF volume between the vascular and interstitial fluid compartment. It is responsible for maintaining the distribution of fluids in the interstitial space and plasma, which affects blood volume and blood pressure. Four primary forces determine fluid movement through the capillary membrane.

(1) Capillary blood pressure (P_c).

(a) Arteriolar end (30 to 37 mm Hg).

(b) Venous end (10 to 17 mm Hg).

(c) Tends to force fluid out into the interstitial space.

(2) Interstitial fluid pressure (P_{if}).

(a) Approximately −3 to 1 mm Hg.

(b) If positive, tends to force fluid into the capillaries.

(c) Excess fluid is removed secondary to lymphatic drainage.

(3) Plasma colloid osmotic pressure (π_p).

(a) Approximately 25 to 28 mm Hg.

(b) Causes osmotic flow of fluid from interstitial space to the plasma.

(c) Is due to plasma proteins trapped in the capillary.

(4) Interstitial fluid colloid osmotic pressure (π_{if}).

(a) Usually 0 mm Hg.

(b) If increased, tends to cause fluid to move into interstitial space.

(c) Caused by protein in interstitial space.

c. Overall fluid movement.

(1) Ultrafiltration.

(a) Bulk movement of fluid from the capillaries to the interstitial areas.

(b) Forces primarily responsible.

(i) Capillary blood pressure.

(ii) Interstitial fluid colloid osmotic pressure.

(2) Resorption.

(a) Bulk movement of fluid from interstitial space into capillaries.

(b) Forces primarily responsible.

(i) Plasma colloid osmotic pressure.

(ii) Interstitial fluid pressure.

(3) Net exchange.

(a) Net exchange pressure = $(P_c) + (\pi_{if}) − (\pi_p + P_{if})$.

(b) Positive net exchange (outward exceeds inward)—ultrafiltration.

(c) Negative net exchange (inward exceeds outward)—resorption.

d. Edema—accumulation of excess fluid in the interstitial areas. This may be caused by the following.

(1) Reduced concentration of plasma proteins.

(a) Loss of plasma proteins (burns).

(b) Protein deficiency.

(c) Reduced protein synthesis by liver (liver disease).

(d) Loss of protein in the urine (kidney disease).

(2) Increased permeability of capillary walls.

(a) Histamine and other mediators of allergic reactions and inflammation.

(b) Leakage of plasma proteins into interstitial space secondary to tissue trauma.

(3) Increased venous pressure.

(a) Congestive heart failure.

(b) Localized edema (pregnancy).

(4) Lymphatic blockage.

    (a) Parasitic infection (elephantiasis).

    (b) Surgical removal of lymph nodes.

G. Veins.

1. Serve as a blood reservoir owing to their distensibility (less smooth muscle and elastin compared with arteries).

2. Increased pooling of blood results in reduced CO.

3. Venous return.

  a. Volume of blood entering each atrium per minute.

  b. Factors affecting venous return.

    (1) Pressure produced by cardiac contraction.

    (2) Sympathetically induced constriction of veins.

    (3) Skeletal muscle activity.

    (4) One-way venous valves.

H. Cardiodynamics and electrophysiology.

1. Anatomic considerations.

  a. Atria—weak and elastic chambers that receive blood from the veins.

  b. Ventricles—heavily muscled chambers.

  c. Endocardium—cells that line the chambers of the heart.

  d. Myocardium—short, branched, interconnected muscle cells joined together by gap junctions. These cells are electrically joined and behave as a single functional unit (syncytium). The heart muscle contracts with an all-or-none contraction.

  e. Epicardium—thin external membrane covering the heart.

  f. Fibrous connective tissue—separates atria from the ventricles.

  g. Valves.

    (1) Atrioventricular (AV)—open passively when the pressure in the ventricle decreases to less than the atrial pressure. This permits blood to enter the ventricle. Closing of AV valves is associated with the first heart sound.

    (a) Tricuspid valve—separates the right atrium and ventricle.

    (b) Bicuspid (mitral) valve—separates the left atrium and ventricle.

    (2) Semilunar—open when the pressure in the ventricle exceeds the pressure in the aorta or pulmonary artery. This permits blood to be pumped out of the ventricles. Closing of these valves is associated with the second heart sound.

    (a) Aortic valve.

    (b) Pulmonic valve.

2. Electrical activity.

  a. Pacemaker—region demonstrating spontaneous electrical activity.

    (1) Sinoatrial (SA) node—cluster of specialized cells with inherent contractile rhythm faster than any other cells in the heart.

    (2) Ectopic pacemaker—pacemaker other than the SA node.

    (3) Pacemaker potential—spontaneous depolarization produced by the slow depolarization current through the membranes. Both fast and slow channels exist. Repolarization is caused by the outward diffusion of potassium ions.

  b. Conducting tissues of the heart.

    (1) AV node—located on the inferior portion of the interatrial septum. These cells conduct more slowly than the atrial cells. As a result of fibrous tissue surrounding this node, it is the only normal pathway between the SA node and the ventricles. The reduced rate of conduction through the AV node is responsible for the atria contracting before the ventricles.

    (2) AV bundle (bundle of His)—specialized muscle fibers that conduct impulses through the interventricular septum. The conduction rate is greatly increased compared with ventricular muscle. Responsible for the simultaneous contraction of the ventricles.

    (3) Purkinje fibers—specialized cardiac muscle fibers that carry impulses to ventricular musculature.

3. Action potential in myocardial cells—the heart has an extremely long refractory period (owing to calcium channels opening and maintaining a prolonged positive membrane potential), which is almost as long as the contraction. Because of this long refractory period, the heart cannot be tetanized.

4. Cardiac innervation.

  a. Parasympathetic stimulation (vagus nerve) is inhibitory because it decreases the rate of spontaneous depolarization in autorhythmic cells. Heart rate is reduced (negative chronotropic effect).

  b. Sympathetic stimulation is stimulatory because it increases the rate of spontaneous depolarization, which results in an increased heart rate (positive chronotropic effect). Sympathetics also produce an increased contractility, which results in a more forceful contraction (positive inotropic effect).

5. Electrocardiogram (ECG)—standardized measurement of potential difference between two points on body surfaces caused by the electrical activity of the heart.

  a. A typical tracing produces a P-Q-R-S-T wave (Figure 2-20).

    (1) P wave is caused by depolarization of the atria.

    (2) QRS complex represents ventricular depolarization.

    (3) T wave is produced by repolarization of the ventricles.

  b. ECG can be used to monitor abnormal heart rate and rhythm.

    (1) Tachycardia—shorter distances between QRS complexes (>100 beats/min).

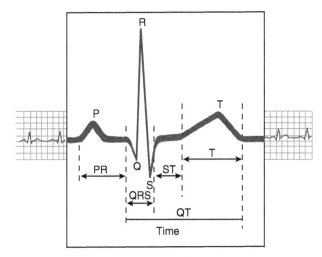

Figure 2-20 Important deflections and intervals of a typical electrocardiogram. *(From Berne RM, Levy MN: Principles of Physiology, ed 4, St. Louis, Mosby, 2006.)*

(2) Bradycardia—longer distances between QRS complexes (<50 beats/min).

(3) Extrasystoles—beats from an ectopic source.

(4) Atrial flutter—very rapid atrial depolarization.

(5) Atrial fibrillation—rapid, irregular uncoordinated atrial depolarization.

(6) Ventricular fibrillation—rapid, uncoordinated ventricular contractions.

(7) Heart block—interruptions of impulses between atria and ventricles.

6. Mechanical events of the cardiac cycle (Figure 2-21).

a. Early diastole (diastole refers to periods of relaxation and filling).

(1) Semilunar valves are closed.

(2) Owing to venous return, atrial pressure is greater than ventricular pressure.

(3) AV valves are open.

(4) Ventricular volume increases (rapidly initially, then slowly).

b. Late diastole.

(1) SA node fires and spreads over the atria (P wave), and atria contract.

(2) Atrial contraction causes an increase in both atrial and ventricular pressure.

c. Early systole (systole refers to periods of contraction).

(1) Ventricle has reached the end-diastolic volume (EDV). This is also referred to as the *preload*.

(2) Impulses pass through the AV node.

(3) QRS complex represents ventricular depolarization and contraction.

(4) Ventricular pressure increases.

(5) AV valves close when pressure in ventricle is greater than pressure in atrium.

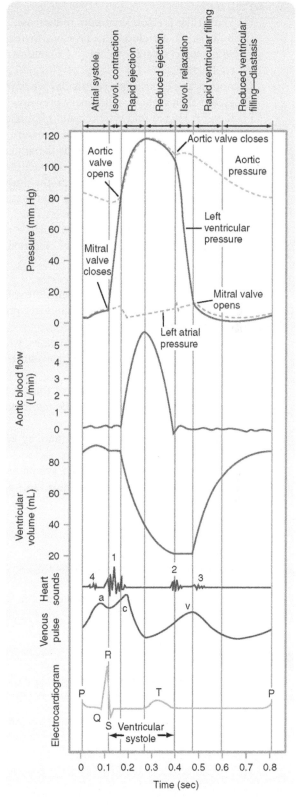

Figure 2-21 Left atrial, aortic, and left ventricular pressure pulses correlated in time with aortic flow, ventricular volume, heart sounds, venous pulse, and the electrocardiogram for a complete cardiac cycle. *(From Koeppen BM, Stanton BA, Berne RM: Berne & Levy Physiology, ed 6. Philadelphia, Saunders, 2010.)*

d. Peak systole.
  (1) Ventricular pressure continues to increase.
  (2) Both valves are closed, so pressure increases with a constant volume (isovolumetric contraction).
  (3) Aortic valve opens when ventricular pressure is greater than aortic or pulmonary pressure.
  (4) Blood is ejected into systemic and pulmonary branches, resulting in increased pressure in these vessels. The *stroke volume* is the amount of blood pumped out with each contraction.
  (5) Ventricular volume decreases to the lowest level in the cycle. This is the end-systolic volume (ESV), also known as the *afterload*.
  (6) T wave, which represents ventricular repolarization, occurs at the end of ventricular systole.
e. Late systole.
  (1) Ventricles start to relax, and when ventricular pressure is less than aortic or pulmonary pressure, the semilunar valves close.
  (2) The pressure in the ventricle decreases, while blood volume remains constant (isovolumetric relaxation).
  (3) When ventricular pressure is less than atrial pressure, the AV valves open, and ventricular filling begins.
7. CO—volume of blood pumped per minute by each ventricle. This depends on the following factors.
  a. Cardiac rate—influenced by SA node, sympathetic stimulation, parasympathetic stimulation, and cardiac control centers.
    (1) SA node.
    (2) Sympathetic stimulation (epinephrine and norepinephrine) (Table 2-6).
      (a) Increases rate of depolarization of SA node.
      (b) Increases electrical conduction in the heart.
  (3) Parasympathetic stimulation (vagus nerve) (see Table 2-6).
      (a) Hyperpolarizes SA node because of enhanced K^+ permeability.
      (b) Decreases rate of spontaneous depolarization.
      (c) Decreases the excitability of the AV node.
  (4) Cardiac control centers in the medulla are influenced by baroreceptors in the aorta and carotid arteries.
  b. Stroke volume—influenced by EDV, total peripheral resistance (TPR), and contractility.
    (1) EDV—volume of blood in the ventricles at the end of diastole. Stroke volume is directly proportional to EDV.
    (2) TPR—frictional resistance to blood flow in the arteries. Stroke volume is inversely proportional to TPR.
    (3) Contractility—strength of ventricular contraction. Stroke volume is directly proportional to contractility.
  c. Stroke volume is also regulated by intrinsic and extrinsic means.
    (1) Intrinsic control—the inherent ability of the heart to vary stroke volume. This is referred to as the *Frank-Starling law of the heart*.
      (a) The strength of ventricular contraction varies directly with EDV.
      (b) Increased stretching of cardiac muscle allows for more advantageous overlapping of actin and myosin, resulting in a more forceful contraction.
    (2) Extrinsic control—factors originating outside the heart that affect stroke volume.
      (a) Contraction strength—increasing sympathetic stimulation and epinephrine from the adrenal medulla increases the amount of calcium available for the sarcomeres. This results in an increased stroke volume.

Table 2-6

Effects of Autonomic Nervous System on the Heart and Blood Vessels

	SYMPATHETIC		PARASYMPATHETIC	
	ACTION	RECEPTOR	ACTION	RECEPTOR
Heart rate	↑	β_1	↓	M_2
Contractility	↑	β_1	↓ (atria only)	M_2
Conduction velocity (AV node)	↑	β_1	↓	M_2
Vascular smooth muscle (skin, renal, and splanchnic)	Constriction	α_1	Dilation (releases EDRF)	M_3
Vascular smooth muscle (skeletal muscle)	Dilation	β_2	Dilation (releases EDRF)	M_3
	Constriction	α_1		

From Costanzo LS: Physiology, ed 3, Philadelphia, Saunders, 2004.

AV, Atrioventricular; *EDRF*, endothelial-derived relaxing factor or nitric oxide; *M*, muscarinic.

(b) Increased venous return.
    (i) Increased sympathetic activity stimulates smooth muscle contractions in venous walls, increasing venous return.
    (ii) Skeletal muscle pump.
    (iii) Pressure difference between thoracic and abdominal muscles.

8. Blood pressure determinants and regulation.
  a. MAP = CO × TPR.
  b. Regulatory mechanisms of the autonomic nervous center (vasomotor center). All are located in the medulla.
    (1) Cardioinhibitory center—parasympathetic innervations to SA and AV nodes of the heart.
    (2) Cardiostimulatory center—sympathetic stimulation to SA and AV nodes of the heart and ventricle.
    (3) Vasoconstrictor system—innervates vasoconstrictor fibers to provide vascular tone (sympathetic system acts on α-adrenergic receptors) (see Table 2-6).
  c. Arterial pressure is regulated (adjusted) by short-term and long-term adjustments.
    (1) Short-term adjustments.
      (a) Baroreceptors—respond to increased blood pressure.
        (i) Located in aortic arch and carotid sinus.
        (ii) Afferent nerves carry signals to vasomotor center via glossopharyngeal and vagus nerves.
        (iii) Efferent pathways in ANS result in decreased sympathetic tone and increased parasympathetic activity.
        (iv) Ultimately produces decreased CO and TPR.
      (b) Bainbridge reflex—produces an increased heart rate owing to stretching of the right atrium.
      (c) Carotid and aortic chemoreceptors.
        (i) Sensitive to decreased O_2, increased CO_2, and decreased pH.
        (ii) Input acts via CNS vasomotor center.
        (iii) Reductions in blood pressure (resulting in reduced flow through these chemoreceptor areas) result in an increase in blood pressure.
      (d) CNS ischemic response.
        (i) Reduced blood flow in CNS produces increased CO_2.
        (ii) Vasomotor center is stimulated to produce increased blood pressure.
    (2) Long-term adjustments—adjustments in body fluid by the kidney.
      (a) Renal function curve.
        (i) Increased blood pressure results in increased renal fluid excretion.
        (ii) Increased fluid loss produces the following.
          1. Less ECF and blood volume.
          2. Less venous return and CO.
          3. Reduced blood pressure.
      (b) Vasopressin (antidiuretic hormone [ADH]).
        (i) Secreted from the pituitary in response to increased osmolarity.
        (ii) Stimulates the kidney to retain water.
        (iii) Ultimately increases blood volume and increases blood pressure.
      (c) Renin-angiotensin system.
        (i) Reduced renal perfusion pressure leads to renin release (Figure 2-22).
        (ii) Aldosterone.
          1. Secreted by the adrenal medulla in response to reduced circulating fluid volume (may be due to chronic sodium depletion) and increased plasma potassium.
          2. Stimulates resorption of sodium and secretion of potassium in the kidney.
          3. Water is reabsorbed passively, resulting in increased blood volume and blood pressure.

9. Coagulation (Figure 2-23).

9.0 Respiration

9.1 Mechanical Aspects

A. Conducting zone—responsible for bringing air into and out of the respiratory zone. These structures include the nasal passages, pharynx, trachea, bronchi, bronchioles, and terminal bronchioles.
1. Lined with mucus and clara cells.
2. Contain smooth muscle, which is innervated by ANS.
  a. Sympathetics—β_2-adrenergic receptors, which produce relaxation and dilation of airways.
  b. Parasympathetics—muscarinic receptors, which produce contraction and constriction of the airways.

B. Respiratory zone—responsible for gas exchange. Structures include the respiratory bronchioles, alveolar ducts, and alveolar sacs.
1. Respiratory bronchioles have clara and innervated smooth muscle.
2. Alveoli exchange O_2 and CO_2 and are composed of three cell types.
  a. Type I—epithelial cells for diffusion (predominant type).
  b. Type II—synthesize surfactant.
  c. Alveolar macrophages—remove foreign material from alveoli.

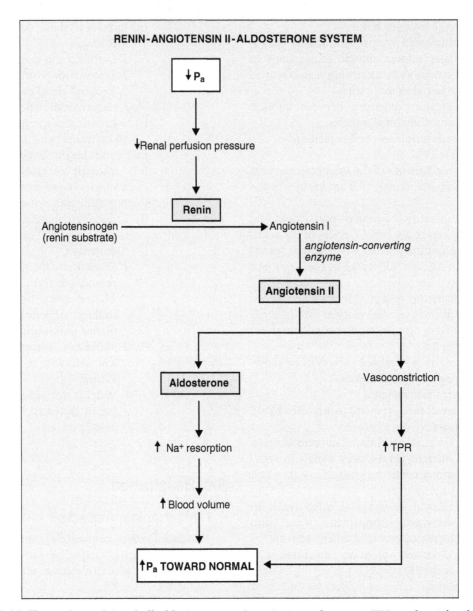

Figure 2-22 The renin-angiotensin II-aldosterone system. P_a, Arterial pressure; *TPR*, total peripheral resistance.

C. Terminology (Figure 2-24).
1. Lung volume.
   a. Tidal volume.
   b. Inspiratory reserve volume.
   c. Expiratory reserve volume.
   d. Residual volume.
2. Lung capacity.
   a. Inspiratory capacity.
   b. Functional residual capacity (FRC).
   c. Vital capacity.
   d. Total lung capacity.
3. Dead space—does not participate in gas exchange.
   a. Anatomic dead space—conducting zone (see previously).
   b. Physiologic dead space—includes anatomic dead space and alveoli that do not participate in gas exchange.

D. Ventilation rate—volume of air moving in and out of the lungs per unit of time.
1. Minute ventilation = tidal volume (mL) × breaths per minute.
2. Alveolar ventilation = (tidal volume − dead space) × breaths per minute.

E. Mechanics and physics of respiration.
1. Inspiration—primarily due to the contraction of the diaphragm. In heavy exercise, the external intercostal muscles and accessory muscles may be used.

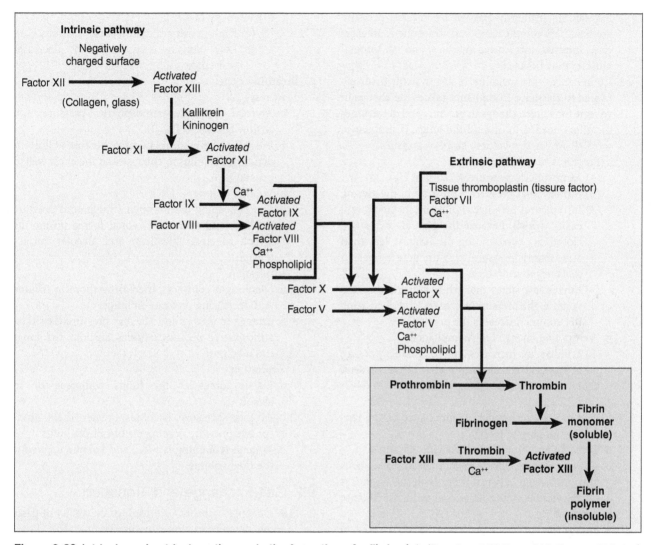

Figure 2-23 Intrinsic and extrinsic pathways in the formation of a fibrin clot. *(From Levy MN, Berne RM, Koeppen BM, et al: Berne & Levy Principles of Physiology, ed 4, Philadelphia, Saunders, 2006.)*

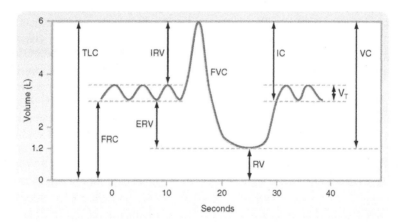

Figure 2-24 The various lung volumes and capacities. *ERV,* Expiratory reserve volume; *FRC,* functional residual capacity; *FVC,* forced vital capacity; *IC,* inspiratory capacity; *IRV,* inspiratory reserve volume; *RV,* residual volume; *TLC,* total lung capacity; *VC,* vital capacity; V_T, tidal volume. *(From Koeppen BM, Stanton BA, Berne RM: Berne & Levy Physiology, ed 6. Philadelphia, Saunders, 2010.)*

2. Expiration—primarily passive by reverse pressure gradient between the lungs and atmosphere. In exercise, internal intercostal muscles and abdominal muscles may be used.
3. Compliance—distensibility of the system; inversely related to elasticity. Compliance relates the change in volume for a given change in pressure and determines the effort needed to distend the lungs. (Compliance = δ V/P, where V = volume and P = pressure).
   a. Pressures to consider.
      (1) Atmospheric pressure = 760 mm Hg.
      (2) Intraalveolar pressure = pressure in the alveoli.
      (3) Intrapleural pressure = pressure in the pleural cavity, which, because the pleural cavity is a closed sac surrounding the lung, is less than atmospheric pressure. Pressure here is referred to as *negative pressure*.
      (4) Boyle's law states that when you increase the volume, the pressure decreases, and decreasing the volume increases the pressure.
   b. Factors that change lung compliance.
      (1) Emphysema increases lung compliance because of loss of elastic fibers. A higher FRC is present.
      (2) Fibrosis decreases lung compliance. A lower FRC exists.
4. Elastance—the reciprocal of compliance or the tendency of the lung to recoil.
   a. Collagen and elastic fibers provide elastance.
   b. Alveolar surface tension resulting from an aqueous film. Attraction between water molecules opposes the expansion of the lungs and tends to collapse the alveoli.
   c. Pulmonary surfactant decreases the surface tension in alveoli, increasing pulmonary compliance and reducing the tendency for the alveoli to collapse.
5. Relationship of pressure and resistance to airflow.
   a. Airflow is directly proportional to the pressure difference between the mouth and nose and the alveoli and is inversely proportional to the resistance of the airways. Q = δ P/R, where Q = flow.
   b. Airway resistance is primarily determined by changes in airway diameter (Poiseuille's law). Changes in lung volume and air viscosity may also change resistance. Three factors must be considered.
      (1) ANS.
         (a) Parasympathetic system causes constriction of smooth muscle and produces increased resistance.
         (b) Sympathetic system produces relaxation and decreases resistance.
      (2) Lung volume.
         (a) High volume—more traction, less resistance.
         (b) Low volume—less traction, more resistance.

   (3) Viscosity of air.
      (a) High density of gas increases resistance.
      (b) Low density (e.g., helium) decreases resistance.
F. Breathing cycle.
   1. At rest.
      a. Alveolar pressure—atmospheric pressure (no airflow because δ P is 0).
      b. Intrapleural pressure is negative because of the tendency of the lungs to collapse and the chest wall to expand.
      c. Volume in lungs—FRC.
      d. Forces keeping alveoli open (transmural pressure gradient and surfactant) equal forces promoting alveoli to close (elasticity and alveolar surface tension).
   2. Inspiration.
      a. Diaphragm contracts, increasing thoracic volume and decreasing pressure in lungs.
      b. Change in airway and alveolar pressure (less than atmospheric pressure) drives air into the lungs (tidal volume).
   3. Expiration.
      a. Elastic forces of the lungs compress air in alveoli.
      b. Alveolar pressure becomes greater than atmospheric pressure, forcing air out of the lungs.
      c. Volume remaining is FRC, and volume expired is the tidal volume.

9.2 Gas Exchange and Transport

A. Gas exchange—occurs as a result of the ability of gases to move down partial pressure gradients.
   1. Partial pressure = total pressure × fractional concentration of dissolved gas.
   2. Partial pressure is the pressure that gas would exert if it occupied the total volume of the mixture.
   3. The diffusion rates of gases depend on the partial pressure differences across the alveoli and the surface area for diffusion (Figure 2-25).
      a. Pulmonary-capillary gas exchange.
         (1) O_2 moves from alveoli (partial pressure of O_2 [Po_2] = 100 mm Hg) to the pulmonary capillaries (Po_2 = 40 mm Hg).
         (2) CO_2 moves from the venous blood (partial pressure of CO_2 [Pco_2] = 46 mm Hg) to the alveoli (Pco_2 = 40 mm Hg).
      b. Tissue-capillary gas exchange.
         (1) O_2 moves from blood (Po_2 = 100 mm Hg) into the cells (Po_2 = 40 mm Hg).
         (2) CO_2 moves from the cells (Pco_2 >46 mm Hg) into the blood (Pco_2 = 40 mm Hg).
   4. Limitations to gas exchange.
      a. Diffusion limited—gas exchange is limited by the diffusion process. Partial pressure is maintained, but exchange cannot occur.

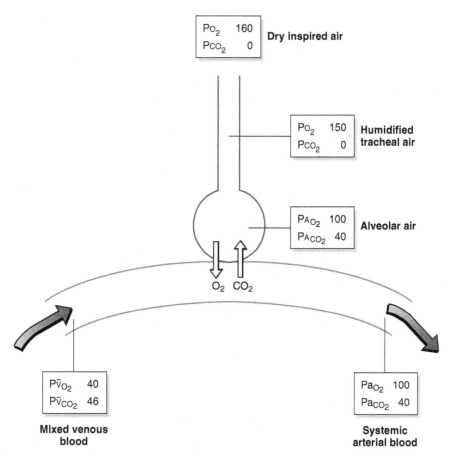

Figure 2-25 Values for Po_2 and Pco_2 in dry inspired air, humidified tracheal air, alveolar air, and pulmonary capillary blood.

(1) Fibrosis—alveolar membrane thickens, increasing the diffusion distance.

(2) Emphysema—surface area for diffusion is decreased.

b. Perfusion limited—gas exchange is limited by flow rate through the pulmonary capillaries. Partial pressure is not maintained because equilibration occurs rapidly.

B. Gas transport.

1. O_2—transported either dissolved or associated with hemoglobin.

a. Dissolved O_2 (2%)—directly proportional to Po_2 (approximately 0.3 mL/100 mL).

b. Hemoglobin O_2 (98%)—responsible for most O_2 transport (20 mL/100 mL). Hemoglobin concentration determines O_2 content of the blood.

c. Hemoglobin–O_2 dissociation curve.

(1) Demonstrates the change in affinity of hemoglobin as each successive O_2 molecule binds to a heme site. This facilitates loading and unloading of O_2 as it is transported through the body.

(a) Leaving the lungs, hemoglobin is almost 100% saturated (bound to four heme groups). Po_2 is 100 mm Hg. The high affinity of hemoglobin at Po_2 greater than 60 mm Hg ensures hemoglobin saturation at different atmospheric pressures.

(b) In tissues (Po_2 = 40 mm Hg), hemoglobin releases O_2, leaving hemoglobin about 75% saturated (O_2 reserve). At lower Po_2, the affinity of hemoglobin for O_2 is less, facilitating the release to tissues.

(2) Changes in hemoglobin–O_2 dissociation curve—reflect a change in affinity of hemoglobin for O_2.

(a) Shift to right—decreased hemoglobin affinity caused by the following.

(i) Increases in Pco_2 or decreases in pH.

(ii) Increases in temperature.

(iii) Increases in 2,3-diphosphoglycerate (2,3-DPG) concentration (product of red blood cell [RBC] glycolysis).

(b) Shift to the left—increased hemoglobin affinity caused by the following.

(i) Decreases in Pco_2 or increases in pH.

(ii) Decreases in 2,3-DPG concentration.

(iii) Fetal hemoglobin—does not bind 2,3-DPG.

(iv) Carbon monoxide poisoning (carboxyhemoglobin).

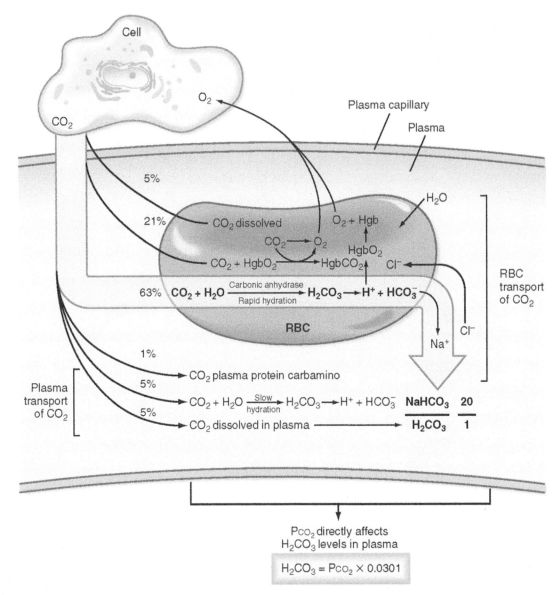

Figure 2-26 Mechanisms of CO_2 transport in blood. The predominant mechanism by which CO_2 is transported from tissue cells to the lung is in the form of HCO_3^-. *RBC*, Red blood cell. *(From Koeppen BM, Stanton BA, Berne RM: Berne & Levy Physiology, ed 6. Philadelphia, Saunders, 2010.)*

(c) Iron in its ferric state (Fe^{3+}); methemoglobin does not bind O_2.

2. CO_2—transported in three forms (Figure 2-26).
   a. Dissolved CO_2—more soluble than O_2.
   b. Carbaminohemoglobin.
   c. Bicarbonate—90% of CO_2 transported in this form.
      (1) CO_2 produced in the tissues diffuses into the plasma and RBCs.
      (2) RBC carbonic anhydrase catalyzes the formation of H_2CO_3, which dissociates into H^+ and HCO_3^-.
      (3) HCO_3^- diffuses out of RBCs (in exchange for Cl^-) and is transported to the lungs where, in

RBCs, CO_2 is regenerated by carbonic anhydrase; this is the reverse of the reaction described in (2).

9.3 Regulation

A. Ventilation/perfusion relationships.
   1. Pulmonary blood flow—pressure and resistance are much lower than systemic circulation. It is regulated primarily by hypoxic vasoconstriction (decreases blood flow owing to poorly ventilated areas of the lung). Thromboxane A_2 from macrophages, leukocytes, and endothelial cells produces vasoconstriction. Prostacyclin is a potent vasodilator. Leukotrienes produce airway constriction.

2. Distribution of pulmonary blood flow—three zones owing to gravitational effects.
   a. Zone I (apex)—highest ventilation/perfusion ratio ($\dot{V}/\dot{Q}$) (see later).
      (1) Lowest blood flow.
      (2) Arterial pressure < alveolar pressure (vessels partially collapsed).
   b. Zone II (middle).
      (1) Blood flow medium.
      (2) Arterial pressure > alveolar pressure > venous pressure.
      (3) Blood flow driven by difference between arterial pressure and alveolar pressure.
   c. Zone III (base)—lowest $\dot{V}/\dot{Q}$ (see later).
      (1) Blood flow highest.
      (2) Arterial pressure > venous pressure > alveolar pressure.
      (3) Blood flow driven by differences between arterial and venous pressures.
3. $\dot{V}/\dot{Q}$—the ratio of alveolar ventilation ($\dot{V}$) to pulmonary blood flow ($\dot{Q}$).
   a. Normal $\dot{V}/\dot{Q} = 0.8$ (this is an average for all three zones).
      (1) Breathing frequency, tidal volume, and CO are normal.
      (2) Po_2 (100 mm Hg) and Pco_2 (40 mm Hg) are normal.
   b. $\dot{V}/\dot{Q}$ is infinite—lack of perfusion (dead space), which can occur in pulmonary embolism.
   c. $\dot{V}/\dot{Q}$ is high—reduced blood flow through the lung.
   d. $\dot{V}/\dot{Q}$ is low—reduced alveolar ventilation.
B. Control of respiration.
   1. CNS.
      a. Medullary respiratory center (reticular formation).
         (1) Inspiratory center—controls the basic rhythm (frequency).
         (2) Expiratory center—inactive during quiet breathing but active during active breathing (exercise).
      b. Apneustic center (pons).
         (1) Stimulates inspiration.
         (2) Produces prolonged inspiration.
      c. Pneumotaxic center (pons).
         (1) Inhibits inspiration.
         (2) Limits tidal volume and respiratory rate.
      d. Cortex.
         (1) Voluntary regulation of breathing.
         (2) Produces hyperventilation or hypoventilation.
   2. Chemoreceptors.
      a. Central chemoreceptors (medulla).
         (1) Increased H^+.
            (a) Acts directly on central chemoreceptors.
            (b) Stimulates breathing (hyperventilation).
         (2) Increased Pco_2.
            (a) Diffuses into the cerebrospinal fluid, combines with H_2O to produce carbonic acid.
            (b) Resulting H^+ acts directly on central chemoreceptors (see previous text).
         (3) Reduced H^+ and CO_2 produce hypoventilation.
      b. Peripheral chemoreceptors (carotid and aortic bodies).
         (1) Decreased Po_2 (<60 mm Hg)—stimulates increased breathing rate.
         (2) Increased arterial Pco_2—stimulates increased breathing rate.
         (3) Increased arterial H^+—stimulates directly and independently of Pco_2.
      c. Other receptors.
         (1) Hering-Breuer reflex.
            (a) Prevents excessive stretching of the lungs.
            (b) Distention of smooth muscle produces decreased breathing frequency.
         (2) Mechanoreceptors.
            (a) Located in joints and muscles.
            (b) Movement stimulates inspiratory center to increase respiration.
            (c) Irritant receptors—located in epithelial cells of the lung. They are stimulated by noxious substances.

10.0 Renal System

A. Body fluids.
   1. Total body water—about 60% of adult body weight. It is distributed in two major compartments.
      a. ICF—within the cells; two thirds total body water.
         (1) Mg^{2+} and K^+ are major cations.
         (2) Proteins and organic phosphates (ATP, ADP, and AMP) are major anions.
      b. ECF—all fluid outside of the cells; one third total body water (e.g., plasma, interstitial fluid).
         (1) Na^+ is major cation in ECF.
         (2) HCO_3^- and Cl^- are major anions.
         (3) Plasma proteins—albumin and globulins are the major plasma proteins.
         (4) Only a small amount of protein is in interstitial fluid under normal conditions.
   2. Body fluid balance.
      a. Control of fluid volume—primarily through water and mineral retention and loss through the kidney. The basic principles essential to understanding fluid movement are the following.
         (1) Volume of body fluid depends on the amount of solute it contains.
         (2) ICF and ECF are in osmotic equilibrium (290 mOsm/L). However, specific ion concentrations differ between compartments (see previous text).
         (3) Equilibration between ICF and ECF occurs through fluid movement, not through the movement of osmotically active molecules.

Table 2-7

Disturbances of Body Fluids

TYPE	EXAMPLE	ECF VOLUME	ICF VOLUME	OSMOLARITY	HEMATOCRIT	PLASMA PROTEIN
Isosmotic volume contraction	Diarrhea	↓	NC	NC	↑	↑
Hyperosmotic volume contraction	Sweating; fever; diabetes insipidus	↓	↓	↑	NC	↑
Hyposmotic volume contraction	Adrenal insufficiency	↓	↑	↓	↑	↑
Isosmotic volume expansion	Infusion of isotonic NaCl	↑	NC	NC	↓	↓
Hyperosmotic volume expansion	High NaCl intake	↑	↓	↑	↓	↓
Hyposmotic volume expansion	SIADH	↑	↑	↓	NC	↓

From Costanzo LS: Physiology, ed 3, Philadelphia, Saunders, 2004.

ECF, Extracellular fluid; *ICF,* intracellular fluid; *NaCl,* sodium chloride; *NC,* no change; *SIADH,* syndrome of inappropriate antidiuretic hormone.

b. Disturbances in body fluid occur under various conditions (Table 2-7).
B. Renal function.
  1. Overview of function.
    a. Regulatory function.
      (1) Composition of body fluids.
      (2) Volume of body fluids.
    b. Endocrine function.
      (1) Activation and secretion of vitamin D (1-25-dihydroxyvitamin D_3).
      (2) Secretion of renin.
      (3) Secretion of erythropoietin.
    c. Excretory function.
      (1) Uric acid.
      (2) Urea.
      (3) Creatinine.
      (4) Foreign substances or drugs.
  2. Functional anatomy.
    a. Vasculature—composed of two sets of capillaries to filter and reabsorb or secrete plasma components.
      (1) Renal arteries.
      (2) Afferent arterioles.
      (3) Glomerular capillaries.
      (4) Efferent arterioles.
      (5) Peritubular capillaries.
      (6) Venules and renal veins.
    b. Tubules.
      (1) Bowman's capsule.
      (2) Proximal tubule.
      (3) Loop of Henle.
      (4) Distal tubule.
      (5) Collecting ducts.
    c. Accessory structures.
      (1) Ureters.
      (2) Bladder.
      (3) Urethra.
  3. Renal activities.
    a. Renal blood flow—volume of blood entering the renal artery (mL/min).
      (1) The amount is directly proportional to the pressure difference between the renal artery and renal vein and indirectly proportional to resistance of the renal vasculature.
      (2) Characterized by autoregulation between 100 and 200 mm Hg blood pressure.
      (3) Sympathetic stimulation and angiotensin II can alter renal blood flow, increasing resistance and reducing renal blood flow. This ultimately results in a reduced glomerular filtration rate (GFR) (see later).
      (4) Measured by clearance of para-aminohippuric acid.
    b. Glomerular filtration—filtration across the glomerular capillaries and through the glomerular membrane, which normally is impermeable to protein. (Approximately 20% of the renal plasma flow is filtered by the glomerulus.)
      (1) GFR—rate at which tubular fluid is produced. This is dependent on several factors.
        (a) Hydrostatic pressures (capillary pressure) in Bowman's capsule—favors filtration.
        (b) Colloid osmotic pressure in plasma—opposes filtration.
        (c) Colloid osmotic pressure in filtrate—favors filtration when present.

(d) Bowman's hydrostatic pressure—opposes filtration.

(e) Permeability of capillaries and glomerular membrane—may oppose or favor filtration.

(f) Renal blood flow—may oppose or favor filtration.

(2) As a result of the combination of these factors, filtration is always favored along the entire length of the glomerular capillaries.

(3) GFR is measured by the clearance of inulin and creatinine, which are filtered but not reabsorbed or secreted by the renal tubules.

c. Tubular resorption—selective removal of filtered solutes from tubule back into the peritubule capillaries.

(1) May be either active (transporters in membranes) or passive (urea).

(2) All glucose is reabsorbed.

(a) Secondary active transport system in the proximal tubule, which depends on the sodium gradient established by the Na^+-K^+-ATPase pump.

(b) Facilitated diffusion also occurs using Na^+ glucose transporter.

(c) Under normal conditions, all glucose is reabsorbed. However, the carrier proteins are saturable and specific. If the transport potential is exceeded (>T_{max} [transport maximum]), glucose appears in the urine.

(3) Most Na^+ is reabsorbed by an active transport system throughout the tubules. Na^+/K^+ ATPase pumps sodium out of the epithelial cells and, once in the interstitial space, establishes a concentration gradient for passive diffusion. Cl^- and water follow passively.

(a) Two thirds in the proximal tubule (not regulated).

(b) One quarter in the loop of Henle (not regulated).

(c) Remainder in the distal and collecting tubules (regulated by aldosterone).

(4) Half of the urea resulting from protein degradation is reabsorbed passively, and the remainder is excreted.

(a) Distal tubule and cortical and outer medullary collecting ducts are impermeable to urea and do not contribute to reabsorption.

(b) ADH or vasopressin (see later) increases urea permeability in the inner medullary collecting ducts, and urea diffuses down a concentration gradient into the inner medulla.

(5) Most filtered K^+ is reabsorbed in the proximal tubule.

(6) Most filtered phosphate is reabsorbed in the proximal tubule and distal nephron. This is inhibited by parathyroid hormone (PTH) (see Section 13, Endocrine System), leading to increased phosphate excretion.

(7) Most filtered calcium is passively reabsorbed in the proximal tubule and loop of Henle. PTH increases Ca^{2+} resorption in the distal tubule.

(8) Most HCO_3^- is reabsorbed in the proximal tubule.

(a) Uses carbonic anhydrase as an intermediate step.

(b) Results in a net reabsorption of bicarbonate and sodium.

(c) At high levels, HCO_3^- is excreted.

(d) Increased P_{CO_2} increases bicarbonate reabsorption.

d. Tubular secretion—selective secretion of plasma constituents into the tubule for excretion in the urine.

(1) K^+ is passively secreted in the distal and collecting tubules via a K^+ Cl^- cotransporter pathway. This accounts for most of the K^+ appearing in the urine.

(a) Aldosterone (released secondary to elevated plasma K^+ or reduced plasma Na^+) stimulates the secretion of K^+ in exchange for Na^+ (see previous text).

(b) Acidosis decreases K^+ secretion because H^+ exchanges for K^+. Alkalosis increases K^+ secretion.

(2) H^+ is excreted with urinary buffers.

(a) Inorganic phosphate is the major buffer involved with urinary excretion of acid.

(b) The net process results in the reabsorption of bicarbonate and secretion of H^+ as $H_2PO_4^-$ (titratable acid).

(c) NH_4^+ (produced from protein and phospholipid metabolism) is also secreted, resulting in an overall loss of H^+.

4. Renal clearance is the volume of arterial plasma that is completely cleared of a particular substance by the kidneys per minute.

a. A substance freely filterable but not secreted or reabsorbed can be used to measure GFR (inulin and creatinine).

b. A substance that is present in the plasma but not excreted has a clearance of 0. Under normal conditions, glucose has a plasma clearance of 0.

5. Corticopapillary osmotic gradient—changes in osmotic characteristics in the interstitial fluid of the kidney with progression through the medulla to the pelvis of the kidney. This osmotic gradient established by the loop of Henle helps to reabsorb water

from the distal ducts and collecting tubules in the presence of ADH (see previous text). This is also known as the *countercurrent mechanism.*

  a. The gradient is established by selectively reabsorbing sodium chloride (NaCl) in the thick ascending limb by Na^+-K^+-$2Cl^-$ cotransporter.

  b. Urea recycling and selective permeability of urea also add to the osmotic gradient in the inner medulla.

6. Osmoregulation—maintaining body fluid osmolarity of approximately 290 mOsm/L. This function is primarily under the control of the kidney.

  a. Hypotonicity—produced when excess water is consumed (osmolarity <290 mOsm/L).

    (1) Inhibits osmoreceptors in hypothalamus.

    (2) Decreases thirst and inhibits secretion of ADH (vasopressin) from posterior pituitary.

    (3) Decreases circulating ADH, which results in decreased water permeability in the distal tubules and collecting ducts.

    (4) Decreased water permeability results in decreased water reabsorption and increased urine volume (decreased urine osmolarity).

    (5) Less water returned to the circulation returns plasma osmolarity to normal.

  b. Hypertonicity—produced by deprivation of water or dehydration (osmolarity >290 mOsm/L).

    (1) Stimulates osmoreceptors in hypothalamus.

    (2) Stimulates thirst and secretion of ADH from posterior pituitary.

    (3) Increased ADH increases water permeability in the distal tubules and collecting ducts.

    (4) Increased water permeability results in increased water resorption and decreased urine volume (increased urine osmolarity).

    (5) More water returned to the circulation returns osmolarity to normal.

7. Urination.

  a. Stretch receptors in the bladder initiate the micturition reflex.

    (1) Sensory fibers enter the spinal cord and return to the bladder through parasympathetic fibers.

    (2) Parasympathetic stimulation causes contraction of the bladder.

  b. Voluntary relaxation of the external sphincter permits flow of urine through the external meatus.

10.1 Acid-Base Balance

A. Concerned with maintaining the normal H^+ concentration in body fluids. This is accomplished in three ways.

1. Intracellular and extracellular buffers.

  a. Buffers resist a change in pH.

  b. Intracellular buffers.

    (1) Organic phosphates (e.g., ATP, ADP, glucose-1-phosphate).

    (2) Proteins—hemoglobin and other proteins with numerous acidic or basic groups.

  c. Extracellular buffers.

    (1) Bicarbonate ion (HCO_3^-/CO_2).

    (2) Phosphate (HPO_4^{-2}/$H_2PO_4^-$).

2. Excretion of CO_2 by respiratory mechanisms (rapid response).

3. Bicarbonate resorption and H^+ excretion by the kidney (slow response).

B. Acid-base disorders.

1. Metabolic acidosis.

  a. Decreased HCO_3^- resulting in decreased pH.

  b. Causes.

    (1) Increased fixed (nonvolatile) acids (lactic acid).

    (2) Metabolic disorders (diabetic production of keto acids).

    (3) Decreased excretion of fixed acids.

    (4) Loss of bicarbonate (diarrhea).

  c. Compensation.

    (1) Increased respiration and loss of CO_2.

    (2) Increased H^+ loss by kidney.

    (3) Infusion of chemical buffers (medical intervention).

2. Metabolic alkalosis.

  a. Increased HCO_3^-—resulting in increased pH.

  b. Causes.

    (1) Loss of fixed acids (vomiting).

    (2) Gain of bicarbonate (ingestion of bicarbonate).

  c. Compensation.

    (1) Retention of H^+ by kidney.

    (2) Retention of CO_2 (reduced respiration).

    (3) Infusion of buffers (medical intervention).

3. Respiratory acidosis—resulting in decreased pH.

  a. Retention of CO_2.

  b. Caused by hypoventilation.

    (1) Depression of respiratory center (medications and drugs).

    (2) Reduced respiratory muscle activity.

    (3) Lung disease.

  c. Compensation.

    (1) Increased bicarbonate resorption in kidney.

    (2) Infusion of chemical buffers.

4. Respiratory alkalosis—resulting in increased pH.

  a. Loss of CO_2.

  b. Caused by hyperventilation (anxiety, fever, poisons).

  c. Compensation.

    (1) Retention of H^+ by kidney.

    (2) Decreased respiration rate.

    (3) Infusion of chemical buffers.

C. Approach for analysis of simple acid-base disorders (Figure 2-27).

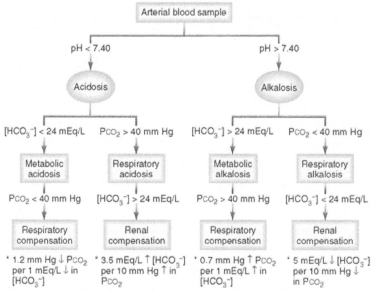

Figure 2-27 Approach for the analysis of simple acid-base disorders. *(From Koeppen BM, Stanton BA, Berne RM: Berne & Levy Physiology, ed 6. Philadelphia, Saunders, 2010.)*

11.0 Oral Physiology

11.1 Oral Cavity

A. Anatomic considerations.
   1. Components—lips, teeth, tongue, hard and soft palate, cheeks, uvula, tonsils, and gums.
   2. Oral mucosa—three types of stratified squamous epithelium.
      a. Lining mucosa—nonkeratinized.
      b. Masticatory mucosa—keratinized or parakeratinized.
      c. Specialized mucosa—taste buds.

11.2 Taste

A. Anatomic considerations.
   1. Taste receptors are modified epithelial cells (not neurons).
   2. Dissolved molecules interact with receptors; stimulate neurons that travel to the cortical gustatory area, hypothalamus, and limbic system.
   3. Pathways depend on localization of receptors.
      a. Posterior one third of tongue—glossopharyngeal and vagus nerves.
      b. Anterior two thirds of tongue—facial nerve.
B. Taste discrimination (Figure 2-28).
   1. Coded by patterns of receptor activity.
   2. Five distinct categories of flavors have been identified. All receptors respond to varying degrees to these primary tastes.
      a. Sweet.
         (1) Produced by certain organic molecules (e.g., glucose, saccharine, aspartame).
         (2) Use G proteins, which activate cAMP second messenger system.
         (3) Blockage of K^+ channels produces depolarization of receptor cell.
      b. Salt.
         (1) Produced by chemical salts (e.g., NaCl, potassium chloride).
         (2) Direct passage of ions through specialized channels is responsible for receptor depolarization.
      c. Sour.
         (1) Produced by H^+ (acids).
         (2) Receptor stimulation results from the blockage of K^+ channels by H^+ resulting in a reduced internal negativity and depolarization.
      d. Bitter.
         (1) Produced by a diverse range of compounds, including many poisonous substances. Few chemical similarities exist when one compares the bitter-tasting chemicals.
         (2) Taste G protein (gustducin) stimulated by the receptor activates a second messenger system to produce a depolarizing potential.
      e. Umami (taste sensation from L-glutamate and aspartate).
         (1) Produced by amino acids, most notably glutamate.
         (2) Use G proteins, which activate a second messenger system responsible for receptor depolarization.
C. Taste abnormalities.
   1. Ageusia—absence of the sense of taste.
   2. Hypogeusia—diminished taste sensation.
   3. Dysgeusia—disturbed sense of taste.

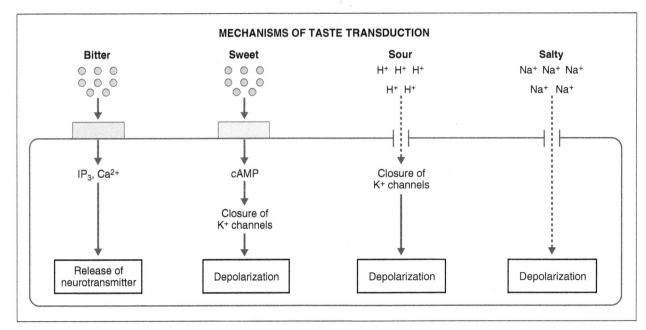

Figure 2-28 Mechanisms of taste transduction.

11.3 Salivary Glands and Secretions

A. Salivary glands—compound tubuloalveolar glands.
  1. Parotid—serous gland produces 20% to 30% of resting saliva volume; produces 90% of stimulated saliva volume.
  2. Submandibular—mixed gland that produces predominantly serous secretions; produces 60% to 70% of resting saliva volume.
  3. Sublingual—mixed gland that produces predominantly mucous secretions; produces 2% to 5% of resting saliva.
B. Saliva—functions in lubrication, solubilization of food, initiating starch digestions, and maintaining oral health.
  1. Salivary composition is dependent on the following structures.
    a. Salivary gland acini.
      (1) Secrete a fluid similar in composition to plasma.
      (2) Fluid contains K^+, Na^+ Cl^-, and HCO_3^- in similar concentrations to plasma.
      (3) Also responsible for secretion of most of the organic components.
    b. Salivary gland ducts.
      (1) Modify the fluid secreted by the acini to produce a more hypotonic fluid.
        (a) Reabsorb Na^+ and Cl^-.
        (b) Secrete K^+ and HCO_3^-.
        (c) Minimal water movement occurs in the ducts.
      (2) Secrete small peptides and growth factors.
      (3) Aldosterone increases Na^+ reabsorption and K^+ secretion.
      (4) As flow rate increases, less reabsorption and secretion occur (Figure 2-29).

2. Composition.
    a. Inorganic components.
      (1) Cations include Na^+ and K^+.
      (2) Anions include Cl^- and HCO_3^-.
      (3) Additional electrolytes are $CaPO_4$, SCN^-, F^-, and $MgSO_4$.
    b. Organic components.
      (1) Amylase—initiates starch digestion.
      (2) Lipase—initiates lipid digestion.
      (3) Proline-rich proteins (acidic and basic).
        (a) Stabilize calcium and hydroxyapatite (aid in supersaturation).
        (b) Play a role in pellicle formation and remineralization.
      (4) Histidine-rich proteins.
        (a) Aid in supersaturation of calcium.
        (b) May have antibacterial effect.
        (c) May have antifungal effect.
      (5) Tyrosine-rich proteins.
        (a) Aid in supersaturation of calcium.
        (b) May have antimicrobial action.
      (6) Cysteine-containing proteins (cystatins).
        (a) Aid in supersaturation of calcium.
        (b) May have antimicrobial activity.
      (7) Statherin.
        (a) Aids in supersaturation of calcium.
        (b) Lubricates teeth.
      (8) Mucous glycoproteins (mucins)—important for protection, lubrication, and oral clearance of microorganisms.
      (9) Salivary peroxidase—catalyzes the oxidation of thiocyanate by H_2O_2 to produce highly reactive oxidizing agents.

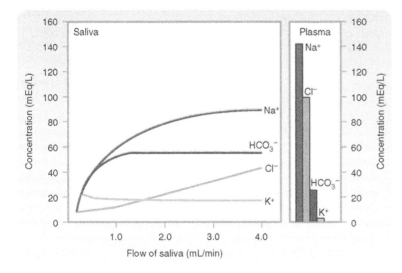

Figure 2-29 Average composition of parotid saliva as a function of salivary flow rate. Saliva is hypotonic to plasma at all flow rates. The bicarbonate (HCO_3^-) level in saliva exceeds the level in plasma except at very low flow rates. *(Redrawn from Thaysen JH, Thorn NA, Schwartz IL: Excretion of sodium, potassium, chloride and carbon dioxide in human parotid saliva. Am J Physiol 178:155, 1954.)*

(10) Lactoferrin—bacteriostatic owing to its ability to bind iron.

(11) Secretory immunoglobulin A (IgA).

    (a) Predominant immunoglobulin in saliva.

    (b) Inhibits bacterial attachment.

(12) Lysozyme—strongly cationic antibacterial molecule.

c. Buffers.

    (1) HCO_3^-.

    (2) Urea.

    (3) Arginine-rich proteins.

3. Regulation occurs through both parasympathetic and sympathetic stimulation.

a. Parasympathetic (cranial nerves VII and IX).

    (1) Muscarinic receptors.

    (2) Second messengers (IP_3, diacylglycerol, and Ca^{2+}).

    (3) Neuropeptides (vasoactive intestinal peptide and substance P) are also released.

    (4) Results in increased volume by increasing acinar and ductal cell transport and vasodilation.

    (5) Failure of parasympathetic stimulation may result in xerostomia and may be restored by muscarinic agonists pilocarpine or cevimeline.

b. Sympathetic (superior cervical ganglion).

    (1) β-Adrenergic receptors.

    (2) Second messenger (cAMP).

    (3) Stimulation produces increased amounts of protein and low volume.

11.4 Mastication

A. Complex, highly coordinated activity that initiates digestion.

B. Movements—characterized as a series of cyclic opening and closing activities involving several muscles that extend from ingestion to swallowing.

1. Muscle activity varies with the stage of mastication and can be interrupted by reflex activity (see text later on).

a. Jaw-opening muscles.

    (1) Mylohyoid.

    (2) Digastric.

    (3) Lateral pterygoid.

b. Jaw-closing muscles.

    (1) Temporalis.

    (2) Masseter.

    (3) Medial pterygoid.

C. Coordination of muscular activity occurs at the level of the brainstem.

1. Trigeminal sensory nucleus—receives sensory input via trigeminal nerve.

2. Trigeminal mesencephalic nucleus—contains afferent cell bodies of afferent fibers from muscle spindles of jaw-closing muscles and cell bodies of periodontal ligament, gingival, and palatal mechanoreceptors.

3. Trigeminal motor nucleus—contains motoneurons that control the muscles of mastication; contain both γ and α motoneurons.

4. Hypoglossal motor nucleus—controls muscles of the tongue.

5. Facial motor nucleus—controls the facial muscles.

D. Control of mastication.

1. Brainstem activity.

a. Responsible for rhythmic movements of mastication.

b. Reflex activity is coordinated in this area.

    (1) Jaw-closing reflex (monosynaptic).

        (a) Tapping the chin stretches muscle spindles in the jaw-closing muscles.

        (b) Masseter and temporalis muscles contract after short latency.

        (c) Stimulation of periodontal ligament and other orofacial receptors produces a similar reflex.

(2) Jaw-opening reflex (polysynaptic)—mechanical stimulation of periodontal ligament or other mechanoreceptors stimulates jaw-opening muscles and inhibits jaw-closing muscles.

2. Cortical motor area.
   a. Responsible for modifications in masticatory motoneuron excitability.
   b. Initiates tongue and orofacial movements.

11.5 Swallowing

A. Movements.
   1. Oral phase.
      a. Tongue forces bolus of food into the pharynx.
      b. Bolus stimulates tactile receptors that initiate pharyngeal phase.
   2. Pharyngeal phase.
      a. Palate is pulled forward, and pharyngeal folds move inward to prevent reflux into nasopharynx.
      b. Larynx moves against epiglottis to prevent food from entering trachea and opens upper esophageal sphincter.
      c. Pharyngeal muscles contract to force bolus of food into the pharynx.
      d. Peristaltic wave is initiated, and respiration is inhibited.
   3. Esophageal phase.
      a. Peristalsis continues (controlled by swallowing center).
         (1) Visceral motoneurons are parasympathetic.
         (2) Neurons of myenteric plexus coordinate the motor activity.
      b. Lower esophageal sphincter relaxes, mediated by vagal inhibitory fibers.
B. Coordination of swallowing occurs in the medulla (via vagus and glossopharyngeal nerves).
   1. Initial (oral) phase is voluntary.
   2. Pharyngeal and esophageal phases are involuntary.

12.0 Digestion

A. Functional considerations of the GI tract.
   1. Histologic considerations.
      a. Mucosa.
         (1) Epithelium—provides protection, secretions, and absorptive capacity.
         (2) Lamina propria—contains glands, blood vessels, nerves, and lymphoid tissue.
         (3) Muscularis mucosa—contains inner circular and outer longitudinal smooth muscle layers.
      b. Submucosa.
         (1) Larger vessels and nerves (Meissner's plexus).
         (2) Connective tissue for distensibility and elasticity.
         (3) No glands except in esophagus and duodenum.

c. Muscularis externa.
   (1) Major smooth muscle layer in the GI tract.
      (a) Inner circular layer.
      (b) Outer longitudinal layer.
   (2) Contains myenteric plexus (Auerbach's plexus).
d. Serosa—important for lubrication and protection.

2. Neuroendocrine considerations.
   a. Basal electrical rhythm.
      (1) Fluctuations in membrane potentials.
      (2) Influenced by mechanical, neural, and hormonal factors.
      (3) Contraction occurs as a unit because of gap junctions.
   b. Intrinsic nerve plexuses—innervate exocrine, endocrine, and smooth muscle cells.
3. Extrinsic nerves (Figure 2-30).
   a. Sympathetic nervous system—inhibitory.
   b. Parasympathetic nervous system—stimulatory.
4. GI hormones.
   a. Released in response to local changes (also CNS activity).
   b. Can be either stimulatory or inhibitory.
5. GI receptors.
   a. Chemoreceptors—sensitive to intestinal contents.
   b. Mechanoreceptors—sensitive to tension and stretch of GI tract.
   c. Osmoreceptors—sensitive to osmotic qualities of intestinal contents.

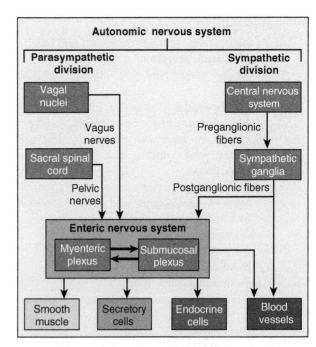

Figure 2-30 Major features of the autonomic innervation of the gastrointestinal (GI) tract. In most cases, the autonomic nerves influence the functions of the GI tract by modulating the activities of the neurons of the enteric nervous system. *(Redrawn from Costa M, Furness JB: Neuronal peptides in the intestine. Br Med Bull 38:247, 1982.)*

6. GI reflexes.
   a. Short reflex—acts locally within the wall.
   b. Long reflex—acts through the CNS via activation of the ANS.
B. Oral cavity and pharynx (see Section 11, Oral Physiology).
C. Esophagus—conduit for food from pharynx to stomach.
   1. Nonkeratinized stratified squamous epithelium.
   2. Only single layer of smooth muscle in muscularis mucosa.
   3. Esophageal glands proper in the submucosa secrete mucus and a serous secretion containing pepsinogen and lysozyme.
   4. Muscularis externa consists of skeletal muscle or smooth muscle or both depending on location.
D. Stomach—function is storage, secretion, mixing, and liquefying food into chyme.
   1. Motility.
      a. Characterized by spontaneous rhythmic depolarization and contractions.
      b. More powerful in antral area.
      c. Receptive relaxation mediated by vagus.
      d. Retropulsion—pyloric muscle contracts pushing chyme back toward stomach body.
   2. Emptying—produced by factors acting through the enterogastric reflex (neuronal and endocrine).
      a. Inhibitory factors.
         (1) Low pH in duodenum.
         (2) Fat in duodenum.
         (3) Hypertonicity in duodenum.
         (4) Distention of duodenum.
         (5) Sympathetic stimulation.
         (6) Intense pain.
      b. Stimulatory factors.
         (1) Parasympathetic stimulation.
         (2) Increased volume and fluidity of gastric contents.
         (3) Forceful peristaltic contractions.
         (4) Absence of segmental contractions in intestine.
   3. Secretion.
      a. Substances secreted.
         (1) Hydrochloric acid (HCl) (from parietal cells).
         (2) Intrinsic factor (from parietal cells) necessary for the binding and absorption of vitamin B_{12}.
         (3) Mucus.
         (4) Pepsinogen (from chief cells) proteolytic enzyme.
         (5) Gastrin (from pyloric glands).
      b. Regulation.
         (1) Cephalic phase.
            (a) Vagally mediated.
            (b) Directly stimulates HCl, pepsinogen, and gastrin release.
         (2) Gastric phase.
            (a) Acts via agents in the stomach.
            (b) Mediated via intrinsic nerves and vagus.

         (3) Intestinal phase.
            (a) Acts via agents in the duodenum.
            (b) Gastrin released is stimulatory.
            (c) Cholecystokinin (CCK), secretin, and gastric inhibitory peptide (GIP) are inhibitory.
            (4) Zollinger-Ellison syndrome—increased gastrin production resulting from pancreatic tumor.
   4. Digestion.
      a. Carbohydrates continue to be digested owing to the presence of salivary amylase.
      b. Protein digestion begins secondary to the conversion of pepsinogen to pepsin (active form is responsible for protein digestion into small peptides).
   5. Absorption of some substances.
      a. Ethyl alcohol.
      b. Aspirin.
E. Small intestine—digests food and absorbs nutrients.
   1. Motility.
      a. Characterized by segmentation.
      b. Initiated by pacemaker cells.
      c. Rate declines along the length of the intestine.
      d. Intensity influenced by several factors.
         (1) Distention.
         (2) Gastrin.
         (3) Neuronal activity.
            (a) Parasympathetics increase segmentation.
            (b) Sympathetics decrease segmentation.
      e. Ileocecal juncture—area between ileum and cecum.
         (1) Ileocecal valve—normally closed, easily opened.
         (2) Ileocecal sphincter—usually constricted.
   2. Secretion.
      a. Brunner's glands—alkaline mucus for protection of intestinal lining.
      b. Enterocytes—large amount of water and electrolytes.
   3. Digestion.
      a. Fat—broken down to monoglycerides and fatty acids in the lumen under the influence of pancreatic lipase.
      b. Protein—broken down to small peptides and amino acids in the lumen owing to the action of pancreatic proteolytic enzymes. Intestinal brush border enzymes further hydrolyze peptide fragments to amino acids.
      c. Carbohydrates—broken down to disaccharides and monosaccharides in lumen (pancreatic amylase) and in intestinal brush border (disaccharidases). Deficiencies of enzymes required for carbohydrate digestion result in GI disorders (lactose intolerance is the inability to metabolize lactose).
   4. Absorption (Table 2-8).
      a. Fat—fatty acids and monoglycerides are absorbed passively (facilitated by bile). Triglycerides are synthesized within the epithelial cells. Chylomicrons

Table 2-8

Summary of Mechanisms of Digestion and Absorption of Nutrients

NUTRIENT	PRODUCTS OF DIGESTION	SITE OF ABSORPTION	MECHANISM
Carbohydrates	Glucose Galactose Fructose	Small intestine	Na^+-glucose cotransport Na^+-galactose cotransport Facilitated diffusion
Proteins	Amino acids Dipeptides Tripeptides	Small intestine	Na^+-amino acid cotransport H^+-dipeptide cotransport H^+-tripeptide cotransport
Lipids	Fatty acids Monoglycerides Cholesterol	Small intestine	Bile salts form micelles in the small intestine Diffusion of fatty acids, monoglycerides, and cholesterol into intestinal cells Reesterification in the cell to triglycerides and phospholipids Chylomicrons form in the cell (requiring apoprotein) and are transferred to lymph
Fat-soluble vitamins		Small intestine	Micelles form with bile salts and products of lipid digestion Diffusion into the intestinal cell
Water-soluble vitamins		Small intestine	Na^+-dependent cotransport
Vitamin B_{12}		Ileum	Intrinsic factor
Bile salts		Ileum	Na^+-salt acid cotransport
Ca^{2+}		Small intestine	Vitamin D–dependent Ca^{2+}-binding protein
Fe^{2+}	Fe^{3+} reduced to Fe^{2+}	Small intestine	Binds to apoferritin in the intestinal cell Binds to transferrin in blood

From Costanzo LS: Physiology, ed 3, Philadelphia, Saunders, 2004.

(lipoproteins and triglycerides) are extruded from the cell and pass into the lymphatic system.

b. Protein—amino acids and small peptides are absorbed and pass into the portal circulation. Amino acids are absorbed by a secondary active transport system.

c. Carbohydrates—monosaccharides are absorbed using a cotransport system (secondary active transport mechanism with sodium). Fructose moves by facilitated diffusion.

d. NaCl and water.
   (1) Active sodium and passive chloride transport occurs throughout the intestine.
   (2) Water moves owing to osmotic pressure changes.

e. Vitamins.
   (1) Both fat-soluble and water-soluble vitamins are absorbed passively. Some specialized mechanisms exist.
   (2) Vitamin B_{12} absorption requires intrinsic factor from gastric mucosa.

f. Iron.
   (1) Active transport from lumen into epithelial cells.
   (2) Reduced iron (ferrous) is more easily absorbed than oxidized form (ferric).
   (3) Absorption is enhanced by vitamin C.
   (4) Transferred in the blood by transferrin or stored within epithelial cells in the form of ferritin.

g. Calcium—primarily an active process stimulated by vitamin D and enhanced by PTH, which increases activation of vitamin D.

F. Large intestine.
   1. Motility.
      a. Characterized by haustral contractions (slow, non-propulsive contractions).
      b. Increased activity (mass movements) moves contents to distal portion of intestine.
      c. Gastrocolic reflex—mass movement stimulated by gastrin release, often after a meal.
      d. Defecation reflex—distention of the rectum caused by mass movement of fecal material.
         (1) Produces relaxation of smooth muscle of internal anal sphincter.
         (2) Produces increased contraction of rectum and sigmoid colon.
         (3) External sphincter relaxation is under voluntary control.
   2. Secretion.
      a. No digestive enzymes are secreted.
      b. Bicarbonate and mucus are produced for protective purposes.

3. Absorption.
   a. Sodium is actively absorbed.
   b. Vitamin K is absorbed.
   c. Water is absorbed passively.
G. Liver.
   1. Function.
      a. Metabolism of nutrients.
         (1) Helps regulate blood glucose, triglyceride, and cholesterol levels.
         (2) Metabolizes amino acids to provide additional sources of energy.
      b. Detoxification and degradation of organic compounds (drugs, hormones, waste products of metabolism).
      c. Synthesis of essential proteins (e.g., clotting factors, albumin).
      d. Storage of nutrients (e.g., glycogen, fat-soluble vitamins).
      e. Activation of vitamin D.
      f. Excretion of cholesterol and bilirubin via bile.
   2. Bile.
      a. Secreted by hepatocytes and stored in the gallbladder.
      b. Composition.
         (1) Bile salts.
         (2) Cholesterol.
         (3) Lecithin.
         (4) Bilirubin.
      c. Water, bicarbonate, and salts are added by the duct cells.
      d. Involved in fat digestion (emulsion) and absorption.
      e. Most is reabsorbed (enterohepatic circulation).
      f. Stimuli for bile secretion.
         (1) Chemical (primarily bile salts).
         (2) Hormonal and neuronal.
            (a) Secretin stimulates bicarbonate secretion from ducts.
            (b) CCK, gastrin, and vagal activity stimulate gallbladder contraction and relaxation of the sphincter of Oddi.
      g. Complications of bile secretion cause gallstones and obstructive jaundice.
      h. Bile acids cause Cl^- secretion (and Na/H_2O) in the intestine.
H. Pancreas.
   1. Endocrine secretion.
      a. Insulin.
      b. Glucagon.
   2. Exocrine secretion.
      a. Proteolytic enzymes.
         (1) Trypsinogen (activated by enterokinase).
         (2) Chymotrypsinogen (activated by trypsin).
         (3) Procarboxypeptidase (activated by trypsin).
      b. Pancreatic amylase.
      c. Pancreatic lipase.
      d. Bicarbonate.
   3. Regulation of secretion.
      a. Secretin.
         (1) Released from the duodenal mucosa in response to low pH.
         (2) Stimulates increased bicarbonate secretion from pancreas.
      b. CCK.
         (1) Released from the duodenal mucosa in response to fat and protein.
         (2) Stimulates increased pancreatic enzyme secretion.
I. Summary of GI hormones (Tables 2-9 and 2-10).
J. Lipoproteins—Transport of dietary and endogenously synthesized lipids throughout the body (Figure 2-31).
   1. Composition—phospholipids, cholesterol, and proteins (apoproteins).
   2. Apoproteins.
      a. Provide structural framework.
      b. Binding sites for receptors.
      c. Activators or coenzymes for lipid metabolism.
      d. Direct the fate of the lipoprotein.
   3. Classes.
      a. Chylomicron—transports dietary triglycerides.
      b. Very-low-density lipoprotein (VLDL)—transports endogenously synthesized triglycerides.
      c. LDL—delivers cholesterol to peripheral tissues; arises from lipolysis of VLDL.
      d. High-density lipoprotein (HDL)—reverses cholesterol transport back to liver.

13.0 Endocrine System

13.1 Pituitary Gland and Hypothalamus

A. Pituitary gland and hypothalamus function in a coordinated fashion to regulate growth; thyroid, adrenal cortex, and reproductive tissues; and overall osmolarity of body tissues.
B. Posterior lobe of pituitary.
   1. Derived from neural tissue (integrated with the hypothalamus).
   2. Secretes ADH (vasopressin) and oxytocin, which are produced by neurons in the hypothalamus and travel to the posterior pituitary via neurons that are part of the hypothalamic-hypophyseal tract.
C. Anterior lobe of pituitary.
   1. Primarily a collection of endocrine cells that are stimulated or inhibited by hormones synthesized in the hypothalamus and delivered to the anterior pituitary by the hypothalamic-hypophyseal portal blood vessels.
   2. Secretes adrenocorticotropic hormone (ACTH), thyroid-stimulating hormone (TSH), growth

Table 2-9

Summary of Gastrointestinal Hormones

HORMONE	HORMONE FAMILY	SITE OF SECRETION	STIMULI FOR SECRETION	ACTIONS
Gastrin	Gastrin-CCK	G cells of the stomach	Small peptides and amino acids	↑ Gastric H^+ secretion
			Distention of the stomach	Stimulates growth of gastric mucosa
			Vagal stimulation (GRP)	↑ Pancreatic enzyme secretion
CCK	Gastrin-CCK	I cells of the duodenum and jejunum	Small peptides and amino acids	↑ Pancreatic HCO_3^- secretion
			Fatty acids	Stimulates contraction of the gallbladder and relaxation of the sphincter of Oddi
				Stimulates growth of the exocrine pancreas and gallbladder
				Inhibits gastric emptying
Secretin	Secretin-glucagon	S cells of the duodenum	H^+ in the duodenum	↑ Pancreatic HCO_3^- secretion
			Fatty acids in the duodenum	↑ Biliary HCO_3^- secretion
				↓ Gastric H^+ secretion
				Inhibits trophic effect of gastrin on gastric mucosa
GIP	Secretin-glucagon	Duodenum and jejunum	Fatty acids	↑ Insulin secretion from pancreatic β cells
			Amino acids	↓ Gastric H^+ secretion
			Oral glucose	

From Costanzo LS: Physiology, ed 3, Philadelphia, Saunders, 2004.

CCK, Cholecystokinin; *GIP,* gastric inhibitory peptide; *GRP,* gastrin-releasing peptide.

Table 2-10

Summary of Gastrointestinal Secretions

SECRETION	CHARACTERISTICS OF SECRETION	FACTORS THAT INCREASE SECRETION	FACTORS THAT DECREASE SECRETION
Saliva	High $[HCO_3^-]$	Parasympathetic (prominent)	Sleep
	High $[K^+]$	Sympathetic	Dehydration
	Hypotonic		Atropine
	α-Amylase and lingual lipase		
Gastric	HCl	Gastrin	H^+ in the stomach
	Pepsinogen	Acetylcholine	Chyme in the duodenum
	Intrinsic factor	Histamine	Atropine
		Parasympathetic	Cimetidine
			Omeprazole
Pancreatic	High $[HCO_3^-]$	Secretin	
	Isotonic	CCK (potentiates secretin)	
	Pancreatic lipase, amylase, proteases	Parasympathetic	
		CCK	
		Parasympathetic	
Bile	Bile salts	CCK (contraction of the gallbladder and relaxation of the sphincter of Oddi)	Ileal resection
	Bilirubin	Parasympathetic	
	Phospholipids		
	Cholesterol		

From Costanzo LS: Physiology, ed 3, Philadelphia, Saunders, 2004.

CCK, Cholecystokinin; *HCl,* hydrochloric acid.

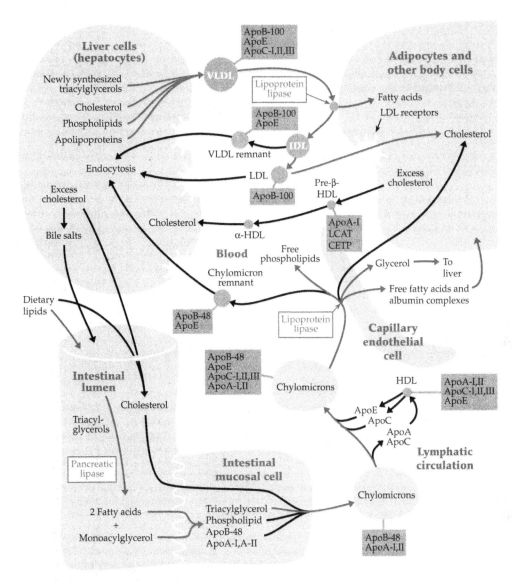

Figure 2-31 Movement of triacylglycerols from liver and intestine to body cells and lipid carriers of blood. *IDL,* Intermediate-density lipoproteins found in human plasma; *LDL,* low-density lipoproteins that have lost most of their triacylglycerols; *VLDL,* very-low-density lipoprotein that contains triacylglycerols, phospholipids, cholesterol, and apolipoproteins B and C. *(From Metzler DE: Biochemistry, ed 2, San Diego, Academic Press, 2003.)*

hormone (GH), follicle-stimulating hormone (FSH), luteinizing hormone (LH), and prolactin.

3. Proopiomelanocortin is the prohormone, which, when hydrolyzed, produces ACTH, melanocyte-stimulating hormone, γ-lipotropin, and β-endorphin.

4. Hypothalamic-releasing hormones.
   a. Thyrotropin-releasing hormone (TRH)—stimulates the release of TSH.
   b. GH-releasing hormone—stimulates the release of GH.
   c. GH-inhibiting hormone (somatostatin).
   d. Corticotropin-releasing hormone (CRH)—stimulates the release of ACTH and β-endorphin.
   e. Prolactin-releasing hormone.
   f. Prolactin-inhibiting hormone (dopamine).

D. ADH (vasopressin).
   1. Responsible for regulation of body fluid osmolarity.
   2. Secreted in response to increased serum osmolarity, pain, nausea, and hypoglycemia.
   3. Release inhibited by decreased serum osmolarity, ethanol, and atrial natriuretic peptide.
   4. Increases permeability of distal tubule and collecting ducts to increase water resorption and return osmolarity to normal (V_2 receptor); also produces contraction of vascular smooth muscle (V_1 receptor).
   5. Diabetes insipidus—caused by the failure of ADH to be secreted (central diabetes insipidus) or failure of renal duct cells to respond to ADH (nephrogenic diabetes insipidus).

E. Oxytocin.
  1. Responsible for milk ejection from the lactating breast and uterine contraction during labor.
  2. Secreted in response to suckling, dilation of cervix, orgasm, and conditioned responses (sight, sound, or smell of the infant).
  3. Inhibited by opioids (endorphins).
  4. Produces contraction of the myoepithelial cells in mammary small ducts and rhythmic contraction of uterine smooth muscle.
F. ACTH.
  1. Responsible for stimulating the conversion of cholesterol to pregnenolone, which serves as a precursor of adrenal steroids. Release is pulsatile and diurnal in nature.
  2. Secreted in response to stress, hypoglycemia, decreased blood cortisol, ADH, and serotonin.
  3. Release is inhibited by increased blood cortisol, opioids, and somatostatin.
  4. Activates cholesterol desmolase, which enhances pregnenolone synthesis; upregulates ACTH receptors and produces hypertrophy and hyperplasia of adrenal tissue.
  5. Cushing's disease results from ACTH hypersecretion.
G. TSH.
  1. Responsible for regulating the growth of the thyroid gland and stimulating the secretion of thyroid hormones (triiodothyronine [T_3] and thyroxine [T_4]).
  2. Secreted in response to TRH (from hypothalamus), which is downregulated by T_3 and T_4.
  3. Activates steps in the synthetic pathway of thyroid hormones and ultimate release.
H. GH.
  1. Important for normal growth and metabolism.
    a. Growth-promoting actions—most are mediated by release of somatomedin. Insulinlike growth factor [IGF] is the newer accepted name for somatomedin.
      (1) Causes hypertrophy and hyperplasia.
      (2) Increases protein synthesis and organ growth.
      (3) Increases linear growth (bone thickness and length).
    b. Metabolic actions.
      (1) Decreases glucose uptake and use (diabetogenic effect).
      (2) Increases lipolysis; increases fatty acids and insulin in blood.
  2. Secreted in response to decreased glucose, fatty acids, fasting, exercise, stress, and sleep.
  3. Inhibited by increased glucose, fatty acids, obesity, somatostatin, IGF, GH, and pregnancy.
  4. Gigantism, characterized by acromegaly and increased linear growth, is produced by GH excess.

I. FSH.
  1. Responsible for stimulating granulosa cells to convert androstenedione to estrogens, which, in combination with FSH, result in positive feedback to produce more estrogen. In males, FSH stimulates spermatogenesis and Sertoli cell function.
  2. Secreted in response to gonadotropin-releasing hormone (GnRH) from the hypothalamus, which is released throughout life and becomes pulsatile at puberty.
  3. Inhibited in males by testosterone and inhibin (glycoprotein secreted by Sertoli cells). In females, in the follicular phase, estradiol inhibits secretion of FSH; however, sharp increases in estradiol before ovulation stimulate FSH release. Progesterone inhibits FSH secretion.
J. LH.
  1. Responsible for stimulating Leydig cells to synthesize testosterone by increasing the activity of cholesterol desmolase (first step in steroidogenesis). LH initiates ovulation, stimulates formation of the corpus luteum, and maintains steroid hormone production throughout the luteal phase of the menstrual cycle.
  2. Secreted in response to GnRH and in midcycle by sharp increases in estradiol.
  3. Inhibited in males by testosterone, which inhibits the release of GnRH and LH from the pituitary. In females, in the follicular phase, estradiol inhibits the secretion of LH. Progesterone inhibits LH secretion from the anterior pituitary.
K. Prolactin.
  1. Responsible for milk production and breast development.
  2. Secreted in response to TRH, estrogen, breastfeeding, sleep, and stress.
  3. Inhibited by dopamine, somatostatin, and prolactin (negative feedback).
  4. High levels prevent ovulation by inhibiting the synthesis and release of GnRH.

13.2 Reproduction

A. Male reproductive system.
  1. Structure of testes.
    a. Seminiferous tubules—responsible for sperm production.
    b. Sertoli cells.
      (1) Provide nutrients for sperm.
      (2) Provide a barrier to the bloodstream to protect developing sperm.
      (3) Secrete fluid to assist sperm transport into epididymis.
    c. Leydig cells—site of synthesis and secretion of testosterone.

2. Testosterone.
   a. Metabolism.
      (1) Synthesized from cholesterol (stimulated by LH).
      (2) 17-β-Hydroxysteroid dehydrogenase responsible for the final conversion of androstenedione to testosterone.
      (3) Small amounts of testosterone are converted to estrogen in some tissue.
      (4) Transported in plasma associated with sex steroid–binding globulin (which is increased by estrogen and decreased by androgens) and albumin.
      (5) Synthesis is inhibited by feedback inhibition by testosterone on the release of LH from the pituitary and GnRH in the hypothalamus. Inhibin, released from the Sertoli cells, also inhibits FSH secretion.
   b. Function.
      (1) Development of male genital tract.
      (2) Development of primary and secondary sex characteristics.
      (3) Spermatogenesis.
3. Dihydrotestosterone.
   a. Metabolism.
      (1) Testosterone in some target tissues must be converted to dihydrotestosterone (active androgen in some tissues) by 5α-reductase.
      (2) Binds in a more stable fashion to DNA and is a more active androgen in some tissues.
   b. Function.
      (1) Fetal differentiation of external genitalia.
      (2) Development of primary and secondary sex characteristics.
      (3) Growth of prostate.
4. Spermatogenesis—requires FSH and LH.
   a. Mitotic division—spermatogonia to spermatocytes.
   b. Meiotic division—spermatocytes become haploid spermatids.
   c. Spermiogenesis—spermatids transformed into mature sperm.
B. Female reproductive system.
   1. Structure of ovary.
      a. Cortex.
         (1) Contains oocytes enclosed in follicles.
         (2) Responsible for steroid hormone synthesis.
      b. Medulla and hilum—remainder of ovary containing a mixture of cell types and blood vessels.
   2. Estrogen and progesterone.
      a. Metabolism.
         (1) Synthesized by ovarian follicles.
         (2) Synthesized from cholesterol (stimulated by LH).

BOX 2-1

Actions of Estrogens on Target Tissues

- Maturation and maintenance of uterus, fallopian tubes, cervix, and vagina
- Responsible at puberty for the development of female secondary sex characteristics
- Required for development of the breasts
- Responsible for proliferation and development of ovarian granulosa cells
- Upregulation of estrogen, progesterone, and LH receptors
- Negative *and* positive feedback effects on FSH and LH secretion
- Maintenance of pregnancy
- Lowers uterine threshold to contractile stimuli
- Stimulates prolactin secretion
- Blocks action of prolactin on the breast

From Costanzo LS: Physiology, ed 3, Philadelphia, Saunders, 2004.
FSH, Follicle-stimulating hormone; *LH,* luteinizing hormone.

BOX 2-2

Actions of Progesterone on Target Tissues

- Maintenance of secretory activity of uterus during luteal phase
- Development of the breasts
- Negative feedback effects on FSH and LH secretion
- Maintenance of pregnancy
- Raises uterine threshold to contractile stimuli during pregnancy

From Costanzo LS: Physiology, ed 3, Philadelphia, Saunders, 2004.
FSH, Follicle-stimulating hormone; *LH,* luteinizing hormone.

---

         (3) Pathway similar to steroid production in adrenal cortex and testes.
         (4) 3-β-Hydroxysteroid dehydrogenase converts pregnenolone to progesterone.
         (5) Aromatase (stimulated by FSH) converts testosterone to 17-β-estradiol.
      b. Function (Boxes 2-1 and 2-2).
   3. Ovarian cycle.
      a. Follicular phase.
         (1) LH stimulates the conversion of cholesterol to androstenedione.
         (2) FSH stimulates the conversion of androstenedione to estrogens.
         (3) Estrogens and FSH (positive feedback) stimulate more estrogen, LH, and FSH receptors.

(4) Elevated estradiol levels cause proliferation of the uterus.

(5) FSH and LH levels are suppressed owing to feedback of estradiol on the pituitary.

(6) Because feedback inhibition of FSH is greater than LH, further follicular development does not occur.

b. Ovulation.

(1) Burst of estrogen causes an LH surge and increased FSH secretion.

(2) LH surge causes ovulation and completion of meiosis of the oocyte.

(3) Estrogen secretion decreases.

c. Luteal phase.

(1) As a result of the LH surge, the corpus luteum develops and begins synthesizing estradiol and progesterone.

(2) These hormones cause feedback inhibition on the hypothalamus to reduce secretion of LH and FSH.

(3) If fertilization does not occur, the corpus luteum degenerates. This results in a sharp decrease in estradiol and progesterone.

(4) Under reduced hormonal stimulation, the endometrium is sloughed (menses).

4. Pregnancy.

a. If fertilization occurs, chorionic gonadotropin (from placenta) maintains the corpus luteum, which continues to secrete estradiol and progesterone.

b. Continued elevated levels of estradiol and progesterone maintain the endometrium, stimulate breast development, and suppress follicular function.

c. Progesterone also is responsible for reducing contractility of the uterus.

5. Parturition.

a. Oxytocin causes uterine contractions as a result of increased receptor sensitivity.

b. The estrogen-to-progesterone ratio increases, which increases the sensitivity of the uterus to contractile sensitivity (fetal growth and uterine distention).

c. Increased prostaglandin production and resulting increased intracellular calcium result in increased contractility.

13.3 Signaling Systems

A. General principles.

1. Mechanisms of communication.

a. Endocrine—involve regulatory substances, which, when released, have effects on targets far removed from the endocrine cells.

b. Paracrine—involve regulatory substances released from cells that are not immediately adjacent to the target cells but are sufficiently close to reach the target cell by diffusion.

c. Autocrine—involve regulatory factors that act on that cell itself or neighboring identical cell.

d. Neurocrine—involve regulatory factors released by neurons in the immediate vicinity of the target cells.

2. Classification of signaling systems.

a. Intracellular hormones.

(1) Lipophilic (nonpolar)—diffuse across membrane.

(2) Bind to intracellular receptors forming complexes that bind to DNA (hormone response element), which activates gene transcription.

(3) Binding domain stabilized by adjacent motifs called *zinc fingers*.

(4) Transported in blood bound to plasma proteins.

(5) Examples include steroid hormones, vitamin D, thyroid hormone, and carotenoids.

b. Extracellular hormones (peptides and proteins).

(1) Hydrophilic (polar)—cannot diffuse across membrane.

(2) Bind to receptors on the cell surface and activate second messenger systems.

(3) Examples—insulin, epinephrine, glucagon, gastrin, and pituitary hormones.

3. G proteins—family of proteins that bind to the inner aspect of the plasma membrane. G proteins bind to seven-transmembrane cell surface receptors and communicate the messages from these stimulated receptors to enzymes, which leads to the production of second messengers. These second messengers act on various cytoplasmic proteins. G proteins can also act on ion channels.

a. Heterotrimeric in nature, having an α, β, and γ subunit.

b. α subunit—has GTPase activity.

(1) Bound to GDP (G protein inactive).

(2) Bound to GTP (G protein active).

c. G proteins can either be stimulatory (G_s) or inhibitory (G_i).

d. Cholera toxin modifies the G_s protein, resulting in a persistent stimulation of adenylate cyclase and production of cAMP.

e. Pertussis toxin modifies G_i, preventing the adenylate cyclase system from being inhibited by G_i, also resulting in abnormally high levels of cAMP.

4. Mechanism of action.

a. Signaling systems that employ adenylate cyclase.

(1) Examples: ACTH, LH, calcitonin, PTH, glucagon, β-adrenergic receptors.

(2) Hormone binds to receptor, producing a conformational change on the α subunit ultimately to exchange the α_s-GDP complex with GTP.

(3) α_s-GTP activates adenylate cyclase, which catalyzes the conversion of ATP to cAMP (α_s-GTP is inactivated by intrinsic GTPase).

(4) cAMP activates protein kinase A, which phosphorylates intracellular proteins.

(5) Phosphorylated proteins produce physiologic activities within the cell.

(6) cAMP is degraded to 5′ AMP by phosphodiesterase.

b. Signaling systems that employ phospholipase C.

(1) Examples: TRH, GH-releasing hormone, angiotensin II, oxytocin, α_1-adrenergic receptors.

(2) Hormone binds to receptor and activates phospholipase C via G protein.

(3) Phospholipase C cleaves PIP_2 (phosphatidylinositol 4,5-diphosphate) to form IP_3 and diacylglycerol.

(4) IP_3 binds to receptors on endoplasmic reticulum to produce Ca^{2+} release and subsequent activation of additional molecules (calmodulin).

(5) IP_3 is dephosphorylated by a cytoplasmic phosphorylase, inactivating the molecule.

c. Signaling systems that employ tyrosine kinase.

(1) Examples: insulin, IGF-I.

(2) Hormone binding causes changes that result in autophosphorylation of the receptor. (In this case, the enzyme is a function possessed by the receptor itself.)

(3) The phosphorylation triggers multiple cellular responses.

(a) Calcium influx.

(b) Increased Na^+/H^+ exchange.

(c) Amino acid and glucose uptake.

d. Signaling systems that employ guanylate cyclase.

(1) Examples: atrial natriuretic peptide, nitric oxide.

(2) Hormone binding results in the stimulation of guanylyl cyclase, which elevates the intracellular concentration of cGMP.

(3) cGMP (second messenger) stimulates cGMP-dependent protein kinases (protein kinase G).

13.4 Pancreas and Parathyroid

A. Pancreatic hormones.

1. Insulin.

a. Structure and synthesis.

(1) Peptide consisting of two chains (α and β).

(2) Synthesized as a prohormone and cleaved to produce the active hormone.

(3) The cleaved peptide (C protein) is used as an indicator of β-cell function.

b. Regulation of secretion.

(1) Stimulants.

(a) Increased concentrations of blood glucose, amino acids, fatty acids, and ketone bodies.

(b) Oral glucose.

(c) Increased levels of glucagons, GH, cortisol, and GIP.

(d) Increased potassium levels.

(e) Cholinergic stimulation (vagal stimulation).

(2) Inhibitors.

(a) Decreased blood glucose.

(b) Fasting.

(c) Exercise.

(d) Somatostatin.

(e) α-Adrenergic agents.

c. Mechanism of action.

(1) Receptor consists of four subunits (two α and two β subunits).

(a) α subunits are surface peptides that contain the recognition site for insulin.

(b) β subunits span the plasma membrane and have tyrosine kinase activity.

(2) Insulin binding to the receptor causes phosphorylation of the β subunits (autophosphorylation) and phosphorylation of target proteins, which have multiple effects within the cell.

(3) The insulin receptor complex is internalized, resulting in downregulation of its receptor (involved in decreased insulin sensitivity in obesity and type 2 diabetes).

(4) Glucose transporters are redistributed to the cell membrane, which results in increased transport of glucose into the cell.

d. Functions—facilitates the use of energy sources in the body. These activities are summarized in Figure 2-32.

2. Glucagon.

a. Structure and synthesis.

(1) Single polypeptide synthesized as a prohormone from a cell of the islets of Langerhans' cells.

(2) Structurally related to other GI hormones (secretin and GIP).

b. Regulation of secretion.

(1) Stimulants.

(a) Fasting and intense exercise.

(b) Reduced plasma glucose.

(c) Increased ingestion of amino acids.

(d) CCK.

(e) Acetylcholine.

(2) Inhibitors.

(a) Insulin and somatostatin.

(b) Increased plasma fatty acids and ketones.

c. Mechanism of action.

(1) Cell membrane receptor activates adenylate cyclase using the G protein, G_s.

(2) The cAMP produced activates protein kinase A, and protein kinase A catalyzes the phosphorylation of enzymes, which mediate the physiologic effects.

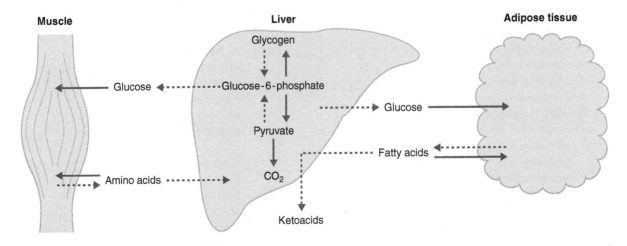

Nutrient	Effect of Insulin on Blood Level
Glucose	Decreased
Fatty acids	Decreased
Ketoacids	Decreased
Amino acids	Decreased

Figure 2-32 Effects of insulin on nutrient flow. *Solid arrows* indicate steps favored by insulin; *dashed arrows* indicate steps inhibited by insulin.

   d. Functions.
      (1) Increases glycogenolysis.
      (2) Increases gluconeogenesis.
      (3) Increases lipolysis.
      (4) Increases ketone body production.
      (5) Inhibits glycogenesis.
3. Somatostatin.
   a. Structure and synthesis.
      (1) Single polypeptide secreted by the δ cells of the islets of Langerhans.
      (2) Secretion is stimulated by the ingestion of all nutrients (glucose, amino acids, and fatty acids) and glucagon.
      (3) Secretion is inhibited by insulin.
   b. Function.
      (1) Inhibits the secretion of insulin and glucagon.
      (2) Serves to modulate the overall effects of a meal on the pancreatic release of insulin and glucagons.
B. Calcium-regulating hormones (PTH, calcitonin, and vitamin D).
   1. Calcium balance—regulated by three organ systems.
      a. Bone—99% of calcium in the body (resorption regulated by PTH and calcitonin).
      b. Kidney—filters and reabsorbs calcium (regulated by PTH).

   c. Intestine—absorption regulated by 1,25-dihydroxycholecalciferol (active form of vitamin D).
      (1) Net absorption and excretion is about 200 mg/day.
      (2) Ionized calcium (Ca^{2+}) is the only biologically active form of the mineral.
      (3) Hypocalcemia (low blood calcium).
         (a) Symptoms include tetany, tiredness, and convulsions.
         (b) Caused by renal failure and reduced 1,25-dihydroxycholecalciferol.
   d. Hypercalcemia.
      (1) Symptoms include lethargy, depression, and cardiac arrhythmias.
      (2) Caused by malignancy or hyperparathyroidism.
   2. PTH.
      a. Structure and synthesis.
         (1) Single-chain polypeptide synthesized in the chief cell of the parathyroid gland.
         (2) Synthesized as a prohormone and cleaved before release.
      b. Regulation of secretion.
         (1) Stimulants.
            (a) Low serum calcium.
            (b) Low serum magnesium.

(2) Inhibitors.

  (a) High serum calcium.

  (b) High serum magnesium.

  (c) Very low serum magnesium.

c. Mechanism of action.

  (1) Cell membrane receptor activates adenylate cyclase using G_s (bone and kidney).

  (2) In intestine, PTH enhances calcium absorption by activation of renal 1α-hydroxylase to form 1,25-dihydroxycholecalciferol, which increases calcium absorption in the intestine.

d. Function—overall effect is to increase serum Ca^{2+} and decrease serum PO_4^{-3}.

  (1) Bone.

    (a) Initially and rapidly activates PTH receptors on osteoblasts to increase bone formation.

    (b) Long-term stimulation of osteoclasts to increase bone resorption mediated by cytokines.

  (2) Kidney.

    (a) Inhibits phosphate reabsorption—in proximal convoluted tubule.

    (b) Stimulates Ca^{2+} reabsorption in the distal convoluted tubule.

    (c) Overall effect is to increase the circulating levels of calcium and reduce the possibility of forming calcium complexes in ECF (reduces phosphate).

  (3) Intestine—increases the absorption of calcium by activating vitamin D.

3. Calcitonin.

a. Structure and synthesis.

  (1) Peptide synthesized in the thyroid gland by parafollicular cells.

  (2) Stored as a prohormone and secreted on stimulation.

b. Regulation for secretion—release is stimulated by increased plasma Ca^{2+}.

c. Mechanism of action—inhibits osteoclastic activity.

d. Function—overall effect is to prevent increases in plasma Ca^{2+}.

4. Vitamin D.

a. Structure and synthesis.

  (1) Vitamin D (cholecalciferol) is obtained in the diet, but most is produced (from cholesterol) in the skin by exposure to sunlight. Unless it is activated by successive hydroxylation, it remains inactive.

  (2) Hydroxylation occurs in two organs.

    (a) The liver hydroxylates cholecalciferol to form 25-hydroxycholecalciferol.

    (b) The kidney hydroxylates 25-hydroxycholecalciferol to 1,25-dihydroxycholecalciferol, which is physiologically active.

    (c) The kidney can also hydroxylate 25-hydroxycholecalciferol to 24,25-hydroxycholecalciferol (inactive form).

b. Regulation of synthesis (Figure 2-33).

  (1) Hydroxylation is regulated by negative feedback mechanisms, which depend on plasma calcium levels and hormones responsible for regulating plasma concentration of calcium.

c. Mechanism of action.

  (1) Overall function of 1,25-dihydroxycholecalciferol is to increase plasma and phosphate concentrations in the blood. This is

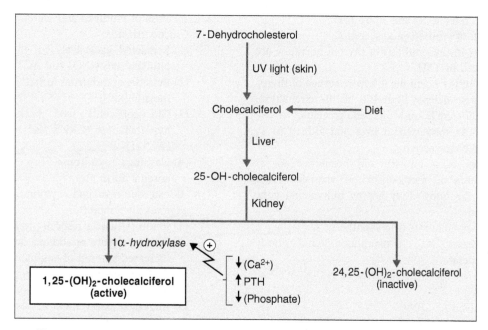

Figure 2-33 Steps involved in the synthesis of 1,25-dihydroxycholecalciferol.

accomplished by stimulation of gene transcription and synthesis of new proteins in three tissues.

    (a) Intestine.

        (i) 1,25-Dihydroxycholecalciferol induces the synthesis of calcium-binding proteins (calbindin D).

        (ii) Calcium also diffuses down an electrochemical gradient and is pumped into the circulation by Ca^{2+}-ATPase on the basolateral membrane.

        (iii) Phosphate absorption is also enhanced by 1,25-dihydroxycholecalciferol.

    (b) Kidney.

        (i) 1,25-Dihydroxycholecalciferol stimulates the reabsorption of both calcium and phosphate ions.

    (c) Bone.

        (i) 1,25-Dihydroxycholecalciferol stimulates osteoclastic activity and bone resorption.

13.5 Adrenal and Thyroid

A. Thyroid hormone.

  1. Structure and synthesis.

    a. Iodide pump (trapping) is present in follicular cells. This pump is regulated by iodide levels in the body (low iodide stimulates the pump).

    b. Iodide is oxidized and attached to tyrosyl residues of thyroglobulin (glycoprotein, which serves as the storage form of thyroid hormones).

    c. Iodotyrosines are coupled to form either T_3 (three iodides) or T_4 (four iodides) and are stored in the peptide linkage (thyroglobulin).

    d. Thyroglobulin is stored as colloid until stimulated to be secreted as T_3 and T_4 by TSH.

  2. Regulation of synthesis and secretion.

    a. All steps in the synthesis of thyroid hormone are stimulated by TSH.

    b. Release of the hormone follows cleavage of thyroglobulin to deliver T_3 and T_4 to the circulation, where they are bound to plasma proteins.

    c. Most T_4 is converted in liver and kidney to T_3 (more biologic activity).

  3. Mechanism of action—thyroid hormones act as a modulator of metabolism on virtually every organ in the body. They act by influencing gene expression.

    a. Basal metabolic rate (increased).

      (1) Increases O_2 consumption and body temperature.

      (2) Due to increased activity of Na^+-K^+-ATPase activity.

    b. Metabolism.

      (1) Potentiates the effects of other hormones on energy metabolism, resulting in increased glycogen breakdown, increased carbohydrate metabolism, and fat metabolism.

      (2) Overall catabolic effect on protein metabolism.

    c. Growth and development.

      (1) Act synergistically with GH and somatomedins to promote bone growth.

      (2) Required for the normal maturation of the CNS in children.

    d. Cardiovascular, respiratory, and sympathomimetic.

      (1) Increased metabolism requires increased activity of respiratory and cardiovascular systems.

      (2) Upregulation of β_1-adrenergic receptors by thyroid hormone mediates this response.

B. Adrenocortical (steroid) hormones.

  1. Structure and synthesis.

    a. Three classes of hormones are synthesized (all from cholesterol).

      (1) Glucocorticoids (21 carbons).

      (2) Mineralocorticoids (21 carbons).

      (3) Androgens (19 carbons).

    b. Rate-limiting step is conversion of cholesterol to pregnenolone.

    c. Because of compartmentalization of the synthetic enzymes, different zones of the adrenal gland specialize in synthetic activity.

      (1) Zona glomerulosa (outermost zone)—secretes mineralocorticoids (aldosterone).

      (2) Zona fasciculata (middle zone)—secretes mainly glucocorticoids (cortisol and corticosterone).

      (3) Zona reticularis (innermost zone)—secretes adrenal androgens (dehydroepiandrosterone and androstenedione).

  2. Regulation of synthesis and secretion.

    a. Glucocorticoids.

      (1) Regulated exclusively by the hypothalamic-pituitary axis (CRH and ACTH).

      (2) Pulsatile and diurnal in nature (highest in the morning).

      (3) Glucocorticoids feed back negatively on hypothalamus (CRH) and anterior pituitary (ACTH).

      (4) Cushing's syndrome (excess secretion of adrenal hormones).

    b. Aldosterone-regulated primarily by renin-angiotensin system.

      (1) Renin release in response to reduction in perfusion pressure or sodium depletion produces increased amount of angiotensin II.

      (2) Angiotensin II acts on the adrenal cortex to increase aldosterone secretion.

      (3) Increased extracellular K^+ also increases aldosterone secretion by acting directly on the adrenal cells.

Table 2-11		
Actions of Adrenocortical Steroids		
ACTIONS OF GLUCOCORTICOIDS	**ACTIONS OF MINERALOCORTICOIDS**	**ACTIONS OF ADRENAL ANDROGENS**
Increase gluconeogenesis	Increase Na^+ reabsorption	Females: presence of pubic and axillary hair; libido
Increase proteolysis (catabolic)	Increase K^+ secretion	Males: same as testosterone
Increase lipolysis	Increase H^+ secretion	
Decrease glucose use		
Decrease insulin sensitivity		
Antiinflammatory		
Immunosuppression		
Maintain vascular responsiveness to catecholamines		
Inhibit bone formation		
Increase GFR		
Decrease REM sleep		

From Costanzo LS: Physiology, ed 3, Philadelphia, Saunders, 2004.

GFR, Glomerular filtration rate; REM, rapid eye movement.

 c. Androgens—regulated by the same mechanisms as glucocorticoids.
 3. Actions of adrenocortical steroids (Table 2-11).
C. Adrenal medullary (catecholamines) hormones.
 1. Structure and synthesis.
  a. Synthesized by a series of steps from tyrosine.
  b. Epinephrine (methylated form of norepinephrine) is the major secretory product.
  c. The adrenal medulla is essentially a sympathetic ganglion, which has secretory cells instead of postganglionic neurons. The catecholamines are secreted directly into the bloodstream to play an important role in the "fight or flight" response.
 2. Regulation of synthesis and secretion.
  a. Catecholamines are stored in granules in chromaffin cells.
  b. Stimulation of the sympathetic nerve to the adrenal gland releases acetylcholine at ganglionic type receptors, which results in the release of catecholamines.
  c. Examples of stress-related factors that result in adrenal medullary secretion.
   (1) Fear, anxiety, and excitement.
   (2) Trauma and pain.
   (3) Hypovolemia.
   (4) Hypoglycemia.
   (5) Hypothermia.
 3. Mechanisms of action—although both epinephrine and norepinephrine are secreted from the adrenal medulla, epinephrine is the main catecholamine. β-Adrenergic receptor stimulation tends to be the major response to adrenal medullary stimulation, even though epinephrine stimulates both α-adrenergic and β-adrenergic receptors.
  a. α-Receptor–mediated.
   (1) Increased gluconeogenesis.
   (2) Decreased insulin secretion.
   (3) Increased vasoconstriction (splanchnic, renal, cutaneous, and genital).
   (4) Increased sphincter contraction (GI and urinary).
   (5) Dilation of pupils.
   (6) Increased sweating.
  b. $β_1$-Receptor–mediated.
   (1) Increased lipolysis and ketosis.
   (2) Increased cardiac contraction and rate.
   (3) Increased glycogenolysis.
  c. $β_2$-Receptor–mediated.
   (1) Increased insulin secretion.
   (2) Increased glucagon secretion.
   (3) Increased K^+ uptake by muscle.
   (4) Increased arteriolar dilation in cardiovascular muscle.
   (5) Increased muscle relaxation in bronchial wall, GI wall, and wall of the urinary bladder.

Acknowledgments

The section editor acknowledges Dr. Kenneth R. Etzel for his contributions as author and editor of the Biochemistry and Physiology section of the first edition. His outstanding efforts provided the foundation for this revision. The section editor would like to thank Dr. Stanley Hillyard for critically reading the renal and respiratory section and Michelle Farnoush for assistance with the cellular and molecular biology section.

Sample Questions

1. Nonsteroidal antiinflammatory agents are pain relievers and antiinflammatories. They are effective because they act to inhibit prostaglandin synthesis by _____.
   A. Inhibiting fatty acid lipoxygenase activity
   B. Inhibiting fatty acid–specific cyclooxygenase activity
   C. Inhibiting fatty acid–specific hydroperoxidase activity
   D. Inhibiting phospholipase A_2

2. The synthesis of all steroid hormones involves which of the following compounds?
   A. Pregnenolone
   B. Progesterone
   C. Aldosterone
   D. Cortisone
   E. Testosterone

3. Lipid micelles are stabilized by which of the following?
   A. Hydrophobic interactions
   B. Hydrophilic interactions
   C. Interactions of lipid and water
   D. Interaction of hydrophobic lipid tails with hydrophobic domains of proteins

4. Which one of the following carbohydrates is a ketose sugar?
   A. Galactose
   B. Fructose
   C. Glucose
   D. Mannose
   E. Glyceraldehydes

5. Mucopolysaccharidoses are hereditary disorders that are characterized by the accumulation of glycosaminoglycans in various tissues as a result of which of the following?
   A. Overproduction (synthesis) of proteoglycans
   B. Deficiency of one of the lysosomal, hydrolytic enzymes normally involved in the degradation of one or more of the glycosaminoglycans
   C. The synthesis of abnormal proteoglycans
   D. The synthesis of highly branched glycosaminoglycan chains

6. Hydrolysis of which of the following compounds yields urea?
   A. Ornithine
   B. Argininosuccinate
   C. Aspartate
   D. Citrulline
   E. Arginine

7. The binding of epinephrine or glucagon to the corresponding membrane receptor has which of the following effects on glycogen metabolism?
   A. Net synthesis of glycogen is increased
   B. Glycogen phosphorylase is activated, and glycogen synthase is inactivated
   C. Glycogen phosphorylase is inactivated and glycogen synthase is activated
   D. Both glycogen synthase and phosphorylase are activated
   E. Both glycogen synthase and phosphorylase are inactivated

8. When an enzyme is competitively inhibited, which of the following changes occur?
   A. The apparent K_m is unchanged
   B. The apparent K_m is decreased
   C. V_{max} is decreased
   D. V_{max} is unchanged

9. Which compound is produced in the hexose monophosphate (pentose phosphate) pathway?
   A. ATP
   B. NADH
   C. NADPH
   D. Fructose 1,6-bisphosphate
   E. Phosphoenolpyruvate

10. During exercise, which of the following is decreased?
    A. Oxidation of fatty acids
    B. Glucagon release
    C. Glycogenolysis
    D. Lipogenesis

11. Increased formation of ketone bodies during fasting is a result of which of the following?
    A. Increased oxidation of fatty acids as a source of fuel
    B. Decreased formation of acetyl CoA in the liver
    C. Decreased levels of glucagon
    D. Increased glycogenesis in muscle

12. Which of the following enzymes found in the liver is involved in gluconeogenesis during the postabsorptive state?
    A. Glucose 6-phosphate dehydrogenase
    B. 6-Phosphogluconate dehydrogenase
    C. Glucose 6-phosphatase
    D. Glucokinase

13. In which one of the following tissues is glucose transport into the cell unaffected by insulin?
    A. Skeletal muscle
    B. Liver
    C. Adipose tissue
    D. Smooth muscle

14. Which of the following genetic diseases results from a deficiency in the liver enzyme that converts phenylalanine to tyrosine?
    A. Albinism
    B. Homocystinuria
    C. Porphyria
    D. Phenylketonuria

15. If the molar percentage of guanine in a human DNA is 30%, what is the molar percentage of adenine in that molecule?
    A. 10%
    B. 20%
    C. 30%
    D. 40%
    E. 50%

16. Which of the following phrases best describes restriction enzymes?
    A. Site-specific endonucleases
    B. Enzymes that regulate RNA
    C. Nonspecific endonucleases
    D. Topoisomerases

17. Which of the following is the coenzyme that serves as an intermediate carrier of one-carbon units in the synthesis of nucleic acids?
    A. Ascorbic acid
    B. Tetrahydrofolic acid
    C. Biotin
    D. Pyridoxine

18. After the production of Okazaki fragments, which of the following is required to close the gap between the fragments?
    A. DNA ligase
    B. DNA polymerase
    C. RNA polymerase
    D. Reverse transcriptase

19. Which of the following is *not* involved in the process of gene cloning?
    A. DNA polymerase
    B. DNA ligase
    C. RNA polymerase
    D. Restriction endonuclease

20. Vitamin K serves as a coenzyme for _____.
    A. The enzymatic hydroxylation of proline to 4-hydroxyproline
    B. The carboxylation of inactive prothrombin to form active prothrombin
    C. The synthesis of nucleic acids
    D. Protein synthesis

21. Chondroitin sulfate is a major component of which of the following?
    A. Bacterial cell walls
    B. Mucin
    C. IgA
    D. Cartilage
    E. Hair

22. Which of the following amino acids is positioned at every third residue in the primary structure of the helical portion of the collagen-α chains?
    A. Glycine
    B. Glutamate
    C. Proline
    D. Lysine
    E. Hydroxyproline

23. Which of the following is *not* involved in the process of mineralization?
    A. Matrix vesicles
    B. Amelogenins
    C. Fluoride
    D. Phosphoryns

24. ATP is used directly for each of the following processes *except* one. Which one is the *exception*?
    A. Accumulation of Ca^{2+} by the SR
    B. Transport of Na^+ from ICF to ECF
    C. Transport of K^+ from ECF to ICF
    D. Transport of H^+ from parietal cells into the lumen of the stomach
    E. Transport of glucose into muscle cells

25. Both active transport and facilitated diffusion are characterized by which of the following?
    A. Transport in one direction only
    B. Hydrolysis of ATP
    C. Transport against a concentration gradient
    D. Competitive inhibition

26. Which of the following statements regarding the ANS is *true*?
    A. The third cranial nerve (oculomotor nerve) carries sympathetic fibers to the smooth muscles of the eye.
    B. The facial and the glossopharyngeal nerves carry the parasympathetic preganglionic fibers for the autonomic innervation to the salivary glands.
    C. The parasympathetic nervous system innervates primarily striated muscle in the body.
    D. The parasympathetic nervous system is organized for diffuse activation and responses.

27. Which of the following responses is due to the stimulation of α-adrenergic receptors?
    A. Slowing of heart rate
    B. Constriction of blood vessels in skin
    C. Increased GI motility
    D. Increased renal blood flow

28. Which of the following is a property of C fibers?
    A. Have the slowest conduction velocity of any nerve fiber type
    B. Have the largest diameter of any nerve fiber type
    C. Are afferent nerves from muscle spindles
    D. Are afferent nerves from Golgi tendon organs
    E. Are preganglionic autonomic fibers

29. The participation of calcium in the contraction of skeletal muscle is facilitated or associated with which of the following?
    A. Calcium release from SR
    B. Calcium binding to the myosin heads
    C. Active transport of calcium out of longitudinal tubules
    D. Uptake of calcium by T-tubules

30. Calcium that enters the cell during smooth muscle excitation binds with which of the following?

A. Calmodulin
B. Inactive myosin kinase
C. Troponin
D. Myosin
E. Actin

31. Which of the following does *not* affect the muscle tension produced during contraction?
    A. Extent of motor unit recruitment
    B. Proportion of each single motor unit that is stimulated to contract
    C. Number of muscle fibers contracting
    D. Frequency of stimulation

32. The pressure in a capillary in skeletal muscle is 37 mm Hg at the arteriolar end and 16 mm Hg at the venular end. The interstitial pressure is 0 mm Hg. The colloid osmotic pressure is 26 mm Hg in the capillary and 1 mm Hg in the interstitial fluid. What is the net force producing fluid movement across the capillary wall?
    A. 1 mm Hg out of the capillary
    B. 3 mm Hg out of the capillary
    C. 12 mm Hg out of the capillary
    D. 3 mm Hg into the capillary

33. A patient has a heart rate of 70 beats/min. Her EDV is 140 mL. Her ESV is 30 mL. Calculate the CO of this patient.
    A. 9800 mL
    B. 2100 mL
    C. 7700 mL
    D. 15,400 mL

34. The velocity of blood flow _____.
    A. Is higher in the capillaries than the arterioles
    B. Is higher in the veins than in the venules
    C. Is higher in the veins than in the arteries
    D. Decreases to zero in the descending aorta during diastole

35. Which of the following does *not* occur to compensate for a decrease in blood pressure to less than normal values?
    A. Increased CO
    B. Increased stroke volume
    C. Increased heart rate
    D. Decreased TPR

36. CO_2 generated in the tissues is carried in venous blood primarily in which form?
    A. CO_2 in the plasma
    B. H_2CO_3 in the plasma
    C. HCO_3^- in the plasma
    D. CO_2 in the RBCs
    E. Carboxyhemoglobin in the RBCs

37. Which of the following is the *most* significant stimulant of the respiratory center?
    A. Decreased blood O_2 tension
    B. Increased blood H^+ concentration
    C. Decreased blood H^+ concentration
    D. Increased blood CO_2 tension

38. The primary factor determining the percent of hemoglobin saturation is _____.
    A. Blood P_{O_2}
    B. Blood P_{CO_2}
    C. 2,3-DPG concentration
    D. The temperature of the blood
    E. The acidity of the blood

39. For which of the following substances would the renal clearance be expected to be the lowest under normal conditions?
    A. Urea
    B. Creatinine
    C. Sodium
    D. Water
    E. Glucose

40. The process of active sodium transport in the ascending limb of the loop of Henle is absolutely essential for which of the following processes?
    A. Regulation of chloride excretion
    B. Regulation of pH in ECF
    C. Regulation of aldosterone excretion
    D. Regulation of water excretion

41. Long-term hypertension is compensated by which of the following renal mechanisms?
    A. Increased circulating ADH (vasopressin)
    B. Increased sympathetic activity
    C. Decreased circulating aldosterone
    D. Increased circulating angiotensin II

42. Which of the following statements regarding tubular secretion in the kidney is *true*?
    A. The secretion of K^+ increases when a person is in acidosis.
    B. The secretion of H^+ increases when a person is in alkalosis.
    C. It is a process that transports substances from the filtrate to the capillary blood.
    D. It accounts for most of the K^+ in the urine.

43. Which of the following statements regarding salivary secretion is *true*?
    A. In general, saliva is more hypertonic than plasma.
    B. As salivary flow increases, bicarbonate concentration decreases.
    C. As salivary flow increases, ionic concentration increases.
    D. Salivary secretion is regulated primarily by hormonal stimulation.

44. Which of the following is the predominant immunoglobulin in whole saliva?
    A. Secretory IgA
    B. Secretory IgG
    C. Secretory IgM
    D. Secretory IgB

45. The pancreas produces enzymes that are responsible for the digestion of dietary compounds. Which of the following foods would *not* be digested by enzymes synthesized and secreted by the pancreas?

A. Carbohydrates
B. Lipids
C. Vitamins
D. Protein

46. Which of the following statements regarding the hormone secretin is *true*?
    A. It is responsible for activating chymotrypsinogen.
    B. It stimulates the release of pancreatic secretion rich in bicarbonate.
    C. It stimulates the release of pancreatic enzymes.
    D. It stimulates the contraction of the gallbladder to release bile.

47. Phospholipase C is an enzyme that plays an important role in the production of second messengers, which produce intracellular responses. Which two second messengers are produced through the action of this enzyme?
    A. cAMP and tyrosine kinase
    B. Acetylcholine and histidine
    C. Adenylate cyclase and protein kinase
    D. 1,2-Diacylglycerol and inositol 1,4,5-triphosphate

48. Hormones secreted by the posterior pituitary gland include which of the following?
    A. Prolactin
    B. FSH
    C. LH
    D. Vasopressin

49. Which one of the following hormones does *not* have its effects mediated through cAMP?
    A. Estrogen
    B. Glucagon
    C. Epinephrine
    D. Norepinephrine

50. A scientist has discovered a new peptide hormone. He thinks it acts through the second messenger system, which uses cAMP. If this is true, which of the following substances should decrease the response of this new peptide hormone in cells?
    A. Adenylate cyclase
    B. MAO inhibitors
    C. Phosphodiesterase
    D. Aspirin

51. Which of the following proteoglycans is present in extracellular space?
    A. Hyaluronic acid
    B. Keratan sulfate
    C. Chondroitin sulfate
    D. Dermatan sulfate
    E. Heparin

52. Porphyrins use which amino acid in their synthesis?
    A. Alanine
    B. Phenylalanine
    C. Cysteine
    D. Glycine

53. Which of the following is an essential amino acid?
    A. Tyrosine
    B. Tryptophan
    C. Proline
    D. Serine
    E. Alanine

54. Aspartame contains aspartic acid and which of the following amino acids?
    A. Phenylalanine
    B. Leucine
    C. Isoleucine
    D. Lysine
    E. Proline

55. Which of the following is the end product of purine degradation in humans?
    A. Urea
    B. Uric acid
    C. Adenosine
    D. Xanthine

56. Which of the following participates in both fatty acid biosynthesis and β-oxidation of fatty acids?
    A. Malonyl CoA
    B. FAD
    C. Acetyl CoA
    D. NAD^+

57. The rate-limiting enzyme in glycolysis is which of the following?
    A. Fructose bisphosphatase
    B. Phosphofructokinase
    C. Phosphoglucose isomerase
    D. Glucokinase

58. The coenzyme essential for normal amino acid metabolism is _____.
    A. Biotin
    B. Tetrahydrofolate
    C. Pyridoxal phosphate
    D. Niacin

59. Which of the following metabolic activities is increased 1 hour after a meal (during the absorptive state)?
    A. Glycogenolysis
    B. Oxidation of free fatty acids
    C. Glucagon release
    D. Glycolysis

60. Which of the following coenzymes are involved in the metabolism of pyruvate to acetyl CoA?
    A. Thiamine pyrophosphate, lipoic acid, FAD, NAD, and CoA
    B. NAD, tetrahydrofolate, lipoic acid, FAD, and vitamin B_{12}
    C. Mg^{2+}, FAD, NAD, and biotin
    D. CoA, niacin, FAD, and ascorbic acid

61. Relative or absolute lack of insulin in humans would result in which one of the following reactions in the liver?

A. Increased glycogen synthesis
B. Increased gluconeogenesis
C. Decreased glycogen breakdown
D. Increased amino acid uptake

62. Which one of the following is elevated in plasma during the absorptive period (compared with the postabsorptive state)?
    A. Chylomicrons
    B. Acetoacetate
    C. Lactate
    D. Glucagon

63. Insulin produces which of the following changes in mammalian cells?
    A. Increase in liver glycogen production
    B. Increase in blood glucose concentration
    C. Decrease in the transport of glucose into muscle
    D. Increase in the transport of glucose into the brain

64. Which of the following describes the function of RNA polymerase?
    A. Translates DNA into protein
    B. Terminates transcription
    C. Removes introns during transcription
    D. Synthesizes RNA $5' \rightarrow 3'$

65. Analysis of DNA fragments (probing) is possibly due to which of the following properties of DNA?
    A. Phosphodiester bonds
    B. Complementary strands
    C. Protein binding
    D. Western blotting

66. The amount of cytosine is equal to the amount of guanine in which of the following molecules?
    A. DNA
    B. RNA
    C. DNA and RNA
    D. mRNA

67. What is the correct general structure of the backbone of DNA and RNA?
    A. Sugar-base-sugar
    B. Bases linked through phosphodiester linkages
    C. Bases linked through hydrogen bonds
    D. Sugars linked through phosphodiester linkages

68. The conversion of information from DNA into mRNA is called _____.
    A. Translation
    B. Transcription
    C. Transduction
    D. Transformation

69. Which of the following mineralized tissues have the greatest percentage of inorganic material?
    A. Enamel
    B. Dentin
    C. Bone
    D. Calculus

70. All of the following are descriptions of collagen *except* one. Which one is the *exception*?

A. Most abundant protein in the body
B. Modifications to procollagen occur in the ECM
C. Incorporates hydroxyproline into the molecule by tRNA
D. Hydroxylation of proline requires vitamin C and molecular O_2

71. Hydroxyapatite _____.
    A. Is weakened if fluoride is substituted for some of the hydroxyl ions
    B. Is a noncrystalline structure
    C. Becomes more soluble if it contains carbonate ion
    D. Is composed of calcium and phosphate in a $1:1$ ratio

72. The type of collagen characteristically found in cartilage is _____.
    A. Type I
    B. Type II
    C. Type III
    D. Type IV

73. Which process transports amino acids across the luminal surface of the epithelium that lines the small intestine?
    A. Simple diffusion
    B. Primary active transport
    C. Cotransport with Na^+
    D. Cotransport with Cl^-

74. Cell membranes typically contain all of the following compounds *except* one. Which one is the *exception*?
    A. Phospholipids
    B. Proteins
    C. Cholesterols
    D. Triacylglycerols
    E. Sphingolipids

75. MAO _____.
    A. Inactivates reduced steroid derivatives
    B. Is not associated with nerves
    C. Inactivates catecholamines by oxidative deamination
    D. Is located in the synapse where it inactivates the neurotransmitter acetylcholine

76. Which one of the following does *not* release acetylcholine?
    A. Sympathetic preganglionic fibers
    B. Sympathetic postganglionic fibers that innervate the heart
    C. Parasympathetic postganglionic fibers to effector organs
    D. Parasympathetic preganglionic fibers

77. Where are the temperature control centers located?
    A. Cerebellum
    B. Hypothalamus
    C. Medulla
    D. Cerebral cortex

78. The energy for skeletal muscle contraction is derived from which of the following processes?

A. Calcium release from sarcoplasmic membranes and binding to troponin
B. Cleavage of ATP by the myosin head
C. Membrane Na^+-K^+-ATPase pump
D. Sodium influx during the action potential

79. Muscle spindle stretching when the patellar tendon is tapped produces which of the following responses?
    A. Muscle contraction within muscle where the spindles are located
    B. Increased sympathetic stimulation of the spindles
    C. Reduction in the number of afferent impulses entering the spinal cord
    D. Inhibition of the stretch reflex

80. The γ motoneurons control which of the following?
    A. Muscle spindles
    B. Iris of the eye
    C. Voluntary muscle fibers
    D. Pyloric sphincter

81. Which of the following would be expected to increase blood pressure?
    A. A drug that inhibits the angiotensin II converting enzyme and the production of angiotensin II (angiotensin-converting enzyme inhibitors)
    B. A drug that inhibits the synthesis of nitric oxide
    C. A drug that blocks vasopressin receptors
    D. Increased stimulation of the carotid baroreceptor

82. Which of the following ions has a higher intracellular concentration compared with the ECF?
    A. Na^+
    B. K^+
    C. Cl^-
    D. HCO_3^-
    E. Ca^{2+}

83. All of the following local chemical factors cause vasodilation of the arterioles *except* one. Which one is the *exception*?
    A. Decreased K^+
    B. Increased CO_2
    C. Nitric oxide
    D. Decreased O_2
    E. Histamine release

84. Increasing the radius of arterioles would increase which of the following?
    A. Systolic blood pressure
    B. Diastolic blood pressure
    C. Viscosity of the blood
    D. Capillary blood flow

85. In which of the following conditions might arterial blood pressure be abnormally increased?
    A. Ventricular fibrillation
    B. Acute heart failure
    C. Anaphylactic shock
    D. Increased intracranial pressure

86. A major function of surfactant is to increase which of the following?

A. Pulmonary compliance
B. Alveolar surface tension
C. The work of breathing
D. The tendency of the lungs to collapse

87. The minimum volume of air that remains in the lungs after a maximal expiration is termed the _____.
    A. Tidal volume
    B. FRC
    C. Residual volume
    D. Vital capacity

88. The center that provides output to the respiratory muscles is located in the _____.
    A. Pons
    B. Medulla
    C. Cerebral cortex
    D. Cerebellum
    E. Hypothalamus

89. Aldosterone _____.
    A. Stimulates Na^+ reabsorption in the distal and collecting ducts
    B. Is secreted by the juxtaglomerular apparatus
    C. Stimulates K^+ absorption in the distal tubule
    D. Stimulates bicarbonate reabsorption in the proximal tubule

90. What happens to net fluid filtration in the glomerulus when plasma protein concentration is decreased?
    A. Net filtration (ultrafiltration) increases
    B. Net filtration (ultrafiltration) decreases
    C. Net filtration remains unchanged
    D. Net filtration ceases

91. Which of the following factors would result in decreased GFR?
    A. A decrease in plasma protein concentration
    B. An obstruction of the tubular system, which would increase capsular hydrostatic pressure
    C. Vasodilation of the afferent arterioles
    D. Inulin administration

92. Which of the following statements regarding tubular reabsorption is *true*?
    A. Most calcium filtered is passively reabsorbed and not regulated under any conditions.
    B. Most urea is reabsorbed passively and is unaffected by regulatory mechanisms.
    C. Glucose is reabsorbed by secondary active transport and facilitated diffusion.
    D. Most filtered phosphate is reabsorbed in the collecting ducts and is unaffected by regulatory mechanisms.

93. Which of the following processes is *not* a true component of swallowing?
    A. Closure of the glottis
    B. Involuntary relaxation of the upper esophageal sphincter
    C. Movements of the tongue against the palate
    D. Esophageal peristalsis

94. Which of the following statements regarding the regulation of GI motility is *true*?
    A. Sympathetic stimulation inhibits motility.
    B. Parasympathetic stimulation inhibits motility.
    C. GI motility is not influenced by the CNS.
    D. GI motility is not influenced by hormones.

95. Which one of the following statements regarding the regulation of GI function is *true*?
    A. The main sympathetic nerve supply to the digestive tract is the vagus.
    B. In general, sympathetic stimulation is excitatory to digestive activity.
    C. Salivary secretion is stimulated by both branches of the ANS, although not to the same degree.
    D. Parasympathetic stimulation of the salivary glands produces a saliva rich in mucus.

96. Which of the following factors does *not* influence the rate at which a meal leaves the stomach?
    A. Acidification of the duodenum
    B. Increasing the tonicity of the intestine
    C. Saline in the duodenum
    D. Lipid in the intestine

97. Which of the following forms of thyroid hormone is most readily found in the circulation?
    A. T_3
    B. T_4
    C. Thyroglobulin
    D. TSH

98. A hormone acts to stimulate its neighboring cell to divide. This hormone would best be described as belonging to which category of hormones?
    A. Paracrine
    B. Autocrine
    C. Endocrine

99. Blood levels of progesterone are highest during _____.
    A. The follicular phase of the ovarian cycle
    B. The luteal phase of the ovarian cycle
    C. Ovulation
    D. Menstruation

100. Glucagon decreases which of the following?
    A. Glycogenolysis
    B. Gluconeogenesis
    C. Glycogenesis
    D. Blood glucose

101. Place the citric acid cycle enzymes in the order in which they participate in the cycle by writing the appropriate number in the blank. All enzymes may not be listed.
    A. α-Ketoglutarate dehydrogenase _____
    B. Malate dehydrogenase _____
    C. Citrate synthase _____
    D. Succinate dehydrogenase _____
    E. Fumerase _____
    F. Isocitrate dehydrogenase _____

102. From the following list, select the defects associated with a vitamin B_{12} deficiency.
    A. Night blindness
    B. Rickets
    C. Pernicious anemia
    D. Scurvy
    E. Neurologic degeneration

103. From the following list, select the secretions produced by the pancreas.
    A. HCl
    B. HCO_3^-
    C. Pepsinogen
    D. Lipase
    E. Amylase
    F. Chymotrypsinogen
    G. Enterokinase

104. From the following list, which actions are *not* attributed to CCK?
    A. Stimulates contraction of the gallbladder
    B. Stimulates pancreatic HCO_3^- production
    C. Inhibits gastric acid secretion
    D. Inhibits pancreatic HCO_3^- production

105. Which one of the following is *not* a polysaccharide?
    A. Amylose
    B. Amylopectin
    C. Acetylglucosamine
    D. Glycogen
    E. Glycosaminoglycan

106. During skeletal muscle contraction, depolarization of the T-tubules produces a conformational change in the dihydropyridine receptor that causes the ryanodine receptors to release Ca^{2+} from the terminal cisternae of the SR. What is this excitation-contraction coupling?
    A. Electromechanical coupling
    B. Electrochemical coupling
    C. Pharmacomechanical coupling
    D. Pharmacochemical coupling

107. From the following categories of taste flavors, which have been identified as acting via G protein–coupled receptors?
    A. Bitter
    B. Sweet
    C. Sour
    D. Salty
    E. Umami

108. During stimulated saliva secretion, the concentration of Na^+ more closely resembles the concentration of Na^+ in the plasma because there is less time for ductal modification of the saliva concentration. Which of the following is *true* regarding this statement?
    A. Both the statement and the reason are correct and related
    B. Both the statement and the reason are correct but not related

C. The statement is correct, but the reason is not correct

D. The statement is not correct, but the reason is correct

E. Neither the statement nor the reason is correct

109. Which one of the following lipoprotein particles is responsible for transporting dietary triacylglycerols to the liver and adipose cells?
    A. VLDL
    B. LDL
    C. HDL
    D. Chylomicron

110. The term *cytosol* refers to which one of the following?
    A. All of the cell outside of the nucleus
    B. The aqueous area between the plasma membrane and the membrane-bound organelles
    C. The contents of the nucleus
    D. The contents of all the organelles

111. Which one of the following is *not* a characteristic of smooth endoplasmic reticulum?
    A. Site of lipid synthesis
    B. Site of calcium storage
    C. Site of protein synthesis
    D. Site of drug detoxification

112. Which organelle is considered the "powerhouse" and generates ATP via oxidative phosphorylation?
    a. Mitochondrium
    b. Lysosome
    c. Nucleus
    d. Ribosome
    e. Golgi apparatus

113. What carrier molecule transfers acyl groups between molecules?
    a. ATP
    b. Biotin
    c. NADPH
    d. CoA
    e. Tetrahydrofolate

114. In which cell structure is rRNA transcribed and assembled?
    A. Cytoplasm
    B. Rough endoplasmic reticulum
    C. Nucleus
    D. Nucleolus
    E. Golgi apparatus

115. Blood and bone marrow are specialized forms of which one of the four primary tissue types?
    A. Epithelial tissue
    B. Connective tissue
    C. Nervous tissue
    D. Muscle tissue

116. What is considered the universal currency of biochemical energy?
    a. cAMP
    b. GTP
    c. ATP
    d. dNTP
    e. TNT

117. A sarcomere spans which of the following lengths?
    A. From I-band to I-band
    B. From A-band to A-band
    C. From H-band to H-band
    D. From Z-disc to Z-disc

118. All of the following statements regarding cardiac muscle fibers are correct *except* one. Which one is the *exception*?
    a. They may contain more than one nucleus.
    b. Terminal cisternae are at the A-band to I-band junctions.
    c. They are connected to one another by intercalated discs.
    d. Cardiac muscle fibers may branch.

119. Fibrous proteins are usually which one of the following?
    a. Enzymes
    b. Globular proteins
    c. Structural proteins
    d. Hormones
    e. Antibodies

120. Which one of the following is the net result of one molecule of glucose proceeding through the glycolytic pathway?
    a. Four ATP, four NADH, four pyruvate
    b. Two ATP, two NADH, two pyruvate
    c. One ATP, one NADH, one pyruvate
    d. Four ATP, two NADPH, two pyruvate
    e. Two ATP, two NADPH, two pyruvate

Host Defense, Microbiology, and Pathology

MICHAEL G. SCHMIDT
NISHA D'SILVA

1.0 Immunology and Immunopathology

The immune system of the human body is an elegant and elaborate defense mechanism tasked with defending the host against all enemies foreign (bacteria, fungi, viruses, and other eukaryotic parasites) and domestic (cancer). It involves two types of immunity. In general, the body's first defense mechanism against infection includes anatomic (e.g., skin, mucosal membranes) or physiologic (e.g., temperature, low pH) barriers. When a pathogen invades this physical barrier, the body has two different types of immune responses: innate (nonspecific) and acquired (specific or adaptive). Innate immunity is the body's early defense against any kind of bodily injury, including trauma or infection. Because this nonspecific immune response has a limited ability to recognize specific antigens, it generally reacts to most pathogens in the same manner. As the innate immune response begins its response to combat invading pathogens, the body mounts an acquired immune response. Acquired immunity involves a highly sophisticated recognition of foreign structures. This ability to learn to identify specific structures allows the body's defenses to act quickly and efficiently in killing specific pathogens. This section is not meant to be all-inclusive, but rather is a guide to help you refresh what you have learned and to focus your thoughts.

1.1 Host Defense Mechanisms

A. Anatomic barriers.
   1. Skin (Figure 3-1).
      a. Acts as a physical barrier to external pathogens.
      b. Langerhans' cells—dendritic cells that are found in the stratum spinosum layer and are important in their ability to initiate the immune system.
      c. Acidic environment of pH 3 to 5 retards growth of microbes.
   2. Mucosal membranes.
      a. Line the gastrointestinal (GI), respiratory, and urogenital tracts.
      b. Various protective mechanisms—for instance, in the stomach and vaginal tract, the pH remains low, discouraging microbial growth. The pulmonary mucosa contains cilia and secretes mucus, clearing the air that enters the respiratory tract.
      c. Lysozyme is an important antimicrobial enzyme that is secreted in saliva and tears.
B. Physiologic barriers.
   1. Temperature—increased body temperature (i.e., fever) inhibits growth of some pathogens.
   2. Low pH—acidic pH of the stomach kills many bacteria and fungi and can inactivate many viruses.
C. Innate immune response.
   1. Acute inflammation.
      a. Early immune response to injury or infection.
         (1) Edema—caused by the increased vascular permeability of endothelial cells. Initially, the arterioles briefly vasoconstrict resulting in vasodilation and increased permeability of the endothelium. Fluid moves from the circulation into the interstitial tissue, resulting in hyperemia and local edema. These actions can be summarized by the four classic signs of inflammation: *tumor* (swelling), *rubor* (redness), *calor* (heat), and *dolor* (pain).
         (2) Complement activation (discussed later in Section 1.1.4, Complement System).
         (3) Release of inflammatory mediators by polymorphonuclear leukocytes or neutrophils (PMNs), basophils, and mast cells.
         (4) Activation of natural killer cells, which resemble cytotoxic T cells. Natural killer cells were

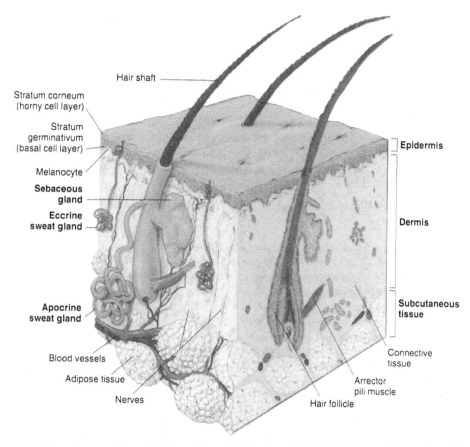

Figure 3-1 Layers and structures of the skin. *(From Henry MC, Stapleton MC: EMT Prehospital Care, ed 4. St. Louis, Mosby, 2010.)*

named as such because they were initially thought not to require activation to kill and lack the "self" makers of the major histocompatibility complex (MHC) class I; they act to destroy cells primarily infected with viruses or tumors.

b. Possible outcomes of acute inflammation.
   (1) Complete resolution.
   (2) Scarring.
   (3) Abscess formation.
      (a) Clinically, if the abscess spreads into the soft tissues, a cellulitis develops.
      (b) Two forms of cellulitis significant in dentistry include Ludwig's angina and cavernous sinus thrombosis.

2. Chronic inflammation.
   a. Usually a more moderate inflammatory response that persists.
   b. Mediators of chronic inflammation include mononuclear leukocytes or macrophages, plasma cells, and lymphocytes.
   c. Example in dentistry: a periapical lesion that persists at the root apex for many years because of continual stimulation of pathogens from inside the tooth.

3. Granulomatous inflammation.
   a. Form of chronic inflammation, characterized by the formation of granulomas.
   b. Granulomas are areas that the immune system "walls off" if phagocytes fail to destroy foreign particles or microbes present in it.
   c. Inflammatory mediators include a dense concentration of macrophages, fibroblasts, lymphocytes, and (less frequently) plasma cells. The continuous activation of macrophages induces them to attach to one another, assuming an epitheliumlike (epithelioid) appearance; they may also fuse with each other to form multinucleated giant cells.
   d. Two types of granulomas.
      (1) Granulomas associated with infectious diseases.
         (a) Tuberculosis (TB) infections (*Mycobacterium*)—granulomas found in infected areas are called *tubercles* and often display central caseous necrosis.
         (b) Fungal infections (*Cryptococcus, Histoplasma, Coccidioides*).
         (c) Syphilis (*Treponema pallidum*)—granulomas seen during syphilis infections are called *gummas*.

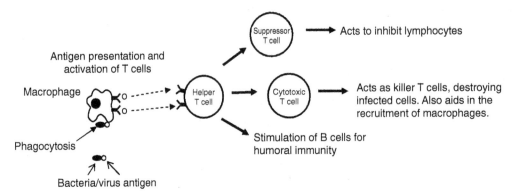

Figure 3-2 Overview of cell-mediated immunity.

(d) Cat-scratch disease (*Bartonella henselae*, formerly *Rochalimaea henselae*)—lymphadenopathy (most frequently seen around the head, neck, and upper limbs) and fever occur often within 1 week of being scratched or bitten by a cat; can also result in bacteremia, endocarditis, bacillary angiomatosis (knotting of capillaries in various organs, resulting in formation of many angiomas).

(2) Granulomas associated with foreign bodies.

(a) Examples: foreign particles (glass, metals), surgical sutures.

D. Acquired immune response.

1. Immunologic attributes of acquired immune response.

a. Specificity—antibody recognition can be as specific as a single amino acid; consider that the influenza vaccine may or may not be effective because the virus can change one amino acid within the hemagglutinin or neuraminidase protein.

b. Diversity—antibodies can recognize billions of unique structures.

c. Memory (i.e., memory B cells).

d. Self and nonself recognition (i.e., MHC).

2. There are two types of specific immune responses: cell-mediated immunity, which is mediated by T cells, and humoral immunity, which is mediated by antibodies that are generated by B cells.

3. Cell-mediated immunity.

a. Mediated by T lymphocytes; distinguished by the presence of T-cell receptor on the cell.

b. T cells cannot directly recognize antigens; antigens are processed and presented to them by antigen-presenting cells (APCs), such as macrophages, dendritic cells, B cells, and endothelial cells. APCs process the antigens into small peptides and present them with a class II MHC molecule to the CD4 receptor on the helper T cell. This activates the helper T cells to release cytokines that cause inflammation and the activation of other T cells, B cells, and macrophages (Figure 3-2).

4. Humoral immunity (antibody-mediated immunity).

a. Branch of the specific immune response serves two purposes.

(1) Targets antigens—the aggregation of antibodies produced by B cells on an antigen specifically identifies, neutralizes, and opsonizes the antigen, making it easier to phagocytize.

(2) Acts as a memory function—allows the immune system to recognize and destroy microbes from previous exposure or infection more efficiently.

b. Antigens are first recognized by macrophages or directly by B cells. Similar to cell-mediated immunity, the macrophage processes and presents the antigens to helper T cells. This causes them to secrete cytokines, interleukin (IL)-4 and IL-5, which results in B-cell stimulation and growth, resulting in the production of specific antibodies against the antigen presented (Figure 3-3).

1.1.1 Wound Healing

A. Primary wound healing.

1. The repair of two well-apposed edges, such as surgical incisions.

2. Timeline of cellular events.

a. First 24 hours—formation of a fibrin clot. Fibronectin, an adhesive molecule found in plasma and on cell surfaces, forms cross-links to stabilize the clot. PMNs migrate to the injured site.

b. Day 1 to 2—basal cells begin to proliferate (i.e., undergo mitosis) to close the epidermal defect.

c. Day 3—proliferation of basal cells continues. Granulation tissue forms at the injured site. Macrophages replace PMNs. Fibroblasts appear and secrete proteoglycans and type III collagen. Neovascularization begins.

d. End of the first week—formation of a scar. Fibroblasts and microphages continue to clean up and remodel the area. Fibroblasts secrete type I collagen. Vascularization and cellular infiltrate largely disappear.

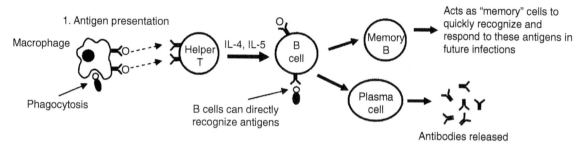

Figure 3-3 Overview of humoral immunity.

3. Secondary wound healing.
   a. Repair of a larger wound with margins that are not well apposed.
   b. Cellular events are similar to primary wound healing except that more granulation tissue is formed and there is a larger inflammatory response. Also, the duration of healing is longer.

1.1.2 Immune Effector Cells

A. T cells.
   1. Important regulators of the immune response.
   2. Involved in both cell-mediated and humoral immunity.
   3. Play a role in type IV delayed hypersensitivity reactions.
   4. Can be categorized by their function—regulatory or effector. The regulatory function is primarily mediated by helper T cells, which have CD4 surface receptors (also called CD4$^+$ T cells). The effector function is primarily mediated by cytotoxic and regulatory T cells, formerly known as *suppressor T cells*, which contain CD8 surface receptors.
      a. CD4$^+$ T cells.
         (1) Recognize class II MHC molecules on antigen-presenting cells (APCs).
         (2) Mainly for the recognition of bacterial antigens.
         (3) Regulatory functions.
            (a) Stimulate B cells to develop into antibody-producing plasma cells.
            (b) Stimulate CD8 cells to become activated cytotoxic T cells.
            (c) Stimulate the actions of macrophages during delayed hypersensitivity reactions.
      b. CD8—cytotoxic and suppressor T cells.
         (1) Recognize class I MHC molecules on APCs.
         (2) Function mainly in recognition of viral or neoplastic antigens.
         (3) Cytotoxic functions are carried out by the following.
            (a) Releasing perforins—destroy cell membranes.
            (b) Inducing apoptosis—programmed cell death.
      c. T-cell maturation occurs in the thymus. There are three developmental stages.
         (1) Immature: CD4$^-$CD8$^-$, a double-negative cell that expresses neither CD4 nor CD8.
         (2) Less mature: CD4$^+$CD8$^+$, a double-positive cell that expresses both CD4 and CD8.
         (3) Mature: CD4$^+$CD8$^-$ or CD4$^-$CD8$^+$, a single-positive cell that expresses either CD4 or CD8.

B. B lymphocytes.
   1. Involved in the humoral immune response.
   2. Perform two important functions.
      a. Responsible for the production and secretion of antibodies.
      b. Are APCs. Antigens are recognized by surface immunoglobulins.
   3. Activated B cells differentiate into the following.
      a. Plasma cells—produce and release monoclonal antibodies.
      b. Memory B cells—circulate for long periods and are able to respond quickly to reexposures.

C. Mononuclear cells—monocytes (in blood) and macrophages (in tissues).
   1. Produced in bone marrow.
   2. Important functions.
      a. Phagocytosis—defense against microbes, removal of cellular debris or breakdown products.
      b. Cytokine production.
      c. Act as APCs.
   3. When monocytes enter tissues, they mature into macrophages.
   4. The body has an extensive network of macrophages known as the *reticuloendothelial system*. These macrophages are fixed and serve different functions, depending on their tissue location. Examples include the following.
      a. Dust cells and heart failure cells in the lungs.
      b. Kupffer's cells in the liver.
      c. Mesangial cells in the kidney.
      d. Macrophages in the lymph nodes.
      e. Splenocytes in the spleen.
      f. Microglia in the CNS.
      g. Histiocytes in connective tissues.
   5. The presence of macrophages indicates chronic inflammation.

6. Phagocytosis.
   a. Occurs in three stages.
      (1) Migration and attachment to site of injury or infection.
      (2) Ingestion—formation of a phagosome.
      (3) Killing—release of enzymes to destroy ingested microbe.
   b. Phagocytosis is a process that initiates with the formation of a membrane-bound vacuole (phagosome) around the foreign particle or microbe. The phagosome fuses with a lysosome, which contains many degradative enzymes, resulting in the formation of a phagolysosome. This process results in the destruction of the microbe.

D. Mast cells.
   1. Contain surface antigen receptors, including IgE. IgE plays an important role in type I immediate hypersensitivity reactions.
   2. Contain dense granules with inflammatory mediators.
      a. Histamine—there are two receptors that bind histamine.
         (1) H_1 receptors—cause increased permeability and vasodilation in capillaries; also cause bronchoconstriction in the lungs.
         (2) H_2 receptors—play a role in gastric acid and pepsin secretion.
      b. Slow-reacting substance of anaphylaxis.
         (1) Leukotriene.
         (2) Actions include bronchoconstriction in the lungs.
         (3) May play an important role as a mediator of asthmatic bronchoconstriction.

1.1.3 Cytokines

A. Cytokines are inflammatory mediators that are released by various cells, such as macrophages or lymphocytes, to regulate immune responses. *Think of cytokines as the words that immune cells use to communicate with each other.*

B. Cytokines secreted from lymphocytes are synonymous with *lymphokines.*

C. Types of cytokines.
   1. Interleukins.
      a. Mediators that affect lymphocytes.
      b. Important interleukins are summarized in Table 3-1.
   2. Interferons.
      a. Mediators that are important for antiviral immunity.
      b. Important interferons are summarized in Table 3-2.

D. Prostaglandins and leukotrienes—mediators of the inflammatory response. Prostaglandins and leukotrienes are metabolites of arachidonic acid. They are

---

Table 3-1

Important Interleukins and Their Actions

CYTOKINE	SOURCE	ACTIONS
IL-1	Macrophages	Stimulate cell activity or production of mediators in various cells, including lymphocytes, macrophages, and endothelial cells. Also cause fever
IL-2	Helper T cells	Activate helper and cytotoxic T cells
IL-3	Activated T cells	Stimulate production of RBCs in bone marrow
IL-4	Helper T cells	Stimulate B-cell growth and production of IgE and IgG
IL-5	Helper T cells	Stimulate B-cell differentiation into plasma cells, activity of eosinophils, and production of IgA

RBCs, Red blood cells.

Table 3-2

Important Interferons (INF) and Their Actions

CYTOKINE	SOURCE	ACTIONS
IFN-α	Leukocytes	Inhibit viral growth
IFN-β	Fibroblasts	Inhibit viral growth
IFN-γ	Helper T cell	Strong activator of macrophages, important in cell-mediated immunity

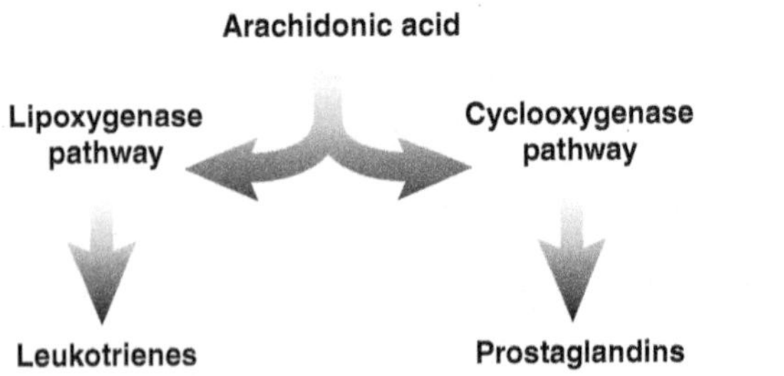

Arachidonic acid

Lipoxygenase pathway ← → Cyclooxygenase pathway

Leukotrienes   Prostaglandins

Figure 3-4 Cyclooxygenase and lipoxygenase pathways.

produced by the cyclooxygenase pathway (prostaglandins) and the lipoxygenase pathway (leukotrienes) (Figure 3-4). General actions of these cytokines include vasoconstriction, bronchoconstriction, and increased inflammatory activity.

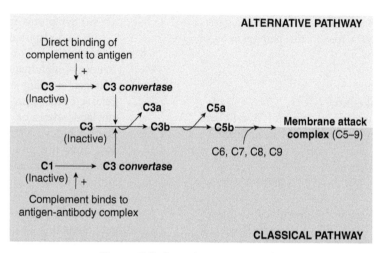

Figure 3-5 Complement cascade.

1.1.4 Complement System

A. Consists of a group of nearly 30 preformed serum and membrane proteins found in serum or on cell surfaces. They become activated through protease activity in a cascading order.
B. Main function is to generate reaction products that enhance antigen clearance and stimulate an inflammatory response. This is achieved by the following actions.
 1. Lysis of foreign body by formation of membrane attack complexes (C5 through C9).
 2. Opsonization—specific complement proteins (C3b), or opsonins, bind to the surfaces of microbes or foreign particles to encourage their phagocytosis.
 3. Chemotaxis of inflammatory mediators—C5a acts to recruit inflammatory cells (i.e., neutrophils) to the site of injury or infection.
 4. Production of anaphylatoxins (C3a, C4a, and C5a)—act to stimulate mast cells in releasing mediators (histamine), resulting in increased vascular permeability (edema), vasodilation, and bronchoconstriction.
C. Complement cascade: two pathways (Figure 3-5).
 1. Alternative pathway—complement becomes activated by direct contact with the microbe or injured site. C3 binds directly to the surface antigen, activating the complement system.
 2. Classical pathway—antibodies first bind to the surface antigen present on the microbe or injured site. Complement (C1) then binds onto the antibody, activating the complement cascade.
 3. The end product of both pathways is the same—the formation of a membrane attack complex. This complex forms directly on the surface of the microbe, "punches a hole in it," and results in cell or microbe lysis.

1.1.5 Immunoglobulins (Antibodies)

A. Antibody effector functions.
 1. Neutralization—by binding directly to the antigen, the antibody neutralizes the antigen by preventing it from further interaction with other cells.
 2. Opsonization—when antibodies bind to an antigen, they act as opsonins to help facilitate host phagocytosis or complement activation.
 3. Activation of the complement system.
B. Antibodies can also cause agglutination of antigens (i.e., antigens clump together). The classic example of this is blood typing, where blood type is determined by agglutination of red blood cells (RBCs) to specific agglutins.
C. Immunoglobulin classes.
 1. IgA.
  a. 15% of antibodies.
  b. Important for the immunity of mucous membranes.
  c. Found in mucosal secretions of the genitourinary, intestinal, and respiratory tracts. It is also found in tears, saliva, and colostrum.
  d. Major action—prevents adhesion of microbes to mucous membranes by binding surface antigens.
 2. IgG.
  a. 75% of antibodies.
  b. Associated with the secondary immune response. (Note: IgM responds first.)
  c. Important for its actions against microbes.
  d. Major actions.
   (1) Activates complement.
   (2) Acts as an opsonin to encourage phagocytosis of bacteria.
   (3) Only antibody that can cross the placenta and is present in newborns.

e. The ability of IgG to activate complement suggests that it likely plays a role in the pathogenesis of adult periodontitis.

3. IgD.
   a. 0.2% of antibodies.
   b. Major actions unknown.
   c. May act as an antigen receptor for B cells and induce the activation of B cells by the antigen.

4. IgE.
   a. 0.004% of antibodies.
   b. Important in its role in type I hypersensitivity reactions.
   c. Acts as antigen receptor for granulocytes, including basophils and mast cells, and stimulates their degranulation.

5. IgM.
   a. 9% of antibodies.
   b. Associated with the body's primary immune response. It is the first antibody to arrive at the site of injury or infection.
   c. Important for its actions against microbes.
   d. Major actions.
      (1) The most efficient immunoglobulin activator of the complement system.
      (2) Acts as an antigen receptor for B cells.

1.2 Hypersensitivity

Hypersensitivity reactions are characterized by exaggerated immune responses that result in injury. There are four types of hypersensitivity reactions.

A. Type I immediate hypersensitivity.
   1. Antibody mediator: IgE.
   2. A hyperresponse of the immune system caused primarily by the production and accumulation of IgE antibody.
   3. The accumulation of IgE requires prior sensitization or exposure to a specific allergen. Reexposure of the allergen causes it to bind to IgE receptors on mast cells, resulting in large releases of inflammatory mediators.
   4. Two subtypes.
      a. Atopic allergies.
         (1) Limited to specific target tissue or organ.
         (2) Family members display a strong hereditary predisposition to allergy sensitization, which may result from a genetic defect affecting the regulation of the IgE response.
         (3) Important examples.
            (a) Asthma.
               (i) Primary inflammatory mediator: slow-reacting substance of anaphylaxis.
               (ii) Symptoms include bronchoconstriction and edema in the lower respiratory tract.
            (b) Hay fever (allergic reaction).
               (i) Primary inflammatory mediator: histamine.
               (ii) Symptoms include rhinitis, teary eyes, and respiratory congestion.
      b. Anaphylaxis.
         (1) Primary inflammatory mediator: histamine.
         (2) Allergen binding of IgE causes a very large release of histamine, which can result in anaphylactic shock, a life-threatening condition that includes severe bronchoconstriction and low blood pressure.
         (3) Treatment—epinephrine (vasoconstrictor, bronchodilator), glucocorticosteroid, antihistamine.

B. Type II antibody-dependent cytotoxic hypersensitivity.
   1. Antibody mediators: IgG and IgM.
   2. The binding of antibodies to cell membrane antigens activates the complement system, resulting in the formation of a membrane attack complex and cell death. Antibodies can also mediate cell destruction by antibody-dependent, cell-mediated cytotoxicity.
   3. Important examples.
      a. Erythroblastosis fetalis.
      b. Blood transfusion reactions.

C. Type III immune complex–mediated hypersensitivity.
   1. Antibody mediator: IgG.
   2. Antigen-antibody interactions result in the formation of immune complexes. These complexes become trapped along the vascular walls, activating complement and the immune response. Damage to the blood vessel walls occurs primarily from phagocytosis of the immune complex by the cells of the reticuloendothelial system.
   3. Important examples.
      a. Arthus reaction.
         (1) Localized type III reaction.
         (2) Injection of an antigen into a patient who already has a high level of circulating antibody (IgG), usually resulting from repeated exposure, leads to formation of localized immune complexes.
         (3) Symptoms include severe swelling and hemorrhaging within a few hours after exposure.
      b. Serum sickness.
         (1) Generalized type III reaction.
         (2) Systemic injection of drug serum (i.e., specific antigens) causes formation of immune complexes throughout the microvasculature.
         (3) Symptoms typically develop within days or weeks after exposure and can include fever, hives, lymphadenopathy, and arthritis.
      c. Other examples of generalized type III reactions.
         (1) Rheumatoid arthritis—autoimmune disease with chronic inflammation of the joints.
         (2) Systemic lupus erythematosus.
         (3) Although the specific antigen is unknown, immune complexes have been found to be deposited in inflamed areas.

D. Type IV delayed (cell-mediated) hypersensitivity.
   1. There are no antibody mediators. Helper T cells are the main mediators in delayed hypersensitivity.
   2. Antigens are presented by APCs to helper T cells. Activated helper T cells release cytokines to activate the immune response, including stimulating macrophages to increase their release of lytic enzymes. Note: the leakage of these enzymes may result in tissue damage.
   3. Symptoms may appear days after exposure (i.e., delayed).
   4. Important examples.
      a. Contact dermatitis.
         (1) Mediated by haptens—small proteins that have antigenic properties. Haptens are unable to initiate an immune response by themselves, unless they can join with a larger body protein.
         (2) Examples: poison ivy or oak, reactions to cosmetics, drugs (penicillin).
      b. Tuberculin (purified protein derivative [PPD]) test—skin test, used to test for *Mycobacterium tuberculosis* exposure.
      c. Rejection of skin graft.

1.3 Immunopathology

A. Bruton's agammaglobulinemia.
   1. Characterized by a deficiency or very low levels of antibodies.
   2. Results from a failure of B cells to differentiate, leading to a decreased concentration of plasma cells and antibody production.
   3. Cell-mediated immunity is unaffected.
   4. Recurrent bacteria-related (pyogenic) infections are common in these patients.
   5. Treatment: administration of IgG.
B. Transient hypogammaglobulinemia.
   1. Seen in infants.
   2. A decreased amount of antibodies is present because of slow antibody production.
   3. Treatment: administration of IgG after the first 6 months.
C. DiGeorge's syndrome.
   1. Characterized by a deficiency of T cells.
   2. Results from a failure of the third and fourth brachial (pharyngeal) pouches to develop normally, leading to a lack of thymus and parathyroid development. Mandibular development is also affected.
   3. Symptoms.
      a. Tetany—caused by hypoparathyroidism hypocalcemia.
      b. Recurrent viral and fungal infections.
D. Severe combined immunodeficiency.
   1. Characterized by a deficiency in both T cells and B cells.
   2. Severe, recurrent, opportunistic infections are common in infants.
   3. Treatment: bone marrow transplantation or gene therapy.
E. Angioedema.
   1. Acquired angioedema is caused by a deficiency of the complement inhibitor, C1-INH, which inhibits the conversion of C1 to C1 esterase. Note: angioedema can also be caused by allergic reactions and may be seen in patients taking certain medications, such as angiotensin-converting enzyme inhibitors.
   2. Symptoms include diffuse, soft tissue swellings in the face, extremities, and pelvic area.
   3. Can be life-threatening.
F. Chronic granulomatous disease.
   1. Results from neutrophils with a defective reduced nicotinamide adenine dinucleotide phosphate oxidase system. This affects the ability of neutrophils to kill microorganisms because they are unable to produce superoxide radicals.
   2. Chronic bacterial infections and the formation of granulomas are common.
   3. Genetic transmission: X-linked.
G. Autoimmune diseases.
   1. Systemic lupus erythematosus (lupus).
      a. Exact cause is unknown.
      b. More common in female patients.
      c. Characterized by the presence of antinuclear antibodies (ANAs). Common ANA findings include anti-DNA, anti-RNA, and anti-Sm antigen. ANAs can form immune complexes in the microvasculature of many organ systems.
         (1) Skin—causing characteristic butterfly rash along the malar and nose area.
         (2) Joints—causing arthritislike symptoms.
         (3) Kidney—most significant problem because it can lead to kidney failure.
         (4) Heart—increased risk of endocarditis because of vegetations found on heart valves.
      d. Raynaud's phenomenon may be seen in patients—a patient's fingertips or toes become white and blue on exposure to cold temperatures, owing to a decrease in blood flow. Note: Raynaud's phenomenon is also seen in patients with CREST syndrome (*c*alcinosis, *R*aynaud's syndrome, *e*sophageal dysmotility, *s*clerodactyly, and *t*elangiectasia) or acrosclerosis.
   2. Scleroderma (systemic sclerosis).
      a. Exact cause is unknown.
      b. Abnormal deposition of collagen leads to the development of fibrosis in certain organs, which can result in organ failure.
      c. Raynaud's phenomenon is common in these patients. Other symptoms may include dysphagia, dyspnea, and myocardial fibrosis.

d. Oral findings include microstomia, or decreased opening of the oral cavity.

2.0 General Microbiology

2.1 Biology of Microbes

2.1.1 Bacteria

A. Background—from every breath we take, from our oral cavity through our digestive system, the surfaces of our bodies, both inside and out, are colonized by bacteria and other microbes. Bacteria outnumber human cells by a factor of 10, reaching an astounding concentration of 100 trillion cells (10^{14}) accounting for 1% to 3% of the body's mass, and are responsible for $4°C$ ($7.2°F$) of the core body temperature.

1. Humans and bacteria—The human microbiome is omnipresent in a complex and dynamic equilibrium with the host, where the collective number of genes and temporal gene expression of the microbial communities outpace the collective genetic contribution of the human genome by at least a factor of 100. Microbes are more friends than enemies to humans providing vitamins, minerals, and other nutritional supplements. It is only now with the advent of deep sequencing technology that we are beginning to appreciate the importance and continuous temporal genetic contributions that the normal flora or human microbiome provide to normal and abnormal physiology of humans.

2. Complexity of the human microbiome—on assessing numbers, types, and distribution from the perspective of location, we learn that there is considerable variation representing different phyla, genera, and species of bacteria based on the niche in which they are found (Figure 3-6). From the low complexity described for skin to the equivalent of an Amazon rainforest–like collection of species found within the digestive system, the varied and distinct niches that make up a human often have greater than 1000 different species and 10,000 strains of microbes contributing to the innate physiology of the host. However, most of what we know of the microbial world results from our study of infections. The next sections provide a perspective of how microbes transition from friends/commensals to enemies/pathogens. It is important to appreciate, especially when considering the role that microbes play in dentistry, that much of what happens in the host is in response to perturbations that disrupt the equilibrium of the local microbiome.

B. Virulence—from friend to enemy.

1. Virulence factors—the pathogenic properties of a given bacterium depend largely on the presence of genes coding for virulence factors either within the bacterial genome or found in extrachromosomal (plasmid) DNA. Common virulence factors include the following.

   a. Adhesins—coded for by plasmids; their distribution among members of a given bacterial species is variable

   b. Capsules—structural units of the bacterium, coded by chromosomal genes and detected in most bacteria within a species.

   c. Toxins—coded for by plasmids; their distribution among members of a given bacterial species is variable.

   d. Enzymes—structural units of the bacterium, coded by chromosomal genes, and detected in most bacteria within a species.

2. Genetic exchange of virulence factors—all the mechanisms of genetic exchange among bacteria can be involved in the transmission of virulence either intraspecifically (between members of the same species or strain) or extra-generally (between members of different genera, e.g., between *Escherichia* and *Shigella*). Lysogeny and plasmid transmission are the best characterized, but some classic examples of transmission of virulence factors involve transformation, the transference of naked DNA from the external medium into a new host, such as the synthesis of antiphagocytic capsules by previously nonencapsulated strains of *Streptococcus pneumoniae*.

   a. Lysogeny has been well documented as a mechanism of transmission of virulence genes. For example, the *Corynebacterium diphtheriae* toxin is produced exclusively in bacteria lysogenized by a temperate bacteriophage that contains the gene for toxin production. Some lysogenized *Escherichia coli* produce cytotoxins identical to the one produced by *Shigella dysenteriae* (Shiga toxins). Different integrated prophages carry the genes coding for the toxins.

   b. Plasmid transmission by conjugation is perhaps the most effective mechanism for transmission of virulence genes. Conjugation is induced by the specialized plasmids encoding *transfer factors* that facilitate the spread of the plasmid amongst members of a bacterial population. These transfer factors code for the expression of the sex pilus and can carry virulence genes themselves, or they may mobilize nonconjugative plasmids carrying the virulence genes. Plasmids carrying virulence genes can be classified as follows.

      (1) Resistance plasmids contain information for resistance to antibiotics. Often multiple genes determining resistance to multiple antibiotics are involved.

      (2) Virulence plasmids may code for exotoxins, adhesins, or invasion factors.

      (3) Enterotoxin-coding plasmids are present in enterotoxigenic *E. coli*. This organism causes

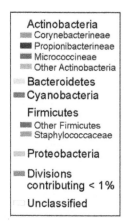

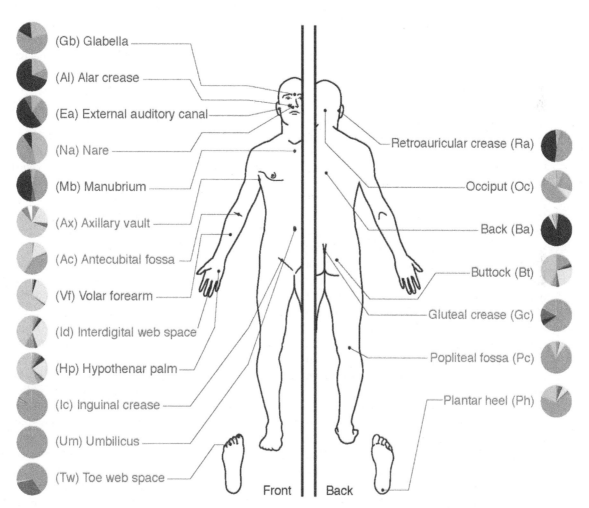

Figure 3-6 Distribution of bacteria by type according to body site. *(Source* http://publications.nigms.nih.gov/findings/jan12/body-bacteria.asp. *Adapted with permission from MacMillan Publishers LTD.* Nature Reviews Microbiology 9:244-53, 2011.)

profuse, watery diarrhea by synthesizing two toxins, heat-labile toxin and heat-stable toxin. Enterotoxigenic *E. coli* also carry adhesion coding plasmids, coding for specific pili known as *colonization factors antigens.*

(4) Invasiveness coding plasmids may determine local or systemic invasion. For example, the

invasion plasmids of *S. dysenteriae* code for several proteins that determine mucosal cell invasion and direct propagation from cell to cell. The systemic invasiveness of some strains of *E. coli* is specified by a conjugative plasmid (ColE1) that codes for a bacteriocin and for an iron-binding protein (siderophore). This siderophore allows *E. coli* to scavenge iron from the blood.

3. Regulation of expression of genes coding for virulence factors.

    a. Stress on bacteria—some virulence factors (e.g., the synthesis of antiphagocytic polysaccharide capsules) are constitutively expressed by all bacteria carrying the necessary glycosidase enzymes. Others may be expressed only when the bacteria face a situation of physiologic stress. This regulation does not apply exclusively to chromosomal genes but also applies to prophage genes. Two common causes of bacterial stress are the following.

        (1) Scarcity of essential nutrients. The regulation of the *tox* gene of *C. diphtheriae* is a classic example of nutrient-related gene regulation. The integrated prophage *tox* gene expression is repressed by an iron-dependent bacterial repressor. When iron becomes scarce at the site of infection, the bacterial repressor becomes inactive, and various bacterial and prophage genes are expressed, including the *tox* gene. The synthesis of diphtheria toxin causes cell death and is the major virulence factor of this bacterium.

        (2) Administration of antibacterial agents. The genome of *E. coli* O157:H7 contains 18 prophages and prophagelike elements including those encoding Shiga toxins 1 and 2. Because of the production of these toxins, *E. coli* O157:H7 has emerged as an important cause of GI disease, including hemorrhagic colitis, and hemolytic uremic syndrome. The production of Shiga toxin by Shiga toxin–producing *E. coli* strains can be modulated by antibiotics such as trimethoprim-sulfamethoxazole, ciprofloxacin, and norfloxacin. Such antibiotics represent an external stress to the bacteria and interfere with bacterial DNA synthesis. Under stressful conditions, bacterial SOS genes are activated, and various bacterial genes, including DNA repair genes, are expressed. The general location of the *stx* gene in the late-phase prophage region and the *recA* dependency of Shiga toxin induction led several investigators to suggest that Shiga toxin production is linked to the phage growth cycle. In other words, the phage "senses" DNA damage and bacteria stress and tries to replicate, expressing all its genes, including Shiga toxins 1 and 2. In *E. coli* O157:H7, the administration of antibiotics may lead to the production of Shiga toxins and consequently to a more severe form of disease.

4. Islands of pathogenicity.

    a. Description—bacteria, bacteriophages, and transposable elements have been around since the beginning of life. The virulence genes that we have just discussed may be encoded on transmissible elements such as plasmids, bacteriophages, or the smallest mobile genetic element, transposons. Over time, as genetic information has been exchanged, selection pressures have been exerted. Through this continued selection pressure, genes that confer a selective advantage to the microorganism have been segregated to a particular region of the bacterial chromosome. This region is easily distinguished in that it often has a very different G+C base ratio than the rest of the genetic material of the bacterium. This genomic region is referred to as a *pathogenicity island* (PAI) because this unique genetic information is most usually found exclusively in the pathogenic strains of a given species.

    b. Occurrences of PAIs—PAIs have been identified in Gram-negative and Gram-positive bacteria and often represent a significant component of the total genetic information (approximately 200 kb). In most cases, PAIs are flanked by specific DNA sequences, such as direct repeats or insertion sequence elements. There is true clinical significance attached to the presence of a PAI in a microorganism. For example, strains of *E. coli* that are uropathogenic, species of *Yersinia* that behave as aggressive facultative intracellular parasites, strains of *Helicobacter pylori* that display particularly high levels of virulence, and highly virulent *Vibrio cholerae* all have PAIs.

    c. Products of PAI-associated genes—some of the best-characterized PAI-associated genes have been found in strains of *Salmonella*. The gene products, invasins, modulins, and effector molecules have been found to facilitate the invasion of host epithelial cells and macrophages. SPI-1 triggers apoptosis in infected cells. SPI-2 promotes intracellular proliferation and systemic spread of the microbe. SPI-3 and SPI-4 facilitate the survival of the invading pathogen with the macrophage. SPI-5 induces intestinal fluid secretion and inflammation. All of these effects primarily depend on the intercellular translocation of the effector molecules from the bacteria to the host cell. Genes associated with the SPI-1 system encode a type III protein secretion system that result in the synthesis of the proteins necessary for the creation of an equivalent of a "molecular syringe" that is directly responsible for the translocation of the proteins into the eukaryotic cell.

5. Role of type III secretion apparatus on the delivery of bacterial effector proteins.

    a. Description—numerous Gram-negative bacterial pathogens use a type III secretion apparatus to deliver virulence effector proteins directly into eukaryotic cells. This multiprotein secretion complex spans both bacterial membranes and has an inner pore believed to be the conduit for delivery of the bacterial proteins. This complex strongly resembles the structure of the bacterial flagellar apparatus. Although the apparatus may be structurally conserved across the Gram-negative domain, the effector molecules translocated into the eukaryotic cell vary widely from species to species, with very different consequences.

b. Mechanisms of virulence—the virulent strains of *Shigella flexneri* carry a large virulence plasmid that also encodes a type III secretion system; some of the proteins injected by the bacteria cause reorganization of the intestinal epithelial cells, which are normally not involved in phagocytosis, so that the cells internalize the bacteria. The internalized bacteria continue releasing proteins that reorganize the cytoskeleton of the epithelial cell, allowing the organism to move freely from cell to cell without exposure to the antibacterial systems in the extracellular environment. As bacteria die and the peptidoglycan is degraded, fragments with meso-diaminopimelic acid are generated, interact with intracellular receptors, and activate nuclear factor κ B, and the epithelial cells release large amounts of IL-8, a chemotactic factor for neutrophils. This results in massive inflammation and tissue damage characteristic of shigellosis. However, in animal models lacking the capacity to release IL-8, *Shigella* disseminates through the bloodstream and causes systemic infection; this is an example of mutual adaptation between bacteria and host, in which bacteria have developed mechanisms that allow their intracellular survival, but the infected cells have a mechanism to detect bacterial components and trigger a massive inflammatory reaction that results in the elimination of the infection, even at the cost of destroying the infected intestinal mucosa. Given the ability of the intestinal mucosa to regenerate quickly, the inflammatory response ends up having a net positive effect.

6. Global regulation of PAIs.
  a. Description—the regulation of the genes within the PAIs is often subject to a phenomenon called *global regulation*. Based on the nutritional status or other environmental stimuli encountered by the cell, a suite of genes or operons or both may be activated, a phenomenon comparable to a response to stress at the bacterial level. This phenomenon is clinically significant when the microorganism perceives itself in a new environment and switches on genes that were switched off when the microbe was outside the patient, resulting in the pathogenic phenotype.
  b. PAIs and colonization—the PAIs often contain the genes that are responsible for encoding the

regulators of the virulence factors associated with PAIs as well as regulators that control genes outside the island. The bacterial stress response may involve both PAI genes and genes regulated by products of the PAIs. Either as a result of the activation of multiple genes in a PAI or as a result of the activation of genes both in and out of the PAI, it is common that several synergistic virulence factors may be activated simultaneously. For example, the PAI associated with *V. cholerae* encodes cholera toxin and the toxin-coregulated pilus (TCP), a type 4 pilus that is an essential intestinal adherence factor. TCP has been shown to be a crucial colonization factor required for adherence of the microorganism in volunteer and animal studies. It has also been shown that TCP mediates interbacterial adherence, and its role in intestinal colonization may be to increase the colonizing mass of bacteria, while some other factor directly binds the bacteria to epithelial cells. This system is coordinated by the *acf* (accessory colonization factor) gene cluster and encodes a regulator located downstream of the *tcp* gene cluster within the *V. cholerae* PAI, and the gene products associated with this are thought to play a role in chemotaxis, assisting in intestinal colonization.

c. Lack of stability of PAIs—the PAIs of pathogenic bacteria are unstable, subject to deletion, duplication, and amplification. PAIs also are often associated with nonessential transfer RNA (tRNA) loci (multicodon amino acids), which may represent target sites for the chromosomal integration of these elements. To date, 75% of the PAIs identified have been associated with tRNA loci. In addition, bacteriophage attachment sites and other cryptic genes are often found on PAIs. Some of the cryptic genes are very similar to phage integrase genes, plasmid origins of replication, or insertion sequence elements strongly suggesting that these particular genetic elements were likely spread horizontally among bacterial populations before their location within the PAI. Whatever the mechanism of maintenance and distribution, the presence of PAIs within virulent bacteria represents a significant clinical concern because they confer to the pathogen a unique set of traits that confer to it a selective advantage in the host.

7. Bacterial biofilms.
  a. Role of hemagglutinin—in addition to PAIs, there are other isolated genetic islands within the chromosomes of bacteria. These may be termed *fitness or persistence islands*. In another example from pathogenic *V. cholerae*, another type 4 pilus, a mannosidase-sensitive hemagglutinin, is encoded by a cluster of 16 genes (16.7 kb) flanked by 7-base-pair direct repeat sequences. This hemagglutinin

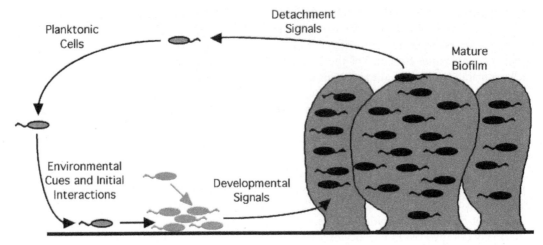

Figure 3-7 Biofilm formation is also seen with other aquatic bacteria, such as *Pseudomonas.*

has been shown not to be involved in intestinal colonization or any other aspect of cholera, suggesting that although this genetic element has the molecular features of a PAI, it is not a PAI because it is not involved in pathogenicity. However, further investigation of this finding revealed that the mannosidase-sensitive hemagglutinin is essential for formation of biofilms on abiotic surfaces leading workers in the field to speculate that this genetic element is an environmental persistence island.

b. Role of exopolysaccharides—in another fitness or persistence island, of *V. cholerae* El Tor, an exopolysaccharide gene product was also shown to be essential for the formation of biofilms leading to the speculation that the fitness or persistence islands in pathogens may be essential for maintenance of *V. cholerae* in an environmental reservoir between epidemics.

c. Role of slime capsules—biofilm formation is also seen with other aquatic bacteria (Figure 3-7), such as *Pseudomonas.* This biofilm formation is particularly a problem in patients with cystic fibrosis, in whom biofilms can be formed in the bronchial tree. The strains involved in biofilm formation have larger slime capsules, and once they establish a successful biofilm, antibiotic therapy becomes ineffective. One additional pathogenic aspect associated with biofilm formation is that different bacterial species frequently become involved in unique symbiotic relationships. The involvement of multiple bacteria in an infection, each one with different antibiotic susceptibility patterns, is another factor that complicates therapy.

8. Quorum sensing.
   a. Description—among the genes that are turned on under special conditions, some determine the ability of the organisms to form complex communities or biofilms. As described in Figure 3-7, Gram-negative biofilms form in an acyl-homoserine lactone–dependent process. The significance of the requirement for this low-molecular-weight molecule is evident from the role it plays in the molecular circuits that coordinate the genes required for the formation of the biofilm. This process is referred to as quorum sensing or autoinduction, in which a quorum or minimum number of cells is needed to switch one or a series of genes on or off, which then results in a particular set of phenotypic responses in the microorganisms. In this way, the microbial community can monitor its own population density and best determine the coordinate expression necessary to survive in a competitive environment.

   b. Mechanism of autoinduction—the process is very elegant and straightforward (Figure 3-8, *A*). Individual bacteria secrete into the environment the quorum sensing molecule or *autoinducer.* In the case of Gram-negative bacteria, this generally is a low-molecular-weight molecule containing an acyl side chain attached to a homoserine lactone (Figure 3-8, *B*); in Gram-positive bacteria, this typically is a low-molecular-weight peptide. The autoinducer diffuses away into the surrounding environment. When the autoinducer encounters another microbe, it diffuses into the cell, where it activates a regulatory molecule that facilitates gene expression. Consequently, the expression is closely controlled by either the population or the extent of diffusion of the autoinducer.

   c. Economics of quorum sensing—from the perspective of cellular economics, quorum sensing makes good sense. Consider the production and release

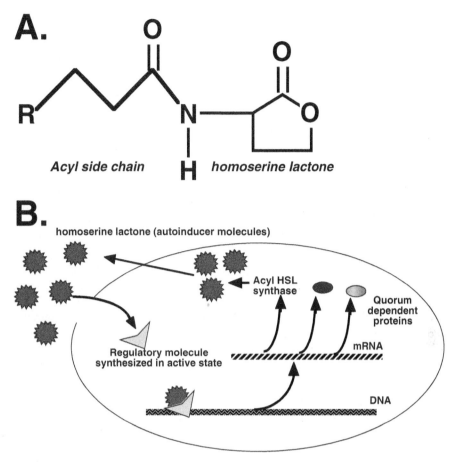

Figure 3-8 A, Structure of a homoserine lactone with attached acyl side chain attached, **B,** Mechanism of autoinduction.

of extracellular enzymes such as DNAses, proteases, and other molecules such as siderophores (an iron-scavenging molecule) and antibiotics and the consequences their production has on the overall fitness of a microbe. If such enzymes or molecules were released by only a few bacteria, their synthesis would be ineffective because of dilution. Similarly, autoinduction might offer the cell a way to determine the extent of diffusion or mixing or both in its local environment. If conditions are such that diffusion or mixing is too great, the concentration of autoinducer would quickly decrease triggering the regulatory circuit not to produce additional molecules of autoinducer.

d. Quorum sensing and disease—from a medical perspective, this is a significant advantage to bacteria because they can tightly control the release of virulence factors into the surrounding tissue until such time as the population has reached a density better able to withstand the defenses mounted by the host. Numerous virulence factors are controlled by this process. In *Pseudomonas aeruginosa*, the extracellular enzymes and toxins elastase, protease,

and exotoxin A are modulated in a quorum-dependent manner. There is increasing evidence that chronic infections are the result of microbial communities and that the bacteria that compose such communities have an inherent ability to monitor and respond to such perturbations within the community. Quorum sensing is only one mechanism that bacteria have in determining the sense of place.

9. Paradigm shift—the implications from quorum sensing to microbial endocrinology and infectious disease.

a. Clinical relevance of biofilms, PAIs, type III secretion, and quorum sensing.

(1) Within the past decade as these concepts have been refined from a molecular microbiologic perspective, the fusion of the disciplines of microbiology, neurosciences, and endocrinology has occurred. The human gut contains more than 100 million neurons, a number equivalent to the number of nerves in the spinal cord. These nerves innervate through all the layers extending down to the microvillus,

which is often in direct contact with microbes. Given the genetic complexity of the flora of the human gut and the realization that the microbial community modulates the endocrine cells of the GI mucosa, investigators have begun to question what role neuroendocrine hormones, such as the catecholamines have on the pathogenesis of infection of an orally acquired pathogen.

(2) Neuroendocrine hormones and bacteria—the range of neuroendocrine hormones and their respective receptors as well as the diversity of microbes that have been found is very large. Insulin was found in *E. coli* in the early 1980s, and it has been postulated that insulin may play a role in the susceptibility of diabetics to infection to *Burkholderia pseudomallei*. Given that innervation of the enteric nervous system of the human GI tract is extensive and that the neuroendocrine hormones are produced by both the nerves themselves and the cells they innervate, it is not surprising that the hormonal environment that the microbe encounters in the gut could play a significant role in determining the path of a pathogenic process. This prevalence would suggest that the interactions in both the host and the microbe can be bidirectional. An observation from the 1930s noted that the administration of adrenaline to a patient resulted in the proliferation of a contaminating microbe. More recent molecular evidence can account for the observation. Noradrenaline increased bacterial growth by providing an essential element, iron, through an interaction with the iron-sequestering proteins of the host, transferrin and lactoferrin, and through the induction of an autoinducer of growth in the bacteria. Consequently, exposure to the human-provided catecholamine provides the necessary stimulus to facilitate the growth of the invading microbe through the induction of the autoinducer of growth.

(3) Cross-communication between hormones and bacteria—more recent work characterizing the colonization potential of the human gut of one agent responsible for bloody diarrhea, *E. coli* O157:H7, has found that in addition to a quorum sensing system (luxS and autoinducer 2), the microbe responds to a eukaryotic signal to activate its virulence genes. This signal is the eukaryotic, gut-synthesized hormone epinephrine. The microbe similarly responded to α- and β-adrenergic receptor antagonists, which resulted in blocking the response to the signal from the host. Consequently, the results imply cross-communication between the *luxS* and autoinducer 2 bacterial quorum sensing system and the epinephrine and norepinephrine host signaling system. Other examples of this cross-communication include the colonization of germ-free mice using high densities of a Gram-negative anaerobe, *Bacteroides thetaiotaomicron*, where the cross-communication has been found to modulate the expression of numerous host genes involved in intestinal functions, including, but not limited to, nutrient absorption, mucosal barrier fortification, and angiogenesis. The class of quorum sensing molecules common in Gram-negative signaling, the acyl homoserine lactones, have been shown to have immunomodulatory activities, including induction of IL-8 production, inhibition of lymphocyte proliferation and tumor necrosis factor (TNF)-α, and limitation of the production of IL-12.

(4) This material is complex because it involves the intersection of the disciplines of microbiology, neurobiology, and mammalian physiology, which requires one to consider that the microbes and host cells are communicating. This is not surprising given the proximity of the microbe and the fact that they share receptors and ligands that are interacting with each other. It is not surprising then the genes from both the host and the microbe are coincident in responding to stimuli from each other. As additional studies are completed, it will be recognized that there is a fine line between symbiosis and pathogenesis.

C. Growth of bacteria.
  1. Measures of growth.
    a. Direct counting—the concentration of the microbes is determined by using a gridded volumetric slide and counting the microbes under a defined number of fields with the aid of a microscope; however, here it is impossible to discriminate live cells from dead unless special dyes are added before counting.
    b. Plating—the concentration of viable cells is enumerated by assessing their ability to form a colony from a single cell on a nutritionally appropriate agar plate.
    c. Turbidimetrically—the scattering of light and reduction to the percentage of light reaching a photomultiplier is related to an increase in cell mass. The value of the optical density can be correlated against cell number by either direct or viable cell enumeration. Direct counting and turbidimetric assessments require at least 100,000 cells/mL.
  2. Growth phases (Figure 3-9).
    a. Phase 1 (lag phase)—bacteria are metabolically active, and the population appears to be growing

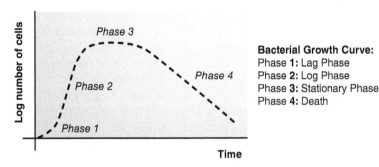

Figure 3-9 Bacterial growth curve.

slowly because the number of cells dividing is only slightly greater than the number of cells dying. Growth can be measured turbidimetrically because the mass of individual cells is increasing.

b. Phase 2 (logarithmic growth)—the population is expanding at an exponential rate. Most bacteria within the population are actively growing; the generation time, the period it takes the population to double, can be determined. Note: penicillins act on actively growing bacteria, and it is during this phase of growth that this phenomenon can be most easily measured because the prevention of cross-linking by penicillin results in death from the lysis of bacterial cells. Consequently, any of the three methods used to measure growth can easily detect the bactericidal activity of this drug.

c. Phase 3 (stationary phase)—the rate of cell division is equivalent to the rate of cell death. The population has reached a steady state, likely as a consequence of nutrient depletion or the accumulation of toxic by-products, or both.

d. Phase 4 (death)—the death of individual cells within the population can be measured by the loss of viability or the spontaneous lysis of dead cells. In general, as resources decrease and toxic wastes increase, bacteria begin to die.

D. Classification of bacteria.

1. Classification by oxygen use.

a. Metabolism—regardless of the terminal electron acceptor (e.g., O_2 or organic acids), bacteria can result in the formation of two toxic molecules: hydrogen peroxide (H_2O_2) and free radicals of oxygen (e.g., superoxide [O_2^-]). Because these molecules are strong oxidants, they are toxic; bacteria have evolved strategies to neutralize their effects (e.g., catalase converts H_2O_2 into water and molecular oxygen, and superoxide radicals may be neutralized by superoxide dismutase). Equations characterizing the neutralization of reactive oxygen species by the bacterial enzymes superoxide dismutase and catalase follow.

Superoxide radical: $2\ O_2^- + 2\ H^+ \rightarrow H_2O_2 + O_2$ catalyzed by superoxide dismutase

Hydrogen peroxide: $2\ H_2O_2 \rightarrow 2\ H_2O + O_2$ catalyzed by catalase

b. Aerobes—require oxygen for growth; molecular oxygen is used as the terminal electron acceptor for metabolism where molecular oxygen is reduced and combined with two protons to form water.

c. Facultative anaerobes—do not require oxygen for growth but may use it when it is present.

d. Anaerobes—do not use molecular oxygen as the terminal electron acceptor, and some lack the enzymes to detoxify toxic oxygen intermediates generated during metabolism. Generally, anaerobes transfer their waste electrons into carbon compounds or molecular hydrogen generating a variety of organic acids or hydrogen gas. This process is referred to as *fermentation.*

e. Note: supragingival plaque consists of mostly aerobes and facultative anaerobes; subgingival plaque consists mostly of anaerobes.

2. Classification by shape.

a. Cocci—round, circular shape.

(1) Diplococci—occur in pairs.

(2) Streptococci—occur in chains.

(3) Staphylococci—occurs in grapelike clusters.

b. Bacilli—rod-shaped.

c. Spirochetes—spiral-shaped.

d. Pleomorphic—bacteria that appear with different, inconsistent shapes.

3. Classification by Gram stain.

a. General characteristics of Gram stain.

(1) Used for identification purposes.

(2) Based on the ability of a microbe to retain the primary stain on reaction with the mordant with subsequent decolorization by 95% ethanol or acetone. Bacteria are classified into two groups.

(a) Gram-positive bacteria—retain the color of the primary stain, crystal violet (violet in color).

(b) Gram-negative bacteria—retain the color of the counterstain, safranin, which stains the cells pink or red. Under some circumstances, carbol fuchsin may be substituted for safranin in the staining of anaerobic microbes. Anaerobes stain best when staining is performed in the absence of oxygen.

(3) May be useful in determining which antibiotic to prescribe.

b. Staining protocol.

(1) Cells from a freshly obtained specimen or a colony less than 24 hours old are attached to a glass slide using mild heat fixation.

(2) Apply the primary stain, crystal violet, to the slide for 1 minute, and rinse with water; all cells are violet in color.

(3) Apply the mordant, Lugol's iodine, to the slide for 1 minute, and rinse with water.

(4) Decolorize the cells with acetone or ethanol— Gram-negative bacteria, with their bimolecular layer of peptidoglycan, are quickly decolorized, whereas Gram-positive bacteria retain the color from the primary stain.

(5) Apply the counterstain with safranin—Gram-negative cells stain red, whereas Gram-positive cells remain violet.

4. Classification by acid-fast staining.

a. Used to assess for the presence of a physical property of certain bacteria—presence of mycolic acids within their cell walls. An example is mycobacteria, which may generate a Gram-variable reaction.

b. Similar to the Gram stain protocol, this is considered a differential stain. The primary stain is carbolfuchsin (acid-fast positive), and the counterstain is methylene blue (acid-fast negative).

(1) Cells from a freshly obtained specimen or a colony suspension less than 24 hours old are attached to a glass slide by allowing them to air dry at 60° C followed by a heat fixation for 10 minutes at 90° C.

(2) The primary stain, carbol fuchsin, is applied, and the slide is held above a flame until steam appears but the liquid does not boil. The hot slide is allowed to cool for 3 to 5 minutes and is rinsed with tap water; all of the bacteria stain fuchsia (reddish or pink colored).

(3) The slide is flooded with 3% hydrochloric acid in isopropyl alcohol (acid alcohol). The slide is allowed to sit for 1 minute with subsequent rinsing with tap water.

(4) The slide is flooded with methylene blue for 1 minute and rinsed with tap water; acid-fast microbes (e.g., mycobacteria) retain the fuchsia color, whereas non–acid-fast bacteria stain blue.

2.2 Bacterial Cell Walls and Their External Surfaces

All bacteria are surrounded by a rigid cell wall except *Mycoplasma*, which have only a cytoplasmic membrane.

A. Cell wall—also known as murein or peptidoglycan, a multilayered structure located external to the cytoplasmic membrane. The cell wall provides structural integrity to the microbe and is responsible for its shape. In all true bacteria (prokaryotes), the cell wall is composed of alternating units of N-acetylmuramic acid (NAM) and N-acetylglucosamine (NAG). The resulting polysaccharide polymer, peptidoglycan, serves to form a molecular corset around the cytoplasm of the cell enabling the cell to withstand great fluxes in osmotic pressures (Figure 3-10). Peptidoglycan is cross-linked through the formation of a peptide bond. There is variability within the amino acid side chain within the peptide, but generally they are linked between the terminal D-alanine (absent from proteins) from one chain to L-lysine or other diamino acids from the other chain. In *Staphylococcus aureus* (Figure 3-11), a pentaglycine bridge (gly_5) is used to cross-link its peptidoglycan. In *E. coli*, a common Gram negative microbe, diaminopimelic acid, the diamino acid in the third position of the peptide, is directly linked to the terminal alanine of another chain strengthening the polymer through cross-linking (see Figure 3-11). Lipoprotein serves to anchor the outer membrane to the cell wall. The periplasmic space between the cytoplasmic and outer membranes contains transport, degradative, and cell wall synthetic enzymes.

1. Cell wall characteristics of Gram-positive bacteria (Figure 3-11, *A*).

a. Thick, multilayer structure composed principally of peptidoglycan.

b. Contains teichoic acid and lipoteichoic acids, which are antigenic, within the peptidoglycan.

2. Cell wall characteristics of Gram-negative bacteria (Figure 3-11, *B*).

a. Thin, generally bimolecular layer of peptidoglycan.

b. In the space between the outer and cytoplasmic membranes, certain species contain enzymes called β-lactamases, which degrade penicillins and other β-lactam drugs.

c. Lipopolysaccharide (LPS) or endotoxin.

(1) Found in the outer membrane.

(2) Causes an immune response by activating macrophages, B cells, and complement.

(3) Toxicity of LPS is attributed to presence of lipid A.

(4) O antigen—outer membrane of LPS; often used for identification purposes.

(5) Found in dental plaque and gingival inflammation.

3. Cell wall characteristics of acid-fast bacteria (Figure 3-12).

a. An unusual cell wall with a high concentration of mycolic acid, which results in an ability to resist decolorization with acid alcohol (i.e., such cells are acid-fast); when Gram staining is done, cells often

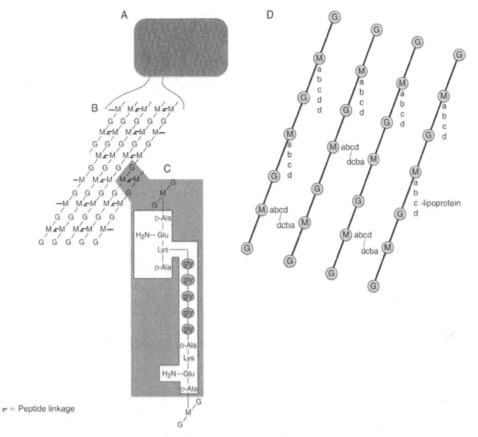

Figure 3-10 A-D, General structure of the peptidoglycan component of the cell wall. (*G,* N-Acetylglucosamine; *Glu,* d-glutamic acid; *gly,* glycine; *M,* N-acetylmuramic acid.) (*A-C,* Modified from Talaro K, Talaro A: Foundations in Microbiology, ed 2. Dubuque, IA, William C Brown, 1996. *D,* Modified from Joklik KJ, et al: Zinsser Microbiology. Norwalk, CT, Appleton & Lange, 1988.)

generate Gram-variable reactions. In addition to the cytoplasmic membrane (Figure 3-12, *A*) and peptidoglycan (Figure 3-12, *B*), the mycobacterial cell wall contains arabinogalactan (Figure 3-12, *C*), mannose-capped lipoarabinomannan (Figure 3-12, *D*), membrane-associated and cell wall–associated proteins (Figure 3-12, *E*), mycolic acids (Figure 3-12, *F*), and glycolipid surface molecules associated with mycolic acids (Figure 3-12, *G*).

B. Specialized structures external to the cell wall.
   1. Capsule.
      a. Gelatinous layer that surrounds the cell walls of certain bacteria; generally made of polysaccharides, but can also be comprised from protein (e.g. the capsule of *Bacillus anthracis*), although the composition varies depending on species.
      b. Functions.
         (1) Antiphagocytic—prevent phagocytosis by macrophages. Often, the presence of a capsule alone may singly confer virulence to the microbe.
         (2) For identification purposes—quelling reaction. When the polysaccharide capsules are treated with antiserum, they swell, allowing them to be identified.

         (3) May play a role in the adherence of bacteria to certain tissues (i.e., caries on the tooth surface).
   2. Spores.
      a. Spores allow certain bacteria to survive through unfavorable environmental conditions. There are two types, exospores and endospores.
         (1) Exospores are external to the vegetative cell and are not found in any clinically significant bacteria.
         (2) Endospores are internal to the cytoplasmic membrane and have a thick, outer layer. It has been suggested that their resistance may be related to dipicolinic acid, a calcium chelator.
      b. Spore-forming bacteria include species from *Bacillus* and *Clostridium*.
   3. Flagella—long, whiplike appendages that generate mobility of bacteria.
   4. Pilli (fimbriae)—fine filaments proteinaceous in makeup that mediate attachment of bacteria to human cells.

2.2.1 Viruses

A. General characteristics.
   1. Basic structure—nucleocapsid; consists of a capsid, or protein coat, and the viral genome, which

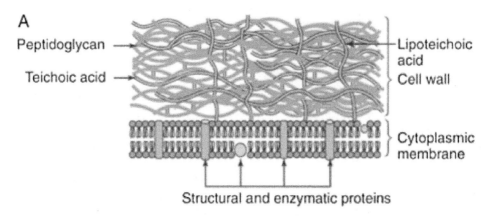

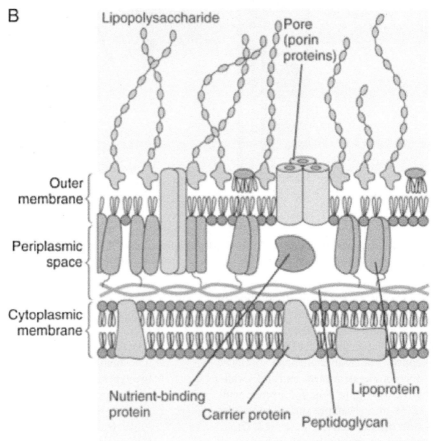

Figure 3-11 **A** and **B,** Comparison of Gram-positive and Gram-negative bacterial cell walls. *(From Murray PR, et al: Medical Microbiology, ed 7. Philadelphia, Saunders, 2013.)*

comprises only one of the following types of nucleic acid: double-stranded DNA or RNA or positive-stranded or negative-stranded RNA or DNA.

2. Some viruses also acquire an outer envelope from the infected host cell. Enveloped viruses are normally more sensitive to environmental conditions (easier to inactivate with desiccation, stomach acids, heat, or detergents) than nonenveloped viruses.

3. Viruses are obligate intracellular parasites and require other organisms for metabolism and reproduction.

B. Replication or growth cycle—seven stages.
1. Attachment—virus binds to the host cell via specific surface proteins.
2. Penetration—virus enters the host cell by receptor-mediated endocytosis, translocation of the entire

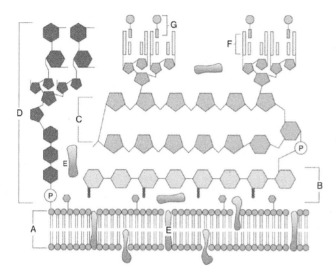

Figure 3-12 A-G, Mycobacterial cell wall structure. *(Modified from Karakousis PC, et al:* Mycobacterium tuberculosis *cell wall lipids and the host immune response. Cell Microbiol 6:105-116, 2004.)*

virus across the plasma membrane, or fusion of its viral envelope with the host membrane.

3. Uncoating of the viral genome—viral nucleic acid separates from its outer protein coat.
4. Early viral protein synthesis—virus may use its own enzymes or host enzymes first to produce proteins needed for viral genome replication.
5. Late viral protein synthesis—structural proteins for the capsid are produced.
6. Assembly of virion—newly synthesized viral genomes and capsid proteins are assembled.
7. Release—progeny virions may be released from the host cell by the following.
   a. Host cell lysis—newly formed viruses are released via lysis of the host cell, leading to host cell death. Note: in cultured cells, the lysis of host cells after viral infections results in the formation of plaques or holes within the lawn of host cells. Such patterns, a consequence of the cytopathic effects manifested by the virus, may be used for identification purposes.
   b. Budding—viruses obtain their outer envelope from the plasma membrane of the host cell. The host membrane contains surface proteins (antigens) or spikes, which the budding virion also acquires onto its outer envelope (Figure 3-13).
C. Detection of viral growth (Figure 3-14).
   1. Eclipse period—time when the virus is actively replicating within the host cell. Virions have yet to assemble.
   2. Latent period—time between the initial viral infection and when the virus can be detected (requires a complete virus).

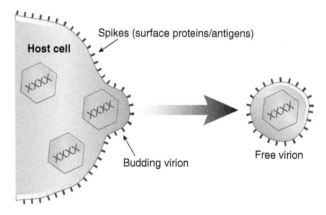

Figure 3-13 Viral budding.

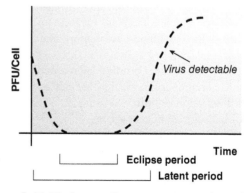

Figure 3-14 Viral growth curve. *PFU,* Plaque-forming units.

D. Viral—bacterial interactions.
  1. Bacteriophages—viruses that infect bacteria.
    a. Virulent phage—infection results in the conversion of host metabolic processes to the sole expression of the phage genome resulting in the death of the host and release of bacteriophages; generally results in the lysis of the host.
    b. Temperate phage—on infection, a genetic circuit specific to the phage genome assesses whether or not to integrate the phage genome within that of the host or proceed with a virulent infection.
  2. Lysogeny—on infection and an affirmative response to a regulatory decision mediated by a phage operon, the bacteriophage nucleic acid is integrated within the host genome. The phage genome remains integrated in so long as the genes necessary and sufficient for the manifestation of a virulent infection are repressed. The infected bacterium retains its normal functioning. The resulting or lysogen-infected host may acquire new phenotypic traits as a result of the infection (e.g., diphtheria toxin in *C. diphtheriae*). This process is called *lysogenic conversion*.

2.2.2 Fungi

A. General characteristics.
  1. Fungi are eukaryotic cells (have a true nucleus).
  2. Cell wall—not all species have a cell wall, but those that do have three layers external to the plasma membrane. The first layer consists of chitin (a polymer of *N*-acetyl-D-glucosamine) followed by a layer of β-1,3-glucan (zymosan) with a final layer of mannoproteins (mannose-containing glycol proteins), which are heavily glycosylated and manifest as the surface of the cell.
  3. Many fungi are dimorphic (i.e., they can exist as two distinct forms, molds or yeasts). Many fungal species that infect humans can grow in these two forms. However, only a subset of pathogenic fungi produce hyphae during an infection; these include the commonly carried yeasts *Candida albicans* and *Candida dubliniensis* and opportunistic fungal pathogens such as *Aspergillus fumigatus* and the common dermatophyte *Trichophyton rubrum* and *Trichophyton mentagrophytes*. Hyphae facilitate invasion of the tissue, viewed by the fungus as support and nutritional matrix.
  4. Spores—some fungi produce spores, and in contrast to bacterial endospores, they are not as recalcitrant to desiccation or heat.
    a. Medically significant spores.
      (1) Blastospores—formed by budding.
      (2) Chlamydospores—have thick walls, making them more resistant to environmental changes.
      (3) Arthrospores—formed from the ends of hyphae.
      (4) Sporangiospores—formed by molds.

B. Immune response.
  1. Fungal infections generally initiate a type IV delayed hypersensitivity reaction.
  2. Formation of granulomas in response to a fungal infection is common.

2.3 Antimicrobials

2.3.1 Antibiotics

A. Inhibitors of bacterial cell wall synthesis—peptidoglycan is a macromolecule unique to prokaryotes. Its biosynthesis makes it an ideal target for antimicrobial therapy because drugs directed against its synthesis have minimal to no consequences on essential host cell functions. Because its biosynthesis is a multistep process, multiple antibiotics have been developed to interrupt its assembly at many of its critical steps (Figure 3-15).
  1. Penicillins.
    a. Bactericidal.
    b. Action—inhibits transpeptidase, the enzyme that catalyzes the final cross-linking step in synthesis of peptidoglycan, a component of the bacterial cell wall.
    c. Adverse reactions to penicillin—hypersensitivity (allergic) reactions (anaphylaxis, skin rashes), seizures, and platelet dysfunction.
    d. Types of penicillins.
      (1) Natural penicillins.
        (a) Effective against Gram-positive bacteria and Gram-negative cocci; limited effect against Gram-negative bacilli bacteria.
        (b) Susceptible to β-lactamases.
        (c) Include penicillin G and penicillin V.
      (2) Extended-spectrum penicillins.
        (a) More effective against Gram-negative bacilli compared with natural penicillins.
        (b) Susceptible to β-lactamases.
        (c) Include amoxicillin and ampicillin.
      (3) Penicillinase-resistant penicillins (antistaphylococcal penicillins).
        (a) Resistant to degradation by β-lactamases.
        (b) Used for treatment of certain strains of *S. aureus* that produce penicillinase.
        (c) Include cloxacillin, dicloxacillin, methicillin, nafcillin, and oxacillin.
  2. Cephalosporins.
    a. Bactericidal.
    b. Broad-spectrum antibiotics.
    c. There are four generations of cephalosporins, with expanded coverage with increasing generation.
    d. Action—similar to penicillins, but they are more resistant to β-lactamases than penicillins are.
    e. Adverse reactions—disulfiramlike reaction with some cephalosporins when alcohol is consumed.
    f. Although cephalosporins are structurally similar to penicillin, patients who are allergic to penicillin

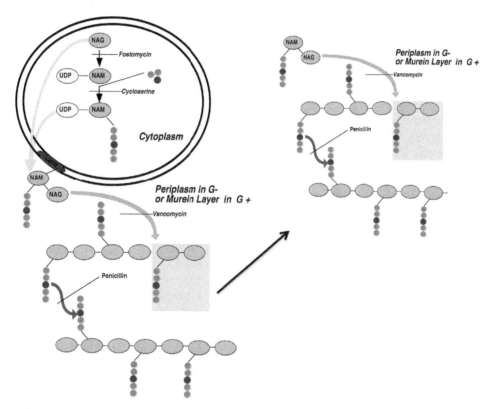

Figure 3-15 Schematic representation of the synthesis of peptidoglycan. The location of the horizontal line represents the site at which the indicated antibiotic targeted to inhibit cell wall biosynthesis acts.

have a 10% chance of being hypersensitive to cephalosporins.
g. Include cephalexin, cefadroxil, and cefazolin.
3. Other inhibitors of cell wall synthesis.
   a. Bacitracin.
      (1) For topical use only.
      (2) Highly nephrotoxic if given systemically.
   b. Vancomycin.
      (1) Produced by *Streptococcus orientalis*.
      (2) Effective against Gram-positive bacteria.
      (3) Has a limited effect against Gram-negative bacteria (*Flavobacterium* is the exception).
      (4) Used for multidrug-resistant bacteria (e.g., methicillin-resistant *S. aureus*) or treatment of endocarditis.
B. Inhibitors of protein synthesis—similar to cell wall biosynthesis, the synthesis of protein by bacteria is a multistep and multienzyme process. The structure of the ribosome (30S/50S bacteria versus 40S/60S ribosomal subunits of eukaryotes and *Archaea*) is distinct to bacteria making it an ideal target for drug development. Consequently, numerous antimicrobials have been developed specifically to target the various biosynthetic steps required to synthesize proteins.
1. Aminoglycosides.
   a. Bactericidal.
   b. Mechanism of action—blocks 30S ribosomal subunit to inhibit protein synthesis.

c. Effective against aerobic bacteria but ineffective against anaerobic bacteria because they require oxygen for transport into bacteria. They are also useful against many Gram-negative rods, TB (streptomycin), and enterococci (gentamicin).
d. Administered by intravenous or intramuscular injection.
e. Adverse reactions.
   (1) Ototoxicity (via damage to eighth cranial nerve)—may result in deafness.
   (2) Nephrotoxicity—may result in permanent kidney damage.
f. Include streptomycin, gentamicin, and tobramycin.
2. Tetracycline.
   a. Bacteriostatic.
   b. Action—blocks 30S ribosomal subunit to inhibit protein synthesis; side effect also found to inhibit matrix metalloproteinases, which are zinc-dependent endopeptidases.
   c. Broad-spectrum antibiotic that targets Gram-positive and Gram-negative bacteria and other microorganisms, such as *Rickettsia*, *Mycoplasma*, and *Chlamydia*.
   d. Adverse reactions.
      (1) Hepatotoxicity, which may result in severe damage to the liver, especially in pregnant women.

(2) Tooth discoloration in developing teeth. Tetracycline should be avoided in pregnant women and young children, until such time as complete eruption of permanent teeth.

3. Macrolides.
   a. Bacteriostatic.
   b. Action—blocks 50S ribosomal subunit to inhibit synthesis of proteins.
   c. Effective in treating mostly Gram-positive bacterial infections but can be used to treat Gram-negative microbes such as *Haemophilus influenzae*, *Legionella pneumophila*, *Mycoplasma*, some *Mycobacterium* species, some *Rickettsia* species, and *Chlamydia*.
   d. Adverse reactions—ototoxicity and GI problems.
   e. Includes erythromycin and clarithromycin.
4. Clindamycin.
   a. Bacteriostatic; can be bactericidal at higher concentrations.
   b. Semisynthetic derivative of lincomycin.
   c. Action—blocks 50S ribosomal subunit to inhibit synthesis of proteins.
   d. Effective in treating anaerobic Gram-positive or Gram-negative bacteria, including *Bacteroides fragilis* and *Fusobacterium*.
   e. Adverse reaction—pseudomembranous colitis, which is caused by overgrowth of *Clostridium difficile* in the gut.
5. Chloramphenicol.
   a. Broad-spectrum antibiotic that is effective against Gram-positive, Gram-negative, aerobic, and anaerobic bacteria.
   b. Used as a last resort because of its toxicity and possible severe adverse reactions.
   c. Adverse reactions—reversible anemia, aplastic anemia, and gray baby syndrome, which can lead to death.
C. Metabolic inhibitors (e.g., inhibitors of folate synthesis).
   1. Both humans and bacteria require folate for the synthesis of DNA precursors. In contrast to bacteria, humans are unable to synthesize their own folic acid; they rely on exogenous folate, via diet or vitamins, to fulfill their requirement for folate. Because bacteria are able to produce their own folic acid, sulfa drugs have a selective effect on them.
   2. Sulfonamides (sulfa drugs).
      a. Bacteriostatic.
      b. Action—synthetic analogues of paraaminobenzoic acid. Sulfonamides competitively inhibit and block the metabolic pathway of folic acid synthesis in bacteria.
      c. Adverse reactions—hemolytic anemia in patients with glucose-6-phosphate dehydrogenase deficiency.

D. Inhibitors of DNA replication.
   1. Quinolones.
      a. Bactericidal.
      b. Action—inhibit DNA gyrase (topoisomerase).
      c. Include ciprofloxacin.
E. Membrane disruption (e.g., chlorhexidine)—the unit membrane is not unique to prokaryotes. Consequently, any agent used to disrupt the integrity of the membrane may have consequences on host tissue. In the example described here, chlorhexidine, it should be considered a chemical antiseptic. In addition to being effective against bacteria, it also has activity against fungi and enveloped viruses.
   1. Broad antimicrobial spectrum.
   2. Present in the only oral wash approved by the U.S. Food and Drug Administration (FDA) that has been registered to make public health claims to decrease supragingival plaque and gingival inflammation associated with gingivitis.
   3. Actions.
      a. Chlorhexidine binds to oral tissues (tooth, mucosa), salivary pellicle, and bacteria, resulting in a persistent, cumulative, antimicrobial effect.
      b. After rinsing, some chlorhexidine remains in the oral cavity where it is gradually released over time. Because chlorhexidine may be neutralized by common toothpaste additives such as sodium lauryl sulfate and sodium monofluorophosphate, it should be used after brushing.

2.4 Sterilization and Disinfection

A. Sterilization.
   1. Inactivation of all microorganisms, including spores, from a substance. Although the process may render the microbe unable to reproduce, the cellular debris is still present and should be considered pyrogenic (able to cause a fever) until it has been certified to be pyrogen-free.
   2. Sterilization techniques are summarized in Table 3-3.
B. Disinfection.
   1. Inactivates most microorganisms but does not include the inactivation of bacterial spores, some viruses, and fungi.
   2. Example: sodium hypochlorite, a surface disinfectant.
      a. Mechanism of action—oxidative destruction of cells.
      b. Advantages—it is a broad-spectrum agent and is inexpensive. It is commonly used as an intracanal irrigant during root canal therapy.
      c. Disadvantages—it is toxic to tissues.
C. Antiseptics.
   1. Disinfectant that can be applied to skin.
   2. Antiseptic agents are summarized in Table 3-4.

Table 3-3

Summary of Sterilization Techniques

	MECHANISM OF ACTION	TEMPERATURE OR TIME REQUIRED	ADVANTAGES	DISADVANTAGES
Dry heat	Coagulation of proteins	160°C for 2 hr	Noncorrosive to metal	Longer time than moist heat
		171°C for 1 hr	Simple method	Can damage heat-sensitive items
Moist heat (autoclave)	Denatures proteins	Wrapped instruments: 121°C (250°F)/15 psi for 15 min	Short time	Can damage heat-sensitive items
		Unwrapped (flash cycle) instruments: 134°C (270°F)/30 psi for 3 min	Very effective and dependable	
Ethylene oxide gas	Alkylating agent that denatures nucleic acids (DNA) and proteins	1-12 hr	Good for heat-sensitive or moisture-sensitive items	Very toxic
				Flammable Long time
2% glutaraldehyde	Alkylating agent that denatures nucleic acids (DNA) and proteins	12 hr	Good for heat-sensitive or moisture-sensitive items	Very toxic
			Noncorrosive to metals	Long time Expensive

Table 3-4

Summary of Antiseptics and Their Actions

	MECHANISM OF ACTION	ADVANTAGES	DISADVANTAGES
2% tincture of iodine	Disruption of cell membranes	Most effective antiseptic	—
Alcohol (70% ethanol)	Dissolution of lipids in cell membranes	Low toxicity	Limited contact time owing to quick evaporation
	Denatures proteins	Effective against most vegetative bacteria, fungi, and viruses	Decreased action against microbes in dried blood or saliva
Quaternary ammonium compounds	Cationic detergents that disrupt cell membranes	Noncorrosive to metals	Are inactivated by anionic detergents Limited antiseptic effect
Formaldehyde	Denatures/precipitates proteins	high-level disinfectant bactericide, tuberculocide, fungicide, virucide and sporicide	Toxic, carcinogenic
Soaps, detergents	Anionic compounds that physically remove microbes	Generally low toxicity	Limited antiseptic effect

3.0 Microbiology and Pathology of Infectious Microbes

3.1 Bacterial Manifestations

3.1.1 Cocci-Shaped, Gram-Positive Bacteria

A. *Streptococcus* belongs to the phylum of Firmicutes.
1. General characteristics.
   a. Cocci-shaped; observed in lines.
   b. Gram-positive.
   c. Facultative anaerobes.
   d. Hemolytic classification.
      (1) α-Hemolytic—incomplete lysis of RBCs; often appears to be green (hence the term *viridans* or green).
      (2) α-Hemolytic bacteria include viridans streptococci, *Streptococcus mutans*, *Streptococcus sanguis*, and *Streptococcus salivarius*.

(a) Bacteria, such as viridans streptococci, are the most common organisms causing subacute endocarditis.

(b) β-Hemolytic—complete lysis of RBCs.

(c) Appear in the clear zone.

(d) β-Hemolytic streptococci are further divided into Lancefield (carbohydrate-based antigen) groups A through U.

(e) β-Hemolytic bacteria include group A (*Streptococcus pyogenes*) bacteria.

(3) γ-Hemolytic—indication of the absence of hemolysis in the RBCs within the indicator.

B. *S. pyogenes.*
1. Hemolytic class—β.
2. Virulence factors.
   a. M protein—important virulence factor.
   b. DNAse—cleaves DNA.
   c. Erythrogenic toxin—causes scarlet fever rash.
   d. Streptolysin O/S (hemolysin)—causes lysis of RBCs and white blood cells (WBCs).
   e. Streptokinase (fibrinolysin)—dissolves fibrin in blood clots by cleaving plasminogen to increase levels of plasmin.
   f. Hyaluronidase—spreading factor that breaks down hyaluronic acid, increasing the ability of the bacterium to spread.
   g. Exotoxin A—causes necrotizing fasciitis by rapidly destroying tissue.
3. Diseases include pharyngitis (i.e., strep throat), rheumatic fever following a streptococcal infection, scarlet fever, impetigo, glomerulonephritis following a streptococcal infection, toxic shock syndrome, and necrotizing fasciitis.

C. Viridans streptococci.
1. Hemolytic class—α.
2. Diseases—endocarditis, caries.

D. *S. pneumoniae.*
1. Hemolytic class—α (though not generally considered diagnostically remarkable).
2. Virulence factors.
   a. Polysaccharide capsule—prevents phagocytosis.
   b. Pneumolysin—a cytolytic toxin.
   c. IgA protease—hydrolyzes IgA to aid in its ability to colonize along the respiratory mucosa.
3. Diseases.
   a. Pneumonia—most common cause of bacterial or lobar pneumonia; classically manifests in four stages.
      (1) Congestion—occurs within the first 24 hours and is characterized histologically by vascular engorgement and intraalveolar fluid, small numbers of neutrophils, and numerous, in this case Gram-positive, encapsulated diplococci.
      (2) Red hepatization or consolidation—vascular congestion persists, with a concomitant recruitment of neutrophils and fibrin. On auscultation, the filling of airspaces with exudate changes the lung sound from one of hollowness to solid or dense sounding.
      (3) Gray hepatization—RBCs disintegrate with persistence of neutrophils and fibrin; the affected lobe still appears consolidated on x-ray.
      (4) Resolution—exudate is digested by enzymes, debris cleared by macrophages and coughing, and the chest sounds clear of consolidation.
   b. Meningitis—inflammation of the meninges. Symptoms include high fever, severe headache, and vomiting or nausea with headache.
   c. Otitis media—earache, the most common cause of otitis media in infants older than 2 months.
4. Dental significance.
   a. Streptococci are the most common bacteria in the oral cavity.
   b. They are cariogenic bacteria for several reasons.
      (1) They lower the pH to promote the demineralization of enamel, which begins between pH 1 and 5, by producing lactic acid.
      (2) They provide a structural component for plaque by producing dextrans. The surface of streptococci contains glycosyl transferase. This enzyme cleaves glucose and fructose from sucrose to form dextrans and fructans, respectively (Figure 3-16).
   c. They provide food for bacteria growth by their production of fructans (levans) from fructose.
   d. They contribute to the adhesion of bacteria to the tooth surface by the production of fructans.
   e. *S. mutans* is the most cariogenic. It contains a polysaccharide glycocalyx coating that allows it to stick firmly to surfaces.
   f. *S. sanguis* is the most common *Streptococcus* species isolated from the oral cavity.
   g. Streptococci are commonly present in Ludwig's angina.

E. *S. aureus.*
1. General characteristics.
   a. Cocci-shaped; arranged in grapelike clusters.
   b. Gram-positive.

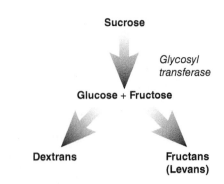

Figure 3-16 Breakdown of sucrose by streptococci glycosyl transferase.

c. Part of normal skin and mucous membranes flora.

d. Causes suppurative or pus-forming (pyogenic) infections, mostly in the form of abscesses.

2. Virulence factors.

a. Protein A—found in its cell wall. It inhibits complement fixation by binding to the Fc portion of IgG, resulting in decreased phagocytosis and opsonization. It can also elicit a hypersensitivity reaction and damage platelets.

b. Coagulase—clots blood (*S. aureus*).

c. Staphylokinase (fibrinolysin)—dissolves blood clots by cleaving plasminogen to increase levels of plasmin.

d. Hyaluronidase—spreading factor that breaks down hyaluronic acid, increasing its ability to spread.

e. β-Lactamases (penicillinase, β-hemolysin)—inactivate penicillin by degrading β-lactam ring. Note: some modified penicillins (penicillinase-resistant penicillins) are resistant to β-lactamases and are more effective in treating penicillinase-producing staphylococci (e.g., dicloxacillin).

f. Toxins—all are exoproteins that can behave as superantigens. Molecules that act as superantigens have the ability to activate 1 in 5 T cells rather than 1 in 10,000 T cells, releasing multiple cytokines. The resulting event is typically referred to as a cytokine storm and may result in profound nonsuppurative effects on the host.

(1) Enterotoxin—causes food poisoning (vomiting, diarrhea).

(2) Exfoliatin—causes staphylococcal scalded skin syndrome, an exfoliative dermatitis in children.

(3) Toxic shock syndrome toxin.

(a) Diseases include food poisoning, endocarditis, and impetigo.

(b) It is often associated with death following viral respiratory infections (e.g., influenza).

3.1.2 Rod-Shaped, Gram-Positive Bacteria

A. *Actinomyces.*

1. General characteristics.

a. Gram-positive—some species may contain mycolic acids in their cell walls, allowing them to stain acid-fast.

b. Strictly anaerobic.

c. Part of normal gut and oral flora.

d. Purulent discharge via the sinus cavities results in particles that resemble sulfur granules; *they are not sulfur* but appear as yellow specks within the purulent exudates.

e. Have branchlike projections that make their appearance similar to fungi but appreciate that they are smaller.

2. Diseases.

a. Root surface caries.

b. Actinomycosis—endogenous, suppurative infection caused by *Actinomyces israelii* or *Actinomyces gerencseriae*. It commonly occurs in the cervicofacial area ("lumpy jaw") and can spread to form abscesses or sinus tracts after minor trauma or dental work. Generally, the clinical condition of "lumpy jaw" is the consequence of a polymicrobial anaerobic infection. Other microbes that may contribute to this include *Propionibacterium propionicum*.

B. *Corynebacterium diphtheriae.*

1. General characteristics.

a. Contains granules that stain metachromatically. Note: in the laboratory, methylene blue stain is used to reveal metachromic granules in bacteria; it stains the cell blue and the granules red.

b. An infection results in the generation of an adherent fibrin-derived pseudomembrane.

2. Virulence factors.

a. Only bacteria that have been infected with a bacteriophage carrying the DNA that codes for the diphtheria toxin are pathogenic. The expression of the toxin is coordinated by the nutritional status of the host and microbe. Symptoms manifest 2 to 7 days after infection.

b. The diphtheria toxin acts to block elongation factor 2 during translation, inhibiting protein synthesis. The toxin follows the common design of many bacterial exotoxins. There are two fragments held together by a disulfide bond. The B fragment ("b" for binding) is the recognition subunit that facilitates entry of the toxin via the heparin-binding Epidermal growth factor (EGF) into the eukaryotic cell. The resultant binding leads to receptor-mediated endocytosis. Once in the endosome, the toxin is split by a protease whereupon the B subunit generates pores within the endosome membrane enabling the A subunit to reach the cytoplasm where it prevents protein synthesis by catalyzing adenosine diphosphate (ADP)–ribosylation of elongation factor 2.

3. Vaccine—toxoid that is part of the diphtheria-pertussis-tetanus (DPT) vaccine.

C. *Lactobacillus.*

1. General characteristics.

a. Produce lactic acid.

b. Part of normal gut, oral, and vaginal flora.

(1) It is the main source of lactic acid in the vagina and responsible for keeping the pH of the environment low, which prevents the growth of some fungi.

(2) *Lactobacillus casei* has been found in deep dental caries.

(3) There are greater than 2000 substrains of *Lactobacillus plantarum* found throughout the

body. Each strain has a unique metabolic attribute that may contribute to the general well-being of the host by producing substances (probiotics) required by the host or substances that confer health to the host.

D. *Listeria.*
  1. General characteristics.
     a. Type species *Listeria monocytogenes*—small pleomorphic rod-shaped psychrophilic (capable of growth at 4° C and 37° C), microaerophilic microbe responsible for listeriosis.
     b. Facultative intracellular parasite (capable of growth inside professional and nonprofessional phagocytic cells); able to spread directly from cell to cell.
     c. Motile at temperatures less than 30° C.
     d. Widely distributed in nature and in numerous animal reservoirs; food is the most common vehicle for transmission of human listeriosis in adults.
        (1) Frequently contaminated foods include unpasteurized milk, cheese made from unpasteurized milk, raw vegetables (coleslaw and other salads), and processed meats (hot dogs and commercially processed cold cuts of turkey or other meats).
        (2) In 10% of humans, the GI tract is colonized by the type species.
     e. Viewed as an opportunistic pathogen in humans causing disease in the very young and immunocompromised.
  2. Virulence factors.
     a. Hemolysin (listeriolysin O)—facilitates survival within professional (macrophage) phagocytic cells by generating a pore within the vacuolar membrane but not the cytoplasmic membrane of the host cell.
     b. Internalins—facilitate entry into nonprofessional phagocytic cells.
     c. Surface protein p104 facilitates adhesion to intestinal cells.
     d. ActA protein—ability to polymerize actin filaments facilitating cell-to-cell movement.
     e. Phospholipases.
  3. Disease.
     a. Meningitis is the most common clinical condition affecting immunocompromised adults and very young children.
        (1) In adults, it is the leading cause of meningitis in patients with cancer with mortality seen in approximately 60% of the cases. Overall mortality in adults is 30%.
        (2) In infants, it is frequently contracted perinatally at birth. It can also be acquired transplacentally, in which case the disease is widely

disseminated throughout the developing fetus. Granulomatous foci may be observed in the liver, spleen, lungs, and CNS. Miscarriage is often associated with intrauterine infections.
     b. Bacteremia (present in the blood) is detected in 25% of cases.
     c. Endocarditis is less frequent and seen in approximately 7% of cases.
  4. Treatment.
     a. For listeriosis, ampicillin with or without an aminoglycoside (gentamicin) remains the best treatment for meningitis caused by *L. monocytogenes*.
        (1) For invasive listeriosis, ampicillin and penicillin, given in daily doses of more than 6 g (2g IV every 4 hours (q4h) (amp); 4 million U, IV q4h (pen)), are equally effective against *L. monocytogenes*. Gentamicin (3 mg/kg/day IV divided 3 times per day (tid)) is often added in patients with compromised immune systems.
        (2) Trimethoprim-sulfamethoxazole, vancomycin, and fluoroquinolones may be substituted in case of penicillin allergies.
        (3) Cephalosporins *are not effective* for treatment of listeriosis.
     b. Prompt treatment of *Listeria* infections in pregnant women is critical to prevent the bacteria from infecting the fetus.
        (1) Amoxicillin and erythromycin are effective oral therapies.
        (2) Ultrasound to monitor the health status of the fetus is recommended.
E. *Propionibacterium.*
  1. General characteristics.
     a. Gram-positive, aerotolerant (not immediately killed by atmospheric concentrations of oxygen) anaerobic rods.
     b. One of the most prominent microbes associated with the flora of the skin of adults; usually undetectable on preadolescents.
     c. Ferments complex carbons (e.g., sebum secreted by sebaceous glands in the follicles of the skin) to propionic acid via transcarboxylase enzymes.
     d. Glows orange when exposed to Wood's lamp (ultraviolet [UV] light).
  2. Disease.
     a. Consumption of sebum and cellular debris by the microbe within the follicles and pores can result in the triggering of an inflammatory response leading to the formation of an abscess (pimple) resulting in acne. This condition is principally caused by *Propionibacterium acnes*.
     b. *Propionibacterium granulosum* is also considered an opportunistic pathogen found in a range of postoperative infections and device-related complications.

3. Treatment.
    a. Susceptible to a wide range of antimicrobials with macrolides and tetracyclines being the drugs of choice.
    b. Susceptible to over-the-counter topical antimicrobials, such as benzoyl peroxide, triclosan, and chlorhexidine gluconate.
    c. Killed by exposure to UV light.

3.1.3 Spore-Forming, Gram-Positive Bacteria

A. *Bacillus anthracis.*
    1. General characteristics.
        a. Rod-shaped.
        b. Aerobic.
        c. Forms a white, ground-glass appearance in colony when recovered from a TSA-blood agar plate.
    2. Virulence factors.
        a. Spores—allow it to survive in the soil for years. Humans can be infected by spores on animal products. The portals of entry include the skin, mucous membranes, and respiratory tract.
        b. Exotoxin with three characteristics—edema factor, protective antigen, and lethal factor.
        c. Aerosol transmission and ability to produce a lethal exotoxin make it a choice for bioterrorism.
    3. Disease—anthrax.
        a. Two types.
            (1) Cutaneous anthrax—10% fatal; clinically observed as a skin lesion or pustule with a dark (eschar) scab. Inflammation is present around the lesion.
            (2) Pulmonary anthrax (woolsorter's disease)—50% fatal; quick onset of fever, muscle pain, respiratory distress, and hemorrhaging lymph nodes leading to necrosis and cyanosis.
        b. Vaccine—purified protective antigen.
B. *Bacillus cereus.*
    1. General characteristics—some strains are harmful to humans; principal manifestation food-borne disease and most often associated with steam table–derived food poisoning where rice is often the vehicle of transmission. As the rice near the surface cools, spores germinate, producing a toxin that is ingested with the rice.
        a. Rod-shaped, endemic, and generally a soil-dwelling β-hemolytic organism.
        b. Facultative anaerobic bacterium.
    2. Virulence factors.
        a. Some strains are psychrotrophic (able to grow at 4° C).
        b. Enterotoxin is highly resistant to heat and to extremes of pH (stable between pH 2 and 11). Ingestion leads to either a diarrheal or an emetic

syndrome, depending on the toxin and concentration ingested.
    (1) Diarrheal form of disease—diarrhea and GI pain manifest within 8 to 17 hours of ingestion of contaminated food.
    (2) Emetic syndrome—vomiting (emesis) generally results from consumption of a sufficient concentration of cereulide toxin that is not inactivated by reheating resulting in vomiting within 1 to 5 hours after consumption of toxin-laced food (generally rice). It is challenging to differentiate *B. cereus* cereulide toxin–mediated food poisoning from enterotoxic staphylococcal food poisoning because of the similarity and timing of symptoms.
C. *Clostridium.*
    1. General characteristics.
        a. Rod-shaped.
        b. Anaerobic.
    2. Virulence factors.
        a. Produce some of the most potent exotoxins that have been identified.
        b. Hyaluronidase—an enzyme that breaks down hyaluronic acid, increasing its ability to spread.
    3. *Clostridium tetani.*
        a. Spores are commonly found in soil.
        b. Exotoxin—tetanus toxin (tetanospasmin); a neurotoxin that inhibits the release of glycine from α-motoneurons in the CNS.
        c. Disease—tetanus (lockjaw) resulting from spastic paralysis.
            (1) Tetanus toxins usually enter the body through an open wound.
            (2) Symptoms include painful muscle contractions, trismus, and spasm of facial muscles. These symptoms continue until death occurs by exhaustion or respiratory failure.
        d. Treatment—antitoxins must be administered as quickly as possible to sequester unbound toxins, an example of passive-active immunity. Antibiotics (penicillin G) should also be administered, and surgical débridement of the infected site is indicated.
        e. Vaccine—consists of tetanus toxoid and should be given about every 10 years. It is part of the DPT vaccine. It can also be administered after infection.
    4. *Clostridium botulinum.*
        a. Spores may be found in canned foods that have been improperly processed or in undercooked foods. On germination, the spores manifest a potent heat-labile but acid-stable neurotoxin. Clostridial proteins "protect" the exotoxin as it transits through the stomach, where it is adsorbed and translocated through the circulatory system.

b. Exotoxin—botulinum toxin.
   (1) A neurotoxin that inhibits the release of acetylcholine in peripheral nerves, leading to loss of motor function (flaccid paralysis).
   (2) Most potent toxin known.
c. Disease—botulism. As with many exotoxin-mediated disease processes, the flaccid paralysis results principally from an intoxication rather than an infection.
   (1) Symptoms include muscle weakness and paralysis, cranial nerve impairment, diplopia, dysphagia and speech impairment, respiratory failure, and death.
d. Treatment—trivalent antitoxins are given, along with respiratory support. These antitoxins are immunoglobulins that act to neutralize the toxins.
e. Infant botulism—occurs when an infant becomes infected after ingesting spores with the toxin being produced and adsorbed through the large intestine. Recovery occurs without intervention.

5. *Clostridium perfringens.*
   a. Spores are commonly found in soil.
   b. Live bacteria are part of the normal gut and vaginal flora.
   c. Exotoxin—α-toxin or lecithinase. This toxin destroys cell membranes by causing cell lysis.
   d. Contains collagenase.
   e. Disease—gas gangrene (myonecrosis).
      (1) Occurs around an improperly treated wound.
      (2) Gas is produced around the infected site by degradative enzymes released after cell lysis. Clinically, pain, swelling, and cellulitis may be observed. Shock and death may ensue from large amounts of tissue destruction.
   f. Treatment—antibiotics (penicillin) should be administered, and surgical débridement and removal of the infected tissues are indicated. Hyperbaric oxygen treatment has been found to be useful.

6. *Clostridium difficile.*
   a. Spores are commonly found in soil, on foods, and within the built environment (in this case the human-made facilities) of hospitals and long-term care facilities; normally transmitted via fecal-oral route. Spores are *not* inactivated by alcohol hand sanitizers.
   b. Not normally considered normal flora; resident as a commensal in 2% to 5% of adult population.
   c. Exotoxins (A or B or both A and B)—on administration of broad-spectrum highly active antimicrobial therapy, *C. difficile* blooms within the gut elaborating a toxin or toxins that result in severe diarrhea and other intestinal disease because the competing bacteria normally resident within the gut have been reduced through the administration of the antimicrobials.

d. Disease presentation—symptoms range from mild flulike conditions to presentations similar to flare of inflammatory bowel disease–associated colitis. Chronic inflammation occurs leading to increased pathology within the large intestine. Mild cases may be treated simply by discontinuing the antibiotic therapy; severe and chronic cases require surgical resection of the necrotic colonic tissue. In some circumstances in which prolonged and chronic disease is evident, and as an alternative to surgery, stool transplantation from a healthy donor has met with increased clinical cure of disease.
e. Treatment—metronidazole is the drug of choice because of cost and comparable efficacy.

3.1.4 Acid-Fast Bacteria

A. *Mycobacterium.*
   1. General characteristics.
      a. Rod-shaped.
      b. Aerobic.
      c. Gram stain challenging because of thick and waxy cell walls, which contain mycolic acids. Acid-fast staining protocol is needed for diagnosis.
   2. *M. tuberculosis.*
      a. Infects reticuloendothelial cells, including macrophages. Because oxygen is required for metabolism, the infection usually occurs in oxygen-rich areas, such as lungs and kidneys.
      b. Cord factor, a surface glycolipid, contributes to pathogenicity.
      c. Disease—TB.
         (1) There is a higher prevalence of TB in individuals with lower socioeconomic status and immunocompromised individuals.
         (2) Disease states.
            (a) Primary TB—asymptomatic. A fibrous nodule may result at the site of infection. Less than 5% of individuals infected progress to the active disease state.
            (b) Secondary TB—reactivation of disease, often owing to compromised immunity.
            (c) Miliary TB—when infection disseminates through the vascular system.
         (3) Important characteristics.
            (a) The host responds to contain the infection by forming granulomas, known as *tubercles*, often with the presence of central caseous necrosis and multinucleated giant cells.
            (b) Ghon complex—the calcified scar that remains after the primary infection; it usually includes the primary lung lesion and its regional lymph node.
         (4) PPD skin test.
            (a) Tests for a delayed hypersensitivity reaction to certain *M. tuberculosis* proteins. A positive TB skin test reports whether or not a

person has been infected with TB or vaccinated with bacille Calmette-Guérin (BCG). It does not tell whether the person has a latent TB infection or has transitioned to active disease. Consequently, further testing such as a chest radiograph, laboratory cultures, or a TB blood test is warranted.

(i) Chest x-rays—a posterior-anterior chest radiograph is generally ordered after a positive PPD test. Lesions may appear anywhere in the lungs and may differ in size, shape, density, and cavitation. When found, the lesions or abnormalities may suggest TB but cannot be used for definitive diagnosis of TB.

(ii) The FDA has approved two interferon-γ release assay tests for TB infection. Briefly, blood is collected and within 8 to 30 hours is processed using the protocols specific to the QuantiFERON-TB Gold In-Tube Test or the T-SPOT.TB test. A positive result demonstrates that there has been an immune response, indicating the presence of TB, whereas a negative test demonstrates that there has not been a recent immune response, indicating the absence of TB.

(5) Treatment—at the present time, 10 drugs are approved for the treatment of TB. The first-line anti-TB agents include isoniazid, rifampin, pyrazinamide, and ethambutol (in combination) and are initially used for 2 months (*initial phase*) followed by a choice of several options for the *continuation phase* for either 4 or 7 months. Patient-centered case management should be used in the development of all treatment strategies to ensure an effective cure.

3. *Mycobacterium leprae*—causes leprosy (Hansen's disease)

a. Affected humanity for greater than 4000 years. It is primarily a chronic infection that manifests through a granulomatous process involving the peripheral nerves and mucosa of the upper respiratory tract. Left untreated, the disease results in progressive and permanent damage to the skin, nerves, limbs, and eyes.

b. Treatment is possible with daily doses of dapsone and monthly doses of rifampicin for 6 months. Multibacillary (lepromatous) forms of the disease require daily dapsone and clofazimine with monthly doses of rifampicin for 12 months.

4. Mycobacteria other than TB or nontuberculous mycobacteria—rapidly growing mycobacteria have emerged in recent years that are of increased clinical concern in the immunocompromised population. The best known is *Mycobacterium avium-intracellulare*

complex, which is a group of species that in a disseminated infection formerly were responsible for significant mortality in patients with AIDS. *M. avium-intracellulare* complex is ubiquitous in its distribution in nature and has been recovered from fresh and salt water, house dust, soil, fecal material of animals and birds, and commercial cigarettes. It can be treated with a cocktail of at least two or three of the following: macrolides (e.g., clarithromycin, azithromycin), rifamycins, ethambutol, clofazime, fluoroquinolines, or aminoglycosides.

3.1.5 Gram-Negative Bacteria

Bacteria that are within the Enterobacteriaceae family account for many of the constituents considered to be resident flora of the human gut microbiome. The type genus is often considered *Escherichia*, and the bacteria within this group generally are operationally defined as Gram-negative, non–spore-forming, facultative anaerobic rods that ferment glucose with the production of acid and gas at 37°C. However, not all of members of the Enterobacteriaceae family are benign, and members of the genera *Salmonella*, *Shigella*, and others are considered to be pathogens when found in the human gut.

A. General characteristics of Enterobacteriaceae.

1. Gram-negative.
2. Rod-shaped.
3. Facultative anaerobes.
4. May be part of normal gut flora.
5. Exchange of genetic material is common, causing the formation of new strains.
6. All species produce *endotoxin*, a toxin kept within the bacterial cell that is released only after destruction of the cell wall. Today, endotoxin and LPS are synonymous where LPS is a major constituent of the outer membrane of most, if not all, Gram-negative cells. The composition of LPS varies among genera with some being more immunogenic than others.
7. Some may produce exotoxins, known as *enterotoxins*.
8. Surface antigens are used to aid in the identification of strains. These include K antigen (capsular antigen), O antigen (somatic antigen), and H antigen (flagella antigen).
9. Species of significance.
   a. *E. coli*.
      (1) Surface traits—O antigen, H antigen (flagella), and pili.
      (2) Virulence factors.
         (a) Capsule—aids in the evasion of host phagocytosis.
         (b) Pili—aids in the attachment of *E. coli* to the intestinal surface.
         (c) Enterotoxin—is released after attachment, clinically causing diarrhea, and may facilitate localized invasion into the wall of the

small intestine. Some strains produce heat-labile and heat-resistant enterotoxins that have moved from *Shigella* to *Escherichia* resulting in the formation of a new strain of *E. coli* 0157H7, which is responsible for hemorrhagic diarrhea with the subsequent development of hemolytic uremic syndrome.

 (3) The most common cause of cystitis and traveler's diarrhea.

 b. *Proteus.*

  (1) Surface trait—O antigen.

  (2) Virulence factors.

   (a) Very motile.

   (b) Produces urease, which hydrolyzes urea to ammonia.

  (3) Disease—cystitis.

 c. *Salmonella.*

  (1) Surface traits—cell wall O antigen, flagella, H antigen, and capsular Vi.

  (2) Diseases—enterocolitis, septicemia, and enteric or typhoid fevers. Note: enterocolitis infections should not be treated with antibiotics. This could prolong the patient's symptoms. The diseases are usually self-limiting.

 d. *Shigella.*

  (1) Surface trait—O antigen.

  (2) Virulence factor—some strains produce neurotoxins.

  (3) Disease—enterocolitis or bacterial dysentery.

  (4) Enterotoxin—is released after attachment, clinically causing diarrhea, and may facilitate localized invasion into the wall of the small intestine.

 e. Other genera belonging to Enterobacteriaceae family.

  (1) The following list of genera have LPS as one of their primary virulence factors, and all may serve as opportunistic pathogens. Some have been implicated in serious disease (e.g., *Klebsiella pneumoniae*, *Yersinia pestis*) and possess unique virulence determinants (e.g., ability to produce copious amounts of mucoid capsule in the case of *Klebsiella*), and all have an ability to participate in interspecies genetic exchange of information via conjugation, transformation, or transduction that may confer increased fitness in a particular niche.

  (2) *Alishewanella, Alterococcus, Aquamonas, Aranicola, Arsenophonus, Azotivirga, Blochmannia, Brenneria, Buchnera, Budvicia, Buttiauxella, Cedecea, Citrobacter, Cronobacter, Dickeya, Edwardsiella, Enterobacter, Erwinia* (e.g., *Erwinia amylovora, Erwinia tracheiphila, Erwinia carotovora*), *Escherichia* (e.g., *E. coli*), *Ewingella, Grimontella, Hafnia, Klebsiella* (e.g., *K. pneumoniae*), *Kluyvera, Leclercia, Leminorella, Moellerella, Morganella, Obesumbacterium, Pantoea, Pectobacterium* (see *Erwinia*), *Candidatus Phlomobacter, Photorhabdus* (e.g., *Photorhabdus luminescens*), *Plesiomonas* (e.g., *Plesiomonas shigelloides*), *Pragia, Proteus* (e.g., *Proteus vulgaris*), *Providencia, Rahnella, Raoultella, Salmonella, Samsonia, Serratia* (e.g., *Serratia marcescens*), *Shigella, Sodalis, Tatumella, Trabulsiella, Wigglesworthia, Xenorhabdus, Yersinia* (e.g., *Y. pestis*), *Yokenella.*

3.1.5.1 Other Gram-Negative Bacteria

A. *Bacteroides.*

 1. General characteristics—type species is *Bacteroides fragilis. B. fragilis* and other members of this genus serve in mutualistic capacity within the host.

  a. Primarily they facilitate the processing and derivation of nutrients from the complex foods ingested.

  b. They represent a substantial fraction of the GI flora (gut) where their numbers may exceed 10^{11} to 10^{12} microbes per Gram of stool.

  c. A diet rich in protein and animal fats favors their support, whereas a diet based principally on plants and carbohydrates results in the selection of a community based on species of *Prevotella.*

  d. Strict anaerobes.

  e. Unusual characteristic is that members of this genus have sphingolipids within their cytoplasmic membranes.

  f. The most common organism found in severe infection below the diaphragm.

 2. Virulence factors.

  a. Generally viewed as an opportunistic pathogen—LPS is poorly antigenic but is present.

  b. Substantial fraction of the type species *B. fragilis* has a potent β-lactamase.

 3. Diseases.

  a. Periodontal disease, including pregnancy gingivitis (hormonal changes result in substantial changes to the selection pressures responsible for normal flora of the oral cavity.

  b. Endogenous infections through mucosal openings.

B. *Bordetella pertussis*—whooping cough.

 1. General characteristics—aerobic, coccobacillus generally capsulated.

 2. Virulence factors.

  a. Pertussis toxin (same in design as diphtheria toxin having A and B fragments, but activity and target are different), hemagglutinin, pili, and capsule.

  b. Transmission is easily accomplished via airborne droplets expelled by coughing or sneezing. Bacteria colonize on the cilia of epithelial cells, causing decreased cilia activity and cell death. Net consequence often called the "cough of 100 days."

3. Disease.
   a. Whooping cough (pertussis).
      (1) Catarrhal stage—incubation period 7 to 10 days, at which time the patient exhibits mild respiratory symptoms including mild coughing, sneezing, and runny nose.
      (2) Paroxysmal stage—after approximately 1 to 2 weeks, the classic cough of high-pitched "whoop" commences. The most notable sign aside from the "whooping" sound is that the patient struggles to inspire after the "fit" of coughing.
      (3) It is responsible for approximately 40 million infections worldwide with approximately 300,000 deaths.
      (4) Vaccination—before vaccination, this disease was responsible for between 10,000 to 20,000 deaths within the United States per year. Vaccination has reduced the annual fatality rate to less than 10 per calendar year.
         (a) Principally administered in concert with the toxoids for immunization against diphtheria and tetanus.
         (b) The pertussis component is acellular and contains chemically inactivated forms of two of the five toxins resident and responsible for disease.
         (c) In addition to vaccination of children, because of a more recent resurgence of whooping cough in young adults and elderly adults, it is recommended that individuals within the respective demographic receive a boost to prevent disease.

C. *Fusobacterium*.
   1. General characteristics.
      a. One of the organisms associated with Vincent's infection, also referred to as *acute necrotizing ulcerative gingivitis*, a mixed infection of oral streptococci, oral treponemes, and fusobacteria.
      b. Strict Gram-negative anaerobe rod distinguished by having one or both ends pointed.
      c. Similar in appearance to *H. influenzae*.
      d. Difficult to culture.
      e. Generates a profound fetor when cultured or when present in an infected site.
      f. Species often indicative of location from which it was isolated.
         (1) *Fusobacterium alocis*—gingival crevice.
         (2) *Fusobacterium gonidiaformans*—colon and genital tract.
         (3) *Fusobacterium mortiferum*—colon.
         (4) *Fusobacterium necrophorum*—oropharynx and colon.
         (5) *Fusobacterium nucleatum*—gingival crevice.
         (6) *Fusobacterium varium*—colon.

2. Disease.
   a. Principally involved with infections of the gum tissue; manifests as an acute infection of the gingiva without involvement of other tissues of the periodontium. On deeper penetration, it is reclassified as necrotizing ulcerative periodontitis.
   b. Treatment involves débridement of the necrotic tissue, improvements to oral hygiene, and the use of oral mouth rinses containing appropriate antiseptics.

C. *H. influenzae*.
   1. General characteristics.
      a. Rod-shaped.
      b. Encapsulated.
   2. Virulence features.
      a. LPS (endotoxin).
      b. IgA protease.
      c. Polysaccharide capsule.
   3. Disease.
      a. *H. influenzae* was mistakenly thought to be responsible for influenza until 1933, when it was demonstrated that flu was result of the influenza virus. However, today, *H. influenzae* is appreciated as the cause of bacterial influenza. Generally, this microbe is considered to be an opportunistic pathogen in that the bacteria generally reside within the host without causing disease.
      b. Meningitis—leading cause in children.
      c. Vaccination has all but eliminated this as a significant disease.

D. *H. pylori*.
   1. General characteristics.
      a. Microaerophilic, helix-shaped (often called a curved rod) microbe 3 μm long and 0.5 μm wide.
      b. This microbe may constitute greater than 50% of the normal flora of the stomach.
      c. Significant surface traits—four to six lophotrichous (having two or more flagella at one end of the microbe) flagella and five major outer membrane protein families.
      d. Similar to other Gram-negative organisms, the outer membrane has LPS.
         (1) The O antigen may be fucosylated and has been shown to mimic the Lewis blood group antigens on the gastric epithelium.
         (2) O antigen is subject to antigenic variation via a process known as *slipped stranded mutagenesis*.
   2. Virulence factors.
      a. Is unique in its ability to thrive in the gastric mucosa overlying gastric mucous cells in the stomach.
      b. Produces urease, which converts urea to ammonia and carbon dioxide. The ammonia produced neutralizes acid in the stomach, increasing the gastric pH.
      c. Has been detected in dental plaque and saliva.

3. Disease.
   (1) Chronic gastritis and peptic ulcers.
   (2) There is an increased risk for developing some stomach cancers, including adenocarcinoma and non-Hodgkin's lymphoma.
E. *Neisseria meningitidis.*
   1. General characteristics.
      a. Typically occur as diplococci.
      b. Oxidase-positive.
      c. Microaerophilic.
      d. Capnophilic.
      e. Presently 13 serogroups have been described: A, B, C, D, E, H, I, K, L, W-135, X, Y, and Z.
         (1) Serogroups B and C have caused most cases of meningococcal meningitis in the United States since the end of World War II; before that, group A was more prevalent.
         (2) More than 99% of meningococcal infections are caused by serogroups A, B, C, 29E, or W-135.
         (3) In Europe and United States, group B is the most predominant agent causing disease.
   2. Virulence features.
      a. LPS (endotoxin).
      b. IgA protease.
      c. Capsule.
      d. Pili for adhesion.
   3. Transmission.
      a. Bacteria in the infected air droplets quickly colonize the mucosal membranes of the nasopharynx and enter the bloodstream to specific sites (e.g., meninges, joints).
   4. Disease.
      a. Meningitis.
         (1) Leading cause of meningitis in people 6 to 60 years old.
         (2) Symptoms include nausea, vomiting, photophobia, altered mental status, and nuchal rigidity.
         (3) May manifest over a period of 2 to 7 days or fulminantly (as if struck by lightning).
         (4) Treatment.
            (a) Because of the poor prognosis if not treated promptly, initial therapy is empiric in nature.
            (b) Until the etiology is certain, treatment should include dexamethasone, a third-generation cephalosporin (e.g., ceftriaxone, cefotaxime), and vancomycin. Acyclovir should be considered based on the results of the initial cerebrospinal fluid (CSF) evaluation. Doxycycline should also be added during tick season in endemic areas and on confirmation of *N. meningitidis.*
            (c) A 7-day course of intravenous ceftriaxone or penicillin is adequate for uncomplicated meningococcal meningitis.

5. Vaccine.
   a. Presently there is a quadrivalent vaccine for serotypes A, C, W-135 and Y.
   b. Suggested for college-aged adults.
   c. Evidence from the literature suggests that complement-mediated serum bactericidal antibody confers protection against meningococcal disease A serum bactericidal antibody titer 1:4 or greater when measured with human complement is generally considered as a marker of protection.
   d. Vaccines against serotype B have been difficult to generate owing to the similarity of the capsular polysaccharide on the type B bacterium to human neural antigens. Absence of a vaccine is concerning because this serotype accounts for greater than 50% of all cases.
F. *Neisseria gonorrhoeae.*
   1. General characteristics.
      a. Typically occur as diplococci.
      b. Oxidase-positive.
      c. Microaerophilic.
      d. Capnophilic.
      e. Nutritionally extremely fastidious, growing on a rich, selective medium such as Thayer-Martin.
   2. Virulence factors.
      a. LPS (endotoxin).
         (1) IgA protease—hydrolyzes IgA, which would otherwise block its attachment to the mucosal surface.
      b. Pili—an important feature because it is antiphagocytic, and pili mediate its attachment to the mucosal epithelium.
   3. Disease—gonorrhea.
      a. The second most common sexually transmitted disease (STD) in the United States. (The most common STD in the United States is chlamydia.)
      b. Although it is commonly asymptomatic, symptoms include urethritis and genital infections.
      c. Consequences include pelvic inflammatory disease and sterility.
      d. Transmission of disease to infants can occur within the birth canal, causing severe ophthalmia that can lead to blindness.
G. *Prevotella.*
   1. General characteristics.
      a. Type species *melaninogenica.*
      b. Principally associated with the microbiome of the oral and vaginal flora.
      c. Strict anaerobe—found deeper rather than shallow within the gingiva and dental sulci.
      d. Rod-shaped.
      e. Bile sensitive.
      f. Saccharolytic.
      g. Pigmented or nonpigmented.
         (1) Type species *melaninogenica* is able to convert hemoglobin to melanin (black pigment).

(2) Evidence of its presence is easily visualized after dental extractions as a black tooth socket.

h. 15% produce a β-lactamase.

2. Role in disease.

a. Commonly associated with infections above the diaphragm.

b. Often associated with bacterially derived halitosis.

c. Often associated with mixed microbial infections.

d. May be associated with mixed anaerobic pneumonia as a consequence of aspiration.

e. May be associated with dental alveolar abscess.

3. Treatment.

a. Dependent on severity of disease, ranging from improvements to hygiene, analgesia, and antibiotics appropriately targeted against the microbes associated with the mixed infection.

G. *Porphyromonas.*

1. General characteristics.

a. Type species *gingivalis.*

b. Gram-negative nonmotile rod.

c. Strict anaerobe.

d. Forms black colonies when grown on solid surfaces.

e. Associated with periodontal disease and dental abscesses.

2. Virulence factors.

a. Gingipan, a protease secreted by *Porphyromonas. gingivalis* facilitates the degradation of cytokines, resulting in an amelioration of the immune response principally through reduced inflammation—play a key role in the collection of nutrients for the microbe and facilitates invasion and colonization of the host.

b. Capsular polysaccharide—capsule-containing strains are more virulent than acapsular forms of the microbe. The presence of the capsular antigen has been found to downregulate cytokine production, especially the proinflammatory cytokines IL-1β, IL-6, IL-8, and TNF-α.

c. Fimbriae—proteinaceous in nature; facilitate attachment. Members of this genus may have two types, long and short.

(1) Short fimbriae are involved in cell-cell adhesion with other dental commensals.

(2) Long fimbriae are long and peritrichous (cover the cell) and play a role in attachment and biofilm formation serving as adhesions to mediate invasion and colonization of host cells.

d. Type strain *Porphyromonas gingivalis* contains the enzyme peptidylarginine deiminase, which is involved in citrullination (a developmental amino acid remarkable for its ability to mediate the expression of genes, particularly in the developing embryo). Citrullination is also important because the presence of citrullinated proteins recruits a response from the immune system leading to the potential to develop autoimmune diseases such as rheumatoid arthritis and multiple sclerosis.

3. Role in disease.

a. The presence of *P. gingivalis* is of concern because there is evidence that it is a "keystone" bacterium in the onset of chronic adult periodontitis. Although its abundance may be low, its establishment and expression of its virulence factors result in a microbial shift of normal microbial flora resident within the oral cavity allowing for uncontrolled growth of the commensal microbial community. The net effect is periodontitis through the disruption of the host tissue homeostasis and adaptive immune response.

H. *Eikenella corrodens* (formerly *Bacteroides corrodens*).

1. General characteristics.

a. Fastidious Gram-negative facultative anaerobic pleomorphic rod.

b. Commensal of the human oral cavity and upper respiratory tract; may be associated with halitosis.

c. Unusual for it to cause an infection.

d. When isolated from infected individuals, most often associated with a mixed infection of facultative and strict anaerobes from the same niche.

2. Medical significance.

a. Infections caused by this microbe are common in the following individuals.

(1) Patients with head and neck cancer.

(2) Individuals with bite infections, especially, a reverse bite-clenched fist injury where the fist of the individual strikes the teeth on the person being punched resulting in broken skin and inoculation of the fist. Left untreated, the infection may damage the underlying tendons of the fighter's hand.

(3) Insulin-dependent diabetics and intravenous drug users who lick the needles before injection resulting in a syndrome termed "needle licker's" osteomyelitis.

(4) Individuals with one of the microbes associated with the HACEK group of microbes implicated in culture-negative endocarditis. The members of this group are considered normal flora of the oropharyngeal flora; they are slow growing, have a preference for an atmosphere enriched in carbon dioxide, and together are responsible for 5% to 10% of cases of infective endocarditis in native values of the heart. They are the most common Gram-negative microbes responsible for endocarditis

in individuals who *do not* use intravenous drugs (both ethical and illicit).

(a) HACEK group.

(i) *Haemophilus* (*Haemophilus parainfluenzae*, *Haemophilus aphrophilus*, *Haemophilus paraphrophilus*).

(ii) *Aggregatibacter* (formerly-*Actinobacillus*) *actinomycetemcomitans* [implicated in destructive periodontal disease], *Aggregatibacter aphrophilus*).

(iii) *Cardiobacterium hominis*.

(iv) *Eikenella corrodens*.

(v) *Kingella* (*Kingella kingae*).

b. Treatment.

(1) The drug of choice for HACEK-implicated endocarditis is a third-generation cephalosporin (ceftriaxone), ampillicin, or low-dose gentamicin.

I. *P. aeruginosa*.

1. General characteristics.

a. Strict aerobic motile (polar flagellum) rod. Type species *aeruginosa* is capable of using nitrate (NO_3^-) as an accessory terminal electron acceptor.

b. Oxidase-positive.

c. Commonly found in soil and water; member of normal skin flora.

d. Easily forms biofilms.

e. Virulence determinants are regulated through quorum sensing (cell-cell, population-dependent communication).

f. Surface traits—flagella, pili, slime layer.

g. Opportunistic pathogen. Infections are a problem for immunocompromised patients. Common infections include wound infections (especially in burn patients), urinary tract infections, pneumonia in cystic fibrosis patients, and septicemia.

h. Resistant to a large number of antibiotics.

2. Virulence factors.

a. Exotoxin A, causes ADP-ribosylation of eukaryotic elongation factor 2 (similar in mode of action to diphtheria toxin) resulting in the inhibition of protein synthesis in the affected eukaryotic cell.

b. Exotoxin S—toxin that is translocated into eukaryotic cells via type III bacterial protein secretion. The toxin has a dual function that affects two different Ras–guanosine triphosphate–binding proteins. (Ras refers to a class of small GTPase proteins.)

c. Ability to form biofilms.

d. Secretes an elastase.

e. Produces fluorescent pigments contained in metachromatic granules. Wounds infected with *P. aeruginosa* can display a bluish green color.

f. Nutritionally resilient; able to survive and use various chemicals as substrates, which makes it

difficult to eliminate these organisms from hospitals and clinics.

3. Disease.

a. Rarely responsible for disease, but under the proper circumstance and conditions, the type species *P. aeruginosa* adheres to tissue surfaces via its flagellum, pili, and exotoxin S where it replicates to an infectious critical mass resulting in the synthesis of additional virulence determinants via quorum sensing leading to further tissue damage and necrosis.

b. Treatment—challenging owing to resistance to many antibiotics. Aminoglycosides, quinolones, cephalosporins, antipseudomonal penicillins (e.g., carbenicillin, piperacillin), carbapenems, and monobactams have been shown to be effective. As with all antimicrobial therapy, it is important to determine sensitivity before long-term application of a specific antibiotic course.

J. Spirochetes.

1. General characteristics.

a. Strict anaerobe, spiral-shaped rod (spirochete) with an axial filament for motility.

b. Unable to culture with routine bacteriologic media.

c. Type species is *T. pallidum*.

2. Disease.

a. Syphilis.

(1) STD that occurs in three stages.

(a) Primary syphilis—an asymptomatic, firm ulcer, known as a *chancre*, forms at the site of the initial infection. The chancre resolves on its own and is infectious (contains viable microbes). Oral lesions may be present. They are most commonly seen on the lips, although they may also be present intraorally.

(b) Secondary syphilis—after a few months, the infection spreads, and signs of a systemic illness, such as fever, malaise, headache, musculoskeletal pain, and lymphadenopathy, are observed. Common signs include a diffuse maculopapular rash (notably on the palms and soles), papules on the skin or mucous membranes, and genital lesions (condylomata lata). These lesions are very infectious and resolve on their own.

(c) Tertiary syphilis—about one third of infected individuals who were never treated progress to this stage. Symptoms include the formation of granulomas (known as *gummas*), cardiovascular damage leading to heart failure or an atherosclerotic aneurysm of the ascending aorta, and CNS impairment.

(2) Treatment—antibiotic therapy. This microbe is sensitive to penicillin, but because other bacterial STDs (e.g., chlamydia and gonorrhea) are often transmitted together, the following antibiotic regimen is recommended for the treatment of syphilis.

(a) Azithromycin, 1 g orally in a single dose, *or*

(b) Ceftriaxone, 250 mg intramuscularly in a single dose, *or*

(c) Ciprofloxacin, 500 mg orally twice a day for 3 days (contraindicated for treating pregnant or lactating women), *or*

(d) Erythromycin, 500 mg orally three times a day for 7 days.

b. Congenital syphilis.

(1) Intrauterine transmission of the disease to infants can occur. This can lead to severe infection, birth defects, or death.

(2) Important signs and symptoms.

(a) Hutchinson's incisors of the anterior teeth and Mulberry molars of the posterior teeth.

(b) Deafness and blindness from interstitial keratitis.

c. Acute necrotizing ulcerative gingivitis.

(1) The oral treponemes in concert with oral streptococci and fusobacteria may lead to the development of acute necrotizing ulcerative gingivitis (see earlier discussion under *Fusobacterium*).

(2) Oral treponemes have also been associated with periodontal disease.

3. *Leptospira.*

a. An aerobic Gram-negative spirochete; the most common zoonotic disease.

(1) Acquired via ingestion of urine-contaminated (pets and rodents) fresh water.

(2) Commonly associated with swimmers who frequent exotic fresh water adventures.

(3) Also known as Weil's syndrome, canicola fever, canefield fever, nanukayami fever, seven-day fever, rat catcher's yellows, Fort Bragg fever, black jaundice, and pretibial fever.

b. Symptoms include high fever, severe headache, chills, muscle aches, and vomiting; may also result in jaundice, red eyes, abdominal pain, diarrhea, or rash.

c. Prevention and treatment.

(1) Doxycycline may be used as a prophylaxis (200 to 250 mg once per week) to prevent infection in high-risk areas or occupations.

(2) Therapeutic drug regimen is complex: doxycycline, 100 mg orally every 12 hours for 1 week, or penicillin, 1 to 1.5 MU every 4 hours for 1 week with the coincident normalization of the hydroelectrolytic balance. Dialysis may be used in serious cases.

4. *Borrelia burgdorferi*—Lyme disease.

a. Tick-borne (ixodid) disease, principally from the bite and deposition of the microbe from the nymph stage (90%) of the tick.

b. Spirochete; challenging to stain.

c. Complex life cycle with humans being an accidental host of what was formerly a zoonotic disease. The adult animal (deer or field mice) is infected by the tick, and nymph infects the human.

d. Widely distributed across the United States.

e. Disease.

(1) Stage 1—initial infection; development of a localized erythema migrans "bull's eye" rash that increases in diameter with time.

(2) Stage 2—dissemination of infection resulting in secondary erythema migrans lesions, neurologic abnormalities, lymphocytic meningitis, carditis, and acute arthritis.

(3) Stage 3—chronic meningitis or meningoencephalitis, encephalopathy, peripheral neuropathy, migratory polyarthritis, and acrodermatitis.

f. Diagnosis.

(1) Isolation and visualization of microbe is very difficult; silver stain and immunofluorescence indicated.

(2) Culture is possible requiring special medium with material recovered from the lesion, blood, or CSF.

(3) Serology.

(a) IgM conversion may not be apparent for 4 or more weeks after infection.

(b) IgG levels may not be sufficiently elevated for 6 to 8 weeks.

(c) Antibody results may be falsely negative very early in infection (on visualization of initial erythema migrans rash).

g. Treatment and prevention.

(1) Stage 1—tetracycline for 10 to 20 days.

(2) Stage 2 and 3—ceftriaxone by parenteral administration.

(3) No vaccine.

K. *Vibrio.*

1. General characteristics.

a. Facultative curved (comma-shaped), oxidase-positive, polarly flagellated marine-associated rod.

b. Number of species associated with food-borne and water-borne disease.

c. Distinct from other prokaryotes in that some species have two independent chromosomes (*V. cholerae*).

2. Disease.

a. *Vibrio* gastroenteritis (principally caused by *Vibrio parahaemolyticus*).

(1) Associated with consumption of raw or undercooked shellfish that results in GI illness within

24 hours of consumption of a sufficient concentration of contaminated seafood. Symptoms include diarrhea, abdominal cramping, headache, upset stomach, vomiting, chills, and fever. The condition generally is limited to approximately 3 days and with appropriate supportive rehydration is generally not severe enough to require hospitalization unless the infected person has a weakened immune system.

(2) *Vibrio vulnificus* in immunocompromised individuals and patients with liver disease or cancer can reach the bloodstream and result in a life-threatening infection (50% are fatal). The incubation period for *V. vulnificus* is 1 to 7 days. In addition to transmission by raw shellfish, *V. vulnificus* can enter the body via a wound when exposed to warm seawater.

b. Cholera (principally caused by toxin-producing strains of *V. cholerae*).

(1) During an infection of the small intestine, toxin-encoding strain secretes cholera toxin, which results in profound watery diarrhea and vomiting. Transmission occurs primarily from the ingestion of at least 100 million *V. cholerae* containing the toxin gene from fecally contaminated water.

(2) An untreated person with cholera may produce 10 to 20 L (3 to 5 gallons) of diarrhea per day.

(3) The term *rice-water diarrhea* is thought to derive from the milk-like opaque nature of the diarrheal fluid resulting from the discharge of sloughed mucus and immature intestinal epithelial cells (enterocytes).

(4) The cholera toxin is an oligomeric complex comprising six protein subunits similar in design to the classic A/B toxin model for bacterial exotoxins. The toxin (CTX or CT) has a single copy of the A subunit and five copies of the B subunit connected via a disulfide bond. The B subunits serve to bind to the GM_1 gangliosides on the surface of the intestinal epithelium cells. On entry into human cells, the A subunit causes permanent ADP-ribosylation of the G_s α subunit of the heterotrimeric G protein resulting in the constitutive expression of cyclic adenosine monophosphate, which leads to the hypersecretion of water, Na^+, K^+, Cl^-, and HCO_3^- into the lumen of the small intestine culminating in rapid dehydration.

(5) Treatment involves oral rehydration therapy generally with Ringer's lactate with added potassium and the continued consumption of food to facilitate recovery of the microbiome and digestive process. Antibiotic therapy (doxycycline) for 1 to 3 days may shorten the course of disease and reduce the severity of symptoms.

c. *V. vulnificus*.

(1) Organism 80 times more likely to spread into the bloodstream in people with immunocompromise, chronic liver disease, or disorders associated with higher iron loads.

(a) Mortality rates of 50% can occur.

(b) Principally acquired from ingestion of contaminated or raw seafood. Oysters harvested from the Gulf of Mexico are especially risky foods.

(2) Responsible for most deaths associated with seafood.

(3) Also results in aggressive, fulminant cellulitis on wound infection in at-risk populations. Wound infections have a 25% mortality. Treatment often involves aggressive resection (often amputation of the affected limb).

3.1.6. Role of Mixed Gram-Negative Infections in Periodontal Disease

Owing to the complexity of the microbiome associated with the human oral cavity, most infections occurring within this space comprise a mixture of bacteria, fungi, and occasionally single-cell protozoa that together result in the development of complex sequelae manifested by the normal physiology and expression of virulence determinants of the mixture of facultative anaerobes and strict anaerobes.

A. Etiology of periodontal disease—bacterial plaque.

1. Consists of 95% bacteria.

2. Bacterial types in supragingival plaque differ depending on diet and saliva composition. Diet and saliva do not affect the makeup of bacteria in subgingival plaque. Subgingival plaque consists mostly of rod-shaped, Gram-negative anaerobic bacteria and spirochetes.

B. Plaque and calculus formation—three phases.

1. Formation of a salivary pellicle—salivary glycoproteins coat the tooth surface, forming a pellicle. This allows plaque to stick to enamel (i.e., bacteria are able to colonize on the pellicle). Plaque usually develops within 24 hours.

2. Plaque maturation—organized bacteria colonization of the pellicle in the following order.

a. Gram-positive, cocci bacteria (mostly streptococci) colonize the pellicle first.

b. Dextrans produced from these bacteria form the structural component of plaque.

c. These bacteria are followed by Gram-negative, rod-shaped anaerobic bacteria, such as *Bacteroides*, *Fusobacterium*, *Porphyromonas*, and *Prevotella*, and finally by filament-type bacteria such as *Actinomyces*.

3. Plaque mineralization (calculus formation)—mineralization of plaque occurs when it becomes supersaturated with calcium and phosphates from saliva. It then mineralizes to form calculus.

3.1.7 Obligate Intracellular Parasites
3.1.7.1 Chlamydial and Rickettsial Organisms
A. *Chlamydia* bacteria.
  1. General characteristics.
     a. Although they are considered bacteria, they are obligate intracellular parasites (i.e., they rely on a host cell to grow and reproduce).
     b. Unique cell cycle—begins when the extracellular, sporelike elementary body enters the cell and transforms into a larger, metabolically active reticulate body. It then undergoes repeated binary fission to form daughter elementary bodies, which are released.
  2. *Chlamydia trachomatis.*
     a. Predominately invades mucous epithelial cells.
     b. Diseases—trachoma, genital infections, inclusion conjunctivitis.
     c. Most common STD in the United States.
     d. Although commonly asymptomatic, symptoms include nongonococcal urethritis, genital or respiratory infections, and conjunctivitis.
     e. Consequences include pelvic inflammatory disease, sterility, and salpingitis.
     f. Transmission of disease to infants can occur within the birth canal, causing inclusion conjunctivitis or pneumonia or both.
     g. Treatment—antibiotic therapy. Choices include sulfonamides, macrolides (azithromycin), and tetracycline.
  3. *Chlamydophila pneumoniae.*
     a. Obligate intracellular pathogen.
     b. Major cause of atypical "walking" pneumonia.
       (1) Elementary body is the principal infectious particle; it travels via droplet secretion from the lung of an infected individual to the lung of a naïve recipient.
          (a) Atypical pneumonia, in contrast to the form caused by streptococci, generally is thought to be milder. It does not generally manifest with the typical respiratory symptoms of lobar pneumonia but rather with more generalized flulike symptoms of fever, headache, and myalgia.
          (b) Treatment—macrolides and tetracyclines.
B. *Rickettsia* bacteria.
  1. General characteristics.
     a. Generally pleomorphic—may range from small cocci 0.1 μm in diameter to rods 1 to 4 μm in length.
     b. Obligate intracellular parasites; cannot be cultured on laboratory media.
     c. Gram-negative but difficult to stain.
     d. Disease transmission usually occurs via arthropod vectors such as ticks, lice, and fleas.
     e. Mainly invade vascular endothelium and smooth muscle cells, causing blood vessel inflammation and necrosis.
  2. *Rickettsia rickettsii*—causes Rocky Mountain spotted fever.
     a. Disease is transmitted by ticks and results in a hemorrhagic rash and hemorrhagic spots.
  3. *Rickettsia prowazekii.*
     a. Causes typhus fever. It is transmitted by lice. Depending on the severity of disease, symptoms can range from a mild rash to skin necrosis and internal organ hemorrhages.
     b. *R. prowazekii* can remain latent in the host and reemerge years later. This reactivation is also known as *recrudescent typhus* or *Brill-Zinsser disease.*
  4. Treatment with a course of tetracycline is generally successful for all forms of rickettsial disease.

3.2 Viruses
3.2.1 Viral Structure, Characteristics, and Life Cycle
A. Viruses are nonliving, replicating obligate intracellular parasites that are able to reproduce only on commandeering the nucleic acid and protein synthetic apparatus of a permissive host. Simply put, they are software, a set of instructions for the cell they infect to implement. Viruses are generally host-specific, have only one form of nucleic acid, are generally classified by the type of nucleic acid used to constitute their genome, and may manifest different pathologies when infecting other hosts (e.g., nonhuman hosts rarely mimic the same human pathology when infected with human-specific viruses). However, as with many things in biology, there are often exceptions to the rules; learning the exceptions helps to learn the rules.
  1. Viruses are smaller than all bacteria and pass through filters that retain bacteria. The exception to this rule is *Mimivirus*, which is a large double-stranded DNA virus with a capsid approximately 600 nm in size (coat of the virus) that is a parasite of *Acanthamoeba polyphaga.*
  2. Viruses are too small to be observed with a traditional light microscope. The resolution of the light microscope is approximately 0.2 μm; the exceptions to this rule are the above-mentioned *Mimivirus* (which stains Gram-positive) and poxviruses.
  3. Viruses contain only one type of nucleic acid, RNA or DNA. Poxviruses are the exception to this rule.
  4. Viruses that cause disease in diverse species are an exception, not the rule. The prominent exception to this rule is influenza A, which can infect mammals

Table 3-5

Main Virus Families and Their Characteristics

VIRUS	NUCLEIC ACID TYPE	STRANDEDNESS	NO. GENETIC SEGMENTS	POLARITY	ENVELOPE
Poxvirus	DNA	Double	1	N/A	No
Herpesvirus	DNA	Double	1	N/A	Yes
Adenovirus	DNA	Double	1	N/A	No
Papovavirus	DNA	Double	1	N/A	No
Hepadnavirus	DNA	Double*	1	N/A	Yes†
Parvovirus	DNA	Single	1	+ and −	No
Picornavirus	RNA	Single	1	+	No
Calicivirus	RNA	Single	1	+	No
Togavirus	RNA	Single	1	+	Yes
Flavivirus	RNA	Single	1	+	Yes
Coronavirus	RNA	Single	1	+	Yes
Retrovirus	RNA	Single‡	2§	+	Yes
Reovirus	RNA	Double¶	10, 11		No
Rhabdovirus	RNA	Single	1	−	Yes
Paramyxovirus	RNA	Single	1	−	Yes
Orthomyxovirus	RNA	Single	8	−	Yes
Arenavirus	RNA	Single	2	−	Yes

*Complex outer protein layer that some authors consider as an envelope.

†Protein-rich envelope.

‡Two identical (+) RNA strands; the genome can be considered single-stranded and consisting of two copies of the same segment.

§Two strands of DNA of unequal length.

¶Replicates as a (−) RNA virus

as diverse as dolphins and humans. Passage through different species influences virulence because replication often selects out an "offspring" with different attributes of virulence based on the requirements necessary for the replication of viral progeny.

5. The main virus families and characteristics that help with differentiation are summarized in Table 3-5.

B. Naked viruses—significantly more resistant to detergents, solvent-based disinfectants, and desiccation; can survive digestion.

C. Enveloped viruses—the viral envelope comes from the infected cell or host and covers the proteinaceous capsid. The lipid bilayer envelope renders the viruses sensitive to desiccation, heat, and detergents; these viruses are easier to sterilize than nonenveloped viruses, have limited survival outside host environments, and typically must transfer directly from host to host.

D. Not all viruses are the same size, and their morphology depends on their programming. Common shapes include icosahedral, helical, and pleomorphic and are not correlated with genome type, morphology, or the presence of a lipid bilayer envelope.

E. The stages of viral replication are attachment, entry, uncoating of the virus (optional), nucleic acid synthesis, virion production, and exit. Not all viruses kill the host; some chronically infect the host allowing their nucleic acid to be maintained by the host. This process is observed in prokaryotic viruses and is referred to as lysogeny; in eukaryotes, it is seen in retroviruses.

1. Viral association with the host is mediated by host-virus interactions generally in the form of a receptor ligand interaction. Mutations within the host or virus prevent infection. The receptor-virus interaction coordinates tissue tropism and ultimate pathology.

2. Viropexis, which refers to entry of the all naked viruses in mammalian cells, is accomplished by endocytosis, with the most common mechanism being mediated by clathrin-coated pits.

3. Enveloped viruses enter via fusion of the viral envelope with plasma membrane or endosomal vesicle membrane.

4. Progeny release is dependent on viral programming; naked viruses (e.g., poliovirus) are released by lysis, whereas enveloped viruses (HIV, herpesvirus) are

Table 3-6			
Viral Diseases with Oral Vesicles			
DISEASE	**VIRUS**	**EXANTHEM**	**ORAL ENANTHEM**
Hand-foot-and-mouth disease	Coxsackie A virus	Vesicles on palms and soles of feet	Herpangina
Herpes labialis	Herpes simplex virus	Localized painful vesicles	"Cold sores"
Chickenpox, shingles	Varicella zoster	Dermatome distribution	Dermatome distribution

released by budding from the plasma membrane or into vesicles that fuse with the plasma membrane.

3.2.2 Clinical Virology

A. Viral exanthem—operationally described as an eruptive disease or its symptomatic skin eruption (rash); generally caused by the inflammation of the skin. All exanthems and enanthems are late manifestations of a viral infection.
  1. Morbilliform is the prototype of a viral exanthema and is the type of rash caused by measles, which results in a blanchable erythematous macule (flat colored area of the skin <1 cm in diameter that generally does not include a change in skin texture or thickness) and papule (opposite of macule, which is a bump on the skin).
  2. Vesicles are a circumscribed fluid-containing elevation (5 to 10 mm) of the skin. Table 3-6 lists viruses that may manifest pathology with oral vesicles.
  3. A bulla is a large vesicle often rounded or irregularly shaped that contains serous or seropurulent fluid.
  4. Pruritic rash is a rash that results in an unpleasant sensation that generally leads to the urge to scratch (itching).
B. Viral enanthem—operationally described as an eruptive disease on a mucosal surface or its symptomatic eruption (open sore in the mouth). Measles results in the development of eruptive sores commonly referred to as Koplik's spots.
  1. Forcheimer's sign—an enanthem consisting of dull red petechiae on the soft palate. This lesion is seen in 20% of patients who contract German (three-day) measles.

3.2.3 DNA Viruses

A. Herpesvirus family (Herpesviridae).
  1. Herpesviruses are known to cause latent infections owing to integration of the genome within the host (recurrence of disease after a latent period).
  2. Basic virion structure—double-stranded DNA, a capsid, a glycoprotein envelope, and a nuclear membrane, which is obtained via budding. Note: herpesviruses derive their virion envelopes from the host nuclear membrane, not the host plasma membrane.
  3. They are usually acquired in childhood, and the initial infection may be asymptomatic.
  4. Herpes simplex virus (HSV) type 1.
    a. Primary herpetic gingivostomatitis.
      (1) Caused by initial exposure to HSV type 1.
      (2) Most often transmitted through saliva.
      (3) Usually occurs in children.
      (4) Symptoms include fever, malaise, and small ulcerations in the oral cavity; commonly asymptomatic.
    b. Acute herpetic gingivostomatitis.
      (1) Usually occurs in children.
      (2) Symptoms are more severe and painful than in primary herpetic gingivostomatitis. Numerous yellowish vesicles form and ulcerate within the oral cavity. The gingiva appears erythematous. Systemic symptoms include fever, malaise, irritability, and regional lymphadenopathy.
      (3) Adult recurrence.
        (a) After the primary infection, the virus remains latent in sensory nerve ganglia. Reactivation occurs at the site of initial infection or in adjacent areas innervated by the infected nerve.
        (b) The most common site of recurrence in adults is along the vermilion border of the lips, known as *herpes labialis* (cold sores). Infection of the eye (herpetic conjunctivitis) is also common.
    c. Treatment—acyclovir, a nucleoside analogue, is an example of a competitive inhibitor. It acts to inhibit viral DNA synthesis and replication. Clinically, it does not cure the disease but often decreases the duration of symptoms and amount of viral shedding.
  5. HSV type 2.
    a. Disease—genital herpes.
      (1) Genital herpes is an STD.
      (2) Symptoms begin as flulike symptoms, followed by severe genital itching and the formation of

painful vesicles that ulcerate. Infectious individuals may be asymptomatic.

    (3) Transmission of disease to infants can occur within the birth canal and may result in CNS impairment, conjunctivitis, or vesicle formation at the site of infection.

  b. Treatment—acyclovir.

6. Varicella-zoster virus (VZV).

  a. Disease—chickenpox is the primary disease; zoster (shingles) is the recurrent form.

    (1) Symptoms include a general vesicular rash. Infected children are highly contagious.

    (2) The administration of aspirin is contraindicated in this and in other childhood viral infections. Aspirin given to infected children increases the incidence of Reye's syndrome, which can cause encephalitis and liver impairment.

    (3) VZV remains latent in the dorsal spinal ganglia. Reactivation of the disease, known as *zoster*, usually occurs at times of reduced immunity. It travels along the dermatome of the infected nerve.

    (4) Treatment—acyclovir or famciclovir.

    (5) Vaccine—live, attenuated virus.

7. Epstein-Barr virus (EBV).

  a. Diseases.

    (1) Mononucleosis ("kissing disease").

      (a) Transmitted through saliva.

      (b) Infects B cells and can remain latent in them after symptoms have resolved.

      (c) Symptoms include pharyngitis, fever, lymphadenopathy, and lethargy. Splenomegaly may also occur. Spontaneous recovery usually occurs in 2 to 3 weeks.

      (d) Laboratory findings include lymphocytosis and the presence of atypical T lymphocytes and heterophile antibodies.

    (2) Burkitt's lymphoma and a B-cell lymphoma that usually occurs in Africa.

      (a) Affects the posterior maxilla or mandible or both.

      (b) Histologic evaluation reveals a characteristic "starry-sky" appearance.

    (3) Hairy leukoplakia—manifests as white, hyperkeratotic lesions found on the tongue; most often seen in immunocompromised patients.

    (4) Nasopharyngeal carcinoma.

8. Cytomegalovirus (CMV), also known as human herpesvirus (HHV) 5.

  a. Most CMV infections are asymptomatic in healthy individuals. Symptomatic CMV infections are commonly seen in immunocompromised patients.

  b. Symptoms may include mononucleosislike symptoms.

  c. CMV can remain latent in lymphocytes or salivary glands cells.

  d. Treatment—ganciclovir or foscarnet, for severe infections in patients with AIDS.

9. HHV 8.

  a. Disease—Kaposi's sarcoma.

    (1) Malignant tumor that mainly affects immunocompromised patients. It is more commonly found in Africa.

    (2) Signs and symptoms include plaquelike or nodular skin and oral lesions. Internal organs also may be affected.

10. Table 3-7 presents a comparison of the relevant clinical features, mode of transmission, site of latency, and ability to cause cancer by the various HHVs.

B. Poxvirus family (Poxviridae).

1. Basic virion structure—double-stranded DNA, a capsid, and envelope.

2. One of the largest and most complex viruses known.

3. Poxviruses.

  a. Smallpox virus (variola virus)—causes smallpox. This is the only disease that has been completely eradicated from the globe as a result of vaccination; frozen stocks remain within few countries (nation state stockpiles). Vaccinia is the strain of poxvirus from which the smallpox vaccine was developed. Members of the military and some health care workers are still vaccinated for smallpox despite its eradication. Vaccination is principally accomplished by scarification. The resulting papule is infectious, and care should be taken to avoid spread among naïve individuals.

  b. Cowpox and monkeypox—principally zoonotic diseases.

  c. Parapoxviruses.

  d. Molluscipoxviruses.

    (1) Molluscum contagiosum—commonly referred to as water warts. This virus is spread person to person or via a fomite (generally contaminated towels, blankets, and toys) contaminated with the virus. There is no known animal reservoir. Common viral disease has a higher incidence in children 1 to 10 years old. Molluscum contagiosum can affect any area of the skin but is most common on the trunk, arms, groin, and legs. It is contagious until the lesions (bumps) are gone. If untreated, some growths may remain for 4 years.

    (2) Treatment.

      (a) Astringent agents (potassium hydrochloride and cantharidin) applied to the surface of the lesion.

      (b) Liquid nitrogen.

      (c) Surgical resection.

Table 3-7

Summary of Human Herpesviruses

VIRUS	CLINICAL FEATURES	SITE OF LATENCY	CAUSES CANCER	MEANS OF SPREAD
HSV 1 and 2	Cold sores, genital herpes*	Nerve ganglia	No	Close contact
VZV	Chickenpox, shingles*	Nerve ganglia	No	Close contact, respiratory
CMV	Mononucleosislike illness, pneumonia, retinitis, birth defects	Monocytes, lymphocytes	Not clear	Saliva, transplacental, tissue grafts
EBV	Mononucleosis	B cells	Burkitt's lymphoma	Saliva
HHV 6 and HHV 7	Roseola infantum, exanthem subitum	T cells	No	Saliva
HHV 8, KSHV	Usually none at acquisition	B cells	Kaposi's sarcoma	Saliva

CMV, Cytomegalovirus; *EBV,* Epstein-Barr virus; *HSV,* herpes simplex virus; *HHV,* human herpesvirus; *KSHV,* Kaposi sarcoma–associated herpesvirus; *VZV,* varicella-zoster virus.

*shingles-Same virus, VSV, results in two different clinical sequalae. Vesicular lesions on the skin often associated with the primary infection in children and a rash in one or two adjacent dermatomes.

C. Adenovirus family (Adenoviridae).
   1. Basic virion structure—double-stranded DNA and a capsid surrounded by fibers, which aid in its attachment to the host cell.
   2. Disease characteristics.
      a. Multiple routes of infection.
      b. Usually mild disease but can be serious.
         (1) Respiratory illnesses (especially in children).
         (2) Conjunctivitis (most common cause of pink eye).
         (3) Pharyngitis.
      c. Viremia and seeding of distant sites may occur.
      d. Persistence with viral shedding often seen in lymphoid tissues for 6 to 18 months without evident disease.
      e. Latency is rare (integration of genome), but when it occurs, disease persists for years.
D. Papovavirus family (Papovaviridae).
   1. Basic virion structure—double-stranded, circular DNA and a capsid.
E. Papillomavirus family (Papillomaviridae)—human papillomavirus (HPV).
   1. Basic virion structure—double-stranded, circular DNA and a capsid; large group of more than 150 related viruses. More than 40 viral subtypes are spread via direct skin-to-skin contact as a consequence of vaginal, anal, or oral sexual acts.
   2. Diseases—papillomas, warts, cervical cancer, and penile cancer. There is an association with head and neck cancer.
   3. STD—Low-risk HPV or high-risk HPV.
   4. Low-risk HPV viral types do not cause cancer but can cause skin lesions (warts) on or around the genitals or anus (e.g., HPV 6 and HPV 11 cause >90% of genital warts).
   5. High-risk HPV or oncogenic HPV can cause cancer. At the present time, there are at least 12 viral types. HPV 16 and HPV 18 are responsible most HPV-related cancers (cervix, anus, oropharyngeal, penis, vulva, and vagina).
   6. More recent evidence indicates high-risk HPV may be associated with oropharyngeal cancer.
   7. Treatment of warts and early carcinomas—surgical elimination or destruction via the application of liquid nitrogen or acid (pyruvic).
   8. Cancer is thought to occur as a consequence of the integration of the high-risk HPV genome of HPV 16 or HPV 18 into the basal layers of the epithelium layer of the affected tissue. On entry, the virus synthesizes proteins. two of which (E6 and E7) interfere with normal cell function facilitating uncontrolled growth of the infected cells within the tissue.
   9. Approximately 50% of high-risk cervical lesions progress to cancer. The process of tumor development takes 10 to 20 years.
   10. Because HPV is not thought to be transmitted hematogenously, having an HPV in one part of the body should not result in infection of another tissue.
   11. The vaccine is based on HPV proteins. Proteins are used to make viruslike particles that correspond to HPV types 6, 11, 16, and 18 or HPV 16 and HPV 18.
   12. Epidemiology.
      a. Extremely common in men and women, likely ubiquitously distributed among the human population.
      b. At any given time, 50% of sexually active women and men are positive by genital swab.

c. Younger women (<25 years old) are less likely to clear the virus from the cervix.

d. Transmission is common among vaginally delivered children.

e. Specimens obtained from the oral cavity demonstrate that 25% of children younger than 5 years old are positive for HPV.

f. Vaccine—two FDA-approved vaccines are available for the prevention of cervical cancer. Vaccines are administered as three separate injections over 6 months.

g. Gardasil (Merck) quadrivalent—protects viral types against HPV types 6, 11, 16, and 18.

h. Cervarix (GlaxoSmithKline) divalent—protects against HPV types 16 and 18.

i. Recommended by the U.S. Centers for Disease Control and Prevention (CDC) for males and females before first sexual encounter or ages 11 to 26.

j. By 2020, as a consequence of vaccination, HPV will be responsible for more oropharyngeal cancers than cervical cancers in the United States.

F. Human parvovirus B19 (*Erythrovirus*)—erythema infectiosum (also called fifth disease).

1. Very small, naked single-stranded DNA virus.

2. Spread via respiratory secretions.

3. Usually mild illness with fever, malaise, and itching.

4. Exanthem is called *erythema infectiosum*, which resembles a "slapped cheek" appearance.

5. Facial erythema spreads to become a lacy rash on the rest of the body.

6. Mild in immunocompetent children.

7. Complications in adults include arthropathy in 50% of those infected with a long duration.

8. Generalized lymphadenopathy and splenomegaly.

9. Rash and joint symptoms likely attributed to immune complex deposition.

3.2.4 RNA Viruses

A. Orthomyxovirus family (Orthomyxoviridae).

1. Influenza virus.

a. Basic virion structure—single-stranded RNA, capsid, and envelope; also contains an RNA-dependent RNA polymerase.

b. Envelope—covered with spikes or peplomers. The peplomers contribute to pathogenicity and can be used for identification purposes. The spikes consist of two proteins, neuraminidase (which aids in the attachment to host cell via specific receptors) and hemagglutinin (which causes the agglutination of RBCs).

c. Influenza viruses are known to show small or large changes in the antigenicity of their hemagglutinin and neuraminidase proteins (i.e., undergo antigenic change), which sometimes can result in a new strain of virus. This property contributes to their capacity to cause devastating epidemics.

d. Influenza can be classified as influenza A, B, or C.

e. Short incubation period—48 hours. An infected patient is able to spread virus approximately 24 hours before the onset of symptoms. The virus is principally transmitted by droplet secretion (coughing and sneezing) and through the handling of contaminated fomites. Virus may remain viable for prolonged periods in the environment.

f. Disease—flu. Principal symptoms include fever, malaise, extreme lethargy (too tired to text), and muscle aches with occasional GI symptoms.

(1) Severe consequences of a flu infection.

(a) Reye's syndrome—a rare but serious reaction that can lead to encephalitis and liver impairment. Aspirin given to children with flulike symptoms increases the incidence of Reye's syndrome.

(b) May also lead to meningitis in young children.

(2) Treatment.

(a) Oseltamivir—oral antiviral that may slow the spread of influenza between cells in the body. Found to be active against influenza A or B. Mechanism of action is through inhibition of neuraminidase, which prevents viral budding from the infected cell. It is recommended that for the drug to limit the course of disease that it be administered within the first 2 days of symptoms.

(b) Amantadine and rimantadine—act to prevent viral replication and are effective only against influenza A. Their effects are greater when given prophylactically, but they can also be administered for treatment.

(3) Vaccine—killed virus, usually consisting of two to three A strains and one B strain.

g. Table 3-8 presents a summary of viruses responsible for influenza.

B. Paramyxovirus family (Paramyxoviridae).

1. Basic virion structure—single-stranded negative RNA, helical nucleocapsid; no icosahedral capsid, enveloped.

2. Contain an RNA-dependent RNA polymerase.

3. General structures resemble the structure of orthomyxoviruses except that they are usually larger in size, have different surface proteins, and have nonsegmented genomes.

4. Measles virus.

a. Disease—measles (rubeola).

b. Transmitted via respiratory droplets.

c. Symptoms—infection begins with flulike symptoms. Koplik's spots (bright erythematous patches with a white, central dot surrounded by bluish

Table 3-8

Influenza Viruses

FEATURE	INFLUENZA A	INFLUENZA B	INFLUENZA C
Genetic segments	8	8	7
Unique proteins	M2	NB	HEF
Host range	Humans, pigs, birds, horses, marine mammals	Humans only	Humans only
Disease severity	Often severe	Occasionally severe	Usually mild
Epidemic potential	Extensive (antigenic shift and drift)	Possible (antigenic drift only)	Limited (antigenic drift only)

Table 3-9

Comparison of Disease Type Mediated by Orthomyxoviruses and Paramyxoviruses

VIRUS	GENERAL CHARACTERISTICS	DISEASE
Influenza A, B, C	Orthomyxovirus Plurisegmented SS(−) RNA genome, enveloped Hemagglutinins and neuraminidase inserted in envelope Nuclear replication	Viral influenza
Parainfluenza virus, types 1-3	Paramyxovirus Monosegmented SS(−) RNA genome, enveloped H and F proteins in envelope Replication in cytoplasm	Common cold Croup Bronchiolitis Pneumonia
Respiratory syncytial virus	Paramyxovirus Monosegmented SS(−) RNA genome, enveloped Combination H-N and F in envelope Replication in cytoplasm	Common cold Bronchiolitis Tracheobronchitis Pneumonia

rings) appear along the buccal mucosa and are virtually diagnostic of the disease. A maculopapular rash follows, covering most of the body.

    d. Vaccine—live, attenuated virus that is part of the measles, mumps, and rubella (MMR) vaccine.

  5. Mumps virus.

    a. Disease—mumps.

    b. Transmitted via respiratory droplets.

    c. Symptoms—infection begins with flulike symptoms followed by infection and swelling of the salivary glands, with the parotid gland most commonly affected. Orchitis, or testicular inflammation, may be present in males.

    d. Consequences include orchitis (testicular inflammation) in postpubertal males. If bilateral, sterility may occur. Meningitis and loss of hearing may occur in children.

    e. Vaccine—live, attenuated virus that is part of the MMR vaccine.

  6. Respiratory syncytial virus (RSV).

    a. Virion surface proteins cause infected cells to fuse (syncytium).

    b. Diseases—RSV is a major cause of lower respiratory infections, including pneumonia and bronchiolitis, in infants.

    (1) Incubation period—2 to 4 days.

    (2) Onset is rhinitis followed by coughing, wheezing, and possible respiratory distress.

      (a) Manifests as a common cold in older children and adults.

      (b) Symptoms in children younger than 1 year old and frail elderly adults include bronchiolitis and pneumonia, listlessness, poor appetite, and atelectasis.

      (c) Fever is variable.

      (d) Prevention—via hygiene and limiting exposure to at-risk populations.

      (e) Treatment—none or ribavirin by aerosol for severe disease.

  7. Parainfluenza viruses.

    a. Diseases—second most common cause of viral respiratory infections, including croup, in children.

  8. Table 3-9 compares orthomyxoviruses and paramyxoviruses.

C. Togavirus family (Togaviridae).
1. Basic virion structure—single-stranded RNA, a capsid, and an envelope with surface proteins, including hemagglutinin.
2. Rubella virus.
   a. Disease—rubella (German measles).
   b. Transmitted via respiratory droplets.
   c. Symptoms—infection begins with flulike symptoms and lymphadenopathy, followed by a rash that progressively spreads from the head and neck to the rest of the body.
   d. Transmission of disease from an infected mother to her fetus can cause birth defects, including heart disease, cataracts, deafness, and brain impairments.
D. Picornavirus family (Picornaviridae).
1. Basic virion structure—single-stranded positive RNA, icosahedral capsid. No envelope is present.
2. Rhinoviruses—cause of the common cold.
   a. More than 115 serotypes.
   b. Very similar to enteroviruses except acid labile and replicate best at 33°C.
   c. Lower temperature typical of nasal epithelium.
   d. Host cell receptor is intracellular adhesion molecule 1.
   e. Lower respiratory infections rare.
   f. Cell injury minimal.
   g. Principal symptoms facilitated by bradykinin production.
   h. Not completely benign—increasing evidence suggests rhinoviruses are the number one cause of acute asthma exacerbations. Repeated rhinoviral infections during childhood have been associated with an increased risk of developing asthma.
3. Poliovirus.
   a. Transmission—fecal-oral route.
   b. Disease—poliomyelitis.
   (1) Symptoms of polio range from completely asymptomatic to CNS impairment leading to paralysis. Note: the virus preferentially replicates in the motoneurons of the anterior horn of the spinal cord; the death of those cells leads to muscle paralysis.
   (2) As a result of successful vaccinations, outbreaks rarely occur in the Western world.
   (3) Two vaccines are available.
      (a) Salk vaccine—consists of a killed virus that is given intravenously.
      (b) Sabin vaccine—consists of a live, attenuated virus that is administered orally.
4. Hepatitis A—discussed later in the hepatitis viruses section.
5. Coxsackievirus (group A and group B).
   a. Basic virion structure—double-stranded RNA and a capsid; also contains an RNA polymerase.
   b. Diseases caused by coxsackievirus A.
   (1) Herpangina ("summer illness")—manifests with intraoral ulcerating vesicles that are seen only in the posterior portion of the oral cavity, including the uvula, anterior pillars, oropharynx, and soft palate. Symptoms also include fever and sore throat.
   (2) Hand-foot-and-oral disease—vesicles, similar to vesicles seen in herpangina, are seen on the oral mucosa or tongue and are not limited to the posterior portion of the oral cavity. Vesicles are also found on the hands and feet.
   c. Diseases caused by coxsackievirus B.
   (1) Pleurodynia, myocarditis, and pericarditis.
6. Enteroviruses—nonpolio enteroviruses are second only to rhinoviruses as the most common viral infections in humans. There are an estimated 10 to 15 million symptomatic infections per year. Transmission is principally fecal-oral through the consumption of contaminated water or food, via direct human contact, or via the handling of a fomite (inanimate object containing a sufficient infectious dose of virus that is subsequently self-introduced). Enteroviruses can cause various diseases and manifestations (Table 3-10).

Table 3-10

Clinical Sequelae Associated with Enterovirus Infections

SYNDROME	COXSACKIE A	COXSACKIE B	ECHOVIRUS, PARECHOVIRUS, ENTEROVIRUS	POLIOVIRUS
Aseptic meningitis, encephalitis	+	+++	+++	++
Paralysis	+	−	+	+++
Exanthems, enanthems	+++	−	+++	−
Pericarditis, myocarditis	−	+++	−	−
Epidemic myalgia	−	+++	−	−
Conjunctivitis	++	−	++	−
Newborn disease	−	+++	−	−

F. HIV.
1. Part of the Retroviridae family (i.e., it is a retrovirus).
2. Basic virion structure.
   a. The nucleocapsid contains single-stranded RNA and three enzymes, reverse transcriptase, integrase, and protease.
   b. Exterior consists of two glycoproteins, gp120 and gp41, which are embedded in the lipid bilayer. This lipid bilayer was obtained from the host cell via budding.
3. Virion characteristics.
   a. HIV genome.
      (1) *gag* gene—codes for core proteins.
      (2) *pol* gene—codes for its three enzymes.
      (3) *env* gene—codes for its two envelope glycoproteins.
   b. HIV enzymes.
      (1) Reverse transcriptase—reverse transcription of RNA to viral DNA.
      (2) Integrase—responsible for integrating viral DNA into host DNA.
      (3) Protease—responsible for cleaving precursor proteins.
4. Pathogenicity.
   a. HIV mainly infects CD4 lymphocytes, or helper T cells. Its envelope protein, gp120, binds specifically with CD4 surface receptors. After entry, viral RNA is transcribed by reverse transcriptase to viral DNA and integrated into the host DNA. New virions are synthesized and released by lysis of the host cell.
   b. The predominant site of HIV replication is lymphoid tissues.
   c. Although HIV mainly infects CD4 helper T cells, it can bind to any cell with a CD4 receptor, including macrophages, monocytes, lymph node dendritic cells, and a selected number of nerve cells. Macrophages are the first cells infected by HIV.
5. HIV infection versus AIDS.
   a. An HIV-infected person has AIDS when he or she has one of the following conditions.
      (1) CD4 lymphocyte count of less than 200.
      (2) The person is infected with an opportunistic infection or other AIDS-defining illness, including, but not limited to, TB, recurrent pneumonia infections, or invasive cervical cancer.
   b. The cause of death in a patient with AIDS is most likely due to an opportunistic infection.
6. Common opportunistic infections associated with AIDS.
   a. Pneumonia caused by *Pneumocystis jiroveci* (formerly *Pneumocystis carinii*).
   b. TB.
   c. Periodontal disease—severe gingivitis, periodontitis, acute necrotizing ulcerative gingivitis, necrotizing stomatitis.
   d. Candidiasis.
   e. Oral hairy leukoplakia (EBV).
   f. Kaposi's sarcoma (HHV 8).
   g. Recurrent VZV infections.
   h. Condyloma acuminatum or verruca vulgaris (warts, HPV)—less common.
   i. CMV infections.
   j. Disseminated herpes simplex, herpes zoster.
   k. Hodgkin's lymphoma and non-Hodgkin's lymphoma.
7. Laboratory diagnosis of HIV.
   a. Enzyme-linked immunosorbent assay (ELISA) test—detects HIV antibodies. False-negative results can occur.
   b. Western blot—detects HIV proteins. There is a 99% accuracy rate when both the ELISA test and Western blot are used to diagnose HIV infection.
   c. Polymerase chain reaction—more sensitive; can amplify and identify the virus at an early stage.
8. Treatment.
   a. Inhibitors of reverse transcriptase.
      (1) Nucleoside analogues.
         (a) Inhibit viral replication via competitive inhibition.
         (b) Examples: zidovudine (AZT), didanosine, lamivudine, stavudine.
      (2) Nonnucleoside inhibitors.
         (a) Act by binding directly to reverse transcriptase.
         (b) Examples: nevirapine, delavirdine.
   b. Protease inhibitor.
   c. "Triple cocktail" therapy—often consists of two nucleoside inhibitors and a protease inhibitor.
G. Hepatitis viruses—this group of viruses (different types) is so named for the principal clinical presentation, which is an inflammation of the liver, or hepatitis.
1. General characteristics of hepatitis.
   a. The general presentation of hepatitis is the same regardless of the infecting virus; however, the time and severity of symptoms may differ.
   b. Symptoms of hepatitis include fever, anorexia, malaise, nausea, jaundice, and brown-colored urine.
   c. Complications of hepatitis infection include cirrhosis, liver failure, and hepatorenal failure.
   d. A summary of these viruses is shown in Table 3-11.
2. Hepatitis A virus.
   a. Symptoms last 2 to 4 weeks.
   b. There is no risk of developing chronic hepatitis in the future.
   c. Incubation period—2 to 6 weeks.
   d. Laboratory diagnosis—ELISA test for IgM antibody.
   e. Vaccine—killed virus.
   f. Prevention—serum immunoglobulins are available.

Table 3-11

Summary of Hepatitis Viruses

	GENOME	FAMILY	TRANSMISSION
Hepatitis A	ssRNA	Picornavirus	Oral-anal
Hepatitis B	dsDNA	Hepadnavirus	Sexual contact Blood (needles) Perinatal
Hepatitis C	ssRNA	Flavivirus	Sexual contact Blood (needles)
Hepatitis D	ssRNA	Deltavirus	Sexual contact Blood (needles)
Hepatitis E	ssRNA	Calicivirus	Oral-anal

ssRNA, Single-stranded RNA, *dsDNA*, double-stranded DNA.

3. Hepatitis B virus ("serum hepatitis").
  a. Symptoms last 2 to 4 weeks, but patients may be asymptomatic.
  b. Incubation period—ranges from 4 to 26 weeks; averages 6 to 8 weeks.
  c. The hepatitis B viral structure has also been named the *Dane particle*.
  d. Infection increases the risk for hepatocellular carcinoma.
  e. Laboratory assay of hepatitis B antigens and antibodies.
    (1) Hepatitis B surface antigen (HBsAg)—present only in acute infection or chronic carriers.
    (2) Hepatitis B surface antibody (HBsAb)—detectable only 6 months after initial infection. HBsAb is present in chronic infections or vaccinated individuals. Note: HBsAb is also produced during acute infections and in chronic carriers; however, it is not detectable via current laboratory methods.
    (3) Hepatitis B core antigen (HBcAg)—present in either acute or chronic infection.
    (4) Hepatitis B e antigen (HBeAg)—present when there is active viral replication. It signifies that the carrier is highly infectious.
    (5) Hepatitis B e antibody (HBeAb)—appears after HBeAg. It signifies that the individual is not as contagious.
  f. Vaccine—contains HBsAg.
  g. Prevention—immunoglobulins (HBsAb) are available.
4. Hepatitis C virus.
  a. Causes 90% of blood transfusion–related hepatitis.
  b. 50% progress to chronic disease.
  c. Increased risk for hepatocellular carcinoma.
  d. Incubation period—ranges from 2 to 26 weeks; averages 8 weeks.
  e. Treatment and prevention—α-interferon is used to treat chronic hepatitis C. No vaccine is available at the present time.
5. Hepatitis D virus—can infect only cells previously infected with hepatitis B.
6. Hepatitis E virus—high mortality rate in infected pregnant women.

3.2.5 Viruses of Diarrhea

A. Types of viruses that mediate diarrhea.
  1. Rotaviruses—most common cause of gastroenteritis in children, which is commonly known as winter gastroenteritis in children younger than 2 years.
    a. Group A rotaviruses cause the majority of the morbidity and mortality in children.
    b. Introduction of vaccines has reduced disease burden by 60% to 70% in developed countries.
    c. Group B rotaviruses cause sporadic but large outbreaks in adults (Adult Rotavirus (ADRV).
    d. Group C rotaviruses result in mild disease in children.
    e. A DNA virus.
  2. Caliciviruses (a RNA virus).
  3. Astroviruses (a RNA virus).
  4. Enteric adenovirus (DNA virus).
    a. Brief incubation periods.
    b. Fecal-oral spread via contaminated food, water, and fomites.
    c. Occurrence of vomiting preceding or with onset of diarrhea—generally termed *acute gastroenteritis*.
  5. Table 3-12 summarizes differentiating characteristics of viruses implicated in diarrhea.

3.2.6 Disease-Causing Viruses and Comparisons

A. Top four viruses that cause respiratory disease in children.
  1. RSV—most common.
  2. Parainfluenza.

Table 3-12

Differentiating Characteristics of Viruses Implicated in Diarrhea

	ROTAVIRUSES	CALICIVIRUSES	ASTROVIRUSES	ENTERIC ADENOVIRUSES
Genome	11 dsRNA segments	ssRNA	ssRNA	dsDNA
Capsid	Naked, double-shelled	Naked, round	Naked, star-shaped	Naked, icosahedral with spikes
Cell culture?	Usually incomplete	No	No	Incomplete
Serotypes	5 in humans	>4	At least 8	Unknown
Site of infection	Duodenum and jejunum	Jejunum	Small intestine	Small intestine
Epidemicity	Epidemic or sporadic	Family, community outbreaks	Sporadic	Sporadic
Ages usually affected	1-24 mo	Older children and adults	Infants, children	Infants, children
Incubation period	1-3 days	0.5-2 days	1-2 days	8-10 days
Duration of diarrhea	4-8 days	1-2 days	3-4 days	7-14 days
Duration of vomiting	1-3 days	1-2 days	3-4 days	7-14 days

dsDNA, Double-stranded DNA; *dsRNA*, double-stranded RNA; *ssRNA*, single-stranded RNA.

3. Rhinovirus.
4. Adenovirus.
B. Common viral causes of pharyngitis.
  1. Coxsackievirus.
  2. Adenovirus.
  3. Picornaviruses.
  4. Orthomyxoviruses.
  5. EBV.
C. Leading causes of meningitis.
  1. *E. coli*—in neonates.
  2. *H. influenzae*—in infants and children.
  3. *N. meningitidis*—in young adults.
  4. *S. pneumoniae*—in older adults.
  5. *L. monocytogenes*—in patients with cancer and immunocompromised individuals.
D. Common causes of nosocomial infections.
  1. *E. coli*.
  2. *S. aureus* and *Staphylococcus epidermidis*.
  3. *Streptococcus faecalis*.
  4. *P. aeruginosa*.
  5. *K. pneumoniae*
  6. *Enterobacter* species.
  7. *Candida* species.
E. Microorganisms that can infect the fetus of an infected mother.
  1. Rubella.
  2. Herpes.
  3. HIV.
  4. Syphilis.
  5. Toxoplasmosis.
  6. CMV.
F. Viral infections that can manifest as swellings in the neck (Table 3-13).

Table 3-13

Viral Infections Manifesting as Swellings of the Neck

VIRUS	VIRUS FAMILY	ETIOLOGY OF SWELLING
Mumps virus	Paramyxoviruses (ssRNA)	Inflammatory infiltrates as a result of cellular necrosis
Human papillomavirus	Papillomaviruses	Tumor formation (usually oropharyngeal region)
Epstein-Barr virus	Herpesviruses	Lymphadenopathy or tumor formation (Burkitt's lymphoma)
Cytomegalovirus	Herpesviruses	Lymphadenopathy
Herpes simplex virus	Herpesviruses	Lymphadenopathy

ssRNA, Single-stranded RNA.

G. Viruses that result in fever and coryza (runny nose) (Table 3-14).
H. Viruses that manifest with fever and altered mental status (Table 3-15).
I. Viruses implicated in gastroenteritis and diarrhea (Table 3-16).
J. Viruses and pregnancy (Table 3-17).
K. Differential guide to diarrhea (Table 3-18).

Table 3-14	
Viral Infections Manifesting as Fever and Coryza	
VIRUS	**DISEASE**
Adenoviruses	Common cold, conjunctivitis
Rhinoviruses	Common cold
Coronaviruses	Common cold, SARS
Orthomyxoviruses	Influenza (flu)
Paramyxoviruses	Measles, mumps, RSV, parainfluenza
Parvovirus B19	Erythema infectiosum, hydrops fetalis
Human herpesvirus 6 and 7	Roseola infantum

RSV, Respiratory syncytial virus; *SARS,* severe acute respiratory syndrome.

Table 3-15	
Viral Infections Manifesting with Fever and Altered Mental Status	
VIRUS	**DISEASE**
Herpes simplex virus	Herpes encephalitis
Enteroviruses	Aseptic (viral) meningitis
Flaviviruses	West Nile, yellow fever, hepatitis C, Dengue fever
Rhabdoviruses	Rabies
Filoviruses	Ebola and Marburg
Bunyavirus,	Crimean-Congo hemorrhagic fever virus, Rift Valley Fever Virus, **Hantavirus** Pulmonary Syndrome (4 Corners Disease)
Arenavirus	Lymphocytic choriomeningitis virus (LCMV)-found to be a cause of aseptic (nonbacterial) meningitis
JC virus	PML

PML, Progressive multifocal leukoencephalopathy.

Table 3-16	
Viral Infections Manifesting as Gastroenteritis with Diarrhea	
VIRUS	**FEATURE**
Rotavirus	Reovirus family
Caliciviruses	Includes norovirus
Enteric adenoviruses	Long persistence
Astroviruses	Little known
Hepatitis A	No diarrhea—nausea and jaundice

Table 3-17	
Viral Infections Resulting in Abnormalities in Pregnancy	
VIRUS	**SYNDROME IN PREGNANCY**
Herpes simplex	Neonatal infection can be fatal (neuroinvasive disease)
Cytomegalovirus	Birth defects including deafness, mental retardation
Varicella zoster	Neonatal infection can be fatal (neuroinvasive disease)
Parvovirus B19	Miscarriage, severe anemia, hydrops fetalis
Rubella (*Rubivirus*)	Congenital rubella syndrome
Hepatitis B	Congenital or neonatal infection
HIV	Congenital or neonatal infection

L. Differential guide to common food poisoning—each year in the United States, approximately 77 million people contract some form of food poisoning. Most cases are self-limiting and can be managed with oral rehydration using an over-the-counter beverage with sufficient electrolytes (e.g., Gatorade™). Table 3-19 presents the various bacteria and parasites with their common presentations and associated foods. Viruses have been intentionally eliminated, not because they cannot cause GI illness but because many of them do not have a GI symptom associated with infection.

3.3 Vaccines

A. Bacterial vaccines.
   1. Active immunity—vaccines that contain killed bacteria or inactive bacterial products, such as capsular polysaccharides, toxoids, or purified proteins.
   2. Passive immunity—vaccines that contain preformed immunoglobulins or antitoxins; can be used for either the treatment or the prevention of certain bacterial diseases.
   3. Bacterial vaccines are summarized in Table 3-20.
B. Viral vaccines.
   1. Active immunity—vaccines that contain live, attenuated viruses; killed viruses; or viral products such as surface antigens. Compared with the other vaccines, immunity from live virus vaccines usually lasts longer.
   2. Passive immunity—vaccines that contain preformed immunoglobulins.
   3. Viral vaccines are summarized in Table 3-21.

3.4 Prions

Although prions are not considered to be microbes and are currently under investigation, they can be disease-causing molecules.

Table 3-18

Differential Guide to Infectious Agents Associated with Diarrhea

MICROBIAL TYPE	WATERY: INFECTION OF PROXIMAL SMALL INTESTINE	DYSENTERY: INFECTION OF THE COLON	ENTERIC FEVER: SYSTEMIC INFECTION
Bacterium	Enteropathogenic *Escherichia coli*	*Salmonella* spp.	*Salmonella* serovar Typhi
Bacterium	Enterotoxigenic *E. coli*	*Shigella* spp.	*Yersinia enterocolitica*
Bacterium	*Bacillus cereus*	*Campylobacter jejuni*	
Bacterium	*Clostridium perfringens*	*Clostridium difficile*	
Bacterium	*Vibrio* spp.	Enterohemorrhagic *E. coli*; enteroinvasive *E. coli*	
Virus	Adenovirus		
Virus	Astroviruses		
Virus	Calicivirus		
Virus	Rotavirus		
Parasite	*Giardia* spp.	*Entamoeba histolytica*	
Parasite	*Cryptosporidium* spp.		

Table 3-19

Differential Guide to Common Food Poisoning

AGENT	TIME TO ONSET OF SYMPTOMS	INVASIVE ±	TOXIN MEDIATED ±	FEVER ±	SYMPTOMS	TYPICAL FOOD IMPLICATED
Clostridium perfringens	8-16 hr	−	+	−	Cramps, diarrhea	Poultry, especially gravy; need to ingest at least 10^8 microbes to cause symptoms
Bacillus cereus	8-16 hr	−	+	−	Cramps, diarrhea	Rice and hot foods that have cooled or improperly refrigerated
Salmonella	16-24 hr	+	+	+	Fever, cramps, diarrhea	Always a pathogen; associated with meats and fecally contaminated ingested vegetable matter
Shigella	16-24 hr	+	+	+	Fever, cramps, diarrhea	Associated with meats and fecally contaminated ingested vegetable matter
Campylobacter	16-24 hr	+	+	+	Fever, cramps, diarrhea	Associated with meats, especially poultry (>90% of raw poultry is colonized with this microbe), and fecally contaminated ingested vegetable matter
Enteroinvasive *Escherichia coli*	16-24 hr	+	+	+	Fever, cramps, diarrhea	Associated with meats and fecally contaminated ingested vegetable matter

Continued

Table 3-19

Differential Guide to Common Food Poisoning—cont'd

AGENT	TIME TO ONSET OF SYMPTOMS	INVASIVE ±	TOXIN MEDIATED ±	FEVER ±	SYMPTOMS	TYPICAL FOOD IMPLICATED
Staphylococcus aureus	1-7 hr	−	+	±	Projectile vomiting and diarrhea; may or may not have fever	Associated with foods that select for its growth (higher salt concentration); generally associated with improperly refrigerated "picnic"-type foods
Bacillus cereus	1-7 hr	−	+	±	Cramps, diarrhea, no fever	Associated with ingestion of improperly maintained foods (e.g., letting foods cool and stand, allowing the spores to germinate generating sufficient toxin to result in symptoms)
Vibrio parahaemolyticus	16-24 hr	+	+	+	Fever, cramps, diarrhea	Associated with seafood
Vibrio vulnificus	16-24 hr	+	+	+	Fever, cramps, diarrhea	Associated with seafood; responsible for high mortality (>50% in immunocompromised patients or patients with iron overloads)
Yersinia enterocolitica	16-48 hr	+	+	+	Presents with appendicitislike symptoms, fever, abdominal tenderness or rigidity, diarrhea (often bloody)	Generally associated with pork and pork products
Enterohemorrhagic *E. coli* (*E. coli* O157:H7)	72-120 hr	+	+	+	Produces higher concentrations of shiga toxin acquired from *Shigella* resulting in bloody diarrhea and HUS; administration of antibiotics can often exacerbate the problem	Associated with meats and fecally contaminated ingested vegetable matter
Clostridium botulinum	18-36 hr	−	+	−	Presents with descending paralysis owing to cranial nerve involvement resulting in initial blurring and double vision followed by nausea, vomiting, diarrhea, and ultimately paralysis	Associated with improperly canned foods; toxin is sensitive to heat

Table 3-19

Differential Guide to Common Food Poisoning—cont'd

AGENT	TIME TO ONSET OF SYMPTOMS	INVASIVE ±	TOXIN MEDIATED ±	FEVER ±	SYMPTOMS	TYPICAL FOOD IMPLICATED
Listeria monocytogenes	3-4 wk after ingestion	+	+	+	Fever, muscle aches, and occasionally, GI symptoms, such as nausea or diarrhea	Associated with processed "lunch" meats, fresh fruit (cantaloupes), and unpasteurized cheeses
Cryptosporidium	1-2 wk after ingestion	+	–	–	Diarrhea lasting <1 wk, generally no fever	Number 1 disease mediated by potable water sources
Giardia	1-2 wk after ingestion	+	–	–	Diarrhea lasting <1 wk, generally no fever; generally produces an oily foul-smelling stool; may last a few days to ≥1 mo	Associated with waters contaminated with animal waste and improperly maintained municipal water supplies
Cyclospora	1-2 wk after ingestion	+	–	–	Diarrhea lasting <1 wk, generally no fever; may last a few days to ≥1 mo. Symptoms include watery diarrhea, with frequent, sometimes explosive, bowel movements; loss of appetite, weight loss, stomach cramps/pain, bloating, increased gas, nausea, vomiting, body aches, headache, fever, and other flu-like symptoms may manifest.	Associated with contaminated fragile fruit (raspberries, blackberries)

GI, Gastrointestinal; *HUS,* hemolytic uremic syndrome.

Table 3-20

Bacterial Vaccines

	CAPSULAR POLYSACCHARIDES	TOXOIDS	KILLED BACTERIA OR PURIFIED PROTEINS	IMMUNOGLOBULINS (PASSIVE IMMUNITY)
Streptococcus pneumoniae	X	—	—	—
Neisseria meningitidis	X	—	—	—
Haemophilus influenzae	X	—	—	—
Corynebacterium diphtheriae	—	X	—	X
Clostridium tetani	—	X	—	X
Bordetella pertussis	—	—	X	—
Clostridium botulinum				X

Table 3-21

Viral Vaccines

	LIVE, ATTENUATED VIRUS	KILLED VIRUS	VIRAL ANTIGENS	IMMUNOGLOBULINS (PASSIVE IMMUNITY)
MMR	X	—	—	—
VZV	X	—	—	X
Adenoviruses	X	—	—	—
Hepatitis A	—	X	—	X
Hepatitis B	—	—	X	X
Poliovirus	X	X	—	—
Influenza		X	—	—
Smallpox virus	X	—	—	—
Rabies virus	—	X	—	X

MMR, Measles, mumps, rubella.

A. General characteristics.
   1. Basically, they are infectious protein particles (atypical viruslike agents).
   2. They do not contain nucleic acid.
   3. They are more resistant to inactivation by radiation or heat than viruses but can be inactivated by hypochlorite and autoclaving.
   4. They exist in two forms—an abnormal prion consists of a β-pleated sheet, and a normal prion consists of an α-helical structure.
   5. Pathogenesis—the abnormal prion is able to induce a structural change in the normal prion so that it also becomes an abnormal prion with a β-pleated sheet.
   6. Transmission—includes inoculation or ingestion of nervous tissue containing the abnormal prion.
B. Diseases caused by prions include Creutzfeldt-Jakob disease, a severe degenerative brain disease caused by the ingestion of beef from a cow infected with mad cow disease.

3.5 Fungi

3.5.1 Identification of Fungi

A. Classification—fungi are identified based on their appearance on agar plates or their appearance under magnification. Biochemical reactions, such as carbohydrate utilization, are sometimes required for definitive identification. They have been broadly classified based on their primary physical state as yeasts, molds, or whether or not they may exist in two physical states under different circumstances (dimorphic fungi).
B. Yeasts—unicellular fungi that when grown on solid media generate waxy or creamy colonies similar in size and shape to bacterial colonies. They divide via asexual reproduction, which can be witnessed under magnification as the budding where a projection from a mature mother cell buds forming a blastoconidium, which is commonly referred to as a daughter cell.
C. Pseudohyphae—under certain conditions some yeasts can elongate their buds resulting in the growth of a long branch that can continue to grow and form other buds, which are separated by constrictions rather than cross-walls. These pseudohyphae are produced mainly by members of *Candida* species. Formation of pseudohyphae is suggestive of the transition from an avirulent form to a virulent form of the fungus.
D. Molds—multicellular fungi that when grown on solid media form fluffy, cottony, woolly, powdery, or suede-like colonies on the surface.
E. Hyphae—are distinct from pseudohyphae and form as a consequence of growth of the mold spore, which produces a long sproutlike or tubelike projection. This projection, or hypha, is the basic structural unit of a mold. The colony (also called a mycelium) is composed of hyphae.
   1. Nonseptate (or coenocytic) versus septate hyphae are useful for identification of the fungus.
      a. Nonseptate molds produce hyphae with few or no septa (cross-walls); Zygomycetes fungi are nonseptate.
      b. All other classes of molds produce septate hyphae (i.e., regular septa within the hyphae).
   2. Hyaline versus dematiaceous—most molds have hyaline (transparent) hyphae. Molds with dematiaceous hyphae produce melanin in their cell walls; they are often called "black fungi."
F. Dimorphic fungi—these are the most highly evolved fungi.
   1. Mold form (natural or infectious form)—in nature, the dimorphic fungi are always molds. A person walks by or otherwise disturbs the soil and inhales

Table 3-22

Summary of Diseases Caused by Dermatophytes

DISEASE	ORGANS AFFECTED	DERMATOPHYTES RESPONSIBLE		
		MICROSPORUM	TRICHOPHYTON	EPIDERMOPHYTON
Tinea pedis (athlete's foot)	Feet	—	X	X
Tinea capitis	Hair, skin	X	X	—
Tinea cruris (jock itch)	Groin	—	X	X
Tinea corporis*	Entire body*	X	X	X
Tinea unguium	Nails	—	X	—
Tinea barbae	Bearded areas	—	X	—

*Common signs are circular (ring-shaped) lesions.

mold conidia, or a person may get a splinter carrying mold conidia on it (traumatic inoculation). The mold form is grown in the laboratory at 25°C.

2. Yeast form (tissue or parasitic form)—in the susceptible host, either the mold is killed immediately by a person's immune system or it transforms itself into a yeast form over the next few days or weeks. The yeast form grows in preferred areas and may migrate from the site of introduction, usually the lung or skin, to other areas of the host producing a systemic infection. The yeast form may be seen in stained tissues or exudates. The yeast form is grown in the laboratory by incubating the isolated mold form at 37°C. The temperature induces the mold to convert to the yeast form.

3. Reproduction in dimorphic fungi.
   a. Asexual—most fungi that infect humans reproduce by asexual spores.
      (1) Conidia—the most common type of spore is a conidium. Conidia are produced on the sides or ends of conidiophores (specialized stalks).
      (2) Arthroconidium (arthrospore)—the simplest spore. The ends of hyphal cells wall off into compartments, which fragment into rectangular spores.
      (3) Microconidia and macroconidia—some fungi, mainly dermatophytes, produce macroconidia (large multicellular spores) and microconidia (small unicellular spores).
      (4) Sporangioconidium (sporangiospore)—nonseptate fungi produce sporangioconidia enclosed within saclike sporangia. Sporangia are produced on sporangiophores (specialized stalks).
   b. Sexual—sexual reproduction occurs when opposite mating types attach and form a zygote. These are generally large brown spores. Sexual reproduction is unusual in human infections but, if present, helps identify the organism.

3.5.2 Human Fungal Diseases (Mycoses)

3.5.2.1 Cutaneous Mycoses (Skin Fungi)

A. Superficial fungal infections occur on the superficial layers of the epidermis.
   1. Dermatophytes.
      a. Dermatophytes are cutaneous fungi that mainly infect keratinized skin, hair, and nails.
      b. Three genera—*Microsporum*, *Trichophyton*, and *Epidermophyton*.
      c. Disease—tinea.
         (1) This group of diseases is classified according to the organ affected.
         (2) These diseases are summarized in Table 3-22.

3.5.2.2 Subcutaneous Mycoses

Subcutaneous mycoses are caused by fungi that grow in soil and are introduced into subcutaneous tissue through trauma.

A. Sporotrichosis.
   1. Dimorphic fungi (*Sporothrix schenckii*)—found on vegetation and usually introduced into skin via thorn punctures; often associated with roses.
   2. Symptoms include local pustule or ulcer with nodules that form along draining lymphatics.
B. Chromomycosis.
   1. Soil fungi (*Cladosporium*).
   2. Symptoms include wartlike lesions with crusting abscesses that extend along the affected lymphatic vessel.
C. Mycetoma.
   1. Soil fungi (*Petriellidium*) enters through wounds on the feet, hands, or back.

3.5.2.3 Opportunistic Fungi

A. *Aspergillus* (molds).
   1. Found mostly on decaying vegetables.
   2. Transmission is via airborne conidia.
   3. Virulence factor—aflatoxin, which inhibits transcription by binding to DNA.

4. It is also a carcinogen that can lead to cancer of the liver.
5. Causes three forms of lung infection.
   a. Allergic bronchopulmonary aspergillosis—characterized by the formation of bronchial mucous plugs in the lungs. Asthmalike symptoms are mediated by a high IgE *Aspergillus* antibody titer.
   b. Aspergilloma—when *Aspergillus* colonize (form "fungus balls") in lung cavities without invasion.
   c. Invasive aspergillosis—*Aspergillus* infection that spreads to other organs; usually occurs in immunocompromised patients.
6. Common species—*Aspergillus fumigatus*, *Aspergillus flavus*, and *Aspergillus niger*.

B. *C. albicans*.
1. Found in the normal gut, oral, and vaginal flora.
2. *C. albicans* may be seen in three forms.
   a. As yeast cells.
   b. Pseudohyphae—not true hyphae but an elongated form.
   c. Chlamydospores—only fungal species to be observed in this form.
3. Disease—candidiasis (thrush).
   a. Overgrowth occurs in immunocompromised patients.
   b. Also occurs with angular cheilitis.
   c. Appears as white patches along the buccal mucosa, palate, or tongue that wipe off when rubbed.
   d. Treatment includes nystatin or azole–derived drugs, such as clotrimazole.

3.5.2.4 Systemic Fungus

A. General characteristics.
1. Most are spore-forming and are transmitted via inhalation of airborne spores.
2. Express dimorphism—exist as yeasts when causing systemic infections and as molds when found in the soil.
   a. *Coccidioides immitis*.
      (1) Spore—arthrospores.
      (2) Disease—coccidioidomycosis, valley fever (in San Joaquin Valley of California), or desert rheumatism (in Arizona).
      (3) Usually asymptomatic, but flulike symptoms may be present.
      (4) Treatment—itraconazole or amphotericin B.
   b. *Blastomyces dermatitidis*.
      (1) Spore—conidia.
      (2) Disease—blastomycosis.
   c. *Histoplasma capsulatum*.
      (1) Spore—two asexual spores, tuberculate macroconidia and microconidia.
      (2) Disease—histoplasmosis. Geographic focus is the Ohio River Valley of the United States and its surrounding areas; also associated with spelunkers.

(3) Note: histoplasmosis may clinically resemble TB because its yeast cells are often found in macrophages.
(4) Treatment—usually no therapy is necessary; oral itraconazole may help with progressive lung lesions.

3.5.2.5 Molds and Fungal Disease

A. General characteristics.
1. Are spore-forming and are transmitted via inhalation of airborne spores.
2. Have a tendency to invade blood vessel endothelium in the paranasal sinuses, bronchi, or intestines. This results in a loss of blood supply, leading to infarction and tissue necrosis.
3. Affect immunocompromised patients.
4. Diseases—mucormycosis, phycomycosis, and zygomycosis.

3.5.2.6 Oral Parasitology

A. In contrast to bacterial and viral infections, parasitic infections often result in a chronic condition that may last months to years. Their prevalence is quite high: 50 million children and 80 million adults are infected with a parasite. Single-celled protozoans are involved in 90% of cases.
B. Classification is based on whether the parasite is within the host, endoparasites (e.g., protozoa, helminthes), or on the surface of the host organism, ectoparasites (e.g., fleas, ticks, lice, barnacles), as well as other criteria such as ports of entry, tissue or organ tropism, attachment site, and growth and nutritional requirements.
C. Parasitic disease potential—the route of exposure, duration of exposure, size of the inoculum, how the parasite attaches to specific cells and organs, whether or not the parasite produces toxins, and how the parasite may evade the immune system of the host all are factors related to severity of the disease caused by each agent.
1. Ports of entry.
   a. Ingestion—examples include *Giardia* species, *Entamoeba histolytica*, *Cryptosporidium* (number one cause of water-borne gastroenteritis in the United States), cestodes, and nematodes.
   b. Penetration—hookworm, *Strongyloides* species, schistosomes.
   c. Transplacental—*Toxoplasma gondii*.
   d. Vector-borne—examples include malaria, *Babesia* species, filariae, *Leishmania* species, and trypanosomes.
D. Parasitic immune evasion—Parasites avoid the immune system via numerous mechanisms, which may include antigenic shift as is the case with *Giardia*, maintaining their life cycle as intracellular parasites, specific tissue tropism with penetration to avoid surveillance or

immunosuppression via the production of specific or nonspecific proteinases.

E. Endoparasites (single cell).

1. Protozoa—80% to 90% of parasitic infections are caused by protozoa.

a. Ameba.

(1) *E. histolytica.*

(a) Humans are the primary host; this represents a true oral parasite.

(b) Fecal-oral transmission—cysts are shed in feces and are consumed by the next recipient.

(c) Generally asymptomatic but when virulent is responsible for amebic dysentery.

(i) Bloody stool, diarrhea, and pain.

(ii) Drugs of choice—metronidazole, iodoquinol, or chloroquine.

(2) *Entamoeba gingivalis.*

(a) Humans and mammals are hosts; this represents a true oral parasite.

(b) Oral-oral transmission through kissing of humans or dogs or through shared eating utensils.

(c) Associated with periodontitis and is correlated with oral hygiene.

(i) Found in only 6% of "clean" mouths.

(ii) Present in 65% of periodontal patients.

(d) Associated with furred tongue.

(e) Generally self-limiting; restoration of hygiene facilitates elimination.

(3) *Trichomonas tenax, Trichomonas hominis, Trichomonas vaginalis.*

(a) Humans and mammals are hosts; this represents a true oral parasite.

(b) Oral-oral transmission through kissing of humans or dogs or through shared eating utensils.

(c) *T. tenax* is associated with the oral cavity, *T. hominis* is associated with the intestine, and *T. vaginalis* is associated with the genital urinary tract.

(d) Trichomoniasis is the disease state, and it represents the most common parasitic disease in the United States with 7.4 million cases per year.

(i) *T. tenax*—oral symptoms, principally nonpathogenic scavenger.

(ii) *T. vaginalis*—characterized by inflammation of the vagina, prostate, or urethra.

(4) *Cryptosporidium.*

(a) Humans and mammals are hosts; this represents a true oral parasite.

(b) Fecal-oral transmission.

(i) *Cryptosporidium* parasites are shed in the stool.

(ii) Found in soil, water, or surfaces contaminated with feces from infected humans and animals.

(c) Principal manifestation, cryptosporidiosis, is diarrhea with cramps or pain, dehydration, nausea, vomiting, fever, and weight loss.

(i) Often affects immunocompromised patients (e.g., patients with AIDS).

(ii) Occasional outbreaks of infections in swimming pools and with interruptions to water-treatment infrastructure.

(d) Treatment—nitazoxanide. Mechanism of action is mediated by interfering with the pyruvate:ferredoxin oxidoreductase enzyme–dependent electron transfer reaction, which is essential to anaerobic energy metabolism.

(5) *Giardia lamblia* and *Giardia intestinalis.*

(a) Humans and mammals are hosts.

(b) Fecal-oral transmission; associated with contaminated fresh water through the ingestion of the cysts.

(c) Giardiasis results from the ingestion of infective cysts. Two trophozoites (feeding) are released and attach to the lumen of the intestine facilitating colonization, which results in encystation allowing the parasite to transit toward the colon. The net consequence is cyst "showers" in stool.

(i) Principal symptoms include dysentery, nausea, and vomiting. There is also a strong correlation with persistent bad breath and belching and smells of sulfur. The stool is often foul-smelling and oily owing to the common obstruction of the bile duct limiting the solubilization of fat as a consequence of reduced bile.

(ii) 2 million new cases per year.

(iii) This is a nationally notifiable disease whose incidence is communicated to the CDC via local or state health departments.

(d) Treatment—several drugs are available, including metronidazole, tinidazole, and nitazoxanide.

(6) *Plasmodium*—malaria.

(a) Four infectious species—*Plasmodium falciparum, Plasmodium vivax, Plasmodium ovale,* and *Plasmodium malariae.*

(b) Humans and the *Anopheles* mosquito are the hosts.

(c) Obligate intracellular parasite—principally the liver and erythrocyte.

(d) Life cycle of the parasite requires two hosts.

(i) Female *Anopheles* mosquito delivers the sporozoite to the human, where it travels via the blood infecting the liver where schizonts rupture releasing the merozoites that undergo asexual multiplication with erythrocytes with subsequent development of a gamete, which is ingested as a blood meal by a female *Anopheles* mosquito where the gamete infects the salivary gland of the insect repeating the cycle of the parasite's life.

(e) Disease within the human manifests with chills, fever, anemia, and jaundice. The pallor of the oral mucosa is altered with vesiculoulcerative lesions occurring in 30% of cases.

(f) Diagnosis requires a skilled technician familiar with the technique of fabricating a thin and thick smear. The parasite is visualized by Giemsa staining or other serologic testing.

(g) Treatment—chloroquine is the drug of choice for nonresistant species.

(7) *T. gondii.*
(a) Obligate intracellular parasitic protozoan.
(b) Responsible for toxoplasmosis.
   (i) Common parasite with more than 33% of the Earth's population having been exposed or chronically infected by this microbe.
   (ii) Can generate a self-limiting flulike condition in healthy adults but is generally asymptomatic.
   (iii) May cause serious and fatal illness in infants and immunocompromised individuals, especially patients with HIV/AIDS with uncontrolled viremia infection.
(c) Acquired by consuming raw or undercooked meat containing tissue cysts of the microbe; ingesting contaminated water, soil, or vegetables; contact with fomites contaminated with oocysts shed by an infected cat (risk from litter box cleaning); or transplacentally from mother to fetus.
(d) Birth defects—*T. gondii* hydrocephalus.
(e) 1.5 million U.S. cases, with 4000 cases of congenital toxoplasmosis per year.
(f) Third leading cause of death resulting from food-borne illness (225,000 cases; 400 deaths).
(g) Diagnosis via serology, polymerase chain reaction, and direct microscopy.
(h) Treatment—pyrimethamine, which serves to block dihydrofolate reductase, given with

sulfadiazine. Side effects include rash and bone marrow suppression.

(8) Trypanosomes—*Trypanosoma brucei* and *Trypanosoma cruzi.*
(a) Unicellular flagellated heteroxenous (requires more than one host similar to malaria) protozoa.
(b) Generally transmitted by a vector, typically a blood-feeding insect.
(c) Fatal human sleeping disease caused by *T. brucei.*
(d) Transmitted by the tsetse fly (*Glossina* species), found only in rural Africa.
(e) Two-stage disease process.
   (i) Stage one—parasite is found in peripheral circulation.
   (ii) Stage two—parasite has invaded CNS.
(f) Depending on the subspecies, two types of sleeping sickness may manifest. Symptoms include fever, headache, muscle and joint aches, and enlarged lymph nodes within 1 to 2 weeks being infected. On invasion of the CNS, mental deterioration and other neurologic problems quickly manifest with death ensuing within months (East African variant). The West African variant has a longer time to death (3 to 7 years).
(g) Treatment is based on the species. The drugs are available only in the United States from the CDC.
(h) Chagas' disease is caused by *T. cruzi* and transmitted by the "kissing" bugs of the subfamily *Triatominae.* It may also be spread through blood transfusion, organ transplantation, ingestion of food contaminated with the parasite, or transplacentally.
   (i) Two-stage disease process—acute stage that commences shortly after becoming infected and chronic stage that persists for years.
      1. Acute stage—duration weeks to months after infection; usually asymptomatic to mild symptoms of fever, fatigue, body aches, headache, rash, loss of appetite, diarrhea, and vomiting. Hallmark marker of disease is Romaña's sign, which refers to swelling of the eyelids on the side of the face in close proximity to the initial site of introduction of the parasite.
      2. Symptoms resolve within 3 to 8 weeks, but despite treatment of the infection, the disease persists and enters the second or chronic stage.

3. Chronic stage—nervous system, digestive system, or heart may be involved. Of individuals who have reached the chronic phase, more than 66% have cardiac damage. Additionally, swallowing difficulties may result leading to malnutrition.

(ii) Mechanism of disease—clinical manifestations are a consequence of cell death in the targeted tissues during the infective cycle resulting in the sequential induction of an inflammatory response.

(iii) Medication necessary for treatment in the United States is only available from the CDC.

(9) *Leishmania.*

(a) The disease resulting from this parasite is confined to southern Europe and parts of the tropics and subtropics of the New and Old World. The most common forms of the disease are the cutaneous form, which can result in severely disfiguring skin lesions, or the visceral form, which may affect the liver, spleen, and bone marrow. It is transmitted via the bite of sandflies, *Phlebotomus* or *Lutzomyia.* Sandflies are two thirds smaller than mosquitoes, their bites are hard to appreciate, and they are most active from dusk until dawn.

(b) The responsible species for disease of humans include *Leishmania tropica, Leishmania major, Leishmania aethiopica, Leishmania infantum,* and *Leishmania donovani.*

(c) The main species in the Western Hemisphere are in either the *Leishmania mexicana* species complex (*L. mexicana, Leishmania amazonensis,* and *Leishmania venezuelensis*) or the subgenus *Viannia.*

(d) Cutaneous leishmaniasis.

(i) The cutaneous lesion results in a sore that generally heals on its own. However, resolution may take months or years, and the sores can leave substantial disfiguring scars.

(ii) Treatment decisions are individualized in consultation with an infectious disease specialist and the CDC. Drugs currently in use may be pentavalent antimony, liposomal amphotericin B, and the aminoglycoside paromomycin sulfate.

(e) Visceral leishmaniasis.

(i) Although the incubation period typically ranges from weeks to months, an asymptomatic condition may result that manifests as clinical disease years to decades after infection. Symptoms include fever, weight loss, enlarged liver and spleen, pancytopenia, and a high protein level with low albumin level.

(ii) Treatment decisions are individualized in consultation with an infectious disease specialist and the CDC.

(f) Mucosal leishmaniasis.

(i) Generally confined to the Western Hemisphere, the mucosal form of the disease is a metastatic consequence of the cutaneous infection. The parasites disseminate from the skin to the nasoorpharyngeal mucosa. The clinical manifestations become evident years to decades after infection.

(ii) Treatment decisions are individualized in consultation with an infectious disease specialist and the CDC.

F. Multicellular parasites.

1. Helminths.

a. Nematodes (roundworms).

(1) *Ascaris lumbricoides* (roundworm).

(a) Most common helminthic infection worldwide.

(b) Largest parasitic nematode (15 to 30 cm).

(c) Acquired from contaminated food or drink.

(d) High parasitic loads result in nutritional deficiencies.

(e) Can bore through the intestinal wall and move to the lungs and exit via breathing passages where they can be swallowed perpetuating the life cycle.

(f) Treatment with anthelmintic medications such as albendazole and mebendazole is administered for 1 to 3 days and is effective.

(2) *Enterobius vermicularis* (pinworm).

(a) Commonly referred to as "daycare itch."

(b) Acquired from contaminated food and fomites (toys), anal to oral route.

(c) Female lays eggs at the anus, cause an itch, scratch contaminates fingers and facilities resulting in spread.

(d) Treatment—anthelmintic medications mebendazole, pyrantel pamoate, and albendazole are simultaneously administered in two doses. A second, single, course is administered 2 weeks later to eliminate possible reinfection.

(3) *Trichuris trichiuria* (whipworm).

(a) Acquired from contaminated food, anal to oral route.

(b) Can cause dysentery and diarrhea.

(c) Female can lay 3000 to 20,000 eggs per day.

(d) Can cause dysentery and diarrhea.

(e) Treatment—anthelmintic medications albendazole and mebendazole are administered for 1 to 3 days and are effective.

(f) The life cycle is common to the three nematodes, where the embryonated eggs are ingested by the human; the larvae hatch within the small intestine, and the adults reside within the lumen of the cecum. The gravid female migrates to the perianal region at night to lay the eggs, which mature within 4 to 6 hours.

b. Cestodes (flatworms)—tapeworms.

(1) *Taenia* is the type genus; species are *Taenia saginata* (beef tapeworm), *Taenia solium* (pork tapeworm), and *Taenia asiatica* (Asian tapeworm). The head of the worm attaches onto the intestinal wall. The worm is acquired through the ingestion of raw or undercooked infected meat.

(2) *Taenia* infections are generally asymptomatic, but worms may grow to lengths greater than 10 m. Larger worms may cause intestinal complications, such as abdominal pain, loss of weight, and an upset stomach. Tapeworm segments are occasionally seen in the stool. In rare cases, the segments may lead to an obstruction of the bile or pancreatic ducts or appendix.

(3) Endemic to the southern United States.

(4) Treatment with oral praziquantel or niclosamide on diagnosis.

c. Trematodes (flukes).

(1) Trematodes are worldwide in distribution and cause various clinical manifestations in humans. They are so named from *trematos*, which literally translates from the Greek as "pierced with holes," and the principal anatomic feature serves to suck material from the host.

(2) The type infection is schistosomiasis, also known as bilharziasis. It infects approximately 200 million people in the tropical zones. This agent is *not* endemic to the continental United States. The parasites live in certain types of freshwater snails, and schistosomiasis is second only to malaria in being considered a devastating parasitic disease. Symptoms associated with this infection depend on the immune response from the host to the egg antigens of the parasite.

(a) Most infected people have none to a few symptoms, but a pruritic rash may develop on the skin within days. Without treatment, symptoms progress to fever, chills, cough, and muscle aches within 1 to 2 months of infection. The parasite can persist within the host for years manifesting as abdominal pain, an enlarged liver, blood in the stool or urine, and problems with urination.

(b) Urinary schistosomiasis—terminal hematuria, dysuria, and frequent urination are the chief complaints associated with the urinary form of this disease. Early signs of infection are the formation of a pseudotubercle, but if the infection persists, radiography reveals nests of calcified ova, often described as sandy patches surrounded by fibrous tissue in the submucosa.

(c) Intestinal schistosomiasis—dysentery, diarrhea, weakness, and abdominal pain are the chief complaints of intestinal schistosomiasis.

(d) Neurologic schistosomiasis—in untreated individuals, eggs rarely may be found in the brain or spinal cord where they can cause seizures, paralysis, or chronic inflammation of the spinal cord.

(e) Diagnosis—stool or urine samples may be examined for the presence of the eggs of the parasite (stool for *Schistosoma mansoni* or *Schistosoma japonicum* and urine for *Schistosoma haematobium*).

(f) Treatment for all forms of this disease is the administration of a 1- to 2-day course of praziquantel.

(3) Swimmer's itch—cercarial dermatitis is an allergic reaction resulting from the fluke cercaria (genera *Gigantobilharzia*, *Orientobilharzia*, and *Trichobilharzia*) penetrating an individual who has been exposed to bathing water, salt or fresh, contaminated with cercariae. The dermatitis generates a pruritic rash with edema from the petechial hemorrhages; the responsible flukes do not develop further in humans.

(4) Intestinal flukes, such as *Fasciolopsis buski*, may cause diarrhea, nausea, vomiting, abdominal pain, and facial and abdominal edema. *F. buski* is acquired via contaminated foods such as unpeeled water chestnuts and is endemic to Australia and Southeast Asia.

4.0 Systemic Pathology

4.1 Cardiovascular Pathology

4.1.1 Infective Endocarditis

Infective endocarditis (most often bacterial endocarditis). Microbial infection of the mural endocardium or the heart valves, most often the mitral and aortic valves.

A. Acute endocarditis.
   1. Usually due to infection of a previously healthy valve by highly virulent organisms (e.g., *S. aureus*).
   2. Often requires surgery rather than antibiotics; despite treatment, death may occur in days to weeks.
B. Subacute endocarditis.
   1. Infection of deformed valves by low-virulence microbes. Infection is most often due to Streptococcus viridans, a normal oral microbe that may be introduced systemically via dental procedures.
   2. It has a long clinical course of weeks to months and is usually cured by antibiotics.
      a. Hallmark is a thrombus or vegetation on a previously normal or abnormal valve. These vegetations contain fibrin, bacteria or other microbes, and inflammatory cells. Complications can arise if embolization of the thrombus occurs, causing septic infarcts. Other complications include valvular dysfunction or abscess formation.
      b. Factors leading to bacteremia predispose to endocarditis. Organism may be from dental or surgical procedures; contaminated needle; or innocuous breaks in the epithelial lining of the skin, oral cavity, or gut.
      c. Valves affected (most to least common)—mitral, aortic, tricuspid (except in intravenous drug users, in whom the tricuspid is most often affected). *S. aureus*, which occurs on the skin, is the most common cause in intravenous drug users.

4.1.2 Atherosclerosis

Atherosclerosis is the most frequent type of arteriosclerosis, which is a thickening of arterial walls and loss of elasticity. It is characterized by intimal plaques that extend into the vessel lumen. Plaques mainly consist of cholesterol, foam cells, and calcium. Plaques eventually calcify, resulting in rigidity and distortion of the arterial walls.
   1. Main complications that can arise from plaques.
      a. Thrombosis can lead to partial or complete occlusion of a vessel; complete occlusion may be catastrophic (e.g., occlusion of coronary artery leading to myocardial infarction).
      b. Hemorrhage into the plaque can result in rapid expansion.
      c. Rupture and embolization—may be catastrophic because of vessel obstruction (e.g., myocardial infarction).
      d. Aneurysms—secondary to weakening of tunica media.
   2. Arteries affected (most to least common)—abdominal aorta, coronary arteries, popliteal arteries, internal carotid arteries, vessels of the circle of Willis.

   3. Risk factors.
      a. Advanced age.
      b. Male gender.
      c. Smoking.
      d. Hypertension.
      e. Hypercholesterolemia (abnormally high low-density lipoprotein).
      f. Diabetes mellitus.
      g. Inflammation, particularly high C-reactive protein.
      h. Genetics (e.g., familial hypercholesterolemia).

4.1.3 Ischemic Heart Disease or Coronary Artery Disease

Ischemic heart disease (IHD) and coronary artery disease (CAD) are generic terms for multiple related clinical syndromes that result from varying degrees of myocardial ischemia, which is the imbalance between demand and supply of oxygenated blood to the heart. IHD is caused by partial or complete interruption of blood supply to the myocardium. IHD is the leading cause of death for men and women in the United States. IHD may present as follows.
   1. Angina pectoris.
   2. Myocardial infarction.
   3. Chronic IHD with heart failure—one of the causes of congestive heart failure (CHF).
   4. Sudden cardiac death—occurs in a person without cardiac symptoms.
A. Causes.
   1. Coronary atherosclerosis—this limits the rate of blood flow and may result in the acute cessation of circulation in the event of a plaque rupture.
   2. Coronary emboli.
   3. Blockage of small myocardial blood vessels.
   4. Low systemic blood pressure (e.g., shock).
B. Risk factors—same as previously listed for atherosclerosis.
C. Angina pectoris—characterized by recurrent spasms of constricting or knifelike chest discomfort.
   1. Stable angina (most common)—occurs with increased cardiac workload; relieved by rest or nitroglycerin.
   2. Unstable angina (uncommon)—pain of increasing frequency triggered by progressively less physical activity; may be a warning sign of imminent myocardial infarction. It is relieved by nitroglycerin or calcium channel blockers.
   3. Prinzmetal variant angina—intermittent chest pain at rest. It is less common than other forms. Decreased oxygenation occurs via vasospasm of coronary arteries.
D. Myocardial infarction—"heart attack."
   1. Ischemia is an imbalance between the supply and demand of oxygen. Severe, prolonged (20 to 30

minutes) ischemia results in necrosis or death of cardiac muscle.
  2. Symptoms.
    a. Chest pain, shortness of breath. Chest pain resulting from myocardial infarction is not relieved by nitroglycerin.
    b. Diaphoresis (profuse sweating), clammy hands.
    c. Nausea, vomiting.
  3. Consequences.
    a. Death.
    b. Arrhythmias (most common *immediate* cause of death).
    c. CHF.
    d. Myocardial rupture, which may result in death from cardiac tamponade.
    e. Thrombus formation on infarcted tissue; may result in systemic embolism.

4.1.4 Congestive Heart Failure

CHF occurs when the heart cannot pump enough blood or needs elevated filling pressure to meet the metabolic needs of the tissues.
A. Left-sided CHF.
  1. May result from nearly any heart disease affecting the left ventricle (e.g., IHD, hypertension, valvular disease, myocardial disease).
  2. Common signs and symptoms.
    a. Dyspnea (shortness of breath) exacerbated by exertion.
    b. Paroxysmal nocturnal dyspnea (severe dyspnea at night leading to a feeling of suffocation).
    c. Orthopnea (shortness of breath when lying down, relieved by standing).
    d. Consequences include pulmonary edema.
B. Right-sided CHF.
  1. The most common cause of right heart failure is left heart failure. It uncommonly occurs in isolation. The same conditions causing left-sided CHF cause right-sided CHF. Another cause is pulmonary hypertension.
  2. Frequently manifests with peripheral edema, especially in the ankles and feet (i.e., dependent edema), enlarged liver or spleen, and distention of the neck veins.

4.1.5 Valvular Disease

A. Generally, there are three types.
  1. Stenosis—inability of the valve to open completely resulting in reduced forward blood flow through the valve.
  2. Regurgitation or valvular insufficiency—valves are unable to close completely, allowing blood to regurgitate.
  3. Prolapse—"floppy" valves; may occur with or without regurgitation. This is the most common valvular defect.

B. Causes.
  1. Mitral valve prolapse—mostly asymptomatic. A few patients (3%) develop complications such as infective endocarditis, mitral insufficiency, stroke, or arrhythmias.
  2. Rheumatic fever—before antibiotic therapy, this was the most common cause of valvular disease.
    a. Usually preceded by a respiratory infection caused by group A streptococci (e.g., strep throat).
    b. All three layers of the heart may be affected. Pathologic findings include Aschoff bodies, which are foci of lymphocytes, scattered plasma cells, and activated macrophages.
    c. Most commonly affects the mitral valve, resulting in mitral valve stenosis, regurgitation, or both.
  3. Infective endocarditis.
    a. Acute pericarditis.
      (1) Characterized by inflammation of the pericardium.
      (2) Causes.
        (a) Infections—viral; bacterial infections include *Staphylococcus*, *Pneumococcus*, and *M. tuberculosis*.
        (b) Myocardial infarction.
        (c) Systemic lupus erythematosus.
        (d) Rheumatic fever.
      (3) Signs and symptoms.
        (a) Pericardial friction rub on cardiac auscultation.
        (b) Angina.
        (c) Fever.
C. Consequences include constrictive pericarditis, which results from fusion and scarring of the pericardium. This may lead to the restriction of ventricular expansion, preventing the heart chambers from filling normally.

4.1.6 Cardiac Tamponade

A. Caused by accumulation of fluid in the pericardium. This severe condition can quickly impair ventricular filling and rapidly lead to decreased cardiac output and death.

4.2 Respiratory Pathology
4.2.1 Pulmonary Infections

A. Pneumonia is an inflammatory process of infectious origin affecting the lung parenchyma. Infection may be bacterial, viral, mycoplasmal, or fungal. It is classified by etiology or clinical setting (e.g., community-acquired, acute, community-acquired atypical, hospital-acquired, aspiration, chronic, necrotizing, and in the immunocompromised host).
  1. Bacterial pneumonia pathogens.
    a. *S. pneumoniae* (most common).
    b. *S. aureus*.

c. *H. influenzae.*

d. *K. pneumoniae.*

e. Anaerobic bacteria from the mouth (aspiration of oral secretions).

B. Viral infections.

1. Influenza.

2. Parainfluenza.

3. Adenoviruses.

4. RSV.

5. Note: viruses can also cause pneumonia. Infection of the interstitial tissues, or interstitial pneumonia, is commonly associated with these types of infections.

C. Common symptoms of pneumonia include fever, dyspnea, and a productive cough (Box 3-1).

D. Anatomically, bacterial pneumonias have two patterns of distribution.

1. Lobar pneumonia.

a. Infection may spread through entire lobe or lobes of lung. Intraalveolar exudates result in dense consolidations.

b. Typical of *S. pneumoniae* infections.

2. Bronchopneumonia.

a. Infection and inflammation spread through distal airways, extending from the bronchioles and alveoli. A patchy distribution involving one or more lobes is observed.

b. Typical of *S. aureus, H. influenzae,* and *K. pneumoniae* infections.

E. Lung abscess—localized area of suppuration.

1. Causes.

a. Complication of bacterial pneumonia (e.g., *Staphylococcus*) infection or bronchiectasis.

b. Aspiration of infectious material (e.g., gingivodental sepsis).

c. Bronchial obstruction (often by cancer).

d. Septic emboli.

2. May be seen in patients with impaired gag reflex (e.g., patients under general anesthesia, alcoholics).

3. Common symptoms include a productive cough with a foul odor, cyanosis, and dyspnea.

F. TB.

1. Caused by *M. tuberculosis.*

2. For progression of disease and disease states, see Section 3.1.4, Acid-Fast Bacteria.

3. Common symptoms—weight loss, anorexia, fever, night sweats, productive cough, and hemoptysis.

4. Treatment—multidrug therapy with drugs such as rifampin, ethambutol, and isoniazid.

4.2.2 Obstructive Lung Diseases

A. Chronic obstructive pulmonary disease.

1. Chronic bronchitis.

a. Caused by narrowing and obstruction of the respiratory airways.

b. Chronic productive cough with hypersecretion of mucus that occurs for at least 3 successive months over 2 consecutive years; no other identifiable cause of cough.

c. Associated with smoking.

d. Consequences.

(1) Dyspnea on exertion.

(2) Mild cyanosis.

(3) Cor pulmonale (enlargement of right side of the heart) with cardiac failure.

2. Emphysema.

a. Caused by the destruction of alveolar walls by proteases that are released by inflammatory cells, accompanied by enlargement of air spaces distal to terminal bronchioles.

b. Effect of smoking—α_1-antitrypsin is normally present in the lung to inhibit the actions of elastase. Smoking inhibits the actions of α_1-antitrypsin and increases the number of inflammatory cells present (Figure 3-17).

c. Lungs show decreased elasticity.

d. Based on anatomic distribution in the lobule, emphysema is subclassified as four types.

Box 3-1

Diseases That Produce a Productive Cough

Pneumonia
Lung abscess
Tuberculosis
Chronic bronchitis
Bronchiectasis
Bronchogenic carcinoma

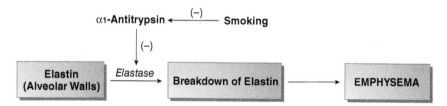

Figure 3-17 Pathogenesis of emphysema: role of elastase, α_1-antitrypsin, and smoking.

(1) Centriacinar—most common; affects central or proximal acini formed by bronchioles. Upper lobes are most severely affected. Causes include smoking.

(2) Panacinar (panlobular)—acini from respiratory bronchiole to terminal alveoli are enlarged; usually occurs in lower zones and anterior margin of lung. It is correlated with α_1-antitrypsin deficiency.

(3) Paraseptal—affects distal part of acini.

(4) Irregular—acini irregularly involved, associated with scarring.

3. Bronchiectasis.
   a. Characterized by permanent dilation of bronchi and bronchioles caused by chronic lung infections and obstruction.
   b. Common symptoms include a productive cough with a foul odor, hemoptysis, dyspnea, orthopnea, and cyanosis.

4. Asthma.
   a. Obstructive lung disease characterized by narrowing of the airways, with recurrent wheezing, breathlessness, chest tightness, and cough. Inflammation of the airways is a major component.
   b. Common symptoms are dyspnea, wheezing on expiration, and coughing.
   c. Two types.
      (1) Atopic asthma.
         (a) Atopic allergy caused by a type I immediate hypersensitivity immune reaction to an allergen.
         (b) Affects children and adults.
      (2) Non-atopic asthma.
         (a) Not caused by an allergic reaction.
         (b) Mostly affects adults.

4.2.3 Pneumoconioses

A. Environmentally related lung diseases that result from chronic inhalation of various substances.

1. Silicosis (stonemason's disease).
   a. Inhalant—silica dust.
   b. Associated with extensive fibrosis of the lungs.
   c. Patients have a higher susceptibility to tuberculosis infections.

2. Asbestosis.
   a. Inhalant—asbestos fibers.
   b. Associated with the presence of pleural plaques, well-circumscribed plaques of collagen.
   c. Consequences.
      (1) Mesothelioma (malignant mesothelial tumor).
      (2) Lung cancer.

3. Anthracosis.
   a. Inhalant—carbon dust.
   b. Usually not as harmful as silicosis or asbestosis.
   c. Associated with the presence of macrophages containing carbon.

4.2.4 Other Lung Diseases

A. Sarcoidosis—systemic disease of unknown etiology.
   1. More common in African-Americans.
   2. Associated with the presence of noncaseating granulomas.

B. Cystic fibrosis.
   1. Transmission—caused by a genetic mutation (nucleotide deletion) on chromosome 7, resulting in abnormal chloride channels.
   2. The most common lethal genetic disease in whites.
   3. Genetic transmission—autosomal recessive.
   4. Affects all exocrine glands. Organs affected include lungs, pancreas, salivary glands, and intestines. Thick secretions or mucous plugs obstruct the pulmonary airways and intestinal tracts.
   5. Ultimately fatal.
   6. Sweat test—sweat contains increased amounts of chloride.

C. Atelectasis.
   1. Characterized by collapse of the alveoli.
   2. May be caused by a deficiency of surfactant or hypoventilation of alveoli.

4.3 Gastrointestinal and Hepatobiliary Pathology

A. Salivary gland pathology.
   1. Sjögren's syndrome.
      a. Autoimmune disease affecting the salivary and lacrimal glands.
      b. Primary Sjögren's syndrome or sicca syndrome—involvement of the salivary and lacrimal glands.
      c. Symptoms.
         (1) Xerostomia—dry mouth from decreased saliva production.
         (2) Keratoconjunctivitis sicca (dry eyes)—from decreased tear production.
         (3) Rheumatoid arthritis and sicca syndrome together—secondary Sjögren's syndrome.
         (4) Enlargement of the salivary or lacrimal glands may also be observed.
      d. Histologically, a dense infiltration of the gland by lymphocytes; epimyoepithelial islands may be observed.
         (1) Warthin's tumor (papillary cystadenoma lymphomatosum)—benign tumor of parotid glands.
         (2) Pleomorphic adenoma.
            (a) Most common salivary gland tumor.
            (b) Benign.
            (c) Prognosis is good after proper surgical excision.
   2. Mucoepidermoid carcinoma.
      a. One of the most common malignant salivary gland tumors.
      b. Most commonly occurs in the parotid glands.

c. Prognosis of tumor depends on grade and stage of disease.

B. Esophagus pathology.

1. Mallory-Weiss syndrome.

a. Characterized by longitudinal lacerations (tears) in the esophagus.

b. Most commonly occurs from severe vomiting (e.g., acute alcohol intoxication).

c. A related condition, known as *Boerhaave syndrome*, occurs when the esophagus ruptures, causing massive upper GI hemorrhage.

2. Esophageal varices.

a. Formation of varices (i.e., abnormally dilated veins secondary to portal hypertension). Causes of portal hypertension include blockage of the portal vein or liver cirrhosis.

b. Rupture of esophageal varices results in massive hemorrhage into the esophagus and hematemesis.

c. Common in patients with liver cirrhosis.

3. Gastroesophageal reflux disease (reflux esophagitis).

a. One of the most common GI disorders. It is caused by the reflux of acidic gastric secretions into the lower esophagus owing to decrease of sphincter tone.

b. Symptoms include dysphagia and substernal pain (heartburn).

c. Although chronic or severe reflux disease is uncommon, consequences of these conditions can lead to Barrett's esophagus, development of a stricture, or hemorrhage.

d. Treatment—diet control, antacids, and medications that decrease the production of gastric acid (e.g., H_2 blockers).

4. Barrett's esophagus.

a. Complication of chronic gastroesophageal reflux disease.

b. Histologic findings include intestinal metaplasia within squamous epithelium of the esophagus.

c. Complications include increased incidence of esophageal adenocarcinoma, stricture formation, or hemorrhage (ulceration).

C. Stomach pathology.

1. Peptic ulcers.

a. Commonly associated with *H. pylori*–induced gastric disease or long-term use of nonsteroidal antiinflammatory drugs.

b. Most common complication is hemorrhage. Note: it is not a precursor lesion of carcinoma of the stomach.

c. Symptoms include epigastric pain or burning that may worsen when eating.

D. Exocrine pancreas pathology.

1. Acute pancreatitis.

a. Caused by early activation of pancreatic enzymes, resulting in autodigestion of the pancreas.

b. Predisposed by excessive alcohol intake or biliary tract disease (gallstones).

c. Laboratory tests show an increase in serum lipase and serum amylase and a decrease in calcium.

d. Symptoms include severe abdominal pain.

E. Liver pathology.

1. Jaundice.

a. Caused by excess conjugated or unconjugated serum bilirubin.

b. Alterations of bile production manifest as yellowness of skin (jaundice), sclerae (icterus), mucous membranes, and excretions.

c. Types and causes.

(1) Hepatocellular jaundice—caused by liver diseases such as cirrhosis and hepatitis.

(2) Hemolytic jaundice—caused by increased degradation of erythrocytes (e.g., hemolytic anemias).

(3) Obstructive jaundice—caused by blockage of the common bile duct either by gallstones (cholelithiasis) or carcinomas involving the head of the pancreas.

2. Cirrhosis.

a. Characterized by abnormal hepatic architecture with excessive scarring and parenchymal nodules.

b. Most commonly caused by alcoholism. Other causes include viral hepatitis, nonalcoholic steatohepatitis, biliary obstruction, hemochromatosis, drugs and chemical agents, and Wilson's disease.

c. Clinical findings.

(1) Portal hypertension.

(2) Formation of arteriovenous shunts including esophageal varices.

(3) An increase in liver enzymes, including alanine aminotransferase and aspartate aminotransferase.

d. Associated with an increased incidence of hepatocellular carcinoma.

3. Wilson's disease.

a. Caused by a decrease in ceruloplasmin, a serum protein that binds copper, resulting in high copper levels.

b. Common organs affected.

(1) Liver, leading to cirrhosis.

(2) Brain (basal ganglia).

(3) Eye—cornea; Kayser-Fleischer rings (greenish rings around the cornea) are observed.

4. Hepatitis—see Section 3.2.4, RNA Viruses.

F. Small bowel pathology.

1. Malabsorption syndromes.

a. A common clinical symptom of all malabsorption syndromes is steatorrhea (excessive fecal fat and bulky stools). There is also a decrease of nutrients absorbed, including fat-soluble vitamins and minerals.

b. Celiac sprue (celiac disease or gluten-sensitive enteropathy).
  (1) Characterized by malabsorption and mucosal lesions of the small intestines.
  (2) Caused by an allergy to gluten (wheat, rye).
  (3) Histology—atrophy of the intestinal villi, intraepithelial lymphocytosis, and crypt hyperplasia.
  (4) Symptoms—weight loss, anemia, fatigue, and diarrhea.
  (5) Complications—T-cell lymphomas.
c. Crohn's disease.
  (1) Chronic inflammatory bowel disease.
  (2) Histologic characteristics.
    (a) Textured, cobblestone appearance of the intestinal mucosa caused by depression of diseased tissue below normal mucosa.
    (b) Presence of transmural edema, inflammation, fibrosis, and noncaseating granulomas.
2. Peutz-Jeghers syndrome.
  a. Disease is characterized by dark, frecklelike spots that appear on the skin, lips, and oral mucosa. Intestinal polyps are also present.
  b. Genetic transmission—autosomal dominant.

G. Large bowel pathology.
  1. Hirschsprung's disease.
    a. Congenital disease.
    b. Caused by a section of aganglionic colon, which failed to develop normally owing to the absence of ganglion cells. This region has no peristalsis resulting in bowel obstruction and distention proximal to the area.
  2. Ulcerative colitis.
    a. Inflammatory bowel disease; related to Crohn's disease but limited to colon and rectum.
    b. Caused by chronic inflammation and ulceration of the colon and rectum.
    c. Histology—inflammation, crypt abscesses, and epithelial metaplasia; granulomas absent.
    d. Symptoms include chronic, bloody diarrhea.
    e. Complications.
      (1) Toxic megacolon.
      (2) Colon cancer.
      (3) Perforation of the colon.

4.4 Genitourinary Pathology

A. Renal pathology.
  1. Glomerulonephritis.
    a. Characterized by inflammation of the glomerulus.
    b. Clinical manifestations.
      (1) Nephrotic syndrome.
        (a) Caused by glomerular disease and by systemic diseases such as diabetes mellitus and amyloidosis.

        (b) Laboratory findings.
          (i) Proteinuria (albuminuria) and lipiduria—proteins and lipids present in urine.
          (ii) Hypoalbuminemia—decreased serum albumin owing to albuminuria.
          (iii) Hyperlipidemia—especially an increase in plasma levels of low-density lipoproteins and cholesterol.
        (c) Symptoms—severe edema, resulting from a decrease in colloid osmotic pressure secondary to a decrease in serum albumin.
      (2) Nephritic syndrome.
        (a) Characterized by inflammation in the glomeruli.
        (b) Classic presentation—poststreptococcal glomerulonephritis. It occurs after a group A, β-hemolytic *Streptococcus* infection (e.g., strep throat.)
        (c) Caused by autoantibodies forming immune complexes in the glomerulus.
        (d) Clinical manifestations—oliguria, hematuria, hypertension, edema, and azotemia (increased concentrations of serum urea nitrogen and creatinine).
  2. Polycystic kidney disease (adult).
    a. Characterized by the formation of cysts with partial replacement of renal parenchyma.
    b. Genetic transmission—autosomal dominant.
    c. Clinical manifestations—hematuria, proteinuria, polyuria, hypertension, palpable renal masses, and progression to renal failure; commonly associated with liver cysts and intracranial berry aneurysms.
  3. Nephrosclerosis.
    a. Disease of the renal arteries caused by chronic hypertension.
    b. Clinical manifestations.
      (1) Benign (arterial) nephrosclerosis.
        (a) Hyaline arteriosclerosis leads to arteriolar narrowing, which decreases renal blood supply to cause glomerular scarring.
        (b) Results in narrowing of the arterioles.
      (2) Malignant nephrosclerosis.
        (a) Caused by malignant hypertension. Common signs of malignant hypertension include severe hypertension, retinal hemorrhages, and hypertrophy of the left ventricle.
        (b) Results in inflammatory changes in the vascular walls, which may lead to rupture of the glomerular capillaries.
  4. Renal tubule diseases.
    a. Acute kidney injury (acute tubular necrosis).
      (1) Characterized by impaired kidney functions owing to the destruction of the renal tubule epithelium.

(2) Caused by various conditions that lead to ischemia of the renal tubules, usually resulting from renal tubular injury or problems with vascular flow. It also can be induced by ingesting toxins or drug-related toxicity (e.g., gentamicin).

(3) Most common cause of acute renal failure.

(4) A reversible condition, although it can be fatal.

b. Pyelonephritis.

(1) Bacterial infection that affects the renal tubules, interstitium, and renal pelvis.

(2) One of the most common renal diseases.

(3) Usually caused by Gram-negative, rod-shaped bacteria that are part of the normal flora of the enteric tract. Most commonly caused by *E. coli,* followed by *Proteus, Klebsiella,* and *Enterobacter.*

(4) The infecting bacteria are usually from the patient's own enteric flora—an example of an endogenous infection.

(5) Usually associated with a urinary tract infection (acute pyelonephritis) or involved with another precipitating condition, such as obstruction (chronic pyelonephritis).

c. Fanconi's syndrome.

(1) Characterized by the failure of the proximal renal tubules to resorb amino acids, glucose, and phosphates.

(2) May be inherited or acquired.

(3) Clinical manifestations include glycosuria, hyperphosphaturia, and hypophosphatemia.

B. Urinary tract pathology.

1. Urolithiasis.

a. Formation of calculi (calcium stones) in the kidney (nephrolithiasis) or urinary tract (urolithiasis).

b. Most common calculi are calcium stones (70%). Others include triple stones, uric acid stones, and cysteine.

c. Signs and symptoms include severe pain, ureteral obstruction, and hematuria.

d. Note: an enlarged prostate can also cause urinary tract obstruction in men.

2. Urinary tract infection.

a. Most often caused by Gram-negative, rod-shaped bacteria that are normal residents of the enteric tract, especially *E. coli.*

b. Clinical manifestations—frequent urination, dysuria, pyuria (increased PMNs), hematuria, and bacteriuria.

c. May lead to infection of the urinary bladder (cystitis) or kidney (pyelonephritis).

4.5 Blood and Lymphatic Pathology

A. Evaluation tests for bleeding.

1. Prothrombin time (PT)—measures extrinsic and common coagulation pathways.

2. Partial thromboplastin time (PTT)—measures intrinsic and common clotting pathways.

3. Platelet counts—measure platelets in anticoagulated blood.

4. Platelet function.

B. Bleeding disorders may be due to the following.

1. Fragility of vessels.

2. Platelet deficiency.

3. Platelet defects.

4. Defects of coagulation.

C. Vessel wall abnormalities.

1. Unlikely to cause severe bleeding problems.

2. Small hemorrhages (petechiae, purpura) in skin and mucous membranes, especially gingiva.

3. Platelet count, bleeding time, and coagulation time (PT, PTT) are normal.

4. Vessel wall abnormalities cause bleeding in the following clinical conditions.

a. Infections such as meningococcemia, septicemia, and infective endocarditis—petechiae and purpuric hemorrhages.

b. Drug reactions—skin petechiae and purpura without thrombocytopenia.

c. Scurvy and Ehlers-Danlos syndrome—microvascular bleeding occurs as a result of collagen defects that weaken vessel walls.

d. Hereditary hemorrhagic telangiectasia—dilated blood vessels that bleed easily because of thin walls. Bleeding usually occurs in the mucous membranes, including tongue, mouth, and nose (epistaxis).

e. Perivascular amyloidosis leads to weak vessel walls, which cause bleeding.

D. Thrombocytopenia (reduced platelet number).

1. Significant cause of generalized bleeding; may manifest as petechiae.

2. Platelet count usually less than 100,000 platelets/μL.

3. Spontaneous bleeding usually occurs at less than 20,000 platelets/μL.

4. PT and PTT time are normal.

5. Causes of thrombocytopenia.

a. Decreased platelet production, which may be due to reduced marrow output.

b. Decreased platelet survival; may be due to autoantibodies or disseminated intravascular coagulation and thrombotic microangiopathies.

c. Sequestration—an enlarged spleen may lead to excessive sequestration of platelets.

d. Dilution—results from large transfusions because prolonged blood storage reduces viable platelets.

E. Platelet defects.

1. Defects in platelet function may be inherited or acquired. Platelet count may be normal.

2. Inherited disorders may be due to defects of adhesion, aggregation, and platelet secretion.

F. Defects of coagulation.
  1. Coagulation defects occur secondary to inherited or acquired deficiencies of coagulation factors. Defects manifest as follows.
    a. Large hematomas.
    b. Prolonged bleeding (e.g., after a tooth extraction).
  2. Inherited disorders—the most common are as follows.
    a. von Willebrand disease.
      (1) This is the most common of all inherited bleeding disorders in humans.
      (2) Leads to secondary defects in platelet adhesion and clotting.
      (3) Genetic transmission is autosomal dominant.
    b. Deficiency of factor VIII (hemophilia A).
      (1) Life-threatening bleeding may occur.
      (2) Inherited as X-linked recessive trait—males and homozygous females are affected.
      (3) Severity of disease varies with factor VIII activity.
      (4) PTT is prolonged; PT is normal.
    c. Deficiency of factor IX (hemophilia B, Christmas disease).
      (1) Clinically similar to hemophilia A.
      (2) Inherited as X-linked recessive trait—males and homozygous females are affected.
      (3) Severity of disease varies with factor IX activity.
      (4) PTT is prolonged; PT is normal.
  3. Disseminated intravascular coagulation—condition in which clots (thrombi) form in the microvasculature using up all available clotting factors, platelets, and fibrin and resulting in problems with bleeding. It represents a complication of other disorders.
  4. Liver disease—results in decreased production of coagulation factors and can lead to bleeding problems.
  5. Vitamin K deficiency.
    a. Causes include malnutrition and malabsorption of fats.
    b. A decrease in clotting factors II (prothrombin), VII, IX, and X is observed.
    c. Prolonged PT.

4.6 Lymphoproliferative Diseases

4.6.1 Leukemia

A. General characteristics.
  1. Leukemia is characterized by the uncontrolled proliferation of abnormal, monoclonal cells. The bone marrow and peripheral blood become saturated with blasts or blastlike cells, which results in decreased production of normal RBCs, WBCs, and platelets in the bone marrow.

Box 3-2

Causes of Gingival Hyperplasia

1. Lymphoproliferative diseases
2. Medications
   Calcium channel blockers
   Phenytoin (Dilantin)
   Cyclosporine

---

  2. General signs and symptoms.
    a. Recurrent infections secondary to decreased normal WBCs.
    b. Severe anemia, pallor, and fatigue secondary to decreased RBCs.
    c. Bleeding problems secondary to decreased platelet production, which exhibits signs such as petechiae.
  3. Uncontrolled growth of leukemic cells causes leukocytosis and accumulation of leukemic cells in other organs, including the spleen (splenomegaly), liver (hepatomegaly), and lymph nodes (lymphadenopathy).
  4. Oral manifestations.
    a. Spontaneous bleeding from mucous membranes.
    b. Gingival hyperplasia (Box 3-2).
    c. Mucosal ulcerations.
B. Acute leukemias.
  1. General characteristics.
    a. Rapid onset of symptoms occurs most often in children or patients older than 60.
    b. Consists of proliferation of immature blast cells.
  2. Signs and symptoms.
    a. Constitutional symptoms—fever, weakness, fatigue, and bleeding.
    b. Pallor from severe anemia.
    c. Bone and joint pain.
    d. Lymphadenopathy—enlarged lymph nodes.
  3. Acute lymphocytic or lymphoblastic leukemia.
    a. Predominantly occurs in children.
    b. Most common malignancy in children.
    c. Blood smear—lymphoblasts appear as null cells.
    d. Prognosis is good with high cure rates.
  4. Acute myeloid leukemia.
    a. Mostly occurs in adults.
    b. Responds poorly to therapy.
    c. Blood smear—Auer rods may be observed in blast cells.
C. Chronic leukemias.
  1. General characteristics.
    a. Consists of proliferation of mature cells (differentiated cells).
    b. Usually less severe than the acute form.
    c. Signs and symptoms similar to acute leukemia except for a slower and more gradual onset. Weight loss is common.

2. Chronic myeloid leukemia.
   a. Characterized by proliferation of myeloid cells (precursor cells of erythrocytes, granulocytes, and platelets).
   b. Associated with Philadelphia chromosome, which results from translocation of chromosomes 9 and 22.
   c. Signs and symptoms—anemia, splenomegaly, and modestly enlarged liver and lymph nodes.
   d. Usually adults, particularly in fifth and sixth decades of life.
3. Chronic lymphocytic leukemia.
   a. Most common leukemia.
   b. Disease course and patient survival are variable.
   c. Characterized by the proliferation of abnormal B lymphocytes, which cannot produce antibodies. The patient is more susceptible to bacterial infections.
   d. Mostly seen in older adults (>60 years old); male predilection (2:1).
   e. Blood smear—lymphoblasts may appear as smudge cells.

4.6.2 Lymphomas

A. Hodgkin's disease.
   1. Characterized by enlarged lymph nodes and the presence of Reed-Sternberg cells (multinucleated giant cells) in lymphoid tissues.
   2. Disease spreads from lymph node to lymph node in a contiguous manner.
   3. Manifests as lymphadenopathy (e.g., cervical and mediastinal lymphadenopathy).
   4. Cause is unknown.
   5. Average age at diagnosis—32 years.
   6. Prognosis of disease depends largely on the extent of lymph node spread and systemic involvement.
B. Non-Hodgkin's lymphoma.
   1. Characterized by tumor occurrence in multiple peripheral lymph nodes.
   2. Tumors do *not* spread in a contiguous manner.
   3. Extranodal involvement is common.
   4. Occurs after age 40.
   5. Example—Burkitt's lymphoma.
      a. Endemic (African) type is commonly associated with EBV infection and a genetic mutation resulting from the translocation of the *C-myc* gene from chromosome 8 to chromosome 14.
      b. The endemic type commonly affects the mandible.
      c. In the United States, it most commonly affects the abdomen.
      d. Histologically, the tumor displays a characteristic "starry-sky" appearance.

4.7 Plasma Cell Pathology

A. Plasma cell myeloma—also known as multiple myeloma.

1. Malignant plasma cell neoplasm that results in the proliferation of monoclonal plasma cells. These tumor cells produce nonfunctional immunoglobulins.
2. Laboratory findings.
   a. Monoclonal immunoglobulins spike.
   b. Bence-Jones proteins in urine.
3. Radiographic findings—characteristic "punched-out" radiolucencies in bones.

4.8 Endocrine Pathology

A. Thyroid pathology.
   1. Hypothyroidism.
      a. May be autoimmune (usually Hashimoto's thyroiditis), congenital, or acquired (myxedema).
      b. Clinical manifestations.
         (1) Hashimoto's thyroiditis.
            (a) Autoimmune disease in which antibodies attack the thyroid gland, causing direct injury to the thyroid.
            (b) Female predilection; 45 to 65 years old.
         (2) Myxedema—hypothyroidism in older children or adults.
            (a) Most commonly caused by treatment for hyperthyroidism such as surgery, irradiation, or drug therapy.
            (b) Iodine deficiency.
            (c) Decreased metabolism, resulting in weight gain and retarded growth.
            (d) Enlarged face, tongue, eyelids, larynx, and hands.
            (e) Mental and physical slowness.
            (f) Decreased heart rate.
            (g) Sensitivity to cold temperature.
         (3) Cretinism—hypothyroidism in infants and young children.
            (a) Causes include embryologic malformation and iodine deficiency.
            (b) Clinical findings include mental retardation and dwarfism.
            (c) Oral findings include macroglossia, prolonged retention of primary teeth, and delayed eruption of permanent teeth.
   2. Hyperthyroidism (thyrotoxicosis).
      a. General signs and symptoms.
         (1) Increased metabolism, resulting in weight loss.
         (2) Irritability, nervousness, and tremor.
         (3) Tachycardia, often with arrhythmia and palpitation.
         (4) Goiter.
         (5) Oral findings include early loss of primary teeth and early eruption of permanent teeth.
      b. Clinical manifestations.
         (1) Graves' disease.
            (a) Autoimmune disease in which antibodies bind to the thyroid-stimulating hormone

Diseases That Can Cause an Increase in Alkaline Phosphatase

Hyperparathyroidism
Paget's disease
Osteosarcoma
Multiple myeloma
Prostate cancer with bone metastases

receptor, resulting in constant stimulation for the release of triiodothyronine (T3) and thyroxine (T4).

  (b) General signs include exophthalmos, or protrusion of eyeballs.

  (2) Plummer's disease.

  (a) May be caused by a nodular growth or adenoma of the thyroid.

  (b) Clinical signs are similar to Graves' disease except no exophthalmos is present.

  c. Dental significance—administration of dental anesthesia with epinephrine to patients with uncontrolled or undiagnosed hyperthyroidism may cause the patient to develop a thyrotoxic crisis.

B. Parathyroid pathology.

  1. Hyperparathyroidism.

  a. General characteristics.

  (1) Hypercalcemia—high levels of serum calcium.

  (2) Hypophosphatemia—low levels of serum phosphate.

  (3) Increased alkaline phosphatase (Box 3-3).

  (4) Osseous changes.

  (a) Extensive loss of bone density.

  (b) Calcifications.

  (c) Kidney stones.

  (5) Radiographic findings of bone include ground-glass appearance.

  b. Clinical manifestations.

  (1) Primary hyperparathyroidism—most commonly caused by a parathyroid adenoma.

  (2) Secondary hyperparathyroidism—usually occurs as a result of chronic renal disease or kidney failure. During renal disease, active vitamin D is not produced, leading to low levels of calcium being absorbed from the intestinal tract. A chronic low level of calcium activates the parathyroid to release parathyroid hormone, resulting in hyperparathyroidism.

  2. Hypoparathyroidism.

  a. Most commonly caused by accidental surgical removal of the parathyroid gland during thyroid surgery.

  b. May be associated with DiGeorge's syndrome, but this is rare.

  c. General findings.

  (1) Hypocalcemia or low levels of serum calcium.

  (2) Increased neuromuscular excitability and tetany secondary to hypocalcemia.

C. Pituitary gland pathology.

  1. Growth hormone (GH) deficiency.

  a. Causes of decreased level of GH.

  (1) Decreased secretion of GH-releasing hormone from the hypothalamus.

  (2) Decreased secretion of GH from the anterior pituitary, also known as *pituitary dwarfism*.

  (3) Decreased response of cells to GH.

  b. Clinical manifestation—dwarfism.

  (1) General signs and symptoms.

  (a) Abnormally short height (failure to thrive).

  (b) Smaller maxilla and mandible.

  (c) Delayed eruption of permanent teeth.

  2. Excessive production of GH.

  a. Gigantism.

  (1) Occurs if increase in GH occurs before the epiphyseal plates have fused.

  (2) Clinical signs include abnormally tall height, enlarged mandible.

  b. Acromegaly.

  (1) Occurs if increase in GH occurs after the epiphyseal plates have fused.

  (2) Clinical signs include gradual enlargement of the hands, feet, and skull. Patients may find that shoes, gloves, and dentures have become too small.

  3. Diabetes insipidus.

  a. Characterized by a deficiency of antidiuretic hormone.

  b. Symptoms include polyuria and polydipsia.

  4. Sheehan's disease.

  a. Characterized by the lack of anterior pituitary functioning, resulting in decreased secretion of follicle-stimulating hormone, luteinizing hormone, thyroid-stimulating hormone, and adrenocortico-tropic hormone (ACTH).

  b. Caused by necrosis of the anterior pituitary after a complicated childbirth.

D. Adrenal (suprarenal) gland pathology.

  1. Adrenal medulla pathology.

  a. Pheochromocytoma.

  (1) Benign tumor formed from adrenal chromaffin cells; 10% become malignant. Note: if the adrenal tumor is formed from extraadrenal paraganglia, it is known as a *paraganglioma*.

  (2) Tumor secretions result in increased epinephrine and norepinephrine.

  (3) Associated syndromes include Sturge-Weber syndrome and multiple endocrine neoplasia type 2a and type 2b.

(4) General signs and symptoms.
  (a) Secondary hypertension.
  (b) Increased heart rate, palpitations.
b. Neuroblastoma.
  (1) Malignant catecholamine-producing tumor formed from immature medullary cells.
  (2) Most common malignant tumor found in children.
  (3) Tumor secretions result in increased epinephrine and norepinephrine.
  (4) Neuroblastomas usually occur sporadically.
2. Adrenal cortex pathology.
  a. Addison's disease—primary adrenocortical deficiency.
    (1) Characterized by a decrease in steroid hormone secretion owing to destruction of adrenal cortex. This results in an increase in production of ACTH from the anterior pituitary. (Pituitary disorders that decrease ACTH secretion produce a syndrome similar to Addison's disease.)
    (2) Clinical findings from decreased cortisol production.
      (a) Darker pigmentation in certain areas (e.g., skin, mucosa) results from increased secretion of melanin by melanocytes that are stimulated by melanocyte-stimulating hormone. The increased levels of melanocyte-stimulating hormone result from increased proopiomelanocortin, which also increases ACTH production.
      (b) Poor response to stress.
      (c) Anemias, GI disturbances, hypotension, and weakness.
    (3) Oral findings include dark pigmentation on the tongue, palate, gingiva, and mucosa.
    (4) Treatment—cortisol or other steroid therapy.
  b. Cushing's syndrome—elevated glucocorticoids
    (1) Exogenous glucocorticoids—majority of cases
    (2) Endogenous glucocorticoid increase
      (a) ACTH dependent—Cushing's disease due to pituitary adenoma
      (b) ACTH independent—adrenal adenoma or carcinoma
    (3) Hypertension, weight gain, fat accumulation—truncal obesity, moon facies.
E. Endocrine pancreas pathology—diabetes mellitus.
  1. General characteristics of diabetes mellitus.
    a. Characterized by hyperglycemia (abnormally high levels of blood glucose).
    b. Hallmark symptoms.
      (1) Polyuria—frequent urination.
      (2) Polydipsia—constant thirst.
      (3) Polyphagia—frequent intake of food.
    c. Complications.
      (1) Retinopathy.

(2) Nephropathy.
(3) Peripheral neuropathy.
(4) Cardiovascular disease—leading cause of death for diabetic patients.
(5) Oral complications of uncontrolled diabetes.
  (a) Increased periodontal disease.
  (b) Increased susceptibility to *Candidiasis*.
2. Two types of diabetes mellitus.
  a. Type 1 diabetes.
    (1) Also known as juvenile-onset or insulin-dependent diabetes mellitus (IDDM).
    (2) Caused by autoimmune destruction of pancreatic β cells, resulting in a complete absence of insulin production.
    (3) The disease usually presents before the age of 20.
    (4) Characterized by severe hyperglycemia and ketoacidosis (ketoacidosis is uncommon in patients with non–insulin-dependent diabetes). Untreated ketoacidosis may result in diabetic coma.
    (5) Treatment—requires insulin and diet control.
  b. Type 2 diabetes.
    (1) Also known as adult-onset or non–insulin-dependent diabetes (NIDDM).
    (2) Caused by a decreased sensitivity of peripheral insulin receptors to insulin, insulin receptor dysfunction, or a decreased production of insulin. In contrast to in type 1 diabetes, insulin is still produced.
    (3) Occurs later in life, usually after the age of 40, but prevalence is increasing in children and teenagers.
    (4) Is commonly seen in obese patients.
    (5) More prevalent than type 1 diabetes.
    (6) Treatment—diet control; may or may not require insulin or other hypoglycemic agent (e.g., metformin, glyburide).
3. Diabetic shock—seen in patients who do not consume enough carbohydrates after an insulin injection. This results in an abnormally low level of glucose in the blood.

4.9 Musculoskeletal Pathology

A. Bone pathology.
  1. Osteoporosis.
    a. Characterized by a decrease in bone mass.
    b. Causes.
      (1) Calcium deficiency, decreased vitamin D, and upregulated parathyroid hormone.
      (2) Decreased level of estrogen, leading to increased bone loss; also known as *postmenopausal osteoporosis*.
      (3) Decreased physical inactivity.
      (4) Advanced age (senile osteoporosis).
      (5) Hyperthyroidism, Addison's disease.

c. Complications include compression fractures, which commonly occur.
2. Vitamin D deficiency.
  a. Vitamin D deficiency results in the failure of new bone to mineralize.
  b. Two types.
    (1) Osteomalacia—vitamin D deficiency in adults. Characterized by defective calcification of osteoid matrix. Contours of bone are unchanged, but bone fractures easily. Patients may also experience diffuse bone pain.
    (2) Rickets—vitamin D deficiency in infants and children. Usually observed in first year of life. Characterized by inadequate calcification and increased thickness in epiphyseal growth plates, resulting in skeletal deformities, including accentuated costochondral junctions (rachitic rosary). Growth retardation may also occur. Rickets is uncommon in the United States because of vitamin D supplementation of milk.
3. Scurvy.
  a. Caused by vitamin C (ascorbic acid) deficiency, leading to impaired osteoid matrix formation.
  b. Clinical findings.
    (1) Bleeding gums, petechiae, subperiosteal hemorrhage.
    (2) Osteoporosis.
    (3) Note: the epiphyseal cartilage is not replaced by osteoid.
4. Osteogenesis imperfecta (brittle bone disease).
  a. Caused by defective formation of type I collagen.
  b. Characterized by fragile (brittle) bones and a deformed skeleton.
  c. Symptoms include fractures and blue ocular sclerae (type I osteogenesis imperfecta).
  d. Oral findings (type I osteogenesis imperfecta) include dentinogenesis imperfecta.
5. Osteopetrosis (Albers-Schönberg disease or marble bone disease).
  a. Caused by abnormal osteoclasts. This results in defective bone remodeling (i.e., abnormally low bone resorption) and increased bone density, which may invade into bone marrow space.
  b. Causes severe defects in infants.
    (1) Anemia and infections—caused by decreased bone marrow.
    (2) Blindness, deafness, paralysis of facial muscles—caused by the narrowing of cranial nerve foramina.
    (3) Life-threatening.
    (4) Oral findings—delayed eruption of teeth.
  c. Disease less severe in adults.
6. Paget's disease (osteitis deformans).
  a. Characterized by abnormal bone remodeling leading to distortion of bone architecture.
  b. Laboratory findings—increased serum alkaline phosphatase.
  c. Radiographic findings—"cotton-wool" appearance.
  d. Complications.
    (1) Osteosarcoma.
    (2) Heart disease.
    (3) Deafness or blindness.
  e. Oral findings.
    (1) Difficult extractions owing to hypercementosis.
    (2) Osteomyelitis.
    (3) Common complaint of edentulous patients is that "dentures no longer fit."
7. Osteomyelitis.
  a. Infection of bone and marrow.
  b. Most commonly caused by *S. aureus*.
  c. Clinical findings include pain and systemic signs of infection (i.e., fever, malaise).
8. Fibrous dysplasia.
  a. Caused by replacement of normal bone with irregular bone interspersed with fibrous connective tissue.
  b. Radiographic findings—ground-glass appearance.
  c. Three types.
    (1) Monostotic—affects one bone (most common); usually asymptomatic.
    (2) Polyostotic (Jaffe-Lichtenstein syndrome)—affects more than one bone. Café au lait pigmentation (brown macules) is observed on trunk and thighs.
    (3) McCune-Albright syndrome—polyostotic fibrous dysplasia, café au lait pigmentation (brown macules), and endocrine abnormalities such as precocious puberty.
  d. In the jaws, the maxilla is more commonly involved than the mandible.
9. Osteochondroses.
  a. Most often caused by osteonecrosis of the epiphyseal plates or the ossification centers in bone. This results in the reossification and sclerosis of the affected areas.
  b. Osgood-Schlatter syndrome is one type of osteochondrosis that affects the tibial tuberosity (i.e., knee). This usually occurs in adolescent boys who play sports.
10. Langerhans' cell histiocytosis (histiocytosis X or Langerhans' cell granuloma).
  a. Group of diseases that exhibit histiocytelike Langerhans' cells and an infiltrate of eosinophils, lymphocytes, plasma cells, and multinucleated giant cells. Langerhans' cells are dendritic cells that occur in the epidermis, bone marrow, lymph nodes, and mucosa.
  b. Most commonly causes bone lesions; however, other tissues can be affected.
  c. Histologic findings—Langerhans' cells containing Birbeck granules and eosinophils.

d. Three types.
  (1) Letterer-Siwe disease—acute, disseminated form that is fatal in infants; involves bone, skin, and viscera.
  (2) Hand-Schüller-Christian disease—chronic, disseminated form that has a better prognosis than Letterer-Siwe disease. It usually manifests before age 5 and is characterized by a triad of symptoms.
    (a) Bone lesions—found in skull, mandible (loose teeth), vertebrae, and ribs.
    (b) Exophthalmos.
    (c) Diabetes insipidus.
  (3) Eosinophilic granuloma of bone—localized, least severe form of the three. Lesions may heal without treatment. One or multiple bones may be involved; no involvement of viscera.
    (a) Most commonly occurs in young adults.
    (b) Lesions in the mandible may cause loose teeth.

11. Bone malignancies.
  1. Osteosarcoma (osteogenic sarcoma).
    a. Most common true primary bone tumor, excluding multiple myeloma and lymphoma.
    b. Findings include an increased serum alkaline phosphatase and radiographic observation of Codman's triangle (lifting of the periosteum by the tumor with subsequent reactive periosteal bone formation).
    c. Occurs in children and adolescents.
  2. Ewing's sarcoma.
    a. Small, blue cell malignant tumor.
    b. Commonly found in long bones (femur) or pelvis.
    c. Usually occurs before age 20.
    d. Symptoms include intermittent pain and swelling.

B. Cartilage pathology.
  1. Achondroplasia.
    a. Caused by delayed or abnormal growth of cartilage, leading to shortened extremities.
    b. Characterized by short stature.
    c. Oral findings—mandibular prognathism.
  2. Osteochondroma.
    a. Bony growths surrounded by cartilage.
    b. Most common benign tumor of the bone.
    c. Occurs in bones of endochondral origin.
    d. Most often found at the distal ends of long bones.
  3. Chondrosarcoma.
    a. Malignant cartilaginous tumor.
    b. Men more frequently affected than women (2 : 1).
    c. Second most common primary bone tumor occurring in bone, excluding multiple myeloma and lymphoma. Osteosarcoma is the most common.
    d. Sites of origin usually include the pelvis, ribs, and shoulder.

C. Joint pathology.
  1. Rheumatoid arthritis.
    a. Cause is autoimmune in nature.
    b. More common in women than men, particularly women 40 to 70 years old.
    c. Characterized by inflammation of the synovial membrane. Granulation tissue, known as *pannus*, forms in the synovium and expands over the articular cartilage. This causes the destruction of the underlying cartilage and results in fibrotic changes and ankylosis. Scarring, contracture, and deformity of the joints may occur. Rheumatoid nodules may occur in the skin.
    d. Clinical symptoms include swollen joints. It can affect any joint in the body.
  2. Osteoarthritis.
    a. Most common disease of joints.
    b. Cause is unknown.
    c. Women more commonly exhibit involvement of knees and hands; men more commonly exhibit hip involvement.
    d. Characterized by degeneration of the articular cartilage and the formation of osteophytes (bony spurs) at the margins of affected areas.
    e. Clinical signs and symptoms.
      (1) Stiff and painful joints affecting joints in the hand (phalangeal joints) and weight-bearing joints.
      (2) Heberden's nodes—nodules at the distal interphalangeal joint.

D. Muscle pathology.
  1. Myasthenia gravis.
    a. Autoimmune disease caused by autoantibodies to acetylcholine receptors at the neuromuscular junctions.
    b. Characterized by muscle weakness or inability to maintain long durations of muscle contractions; this worsens during exercise but recovers after rest.
    c. Affects various muscle groups.
      (1) Eyes—diplopia (double vision), ptosis (drooping eyelids).
      (2) Neck—dysphagia, problems swallowing or speaking.
      (3) Extremities—arms and legs.
    d. Treatment—cholinesterase inhibitors (neostigmine), antiimmune therapy.
  2. Muscle tumors.
    a. Rhabdomyoma—benign tumor of skeletal muscle.
    b. Leiomyoma.
      (1) Benign tumor of smooth muscle.
      (2) Most common tumor found in women.
      (3) Usually affects the uterus, although it can occur anywhere.
    c. Rhabdomyosarcoma.
      (1) Malignant tumor of skeletal muscle.

(2) Most common soft tissue sarcoma found in children.

(3) Usually affects head and neck region—orbit, nasal cavity, and nasopharynx.

4.10 Skin Pathology

4.10.1 Skin Lesions

A. Seborrheic keratosis.
   1. Round, brown-colored, flat plaque.
   2. Most often seen in middle-aged to older adults.
   3. Benign lesion.
B. Verruca vulgaris.
   1. Commonly known as *warts*.
   2. Caused by HPV.
   3. Warts can be seen on skin or as an oral lesion (vermilion border, labial mucosa, or tongue).
   4. Transmitted by contact or autoinoculation.
   5. Benign lesions.
C. Actinic keratosis.
   1. Dry, scaly plaques with erythematous base.
   2. Similar to actinic cheilosis, which occurs along the vermilion border of the lower lip.
   3. Caused by sun damage to the skin.
   4. Premalignant.
D. Melanocytic nevus (pigmented nevus).
   1. Commonly known as a *mole*.
   2. Benign, pigmented tumor of melanocytes, found deep within connective tissue.
   3. Types of skin nevi.
      a. Junctional nevus—nevus cells at the dermoepidermal junction.
      b. Compound nevus—nevus cells in both the epidermis and the underlying dermis.
      c. Intraepidermal nevus—nevus cells in the dermis.
E. Psoriasis.
   1. Characterized by skin lesions that appear as scaly, erythematous plaques.
   2. Caused by rapid proliferation of the epidermis.
   3. Etiology is unclear.
F. Keloids.
   1. Characterized by progressively enlarging scar.
   2. Caused by an abnormal accumulation of collagen at the site of injury.
   3. More common in African-Americans.

4.10.2 Skin Diseases with Oral Manifestations

A. Erythema multiforme.
   1. Erythematous, ulcerative lesions on the skin and oral mucosa.
   2. Skin lesions are round and may have a "bull's-eye" or targetlike appearance.
   3. Can result from drug reaction or infection.
   4. In severe cases, known as Stevens-Johnson syndrome or erythema multiforme major, lesions are seen on the skin, oral mucosa, eye, and genital area.
   5. Treatment—corticosteroids in severe cases.

B. Pemphigus vulgaris.
   1. Ulcerative lesions on the skin and oral mucosa.
   2. Autoimmune disease in which patients have autoantibodies against desmosomal attachment between epithelial cells in skin or oral mucosa.
   3. Histologically characterized by acantholysis, in which epidermal cells appear to detach from each other and become rounded (Tzanck's cells).
   4. Can be life-threatening if untreated.
   5. A positive Nikolsky sign is observed. Because of sloughing of the epidermis, a red blister forms after pressure is applied to affected skin.
   6. Treatment—corticosteroids.
C. Mucous membrane pemphigoid.
   1. Ulcerative lesions on skin and oral mucosa.
   2. Autoimmune disease in which patients have autoantibodies against components of the basement membrane.
   3. Histologically, the entire epithelium appears to separate from the connective tissue. There is no acantholysis.
   4. A positive Nikolsky sign is observed.
   5. Complications in some patients include blindness resulting from ocular lesions that scar.
   6. Treatment—corticosteroids.
D. Lichen planus.
   1. Skin lesions appear as a cluster of purple, itchy, polygonal papules. There are two types of oral lesions, reticular and erosive lichen planus. Reticular lichen planus is characterized by intersecting white lines known as *Wickham's striae*, most often seen along the buccal mucosa. Erosive lichen planus is less common and exhibits erythematous, ulcerated areas. On the gingiva, this appearance is termed *desquamative gingivitis*.
   2. Histologically characterized by saw-tooth rete ridges and the presence of Civatte bodies.
E. Peutz-Jeghers syndrome.
   1. Lesions appear as small, melanotic, and frecklelike. They can be found on the skin, oral mucosa, lips, feet, and hands.
   2. May also occur with intestinal polyps. Patients may develop a GI carcinoma.
   3. Genetic transmission—autosomal dominant.

4.11 Genetic Diseases

A. Lysosomal (lipid) storage diseases.
   1. Genetic transmission—autosomal recessive.
   2. This group of diseases is characterized by a deficiency of a particular lysosomal enzyme or of a protein required for lysosome function. This deficiency results in an accumulation of the metabolite, which would have otherwise been degraded by the presence of normal levels of the enzyme or protein.

3. Diseases.
   a. Gaucher's disease.
      (1) Deficient enzyme—glucocerebrosidase.
      (2) Metabolite that accumulates—glucocerebroside.
      (3) Important cells affected—macrophages.
   b. Tay-Sachs disease.
      (1) Deficient enzyme—hexosaminidase A.
      (2) Metabolite that accumulates—G_{M2} ganglioside.
      (3) Important cells affected—neurons.
      (4) Symptoms include motor and mental deterioration, blindness, and dementia.
      (5) Prevalent among Jews, particularly Ashkenazi Jews.
   c. Niemann-Pick disease.
      (1) Deficient enzyme—sphingomyelinase.
      (2) Metabolite that accumulates—sphingomyelin.
      (3) Important cells affected—neurons and phagocytic cells.
B. Glycogen storage diseases (glycogenoses).
   1. Genetic transmission—autosomal recessive.
   2. This group of diseases is characterized by a deficiency of a particular enzyme involved in either glycogen production or degradative pathways.
   3. Diseases.
      a. von Gierke's disease (type I).
         (1) Deficient enzyme—glucose-6-phosphatase.
         (2) Major organ affected by buildup of glycogen—liver and kidney.
      b. Pompe's disease (type II).
         (1) Deficient enzyme—lysosomal glucosidase (acid maltase).
         (2) Major organ affected by buildup of glycogen—heart.
      c. Cori's disease (type III).
         (1) Deficient enzyme—debranching enzyme (amylo-1,6-glucosidase).
         (2) Organs affected by buildup of glycogen—varies between the heart, liver, or skeletal muscle.
      d. Brancher glycogenosis (type IV).
         (1) Deficient enzyme—branching enzyme.
         (2) Organs affected by buildup of glycogen—liver, heart, skeletal muscle, and brain.
      e. McArdle's syndrome (type V).
         (1) Deficient enzyme—muscle phosphorylase.
         (2) Major organ affected by buildup of glycogen—skeletal muscle.
C. Connective tissue diseases.
   1. Marfan's syndrome.
      a. Genetic transmission—autosomal dominant.
      b. Characterized by a defective microfibril glycoprotein, fibrillin.
      c. Clinical findings—tall stature; joints that can be hyperextended; and cardiovascular defects, including mitral valve prolapse and dilation of the ascending aorta.

   2. Ehlers-Danlos syndrome.
      a. Genetic transmission—autosomal dominant or recessive.
      b. This group of diseases is characterized by defects in collagen.
      c. Clinical findings—hypermobile joints and highly stretchable skin. The skin also bruises easily. Oral findings include Gorlin's sign (touch the tip of the nose with the tongue) and possible temporomandibular joint subluxation. The oral mucosa may also appear more fragile and vulnerable to trauma.
D. Birth defects and chromosome abnormalities.
   1. General chromosome abnormalities.
      a. The normal human cell contains 46 chromosomes, including 22 homologous pairs of autosomes and one pair of sex chromosomes (XX for female and XY for male). A somatic cell is diploid, containing 46 chromosomes. Gametes are haploid, containing 23 chromosomes.
         (1) Aneuploidy.
            (a) Any deviation in the number of chromosomes, whether fewer or more, from the normal haploid number of chromosomes.
            (b) Nondisjunction—a common cause of aneuploidy. It is the failure of paired chromosomes to pass to separate cells during meiotic or mitotic cell division.
            (c) Often seen in malignant tumors.
         (2) Deletion—loss of a sequence of DNA from a chromosome.
         (3) Translocation—the separation of a part of a chromosome and the attachment of the area of separation to another nonhomologous chromosome.
   2. Abnormalities in chromosome number.
      a. Trisomy 21 (Down syndrome).
         (1) Most common chromosomal disorder.
         (2) Disorder affecting autosomes. It is generally caused by meiotic nondisjunction in the mother, which results in an extra copy of chromosome 21 or trisomy 21.
         (3) Risk increases with maternal age.
         (4) Clinical findings include mental retardation and congenital heart defects. There is also an increased risk of developing acute leukemia and an increased susceptibility to severe infections.
         (5) Oral findings—macroglossia, delayed eruption of teeth, and hypodontia.
      b. Trisomies 18 and 13.
         (1) Trisomy 18 (Edwards' syndrome)—characterized by an extra copy of chromosome 18.
            (a) Oral findings—micrognathia.
         (2) Trisomy 13 (Patau's syndrome)—characterized by an extra copy of chromosome 13.
            (a) Oral findings—cleft lip and palate.

(3) Meiotic nondisjunction is usually the cause of an extra chromosome in both of these trisomies.

(4) Clinical findings for both of these trisomies are usually more severe than trisomy 21. Most children with these diseases die within months after birth secondary to manifestations such as congenital heart disease.

c. Klinefelter's syndrome.

(1) One of the most common causes of male hypogonadism.

(2) Characterized by two or more X chromosomes and one or more Y chromosomes. Typically, there are 47 chromosomes with the karyotype of XXY.

(3) The cause is usually meiotic nondisjunction.

(4) Clinical findings include atrophic and underdeveloped testes, gynecomastia, tall stature, and a lower IQ.

d. Turner's syndrome.

(1) One of the most important causes of amenorrhea.

(2) Characterized by having only one X chromosome, with a total of 45 chromosomes and a karyotype of XO.

(3) Clinical findings include underdeveloped female genitalia, short stature, webbed neck, and amenorrhea. Affected females are usually sterile. In contrast to other chromosomal disorders, this disorder is usually not complicated by mental retardation.

e. Mandibulofacial dysostosis (Treacher Collins syndrome).

(1) Genetic transmission—autosomal dominant.

(2) Relatively rare disease that results from abnormal development of derivatives from the first and second branchial arches.

(3) Clinical findings include underdeveloped zygomas and mandible, downward slanting palpebral fissures, and deformed ears. Oral findings include cleft palate and small or absent parotid glands.

4.12 Nervous System

4.12.1 Infections

A. Bacterial meningitis (pyogenic, suppurative infections).

1. Common causes.

a. *E. coli* in newborns.

b. *H. influenzae* in infants and children.

c. *N. meningitidis* in young adults.

d. *S. pneumoniae* and *L. monocytogenes* in older adults.

2. Clinical findings—severe headache, irritability, fever, and stiff neck.

a. A spinal tap shows CSF that is cloudy or purulent and is under increased pressure. There is also an increase in protein and a decrease in glucose levels.

3. Can be fatal if left untreated.

B. Viral meningitis.

1. Can be caused by many different viruses, including EBV, HSV, and VZV.

2. CSF from a spinal tap differs from that seen in a bacterial infection. It shows higher levels of protein and normal levels of glucose.

C. Demyelinating and degenerative diseases.

1. Multiple sclerosis.

a. Demyelinating disease that primarily affects myelin (i.e., white matter). This affects the conduction of electrical impulses along the axons of nerves. Areas of demyelination are known as *plaques*.

b. Most common demyelinating disease.

c. Onset of disease usually occurs between ages 20 and 50; more common in women (2 : 1).

d. Disease can affect any neuron in CNS, including the brainstem and spinal cord. The optic nerve (vision) is commonly affected.

2. Amyotrophic lateral sclerosis (Lou Gehrig's disease).

a. Characterized by rapid degeneration of motor neurons in the spinal cord and corticospinal tracts.

b. Slightly more common in men than women, in their 40s or later.

c. Clinically, the disease results in rapidly progressive muscle atrophy secondary to denervation. Other symptoms include fasciculations, hyperreflexia, spasticity, and pathologic reflexes. Death usually occurs within a few years from onset, usually by respiratory infection.

3. Alzheimer's disease.

a. Most common cause of dementia in older adults.

b. Characterized by degeneration of neurons in the cerebral cortex.

c. Histologic findings include amyloid plaques and neurofibrillary tangles.

d. Clinically, the disease takes years to develop and results in the loss of cognition, memory, and ability to communicate. Symptoms at the terminal stage include motor problems, contractures, and paralysis.

4. Parkinson's disease.

a. Characterized by the degeneration of neurons in the basal ganglia, specifically, the substantia nigra as well as the locus caeruleus.

b. Histologic findings in affected neurons include Lewy bodies.

c. Clinically, the disease affects involuntary and voluntary movements. Tremors are common. Symptoms include pin-rolling tremors, slowness of movements, muscular rigidity, and shuffling gait.

5. Huntington's disease.

a. Causes dementia.

b. Genetic transmission: autosomal dominant.

c. Characterized by degeneration of striatal neurons, affecting cortical and basal ganglia function.

d. Clinically, the disease affects both movement and cognition and is ultimately fatal.

4.13 Further Reading

Students are referred to the following texts for further study of pathology.

Kumar V, et al, editors: Robbins and Cotran Pathologic Basis of Disease, ed 8. Philadelphia, Saunders, 2010.

Neville BW, et al, editors: Oral and Maxillofacial Pathology, ed 3, Philadelphia, Saunders, 2009.

5.0 Growth Disturbances

5.1 Neoplasms—Etiology, Epidemiology, and Biology

A. Neoplasms are new and abnormal masses that grow more than the adjacent normal tissue. Neoplasms may be benign or malignant.

B. Benign versus malignant tumors.

1. Malignant neoplasms (cancer) are invasive (able to infiltrate past the basement membrane into adjacent tissues) and are able to metastasize to other related or nonrelated parts of the body. Benign tumors are self-limiting, usually well-circumscribed, expansive, noninvasive tumors that do not metastasize. However, they can be harmful if their growth impinges on surrounding structures. Generally, the names of benign tumors end with "oma." Malignant epithelial tumors end with "carcinoma" and malignant mesenchymal tumors end with "sarcoma."

2. Benign tumors—general characteristics.

a. Rate of growth—slow. Regression of the lesion is possible.

b. Are usually well-circumscribed noninvasive and may be surrounded by a capsule made of condensed connective tissue.

c. It is uncommon for them to recur after surgical resection.

d. Histologic features.

(1) Differentiated cells that resemble normal cells.

(2) Nuclear-to-cytoplasmic ratio is appropriate.

(3) Low mitotic activity.

3. Malignant tumors—general characteristics.

a. Nomenclature—malignant neoplasms are named according to their presumed cellular origin and their morphologic appearance. For example, a tumor of epithelial origin (carcinoma) that is observed in a glandular growth pattern is called an *adenocarcinoma.*

b. General names of malignant tumors.

(1) Carcinoma—develops from epithelial cells.

(2) Sarcoma—develops from mesenchymal cells.

c. Rate of growth varies from slow to rapid.

d. Usually invade the surrounding structures (i.e., unencapsulated).

e. May recur after surgical resection. Recurrence may be due to stem cells, a small population of immortal cells that may regenerate the original tumor.

f. Histologic features.

(1) Anaplasia—there is a loss of differentiation in these cells.

(2) Pleomorphism—cells and their nuclei can appear in various forms and shapes.

(3) Prominent nucleoli.

(4) Hyperchromatism—dark-staining nuclei.

(5) High nuclear-to-cytoplasmic ratios.

(6) Increased mitotic activity; atypical mitoses.

(7) May be aneuploid (have an abnormal number of chromosomes).

C. Premalignant lesions—for example, epithelial dysplasia of surface oral epithelium, a precancerous lesion that carries the risk for developing into squamous cell carcinoma (SCC).

1. Epithelial dysplasia (mild, moderate, or severe)—a precancerous lesion with changes in appearance and organization of cells that are restricted to the surface epithelium. The risk of developing into SCC varies with the severity of dysplasia. In other words, it is a lesion with the potential to invade but has not yet invaded.

2. Carcinoma in situ—precancerous changes involve the full thickness of epithelium. There is no invasion of the basement membrane. The likelihood of invasive growth is high.

D. Carcinogenesis—environmental and patient-related factors (age, genetic disorders) may contribute to the development of cancer.

1. Environmental factors.

a. Geographic location—it has been shown that where a person lives can affect the likelihood of developing certain types of cancer. For example, people living in Japan are eight times more likely to die of stomach cancer than people living in the United States.

b. Chemical factors—examples include smoking and asbestos.

c. Radiation—an example includes UV radiation from the sun, which increases risk for SCC and basal cell carcinoma (BCC).

d. Viral infections—examples include links between HPV and cervical cancer, HPV and oropharyngeal cancer, and hepatitis B and hepatocellular carcinoma.

2. Age—somatic mutations (changes in genes after birth) accumulate as an individual ages. Somatic mutations and the decrease in immunocompetence with age favor the development of tumors in older rather than younger people.

3. Genetic disorders—some individuals may be predisposed to cancer because of inherited genetic

mutations. For example, individuals with Peutz-Jeghers syndrome, with autosomal dominant inheritance, are predisposed to develop GI carcinoma.

E. Ultimately, carcinogenesis, regardless of whether it is due to environmental or patient-related factors, involves changes in four groups of normal regulatory genes.

1. Proto-oncogenes—promote cell growth. Oncogenes are the constitutively active counterparts of proto-oncogenes.
2. Tumor suppressor genes—inhibit cell growth. Mutations in these genes remove the inhibitory effects, causing increased and uncontrolled cell proliferation.
3. Genes that regulate apoptosis (programmed cell death)—basically, these may act as either proto-oncogenes or tumor suppressor genes.
4. Genes that regulate DNA repair.

F. Phenotypic changes of cancer.
1. Growth.
2. Refractory to growth inhibitory signals.
3. Survival.
4. Stemness.
5. Angiogenesis.
6. Invasion and metastasis.
7. DNA repair defects.

G. The genetic damage of cancer-associated genes may involve a single gene (e.g., point mutations) or large sections of the chromosome (e.g., translocations).

5.2 Specific Neoplasms

For lymphoproliferative diseases and other neoplasms, refer to the specific sections in Section 4, Systemic Pathology.

A. Oral cancer—SCC.
1. SCC is the most common oral cancer, accounting for 90% of the cases. It is a tumor derived from keratinocytes.
2. It carries a poor prognosis.
3. Males are two times more likely to be affected than females, especially men older than age 50.
4. Metastasis of oral SCC most commonly spreads via the lymphatic system to the cervical lymph nodes.
5. Risk factors.
   a. Smoking.
   b. Some types of smokeless tobacco.
   c. Excessive alcohol consumption.
   d. Nutritional deficiencies (e.g., iron, vitamin A).
6. High-risk sites.
   a. Lower vermilion border of the lip. UV radiation is an important risk factor at this site.
   b. Posterior lateral and ventral surface of the tongue—most common intraoral site.
   c. Floor of the mouth.
   d. Soft palate.

B. Skin cancer—most common type of cancer in the United States.

1. SCC.
   a. Tumor of keratinocytes.
   b. Related to sun-exposed skin, or UV radiation.
   c. Males are more commonly affected than females.
   d. Commonly occurs as an indurated, crusting ulcer with raised margins.
   e. Risk of metastasis is lower than intraoral SCC.
2. BCC.
   a. Tumor of basal cells.
   b. Involves sun-exposed areas, frequently the head and neck.
   c. Most common type of skin cancer.
   d. Carries a good prognosis because it metastasizes slowly.
   e. BCCs are also seen in patients with a diagnosis of nevoid BCC syndrome (Gorlin-Goltz syndrome). The most common features of this syndrome are multiple BCCs, odontogenic keratocysts (also termed *keratocystic odontogenic tumors*), epidermal cysts of the skin, calcifications of the falx cerebri, palmar and plantar pitting, occult spina bifida, mild ocular hypertelorism, and rib anomalies.
3. Malignant melanoma.
   a. Tumor of melanocytic origin, primarily associated with UV radiation.
   b. Most lethal form of skin cancer.
   c. Intraoral melanomas are rare.

C. Bronchogenic carcinoma (lung cancer).
1. Leading cause of cancer-related death in men and women.
2. Most important risk factor—smoking.
3. Types of lung cancer.
   a. Adenocarcinoma—most common.
   b. SCC—occurs in the peripheral portion of the lung.
   c. Small (oat) cell carcinoma.
   d. Large cell carcinoma.
4. Sites of distant metastasis—brain, bones (bone marrow), liver, and adrenal gland.
5. Survival—poor prognosis. The 5-year survival rate is 15%. Most lung cancers are diagnosed at a late stage.

D. Colorectal cancer.
1. Colon adenocarcinoma is the most common cancer of the GI tract.
2. Most common type—adenocarcinoma.
3. Often develops from adenomas.
4. Common symptoms include blood in stools, fatigue, cramping in lower left quadrant, and alteration in bowel habits.

E. Breast cancer.
1. Most common form—adenocarcinomas arising from the ductal epithelium.
2. The second most common cause of cancer-related deaths in women. As a result of enhanced screening and detection, mortality is slowly declining.
3. Approximately 50% of tumors have estrogen-receptor proteins.

4. Hormonal and genetic factors are the major risk factors. Risk increases with age, positive family history, and early menarche.
F. Prostate cancer.
  1. Most common form—adenocarcinomas arising from the glandular epithelium.
  2. The incidence of prostate cancer increases with advancing age.
  3. Laboratory findings include higher levels of prostate-specific antigen.
  4. Patients with prostate cancer with osteoblastic metastases have a very poor prognosis.

Sample Questions

1. All of the following cells are associated with chronic inflammation *except* one. Which one is the *exception*?
   A. Macrophages
   B. Neutrophils
   C. T lymphocytes
   D. B lymphocytes
   E. Plasma cells
2. Dust cells can be found in the _____.
   A. Brain
   B. Heart
   C. Lungs
   D. Liver
   E. Spleen
3. Which of the following mediators aid in the killing of intracellular bacteria?
   A. Histamine
   B. IL-2
   C. Catalase
   D. IgG
   E. Lysozyme
4. The class of antibodies that plays an important role in type I hypersensitivity reactions is _____.
   A. IgA
   B. IgD
   C. IgE
   D. IgG
   E. IgM
5. DiGeorge's syndrome is characterized by a deficiency of _____.
   A. B lymphocytes
   B. T lymphocytes
   C. Both B and T lymphocytes
   D. Antibodies
   E. Complement inhibitor
6. Which of the following is the *most* common cause of subacute endocarditis?
   A. *Staphylococcus aureus.*
   B. *Staphylococcus epidermidis.*
   C. *Streptococcus. pneumoniae.*
   D. *Streptococcus. pyogenes.*
   E. *Streptococcus viridans*

7. Aschoff bodies are observed in which of the following conditions?
   A. Acute myelogenous leukemia
   B. Pheochromocytoma
   C. Osteopetrosis
   D. Rheumatic fever
   E. Scleroderma
8. Endotoxin consists of _____.
   A. Coagulase
   B. Hyaluronidase
   C. LPS
   D. Lactic acid
   E. M protein
9. All of the following conditions are commonly associated with a group A, β-hemolytic streptococcal infection *except* one. Which one is the *exception*?
   A. Scarlet fever
   B. Toxic shock syndrome
   C. Pharyngitis
   D. Endocarditis
   E. Impetigo
10. Karyotyping can be used to diagnose which of the following diseases?
   A. Klinefelter's syndrome
   B. Multiple myeloma
   C. Niemann-Pick disease
   D. Pemphigus
   E. Peutz-Jeghers syndrome
11. In pemphigus, autoantibodies are directed against which of the following structures?
   A. Acetylcholine receptor
   B. Sarcomere
   C. Epidermis
   D. Thyroid follicle
   E. Lysosomes
12. Which of the following is a major complication of chronic bronchitis?
   A. Myxedema
   B. Pneumothorax
   C. Emphysema
   D. Pernicious anemia
   E. Malignant transformation
13. Which of the following cells are defective in chronic granulomatous disease?
   A. Neutrophils
   B. Lymphocytes
   C. Plasma cells
   D. Killer T cells
   E. Macrophages
14. Which of the following describes cells that are abnormal in appearance and may become premalignant?
   A. Aplasia
   B. Dysplasia
   C. Karyomegaly
   D. Pleomorphism
   E. Metaplasia

15. HIV binds directly to the surface receptors of CD4 lymphocytes with _____.
    A. Reverse transcriptase
    B. Integrase
    C. Hemagglutinin
    D. gp120
    E. Protease

16. Which of the following microbes is the *most* common cause of gastroenteritis in children?
    A. Reoviruses
    B. Picornaviruses
    C. Togaviruses
    D. Paramyxoviruses
    E. Orthomyxoviruses

17. A cotton-wool appearance may be used to describe the radiograph of a patient with _____.
    A. Osteopetrosis
    B. Osteitis deformans
    C. Peutz-Jeghers syndrome
    D. Seborrheic keratosis
    E. Osteogenesis imperfecta

18. An autoclave sterilizes dental instruments by causing which of the following?
    A. Coagulation of proteins
    B. Denaturing of proteins
    C. Precipitation of nucleic acids
    D. Disruption of cell membranes
    E. Dissolution of lipids

19. Ehlers-Danlos syndrome is a disease affecting _____.
    A. Bone
    B. Connective tissue
    C. Muscle
    D. Joints
    E. Glycogen synthesis

20. An increase in alkaline phosphatase may be seen in all of the following conditions *except* one. Which one is the *exception*?
    A. Hyperparathyroidism
    B. Osteoporosis
    C. Osteitis deformans
    D. Adenocarcinoma of the prostate with bone metastases
    E. Multiple myeloma

21. The most common cause of death in diabetic patients is _____.
    A. Peripheral neuropathy
    B. Pancreatic cancer
    C. Cardiovascular disease
    D. Kidney failure
    E. Opportunistic infections

22. Neuraminidase is produced by _____.
    A. Influenza virus
    B. Hepatitis C viruses
    C. HIV
    D. Measles virus
    E. Rubella virus

23. Which of the following skin lesions is *most* likely premalignant?
    A. Verruca vulgaris
    B. Keloids
    C. Seborrheic keratosis
    D. Actinic keratosis
    E. Compound nevus

24. The most prominent mechanism of spread of hepatitis A virus is by which of the following routes?
    A. Fecal -Oral
    B. Respiratory
    C. Sexual contact
    D. Perinatal
    E. Insect vectors

25. Accumulation of fluid in the pericardium occurs *most* often with which of the following conditions?
    A. Unstable angina
    B. Cardiomyopathy
    C. Myocarditis
    D. Acute pericarditis
    E. Tamponade

26. The most common cause of pyelonephritis is _____.
    A. *Staphylococcus. aureus*
    B. *Vibrio. cholerae*
    C. *Escherichia. coli*
    D. *Helicobacter. pylori*
    E. *Bordetella. pertussis*

27. Polycystic kidney disease is most commonly associated with _____.
    A. Renal cell carcinoma
    B. Peripheral neuropathy
    C. Urolithiasis
    D. Berry aneurysm
    E. Non-Hodgkin's lymphoma

28. SCC is the most common oral cancer. It is a tumor of _____.
    A. Melanocytes
    B. Basal cells
    C. Fibroblasts
    D. Keratinocytes
    E. Macrophages

29. Tinea pedis, commonly known as athlete's foot, is a fungal infection that is caused by which of the following dermatophyte(s)?
    A. *Microsporum*
    B. *Trichophyton*
    C. *Epidermophyton*
    D. Both A and B
    E. Both B and C

30. Fibrotic and thickened heart valves that result in a reduction of blood flow through the valve characterize which of the following?
    A. Stenosis
    B. Regurgitation
    C. Insufficiency

D. Prolapse

E. Ischemia

31. Cystic fibrosis is a hereditary disorder that results from defective _____.

A. Collagen

B. Lysosomal enzymes

C. Chloride channels

D. Fibrillin

E. Myelin

32. The *most* common mutation accounting for the pathogenesis of trisomy 21 is _____.

A. Chromosome translocation

B. Meiotic nondisjunction

C. Mitotic nondisjunction

D. Single deletion

E. X-linked inheritance

33. An endocrine disorder that causes an early loss of primary teeth and the early eruption of secondary teeth is _____.

A. Myxedema

B. Hashimoto's thyroiditis

C. DiGeorge's syndrome

D. Plummer's disease

E. Dwarfism

34. Which of the following is not a feature of poststreptococcal glomerulonephritis?

A. Hematuria

B. Hypertension

C. Edema

D. Polyuria.

35. The *most* common cause of osteomyelitis is _____.

A. *Streptococcus. pyogenes*

B. *Staphylococcus. aureus*

C. *Lactobacillus. casei*

D. *Pseudomonas. aeruginosa*

E. *Escherichia. coli*

36. All of the following are histopathologic features of malignant cells *except* one. Which one is the *exception*?

A. Anaplasia

B. Pleomorphism

C. Aneuploidy

D. Large nuclei

E. Low nuclear-to-cytoplasmic ratio

37. Which of the following best describes anaplastic cells that have not invaded the basement membrane and are confined within their epithelium of origin?

A. Fibrous dysplasia

B. Hyperplasia

C. Metaplasia

D. Sarcoma

E. Carcinoma in situ

Test items 38-42 refer to the following scenario.

A 43-year-old man presents for an emergency dental appointment complaining of a burning sensation in his mouth. On examination, white plaques are observed along the oral mucosa. The patient otherwise appears healthy. There is no history of systemic illness, but the patient stated that he had a blood transfusion more than 10 years ago following a car accident. The dentist referred the patient to emergency department for further tests.

38. On further evaluation, the physician requests an HIV and hepatitis test. The laboratory performed both an ELISA test and Western blot, revealing that the patient is HIV-positive. The Western blot is used to identify which of the following?

A. Antibodies

B. DNA

C. RNA

D. Proteins

E. Plaque-forming units

39. Given the patient's history, if the patient was later given a diagnosis of active hepatitis, which of the following would *most* likely be the causative agent?

A. Hepatitis A

B. Hepatitis B

C. Hepatitis C

D. Hepatitis D

E. Hepatitis E

40. Which of the following would the physician likely prescribe for the patient's intraoral infection?

A. Amoxicillin

B. Vancomycin

C. Ciprofloxacin

D. Nystatin

E. Chlorhexidine

41. All of the following molecules may be found within the nucleocapsid of HIV *except* one. Which one is the *exception*?

A. Reverse transcriptase

B. Integrase

C. Neuraminidase

D. Protease

E. Ribonucleic acid

42. The patient is referred to an infectious disease specialist and placed on HAART. The patient is admitted to the emergency department 2 years later with a dry cough and shortness of breath. His temperature is 101° F. The *most* likely cause of the patient's pneumonia is _____.

A. *Staphylococcus. aureus*

B. *Haemophilus. influenzae*

C. *Pneumocystis. jiroveci (carinii)*

D. *Klebsiella. pneumoniae*

E. *Streptococcus. pneumoniae*

Test items 43-45 refer to the following scenario.

A mother brings her 6-year-old daughter in for an examination because she noticed brown macules on her daughter's leg. The macules have jagged edges but do not appear raised. The mother is worried that her daughter may have a malignancy. After further evaluation and tests, the macules are identified as café au lait spots.

43. Café au lait spots are seen in conjunction with poly-ostotic fibrous dysplasia and endocrine abnormalities in which of the following disorders?
    A. McCune-Albright syndrome
    B. Stevens-Johnson syndrome
    C. Marfan's syndrome
    D. Gorlin-Goltz syndrome
    E. Peutz-Jeghers syndrome

44. The patient's radiographs could be described as having what type of characteristic appearance?
    A. Cotton-wool
    B. Ground-glass
    C. Cobweb
    D. Soap bubble
    E. Starry sky

45. A bone biopsy specimen was taken from the patient. Which of the following would *most* likely be observed under the microscope?
    A. A dense inflammatory infiltrate
    B. Fibrous tissue
    C. Pleomorphic cells
    D. Metastatic calcifications
    E. Giant cells

Test items 46-49 refer to the following scenario.

A 6-year-old boy presents with a history of severe epistaxis. For the past 3 years, the patient has experienced these nosebleeds, often without any apparent cause. The patient is otherwise in good health, but his mother has noticed that he "bruises easily." Laboratory tests are ordered.

46. The laboratory test results show a normal PT but a prolonged PTT. A prolonged PTT suggests that the patient has an abnormality affecting which component of the coagulation cascade?
    A. Activation of platelets
    B. Activation of thromboplastin
    C. Activation of plasminogen
    D. Intrinsic pathway
    E. Extrinsic pathway

47. The diagnosis of hemophilia A is made. This disease is caused by a deficiency of _____.
    A. Factor V
    B. Factor VII
    C. Factor VIII
    D. Factor IX
    E. Factor X

48. Which of the following describes the hereditary transmission of this disease?
    A. Autosomal dominant
    B. Autosomal recessive
    C. X-linked
    D. It is not genetically transmitted

49. The clinical presentation of hemophilia B is indistinguishable from hemophilia A. Which of the following best describes the laboratory method needed to distinguish these two conditions?
    A. Bleeding time
    B. Assay of coagulation factor levels
    C. Assay of von Willebrand's factor
    D. Blood smear
    E. Platelet count

50. An infection by which of the following bacteria may result in the formation of gummas?
    A. *Mycobacterium tuberculosis.*
    B. *Neisseria gonorrhoreae.*
    C. *Treponema pallidum.*
    D. *Bordetella pertussis.*
    E. *Streptococcus. pyogenes.*

51. Which of the following receptors are recognized by CD8 lymphocytes?
    A. Class I MHC molecules
    B. Class II MHC molecules
    C. Surface IgE
    D. Surface IgM
    E. Histamine receptor

52. Which of the following cytokines stimulates B lymphocytes to differentiate into plasma cells?
    A. IL-1
    B. IL-2
    C. IL-3
    D. IL-4
    E. IL-5

53. All of the following symptoms are mediated by antibodies *except* one. Which one is the *exception*?
    A. Arthus reaction
    B. Tuberculin reaction
    C. Asthma
    D. Erythroblastosis fetalis
    E. Serum sickness

54. Which of the following is released by mast cells after antigen binding?
    A. IgE
    B. Lysozyme
    C. IL-4
    D. Leukotriene
    E. Interferon

55. Symptoms of a myocardial infarction include all of the following *except* one. Which one is the *exception*?
    A. Angina
    B. Diaphoresis
    C. Fever
    D. Vomiting
    E. Dyspnea

56. A positive quelling reaction can be observed in bacteria with a _____.
    A. Thick peptidoglycan layer
    B. Capsule
    C. Flagella
    D. Cell wall that contains teichoic acid
    E. Glycocalyx coating

57. Which of the following groups of microorganisms produce dipicolinic acid?
    A. *Actinomycetes*
    B. *Histoplasma*
    C. *Streptococcus*
    D. *Staphylococcus*
    E. *Clostridium*

58. Which of the following consists of glucose molecules linked together that act as the structural component of plaque?
    A. Fructose
    B. Sucrose
    C. Levans
    D. Dextrans
    E. Fructans

59. The *most* common cause of bacterial meningitis in newborns is _____.
    A. *Staphylococcus aureus*
    B. *Streptococcus pneumoniae*
    C. *Escherichia coli*
    D. *Haemophilus influenzae*
    E. *Listeria monocytogenes*

60. All of the following can be found in the cell wall of a Gram-negative bacterium *except* one. Which one is the *exception*?
    A. Endotoxin
    B. A thin layer of peptidoglycan
    C. Lipopolysaccharide
    D. Teichoic acid
    E. O antigen

61. What type of vaccine is used for *Clostridium tetani*?
    A. Capsular polysaccharides
    B. Toxoids
    C. Killed bacteria
    D. Immunoglobulins
    E. No vaccine is available

62. The class of antibodies that plays an important role in mucosal immunity is _____.
    A. IgA
    B. IgD
    C. IgE
    D. IgG
    E. IgM

63. The presence of which of the following in a patient's serum indicates that the patient is a highly infectious hepatitis B carrier?
    A. HBsAg
    B. HBsAb
    C. HBcAg
    D. HBeAg
    E. HBeAb

64. All of the following microbes are associated with infections secondary to HIV infection *except* one. Which one is the *exception*?
    A. *Pneumocystis jiroveci*
    B. Epstein-Barr virusEBV

C. Coxsackievirus
D. *Mycobacterium tuberculosis*
E. *Candida albicans*

65. Rheumatoid arthritis is characterized by inflammation of the _____.
    A. Articular capsule
    B. Articular cartilage
    C. Cortical bone
    D. Perichondrium
    E. Synovium

66. The *most* common form of breast cancer is _____.
    A. Adenocarcinoma
    B. Teratoma
    C. Follicular lymphoma
    D. Sarcoma
    E. Squamous cell carcinoma

67. Which of the following antimicrobials is bacteriostatic and inhibits protein synthesis in bacteria?
    A. Streptomycin
    B. Penicillin V
    C. Ciprofloxacin
    D. Cephalexin
    E. Tetracycline

68. Which of the following may be observed in a child with rickets?
    A. Dark pigmentation on the oral mucosa
    B. Early eruption of teeth
    C. Hutchinson's incisors
    D. Abnormal dentin
    E. Macroglossia

69. In 2% glutaraldehyde, which of the following times is minimally sufficient for achieving sterilization?
    A. 15 minutes
    B. 1 to 2 hours
    C. 6 hours
    D. 12 hours

70. An 8-year-old boy presents with macroglossia and delayed eruption of his primary teeth. Of the following choices, which one is *most* likely?
    A. Plummer's disease
    B. Osteochondroses
    C. Cretinism
    D. Wilson's disease
    E. Mallory-Weiss syndrome

71. Which of the following bacteria would be expected to colonize first onto plaque?
    A. *Streptococcus*
    B. *Bacteroides*
    C. *Fusobacterium*
    D. *Actinomyces*
    E. *Prevotella*

72. The hereditary transmission of Peutz-Jeghers syndrome is _____.
    A. Autosomal dominant
    B. Autosomal recessive
    C. Sex-linked dominant

D. Sex-linked recessive

E. Not genetically transmitted

73. Which of the following structures is the most common intraoral site for cancer?
    A. Soft palate
    B. Tongue
    C. Lower lip
    D. Floor of mouth
    E. Buccal mucosa

74. The presence of Auer rods in a peripheral blood smear suggests which of the following conditions?
    A. Acute lymphocytic leukemia
    B. Acute lymphoblastic leukemia
    C. Acute myelogenous leukemia
    D. Chronic lymphocytic leukemia
    E. Hodgkin's lymphoma

75. The most significant complications of Barrett's esophagus is _____.
    A. Varices
    B. Stricture
    C. Hemorrhage
    D. Adenocarcinoma
    E. Ulceration

76. The presence of M-protein antibodies suggests immunity to infection by which type of bacteria?
    A. *Streptococcus pyogenes.*
    B. *Streptococcus viridans.*
    C. *Streptococcus sanguis.*
    D. *Staphylococcus aureus.*
    E. *Lactobacillus casei.*

77. Hemorrhagic infarction and tissue necrosis suggest which of the following?
    A. Aspergillosis
    B. Blastomycosis
    C. Histoplasmosis
    D. Mucormycosis
    E. Toxoplasmosis

78. Which of the following is usually *least* malignant?
    A. Acute lymphoblastic leukemia
    B. Acute lymphocytic leukemia
    C. Acute myelogenous leukemia
    D. Chronic lymphocytic leukemia
    E. Chronic myelogenous leukemia

79. Lung carcinoma is a complication *most* characteristic of which of the following conditions?
    A. Silicosis
    B. Asbestosis
    C. Anthracosis
    D. Sarcoidosis
    E. Bronchiectasis

80. Which of the following disorders is *least* likely to be included in the differential diagnosis of a patient with jaundice?
    A. Hepatitis
    B. Hemolytic anemia
    C. Cholelithiasis

D. Glomerulonephritis

E. Carcinoma of the pancreas

81. A productive cough may be seen in all of the following conditions *except* one. Which one is the *exception*?
    A. Pneumonia
    B. Lung abscess
    C. Bronchiectasis
    D. Asthma
    E. Bronchogenic carcinoma

82. Antinuclear antibodies are seen in the serum samples from patients with _____.
    A. Hypogammaglobulinemia
    B. Chronic granulomatous disease
    C. Systemic lupus erythematosus
    D. Multiple myeloma
    E. Pheochromocytoma

83. Nephrolithiasis is *most* likely to be associated with which of the following conditions?
    A. Hyperparathyroidism
    B. Myxedema
    C. Pyelonephritis
    D. Wilson's disease
    E. Thrombocytopenia

84. An infant with osteopetrosis has dysfunctional _____.
    A. Chondrocytes
    B. Osteoblasts
    C. Osteoclasts
    D. Fibroblasts
    E. Lymphocytes

85. All of the following factors play a role in the virulence of the microbe that causes whooping cough *except* one. Which one is the *exception*?
    A. IgA protease
    B. Hemagglutinin
    C. Exotoxin
    D. Capsule
    E. Pili

86. T-cell lymphoma is *most* likely to occur in a patient with which of the following conditions?
    A. Chronic granulomatous disease
    B. Myasthenia gravis
    C. Osteochondroma
    D. Wilson's disease
    E. Celiac sprue

Test items 87-92 refer to the following scenario.

A 60-year-old homeless man who lives in a community shelter presents with history of coughing for the past 6 months. He has a slight fever, hemoptysis, and productive cough with a yellowish sputum discharge. After further examination and tests, the patient is given a diagnosis of active TB.

87. When the sputum samples were taken to the laboratory, what test did the physician order to be performed to help make the diagnosis?

A. Gram stain
B. Acid-fast stain
C. Spore stain
D. PPD test (tuberculin test)
E. Voges-Proskauer test

88. After 2 weeks, the bacterial cultures came back from the laboratory confirming the initial diagnosis, positively identifying the organism *Mycobacterium tuberculosis*. This microbe is known to infect which of the following cells?
A. Fibroblasts
B. Basal cells
C. Type I pneumocytes
D. Macrophages
E. Erythrocytes

89. Which of the following is a glycolipid found on the surface of *Mycobacterium. tuberculosis* that plays a role in its pathogenesis?
A. Cord factor
B. O antigen
C. Protein A
D. Exotoxin A
E. Lecithinase

90. Because the patient was living in a homeless shelter, the tuberculin test was administered to all of the staff and residents living at the shelter. This test is based on a delayed type hypersensitivity reaction that is mediated by _____.
A. Only IgG
B. IgG and IgM
C. IgE
D. T cells and macrophages
E. Mast cells and basophils

91. Which of the following is the *most* appropriate drug used in combination therapy for TB to treat the patient?
A. Amoxicillin
B. Clindamycin
C. Cephalosporin
D. Tetracycline
E. Rifampin

92. After 3 weeks, the patient was feeling "much better" and was discharged from the hospital, although he remained on his drug therapy for another 6 months. Which of the following best describes the calcified scar that later formed in the affected lung parenchyma and hilar lymph node?
A. Gumma
B. Chancre
C. Metastatic calcifications
D. Tubercle
E. Ghon complex

Test items 93-97 refer to the following scenario.
A 55-year-old man presents with malaise and dyspnea. He has a low-grade fever and reports that his shortness of breath has increased steadily over the past week and a half. He has a history of rheumatic fever and denies ever using recreational drugs. He is currently being treated by a dentist for full-mouth reconstruction.

93. On further examination, a heart murmur was detected. Given the patient's past medical history, which heart valve is *most* likely affected?
A. Mitral valve
B. Tricuspid valve
C. Aortic valve
D. Pulmonary valve

94. Before the patient's development of rheumatic fever, he likely had which of the following conditions?
A. Cystitis
B. Pharyngitis
C. Food poisoning
D. Thrombocytopenia
E. Meningitis

95. After further evaluation and tests, a diagnosis of subacute endocarditis is made. If the infecting microbe was cultured in the laboratory, the results would *most* likely show that this microbe is positive for _____.
A. α-Hemolysis
B. β-Hemolysis
C. γ-Hemolysis
D. Coagulase
E. Lecithinase

96. Which of the following is the *most* likely complication that may occur from the vegetations forming on the patient's defective heart valve?
A. Myocardial infarction
B. Hemorrhage
C. Petechiae
D. Cor pulmonale
E. Embolus

97. After the diagnosis is made, the patient is immediately prescribed high-dose, intravenous antibiotics. One of the antibiotics that is administered to the patient is streptomycin, an aminoglycoside. The antimicrobial effect of streptomycin is to inhibit the synthesis of _____.
A. The bacterial cell wall
B. Folate
C. Proteins
D. Nucleic acids
E. β-Lactamase

Test items 98-100 refer to the following scenario.
A 3-year-old African girl presents in the emergency department with a palpable mass in the lower right mandible. She is currently in the United States visiting relatives with her parents. Her mother claims that a few days ago she noticed a growing mass in her daughter's jaw. There appears to be slight swelling around the area, although it is painless and not tender to the touch. After further examination, a biopsy

specimen was taken, and the diagnosis of Burkitt's lymphoma was made.

98. Burkitt's lymphoma is a malignancy that affects which of the following cells?
A. Macrophages
B. T lymphocytes
C. B lymphocytes
D. Neutrophils
E. Keratinocytes

99. The pathology report reveals a characteristic pattern of tumor cells that is classically associated with Burkitt's lymphoma. Which of the following describes this histopathologic pattern?
A. Honeycomb
B. Cobweb
C. Cotton-wool
D. Sun ray
E. Starry sky

100. The African form of Burkitt's lymphoma has been linked to the Epstein-Barr virus. This virus is also responsible for which of the following diseases?
A. Mononucleosis
B. Shingles
C. Chickenpox
D. Kaposi's sarcoma
E. Herpangina

101. Pili (fimbriae) are important virulence factors for several microbes. A common property of pili that is almost universally ascribed to their ability to function as a virulence factor is their _____.
A. Monomeric structure
B. Dissociation at low pH
C. Ability to attach to surfaces
D. Participation in transduction
E. Enzyme activity

102. The presence of a type III secretion system in some bacteria is considered to facilitate virulence and invasion of the host. Why?
A. Microbes use this method of export to secrete the quorum-sensing autoinducer into the surrounding environment, facilitating host cell death.
B. Microbes use this system to inject bacterial proteins into the eukaryotic cell, facilitating an invasion.
C. Microbes use this system to facilitate global regulation of bacterial processes through the export of quorum-sensing molecules
D. Microbes use this system to facilitate global regulation of the microbiome of the host.

103. Secretory IgA is commonly associated with mucosal surfaces. Its primary mode of activity in serving to protect the host is to _____.
A. Kill the microbe or pathogen through directly facilitating lysis
B. Facilitate the phagocytosis of the microbe or pathogen through its direct binding
C. Prevent the microbe or pathogen from adhering to the mucosal surfaces
D. Facilitate the ability of the microbe or pathogen to adhere to the mucosal surfaces
E. Coordinate the induction of secreted cytokines from mucosal surfaces

104. A 55-year-old man with uncontrolled type 2 diabetes presents to the emergency dental clinic with acute and massive necrotizing lesions associated with his palate. This is *most* likely the consequence of _____.
A. Aspergillosis
B. Cryptococcosis
C. Fulminant candidiasis
D. Histoplasmosis
E. Mucormycosis

105. In the process of performing a Gram stain, the decolorization step was inadvertently omitted from the protocol. What consequence would this omission have on the clinical assessment of the specimen under evaluation?
A. The Gram stain reaction for Gram-positive cells would be affected and appear pink.
B. The Gram stain reaction for Gram-negative cells would be unaffected and appear pink.
C. The Gram stain reaction for Gram-negative cells would be affected and appear purple.
D. The Gram stain reaction for Gram-positive cells would be unaffected and appear pink.

106. A 26-year-old junior dental student who returned from a Peace Corps mission to Honduras last August is admitted with a 2-month history of increasing malaise, easily fatigued, weakness, and weight loss. She also reports a history of febrile episodes accompanied by sweating and shaking chills starting about 2 months ago and a dark discoloration of her urine in the past 2 weeks. Physical examination reveals pale oral mucosa and conjunctivae. Laboratory tests show marked anemia with increased reticulocytes in the peripheral blood and cells with the appearance in the figure. This patient's anemia is most likely a consequence of _____.

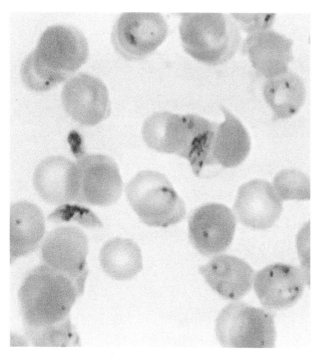

A. Allergic reaction to insect venom
B. Complement mediated lysis of RBCs
C. Invasion of RBCs by *Plasmodia* parasites
D. Persistent intestinal bleeding caused by *Trichuris* species
E. Phagocytosis of RBCs by *E. histolytica*

107. A mother and her 6-year-old son present to the clinic inquiring how to resolve the teeth discoloration illustrated in the figure. Use of which antibiotic would you likely find in the history of the patient or in the gestational history of the mother to account for the intrinsic staining of his teeth?

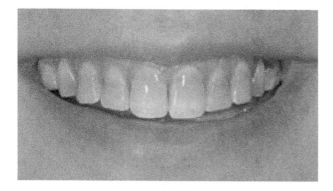

A. Ampicillin
B. Azithromycin
C. Chloramphenicol
D. Doxycycline
E. Streptomycin

108. A patient in the clinic shows the dental malformation illustrated in the figure. These malformed teeth are characteristic of a disease that is acquired by which route of transmission?

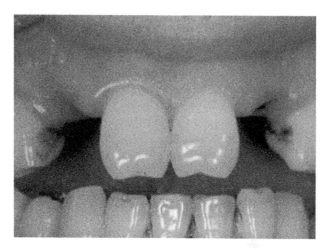

A. Fecal-oral
B. Respiratory
C. Tick-borne
D. Contact with infected animal products
E. Transplacental

109. A 33-year-old woman with mitral stenosis experiences a deterioration of cardiac function a few weeks after having had some dental work done at a free clinic. She is admitted to the university hospital for valve replacement. The pathologic examination of the resected mitral valve shows abundant vegetations from which an α-hemolytic, catalase-negative, Gram-positive coccus, resistant to bacitracin, bile, and optochin, is typed as group H in the Lancefield system. Questioned about her past medical history, the patient states that she was in good health until age 15, when she started having heart problems after a severe sore throat. What are the characteristics of the infectious agent most likely to have been responsible for the sore throat and subsequent heart valve abnormality?

Characteristic	A	B	C	D	E
Bacitracin sensitivity	+	−	−	−	−
Bile solubility	−	−	−	−	+
Hemolysis in agar	β	β	α	α oρ γ	α
Optochin sensitivity	−	−	−	−	+

A. A
B. B
C. C
D. D
E. E

110. A malnourished 50-year-old man with alcoholism and severe dental caries has a 2-week history of malaise and right-sided chest pain. He was found unconscious near a bar with evidence of having vomited 3 weeks ago. He was sent to a homeless center, but he is brought to the emergency department with fever and has a cough productive of foul-smelling, purulent sputum. X-ray film of the chest shows a fluid-filled cavity, 2 cm in diameter, in the upper lobe of the right lung. What is the *most* likely source of the organism causing this infection?
    A. Bacteria in the bloodstream
    B. Gastric contents
    C. Infectious aerosolized secretions
    D. Refluxed intestinal contents
    E. The gingivodental sulcus

111. Based on your interpretation of the graph, select the letter that corresponds to the addition of a bactericidal antibiotic at 3 hours.

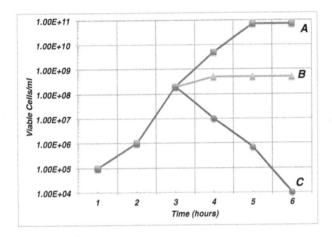

    A. A
    B. B
    C. C
    D. Either B or C
    E. Unable to assess given data provided

112. A child presents with lesions on her face as shown in the figure. Similar lesions could be seen on her legs. A fragment of one of the crusts and the fluid below were sent for culture. The standard of care requires the child be treated with an antibiotic. Culture with subsequent Gram stain of the lesions reveals Gram-positive cocci that are β-hemolytic and catalase-negative. What is the *most* likely non-suppurative complication that may affect this child?

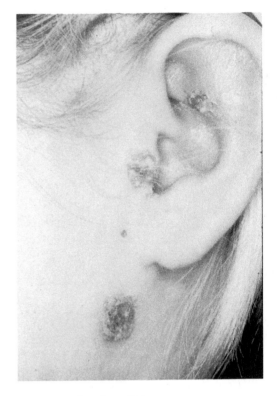

    A. Bacterial endocarditis
    B. Forcheimer's sign
    C. Glomerulonephritis
    D. Osteomyelitis
    E. Scarlet fever

113. A 35-year-old man is seen in the emergency department because of marked shortness of breath. Physical examination shows bilateral anterior cervical and axillary adenopathy and a temperature of 103°F (39.4°C). Chest x-ray shows bilateral interstitial pneumonia. A bronchoalveolar lavage sediment stained with methenamine silver is shown in the figure. Which is the *most* likely diagnosis?

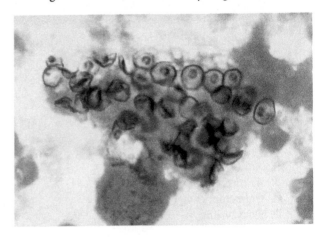

    A. Anaerobic abscess of the lung
    B. Pneumococcal pneumonia
    C. *P. jiroveci* pneumonia
    D. Pulmonary TB
    E. RSV

114. A 4-year-old child presents with fever, cough, conjunctivitis, loss of appetite, and lesions on the oral mucosa as shown in the figure. What is the *most* likely diagnosis?

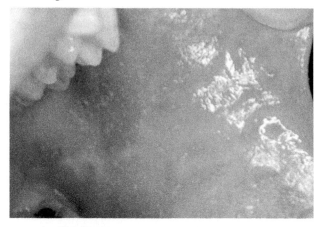

    A. Chickenpox
    B. Herpangina
    C. Measles
    D. Mumps
    E. Roseola infantum (exanthem subitum)

115. A 1-month-old boy with severe diarrhea and dehydration is brought to the emergency department. There are no leukocytes or blood in his stool. Which of the following best describes the pathogen that is causing the diarrhea?
    A. Double-stranded, segmented RNA virus with a double capsid
    B. Gram-negative rod that does not ferment lactose
    C. Gram-positive, spore-forming rod
    D. Pear-shaped protozoan with two nuclei and four pairs of flagella
    E. A single-stranded, enveloped RNA virus

116. A 21-year-old woman with systemic lupus erythematosus receiving treatment with immunosuppressive drugs presents with symptoms of meningitis. CSF protein is elevated, and glucose is low. The Gram stain shows no organisms. The result of an India ink preparation is shown in the figure. This organism is *most* likely _____.

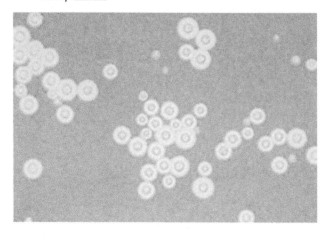

    A. Coxsackie B virus
    B. *Cryptococcus neoformans*
    C. *H. capsulatum*
    D. *N. meningitidis*
    E. *S. pneumoniae*

117. A 24-year-old woman employed at a day care center is referred for investigation of diarrhea and weight loss. The patient complains of intermittent diarrhea and flatulence, some days feeling well, some days passing three to four foul-smelling and greasy-looking stools. She has lost 10 lb since the symptoms started 3 months ago. Stool studies showed increased total fat content. A parasitologic examination of the stool revealed the organisms shown in the figure. The organism in the figure is _____.

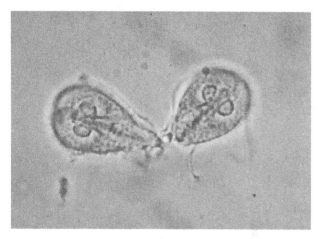

    A. *Entamoeba coli*
    B. *E. gingivalis*
    C. *E. histolytica*
    D. *G. lamblia*
    E. *Naegleria fowleri*

118. Which of the following antiseptics commonly used in formulations for oral rinses has a persistent antimicrobial effect?
    A. Alcohol
    B. Chlorhexidine gluconate
    C. Hydrogen peroxide
    D. Domiphen bromide
    E. Phenol

119. A 29-year-old pregnant women presents for her routine 6-month oral hygiene visit. On examination, you discover that she has developed gingivitis since her previous visit. The microorganism *most* likely associated with her inflamed gingiva is _____.
    A. *Lactobacillus plantarum*
    B. *Prevotella intermedia*
    C. *Porphyromonas. gingivalis*
    D. *Streptococcus mutans*
    E. *Streptococcus sanguis*

120. A 22-year-old woman developed a urinary tract infection during her honeymoon. At the time she

sought medical advice, she was febrile and complained of dysuria and flank pain; her urine was cloudy and contained granular casts. Urine culture yielded a glucose-fermenting, indole-positive, urease-positive, highly motile Gram-negative bacillus. Which organism is *most* likely responsible for the symptoms described by this patient?

A. *Chlamydia trachomatis*
B. *Escherichia coli*
C. *Proteus vulgaris*
D. *Shigella flexneri*
E. *Ureaplasma urealyticum*

121. Match the term with the appropriate definition.

A. Fibroma _____   1. Benign or malignant tumor
B. Osteosarcoma   2. Malignant neoplasm of
   _____   bone
C. Hematoma   3. Benign neoplasm of fibrous
   _____   tissue origin
D. Squamous   4. Variably sized mass of
   papilloma   blood in the tissues, usually
   _____   secondary to trauma
E. Neoplasm   5. Benign neoplasm of
   _____   epithelial origin with
                          fingerlike projections

122. Order the development and progression of oral SCC. Order each letter in sequence, with the initial lesion first.

A. Metastatic SCC
B. Epithelial dysplasia or carcinoma in situ
C. Primary SCC

Dental Anatomy and Occlusion

STANLEY J. NELSON

OUTLINE

This section reviews the basic courses in dental anatomy and occlusion important for a foundation in the study and practice of dentistry. The coverage of these subjects is not exhaustive but should reflect what fundamental information has already been covered early in the dental curriculum. Insofar as possible, the material is based on an evidence-based paradigm that is consistent with the highest level of external evidence, recognizing that the application of such evidence has to be based on appropriate clinical expertise as well as meeting the needs of individual patients. The test questions should be viewed as a learning experience. The basis for answers may be found as needed in the References.

1.0 Introduction to Dental Anatomy

Dental anatomy requires special terminology and nomenclature for communication, for learning, and for clinical and insurance record keeping in the dental office. The term *dental anatomy*, as used here, is an inclusive term for considering the morphologic features of the human primary and permanent dentitions, including their pulp cavities and root canals; pertinent information about the development, calcification, and eruption or emergence of the teeth; and the clinical relevance of these odontologic features to their function and esthetics.

Tables in this section provide information on the dimensions and chronologies of the teeth and, in context, frequency variations in eruption sequences, number of roots and root canals, and variations in tooth size and form. Collections of samples that make up these data come largely from Euro-American populations, sometimes limited because of the problem of obtaining data from other populations, access to in utero material, and statistical methods of incorporating diverse data into a common table derived from various sources. For example, prevalence data on a major anatomic variant of the two-rooted mandibular (i.e., one with an additional distolingual and third root) suggest differences between specific populations regarding the prevalence of this variant of the mandibular first molar, which is of special interest for endodontic therapy. Differences in data on tooth eruption and tooth dimensions may not appear to be significant; however, differences in data found in various textbooks and journals need to be addressed. An example of such differences may be seen in the answers to some of the questions. Sexual, racial, and individual variations in dentofacial patterns reinforce the need to consider interceptive extraction or space-regaining therapy carefully for each patient because of the unpredictability of crowding behavior during the transition from mixed to permanent dentition. The effect of racial origin should be considered when using dental sclerosis as a means of age determination in forensic cases.

A. Terminology.

It is not unusual in the literature to find that more than one term is used to describe a particular dentition (e.g., *primary* or *deciduous* dentition and *permanent* or *succedaneous* dentition), recognizing that the term *deciduous* can mean "not permanent, transitory," and the term *permanent* does not indicate that all the teeth that succeed the primary dentition will not be lost because of disease or injury. In context, both terms for each dentition should present no problem; however, consistent use of a term is important and should reflect the requirements or traditions of a particular journal, dental association, or specialty.

The term *occlusion* can be defined simply as the contact relationship of the teeth in function and parafunction. The contacting interface between the teeth of opposing dental arches may be considered from the standpoint of a static, functional, or parafunctional morphologic tooth contact relationship. Such relationships reflect numerous factors concerned with the development and stability of occlusion.

Changes do occur in terminology; however, they occur in the literature over time, and the reader must be aware of some of the past as well as newer terms that may conceptually relate differentially to the same aspect of occlusion (e.g., *working side contacts* [older term] versus *laterotrusive contacts* [newer term]); the literature may exhibit several terms that reflect various conceptual views of occlusal relationships. For example, in the Glossary of Dental Terms for the National Board Dental Examination, *centric relation* has been defined conceptually as a position of the mandible with the condyles in a specified location that is independent of tooth contact; however, also included is a synonym for centric relation—*retruded contact position*. The term *retruded* has related historically to a concept of centric relation and occlusal contact in which the condyles were thought to be in a most retruded position (Figure 4-1, *A*) compared with the position of the condyles that is now currently held (Figure 4-1, *B*). *Centric relation contact* and *centric relation occlusion* are also terms that have been used to describe tooth contacts that occur when the temporomandibular joints (TMJs) are positioned in centric relation. A candidate for the National Board Dental Examination should be aware of the current terminology appropriate for the test discipline.

B. Formulas for human and nonhuman dentitions.

The number and denomination of mammalian teeth are expressed in formulas that reflect the differences between human dentitions (Figure 4-2) and nonhuman dentitions. The denomination of each tooth may be represented by the first letter in its name (*I* for incisor, *C* for canine, *P* for premolar, and *M* for molar). A notation expressing the number of such teeth in the upper and lower jaws follows these denominations. The formulas include one side only. The dental formula (10 teeth on one side) for the primary or deciduous dentition in humans is indicated as:

$$1 \frac{2}{2} \: C \: \frac{1}{1} \: M \: \frac{2}{2} = 10$$

Similarly, a dental formula for the permanent or succedaneous human dentition reflects the addition of two maxillary and mandibular premolars and the addition of one maxillary and one mandibular third molar. The dental formula (16 teeth on one side) for the human permanent dentition is indicated as:

$$1 \frac{2}{2} \: C \: \frac{1}{1} \: P \: \frac{2}{2} \: M \: \frac{3}{3} = 16$$

The dental practitioner is expected to be able to differentiate the human dentition from the more common nonhuman dentitions. Occasionally, it is necessary to communicate with veterinarians and with attorneys dealing with bite wounds and the identification of human and animal remains in forensic matters. The formula (21 teeth on one side) for a dog (collie) is indicated as:

$$1 \frac{3}{3} \: C \: \frac{1}{1} \: P \: \frac{4}{4} \: M \: \frac{2}{3} = 21$$

It is not unusual for dentists to be interested in some of the morphologic traits used in anthropologic studies (e.g., Carabelli's trait, peg-shaped incisors, enamel extensions, shoveling). Because of keyboard limitations, notations in anthropologic tables are often limited to di_1, di_2, dc, dm_1, and dm_2 for the deciduous dentition and to I_1, I_2, C, P_1, P_2, M_1, M_2, and M_3 for the succedaneous dentition.

C. Terms of orientation.

Terms of orientation in dental anatomy generally indicate place, direction, and extent and include such terms as *mesial, distal, facial, buccal, lingual,* and *anterior/posterior* (Figure 4-3). Abbreviations related to tooth orientation include: *B,* buccal; *D,* distal; *DB,* distobuccal; *M,* mesial; *MB,* mesiobuccal; *L,* lingual; *DL,* distolingual; *ML,* mesiolingual; *MM,* mesiomarginal; and *CR,* cusp ridge. Abbreviations related to permanent

Figure 4-1 A, Incorrect assumption about the normal position of the disc-condyle assembly. **B,** Correct position of the disc-condyle assembly in centric relation. *(From Nelson SJ, Ash MM: Wheeler's Dental Anatomy, Physiology, and Occlusion, ed 9. St. Louis, Saunders, 2010.)*

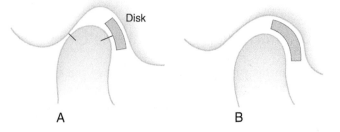

A   B

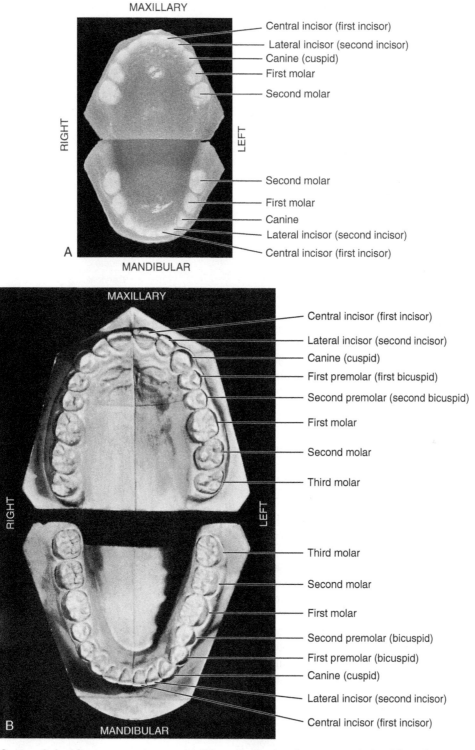

Figure 4-2 A, Casts of deciduous, or primary, dentition. **B,** Casts of permanent dentition. *(From Nelson SJ, Ash MM: Wheeler's Dental Anatomy, Physiology, and Occlusion, ed 9. St. Louis, Saunders, 2010.)*

tooth identification in tables include: *CI,* central incisor; *LI,* lateral incisor; *C,* canine; P_1, P_2, first and second premolars; and M_1, M_2, M_3, first, second, and third molars. All the teeth can be identified by one or more numbering systems. The universal system, which is

considered later, is used in this text except where otherwise indicated.

D. Division into thirds, line angles, and point angles.

The crowns and roots of teeth have been divided into thirds to help understand the location of certain

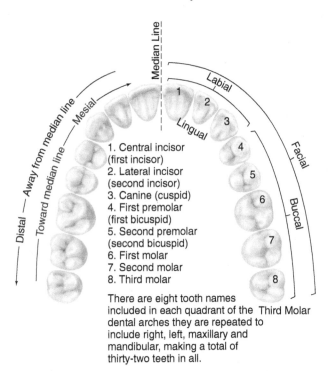

Figure 4-3 **Application of nomenclature.** Tooth numbers indicate left maxillary teeth. Tooth surfaces related to the tongue (lingual), cheek (buccal), lips (labial), and face (facial) apply to four quadrants and the upper left quadrant. The teeth or their parts or surfaces may be described as being away from the midline (distal) or toward the midline (mesial). *(From Nelson SJ, Ash MM: Wheeler's Dental Anatomy, Physiology, and Occlusion, ed 9. St. Louis, Saunders, 2010.)*

Within the figure:

1. Central incisor (first incisor)
2. Lateral incisor (second incisor)
3. Canine (cuspid)
4. First premolar (first bicuspid)
5. Second premolar (second bicuspid)
6. First molar
7. Second molar
8. Third molar

There are eight tooth names included in each quadrant of the dental arches they are repeated to include right, left, maxillary and mandibular, making a total of thirty-two teeth in all.

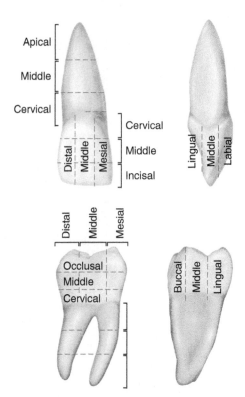

Figure 4-4 **Division into thirds.** *(From Nelson SJ, Ash MM: Wheeler's Dental Anatomy, Physiology, and Occlusion, ed 9. St. Louis, Saunders, 2010.)*

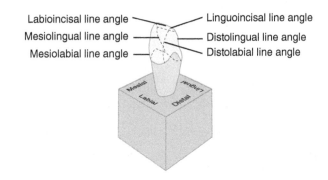

A

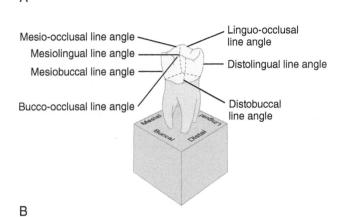

B

Figure 4-5 **Line angles. A,** Anterior teeth. **B,** Posterior teeth. *(From Nelson SJ, Ash MM: Wheeler's Dental Anatomy, Physiology, and Occlusion, ed 9. St. Louis, Saunders, 2010.)*

anatomic features (Figure 4-4). The junctions of crown surfaces are described as line angles (two surfaces) and point angles (three surfaces) (Figure 4-5). Although an actual linear angle may occur on a tooth as a result of fracture or wear, the terms *line angle* and *point angle* are used mostly as descriptive terms to indicate location. An example of this is deciding whether a patient should be charged for a two-surface restoration (mesial-occlusal or distal-occlusal) or three-surface restoration (mesial-occlusal-buccal or distal-occlusal-buccal) when caries crosses the buccal line angles.

E. Anatomic landmarks.

A labial view of a maxillary central incisor (Figure 4-6) shows several of the landmarks relative to the tooth. Anatomic landmarks include the terms *crown, root, apex, incisal edge, cervical line, pulp chamber, pulp horn, pulp (root) canal, fissure, cusp, apex,* and *bifurcation (furcation)* as indicated in the labiolingual sections shown in Figure 4-7.

The primary and permanent teeth are divided for discussion purposes into the crown and root, which is a division marked on the tooth surface by the *cervical line.* This line is the junction between the enamel covering the crown of the tooth and the cementum covering

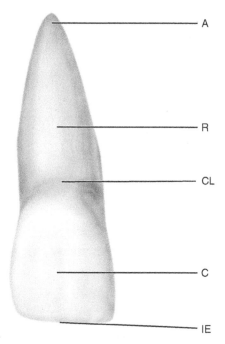

Figure 4-6 Maxillary central incisor (facial aspect). *A,* Apex of root; *C,* crown; *CL,* cervical line; *IE,* incisal edge; *R,* root. *(From Nelson SJ, Ash MM: Wheeler's Dental Anatomy, Physiology, and Occlusion, ed 9. St. Louis, Saunders, 2010.)*

the root. It is referred to as the *cementoenamel junction (CEJ)*. It may occur in several forms, including the enamel overlapping the cementum, an end-to-end approximating junction, the absence of connecting enamel and cementum so that the dentin is an external part of the surface of the root, and an overlapping of the enamel by the cementum. These different junctions have clinical significance in the presence of disease (e.g., gingivitis, recession of the gingiva with exposure of the CEJ, depth of gingival crevice, and level of attachment of the supporting periodontal fibers; cervical sensitivity, caries, and erosion; and placement of margins of dental restorations).

1. CEJ.
   a. The CEJ is a significant landmark for probing the depth of the gingival crevice and the level of the attachment of periodontal fibers to the cementum in the presence of periodontal diseases. Using a periodontal probe (Figure 4-8, *A*), it is possible to relate the position of the gingival margin and the level of attachment to the CEJ (Figure 4-8, *B*).
   b. The clinician should be able to envision the CEJ of each tooth and relate it to areas of risk (e.g., pathologically deepened crevice and loss of attachment or an enamel projection into the bifurcation of a

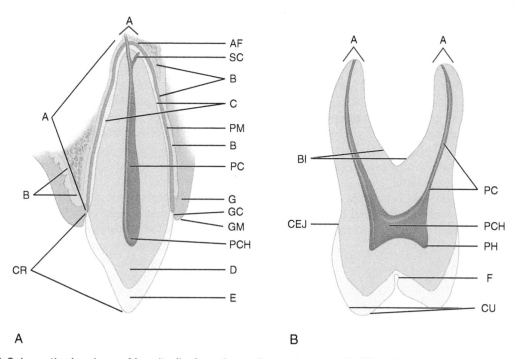

Figure 4-7 Schematic drawings of longitudinal sections of an anterior tooth **(A)** and a posterior tooth **(B)**. *A,* Apex; *AF,* apical foramen; *B,* bone; *BI,* bifurcation of roots; *C,* cementum; *CEJ,* cementoenamel junction; *CR,* crown; *CU,* cusp; *D,* dentin; *E,* enamel; *F,* fissure; *G,* gingiva; *GC,* gingival crevice; *GM,* gingival margin; *PC,* pulp canal; *PCH,* pulp chamber *PH,* pulp horn; *PM,* periodontal ligament; *SC,* supplementary canal. *(From Nelson SJ, Ash MM: Wheeler's Dental Anatomy, Physiology, and Occlusion, ed 9. St. Louis, Saunders, 2010.)*

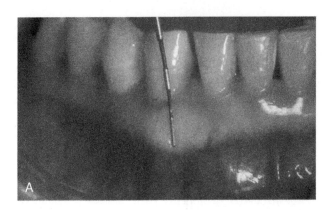

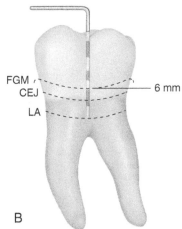

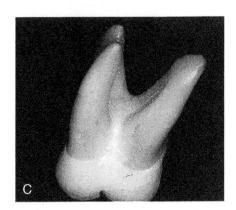

Figure 4-8 A, Periodontal probe divided into 3-mm segments. **B,** Probe at the level of attachment (*LA*). The probe indicates a pathologically deepened crevice of 6 mm and a loss of attachment of 3+ mm. **C,** Enamel projection into the bifurcation of a mandibular molar. *CEJ,* Cementoenamel junction; *FGM,* free gingival margin. (**A,** *From Perry DA, Beemsterboer PL: Periodontology for the Dental Hygienist, ed 3. St. Louis, Saunders, 2007.* **B** *and* **C,** *From Nelson SJ, Ash MM: Wheeler's Dental Anatomy, Physiology, and Occlusion, ed 9. St. Louis, Saunders, 2010.*)

mandibular molar [Figure 4-8, *C*]). Enamel projections into buccal and lingual bifurcations are considered to increase vulnerability to the advance of periodontal disease. The CEJ (and its *location* and *nature*) is more than a descriptive term used simply to describe some aspect of tooth morphology; the CEJ has clinical significance.

   c. The distance from the alveolar bone or alveolar bone crest to the CEJ or enamel is about 1.5 mm in a normal periodontium.

  2. Occlusal landmarks—all landmarks on a tooth should be recognized and identified by name. The landmarks on Figure 4-9 include the following.

   a. Cusp.
   b. Buccocervical ridge.
   c. Cingulum.
   d. Marginal ridge.
   e. Fossa.
   f. Oblique ridge.
   g. Developmental groove.
   h. Transverse ridge.
   i. Supplemental groove.
   j. Triangular ridge.

It is necessary to know how morphologic features relate to contact relations in functional jaw movements and

in jaw closure (e.g., the occlusal contact relation of the mesial buccal cusp of the right mandibular first molar with the central fossa of the maxillary right first molar when the mandible is closed into the maximal intercuspal [clenching] position). These and other morphologic features as well as the positions of the teeth may be related to the development of occlusal stability and oral motor behavior as the occlusion develops.

E. Tooth numbering systems.

    Practitioners need to be able to designate easily (using an acceptable tooth identification system) which tooth or teeth are being considered for diagnosis and treatment and to indicate the identity of a tooth or teeth in dental and insurance records. In the dental office, the dentist, the hygienist, the dental assistant, and the front office assistant have to be knowledgeable about the tooth identification system used in their office and systems used elsewhere for purposes of referral and for reading pertinent professional literature.

1. Universal system.

    In 1968, the American Dental Association recommended the universal numbering system; however, because it does not have universal usage, there are calls to change it. Even so, the notation of one letter for each tooth in the primary dentition and one

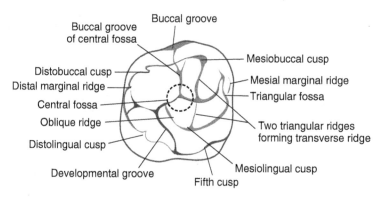

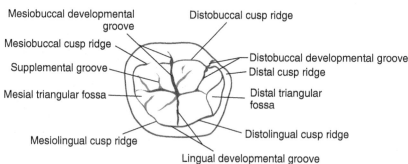

Figure 4-9 Occlusal landmarks on maxillary and mandibular molars.

number for each tooth in the permanent dentition has made its use favored in the United States. An overview of the primary dentition and its universal numbering is shown in Figure 4-10. A simplified scheme to show the letter notations for the 20 primary teeth in four quadrants follows.

Midsaggital Plane

Right   A B C D E F G H I J   Left

          T S R Q P O N M L K

As shown, the right maxillary central incisor is indicated with the letter *E*. Similarly, the left mandibular left central incisor is indicated with the letter *O*. There is no provision for supernumerary teeth. An overview of the permanent dentition and its universal numbering is shown in Figure 4-11. A simplified notation scheme for the permanent dentition follows.

1	2	3	4	5	6	7	8	9	10	11	12	13	14	15	16
32	31	30	29	28	27	26	25	24	23	22	21	20	19	18	17

A single number is used to represent each tooth in the permanent dentition (normally 32 teeth). For example, the right maxillary first molar is indicated in the universal system with the number *3*, and the left mandibular first molar is indicated with the number *19*. There is no provision for numbering

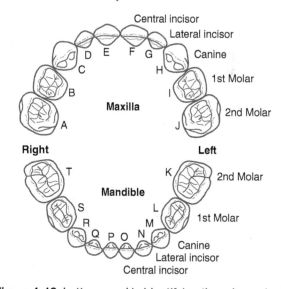

Figure 4-10 Letters used in identifying the primary teeth.

supernumerary teeth and no specific indications for missing teeth that have been replaced with restorative treatment. However, there have been suggestions for such additions.

2. Symbolic system.

Credit for a symbolic system for tooth numbering is given to two dentists and can be referred to as the Zsigmondy/Palmer notation system. However, in the United States, the system is usually referred to as the Palmer system. In this symbolic system, the

Permanent Dentition

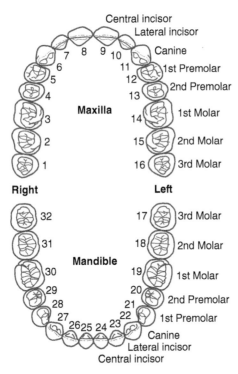

Figure 4-11 Names and numbers of the permanent teeth used in the universal numbering system.

arches are divided into four quadrants, as shown in the following depiction of the entire primary dentition. The Palmer notation for the primary dentition follows.

$$\begin{array}{ccccc|ccccc} E & D & C & B & A & A & B & C & D & E \\ \hline E & D & C & B & A & A & B & C & D & E \end{array}$$

For a single tooth, such as the primary maxillary right central incisor, the designation is A|. For the maxillary left central incisor, the notation is given as |A. This numbering system presents difficulties when an appropriate font is unavailable for keyboard recording of these notations.

The Palmer notation for the permanent dentition divides the arches into four quadrants with eight or more teeth in each quadrant. With a complement of 32 teeth, the entire dentition would appear as follows.

$$\begin{array}{cccccccc|cccccccc} 8 & 7 & 6 & 5 & 4 & 3 & 2 & 1 & 1 & 2 & 3 & 4 & 5 & 6 & 7 & 8 \\ \hline 8 & 7 & 6 & 5 & 4 & 3 & 2 & 1 & 1 & 2 & 3 & 4 & 5 & 6 & 7 & 8 \end{array}$$

The notation for the right permanent maxillary central incisor is 1|. The notation for the right permanent maxillary first molar is 6|. The Palmer notation system is used frequently in the orthodontic literature.

3. Fédération Dentaire Internationale (FDI) system.

The FDI recommends a 2-digit system for the primary and permanent dentitions. This system has been adopted by the World Health Organization (WHO) and is accepted by other organizations and in research and public health journals. The FDI system of notation for the primary dentition follows.

Upper right					Upper left				
55	54	53	52	51	61	62	63	64	65
85	84	83	82	81	71	72	73	74	75

The number *5* indicates the right maxillary quadrant; number *6*, the left maxillary quadrant; number *7*, the left mandibular quadrant; and number *8*, the right mandibular quadrant. Teeth for each quadrant are numbered from *1* to *5*, beginning with the central incisors. The right and left maxillary central incisors of the primary dentition would be numbered *51* and *61*, and the left and right mandibular central incisors would be numbered *71* and *81*. The FDI system for the permanent dentition follows.

Upper right								Upper left							
18	17	16	15	14	13	12	11	21	22	23	24	25	26	27	28
48	47	46	45	44	43	42	41	31	32	33	34	35	36	37	38

In the permanent dentition, the first digit indicates the quadrant, and the second digit indicates the tooth in that quadrant. Numbers that indicate the quadrant are as follows. The right maxillary quadrant is *1*, the left maxillary quadrant is *2*, the left mandibular quadrant is *3*, and the right mandibular quadrant is *4*. The teeth in each quadrant are numbered from *1* to *8*. The right maxillary central incisor is indicated by the double digit *11* (pronounced "one-one," not "eleven"); the left maxillary central incisor, *21*; the left mandibular central incisor, *31*; and the right mandibular central incisor, *41*. For several reasons, it is important that practitioners know the FDI system, including its use in the international literature.

2.0 Development of Human Dentitions

Knowledge of the development of the teeth and their emergence in the oral cavity is applicable to clinical practice and other areas such as anthropology, demography, forensics, and paleontology, which are referred to only briefly here. Although the References can be used to broaden the scope of reader interest, only the areas considered to be basic for the practice of dentistry are reviewed here.

A. Morphogenesis of the teeth.

The interactive mechanisms of patterning, morphogenesis, and cytodifferentiation during organogenesis are studied in Oral Embryology. Tooth development involves interactions between epithelium and mesenchyme, with the formation of a budlike epithelial structure that becomes convoluted into a *cap* and *bell* stage. Subsequently, epithelial and mesenchymal cells, such as *dental papilla*, differentiate into enamel-secreting ameloblasts and dentin-secreting odontoblasts. These stages of early tooth development are well defined histologically; however, the importance of molecular genetics and signaling pathways in tooth morphogenesis has been demonstrated only more recently in the formation of different shapes of teeth (morphogenesis) and their correct position in the jaws (patterning).

These intercellular signaling networks are composed of proteins, including ligands, receptors, and transcription factors. The outcome of these intricate mechanisms during the development of the teeth generally leads to the right shape of teeth in the right place; however, morphologic variability and dental malformations do occur, which may be of significant clinical importance.

B. Timing of human dentitions development.

The timing of chronologic events in the development of the dentitions has been historically difficult to ascertain because of the lack of adequate documentation of the sources of information. Tables of dental chronologies reflect an abbreviated version of a long history of accumulated successive compilations and revisions of chronologies of the primary teeth, which is also true for the permanent dentition. Such chronologies have some deficiencies in population sampling and collection methods, and incorporating revised data based on making critical choices from available sources is associated with methodologic errors. More recent partial chronologies of dental development reflect the use of statistical methods that provide three different types of formation data: age of attainment chronologies based on tooth emergence, age of prediction chronologies based on being in a stage of development, and maturity assessment scales used to assess whether a subject of known age is ahead of or behind compared with a reference population. These types of chronologies are used when more precise information about a particular aspect of dental development is needed for research and surgical procedures.

1. Dental age.

Dental age is usually based on the formation or emergence of the teeth as well as simply counting the number of teeth, the presence of permanent teeth, and the amount of root resorption of the primary teeth. Looking into the mouth and noting which teeth are present is a simple way to approximate the age of young children and adolescents. The dentition may be considered the best physiologic indicator of chronologic age in juveniles.

C. Eruption or emergence of the teeth.

The term *eruption* has been defined historically as the emergence of the tooth into the oral cavity; however,

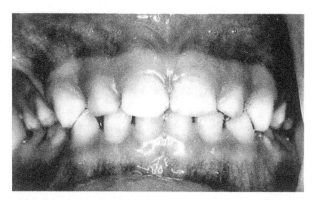

Figure 4-12 Primary dentition in a 5-year-old child. *(From Ash MM, Ramjford SP: Occlusion. Philadelphia, Saunders, 1995.)*

it has been considered more recently to mean continuous tooth movement from the dental tooth bud to occlusal contact. The term *emergence* is thought to be more specific for the emergence of the teeth through the alveolar gingiva.

3.0 Chronology of Primary Dentition

The *primary dentition* (Figure 4-12) is considered to be clinically complete when the second primary molars are in occlusion at about the mean age of 29 months, keeping in mind that the completion of the roots of the canines occurs at about 3.25 years of age. The emergence of the permanent first molars signals the start of the *mixed dentition* period, which is considered to have been completed when all the primary teeth are lost and only the succeeding permanent (succedaneous) teeth are present.

The chronology of the primary dentition is summarized in Table 4-1. The universal numbering system for the primary teeth is used as well as general indications of primary incisors, canine, and molars, i1, i2, C, m1, and m2. The dimensions for the primary dentition are provided in Table 4-2.

4.0 Morphology of Primary Teeth

Detailed coverage of the individual morphology of the primary teeth is beyond the scope of this review, and the reader is invited to consider the material in the References. However, it is anticipated that the present coverage of aspects of morphology for identification and function of the primary dentition will provide a reminder of the important details that have already been considered in the dental curriculum.

A. Schematic views of primary dentition—schematic views of the primary dentition are shown in Figures 4-13 to 4-20. Facial, lingual, mesial, and incisal or occlusal views of the incisors, canines, and molars are illustrated.

Table 4-1

Chronologies of the Primary Dentition

TOOTH		FIRST EVIDENCE OF CALCIFICATION (WEEKS IN UTERO)	CROWN COMPLETED (MONTHS)	EMERGENCE (MEAN AGE) (MONTHS)	ROOT COMPLETED (YEARS)
Upper					
i1	E, F	14	1½	10	1½
i2	D, G	16	2½	11	2
C	C, H	17	9	19	3¾
m1	B, I	15	6	16	2½
m2	A, J	19	11	29	3

Maxillary Teeth

Right A B C D E | F G H I J Left

T S R Q P | O N M L K

Mandibular Teeth

TOOTH		FIRST EVIDENCE OF CALCIFICATION (WEEKS IN UTERO)	CROWN COMPLETED (MONTHS)	EMERGENCE (MEAN AGE) (MONTHS)	ROOT COMPLETED (YEARS)
Lower					
i1	P, O	14	2½	8	1½
i2	Q, N	16	3	13	1½
C	R, M	17	9	20	3¾
m1	S, L	15½	5½	16	2¼
m2	T, K	18	10	27	3

From Ash MM, Nelson SJ: Wheeler's Dental Anatomy, Physiology, and Occlusion, ed 8. Philadelphia, Saunders, 2003.

Table 4-2

Measurements of the Primary Teeth*

		CROWN HEIGHT	ROOT LENGTH	MD CROWN DIAMETER	FL CROWN DIAMETER	MD CERVIX DIAMETER	FL CERVIX DIAMETER
Maxillary Teeth			A B C D E	F G H I J				
CI	E │ F	6.0	10.0	6.5	5.0	4.5	4.0
LI	D │ G	5.6	11.4	5.1	4.0	3.7	3.7
C	C │ H	6.5	13.5	7.0	7.0	5.1	5.5
m1	B │ I	5.1	10.0	7.3	8.5	5.2	6.9
m2	A │ J	5.7	11.7	8.2	10.0	6.4	8.3
Mandibular Teeth			T S R Q P │ O N M L K				
CI	P │ O	5.0	9.0	4.3	4.0	3.0	3.5
LI	Q │ N	5.2	10.0	4.1	4.0	3.0	3.5
C	R │ M	6.0	11.5	5.0	4.8	3.7	4.0
m1	S │ L	6.0	9.8	7.7	7.0	6.5	5.3
m2	T │ K	5.5	11.3	9.9	8.7	7.2	6.4

FL, Faciolingual; *MD*, mesiodistal.

*Average measurements (in mm) adapted from Black GV (Cited by Ash MM, Nelson SJ: Wheeler's Dental Anatomy, Physiology, and Occlusion, ed 8. Philadelphia, Saunders, 2003). A │ J to T │ K = universal numbering system for primary teeth.

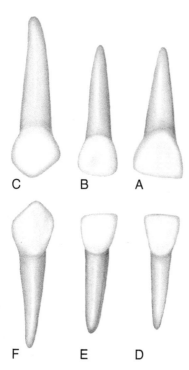

Figure 4-13 Primary right anterior teeth, labial aspect. **A,** Maxillary central incisor. **B,** Maxillary lateral incisor. **C,** Maxillary canine. **D,** Mandibular central incisor. **E,** Mandibular lateral incisor. **F,** Mandibular canine. *(From Nelson SJ, Ash MM: Wheeler's Dental Anatomy, Physiology, and Occlusion, ed 9. St. Louis, Saunders, 2010.)*

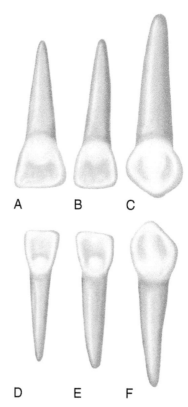

Figure 4-14 Primary right anterior teeth, lingual aspect. **A,** Maxillary central incisor. **B,** Maxillary lateral incisor. **C,** Maxillary canine. **D,** Mandibular central incisor. **E,** Mandibular lateral incisor. **F,** Mandibular canine. *(From Nelson SJ, Ash MM: Wheeler's Dental Anatomy, Physiology, and Occlusion, ed 9. St. Louis, Saunders, 2010.)*

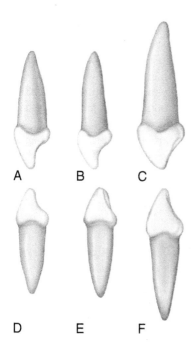

Figure 4-15 Primary right anterior teeth, mesial aspect. **A,** Maxillary central incisor. **B,** Maxillary lateral incisor. **C,** Maxillary canine. **D,** Mandibular central incisor. **E,** Mandibular lateral incisor. **F,** Mandibular canine. *(From Nelson SJ, Ash MM: Wheeler's Dental Anatomy, Physiology, and Occlusion, ed 9. St. Louis, Saunders, 2010.)*

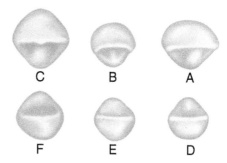

Figure 4-16 Primary right anterior teeth, incisal aspect. **A,** Maxillary central incisor. **B,** Maxillary lateral incisor. **C,** Maxillary canine. **D,** Mandibular central incisor. **E,** Mandibular lateral incisor. **F,** Mandibular canine. *(From Nelson SJ, Ash MM: Wheeler's Dental Anatomy, Physiology, and Occlusion, ed 9. St. Louis, Saunders, 2010.)*

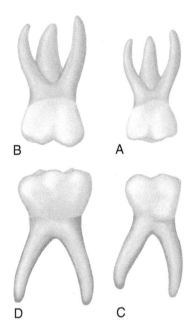

Figure 4-17 Primary right molars, buccal aspect. **A,** Maxillary first molar. **B,** Maxillary second molar. **C,** Mandibular first molar. **D,** Mandibular second molar. *(From Nelson SJ, Ash MM: Wheeler's Dental Anatomy, Physiology, and Occlusion, ed 9. St. Louis, Saunders, 2010.)*

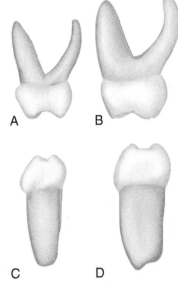

Figure 4-19 Primary right molars, mesial aspect. **A,** Maxillary first molar. **B,** Maxillary second molar. **C,** Mandibular first molar. **D,** Mandibular second molar. *(From Nelson SJ, Ash MM: Wheeler's Dental Anatomy, Physiology, and Occlusion, ed 9. St. Louis, Saunders, 2010.)*

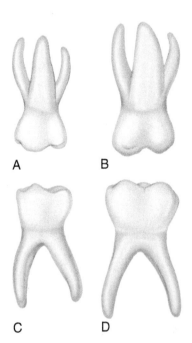

Figure 4-18 Primary right molars, lingual aspect. **A,** Maxillary first molar. **B,** Maxillary second molar. **C,** Mandibular first molar. **D,** Mandibular second molar. *(From Nelson SJ, Ash MM: Wheeler's Dental Anatomy, Physiology, and Occlusion, ed 9. St. Louis, Saunders, 2010.)*

B. Identification characteristics of primary teeth—compared with the permanent teeth, the primary teeth have the following identifying differences.
   1. General characteristics.
      a. Smaller in overall size and crown dimensions.
      b. Whiter in color than permanent teeth.
      c. Markedly more prominent cervical ridges.
      d. Molar roots widely flared, especially maxillary molars.
      e. Molar roots thin, ribbon-shaped; wider buccolingually.
      f. Root trunks narrow or absent.
      g. Crowns frequently abraded.
      h. Large pulp chambers.
      i. Thinner enamel covering.
      j. Roots often partially resorbed.
   2. Identifying characteristics of primary maxillary and mandibular first molars.
      a. Maxillary first primary molar.
         (1) Three roots.
         (2) Generally three cusps (occasional small distolingual cusp).
         (3) Prominent buccal cervical ridge (buccal mesial half).
         (4) Buccal height of contour is at cervical third of crown.
         (5) Lingual height of contour is at middle third of crown.

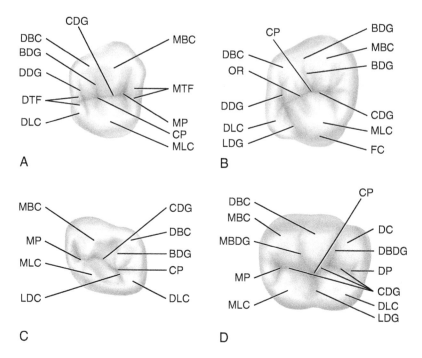

Figure 4-20 **A,** Maxillary first molar. **B,** Maxillary second molar. **C,** Mandibular first molar. **D,** Mandibular second molar. *BDG,* Buccal developmental groove; *CDG,* central developmental groove; *CP,* central pit; *DBC,* distobuccal cusp; *DBDG,* distobuccal developmental groove; *DC,* distal cusp; *DDG,* distal developmental groove; *DLC,* distolingual cusp; *DP,* distal pit; *DTF,* distal triangular fossa; *FC,* fifth cusp; *LDC,* lingual developmental groove; *LDG,* lingual developmental groove; *MBC,* mesiobuccal cusp; *MBDG,* mesiobuccal developmental groove; *MLC,* mesiolingual cusp; *MP,* mesial pit; *MTF,* mesial triangular fossa; *OR,* oblique ridge. *(From Nelson SJ, Ash MM: Wheeler's Dental Anatomy, Physiology, and Occlusion, ed 9. St. Louis, Saunders, 2010.)*

(6) Mesiobuccal root size is wider buccolingually than distobuccal root. Lingual root is longest and most divergent.

(7) Mesiobuccal cusp is largest.

(8) Smallest molar mesiodistally.

(9) Distal marginal ridge thin and poorly developed.

b. Mandibular first primary molar.

(1) Two roots.

(2) Four cusps.

(3) Rhomboidal occlusal outline.

(4) Mesiobuccal cusp is largest and best developed.

(5) Very prominent buccal cervical ridge along the mesial half of buccal surface.

(6) Buccal height of contour on cervical third of crown; lingual height on middle third.

5.0 Chronology of Permanent Dentition

The permanent dentition of 32 teeth is completed by 18 to 25 years of age (Table 4-3). This table suggests the complexity of bringing together all the biologic mechanisms at the right time and place to provide the appropriate relationships between tooth form and jaw movements, tooth form and supporting structures of the teeth, and the alignment of the teeth and their contact relationships with adjacent teeth and opposing teeth in opposing arches, all in such a way as to stabilize the occlusion and protect the supporting structures of the teeth. The dimensions for the permanent dentition are provided in Table 4-4.

6.0 Morphology of Permanent Teeth

A schematic representation of the permanent dentition is shown in Figure 4-21. In Table 4-5, the teeth of each side of the arches are indicated with their universal system numbers.

A. Incisors—some type traits and other characteristics.

B. Canine—some type and arch traits and other characteristics.

C. Premolars—type traits and other characteristics.

D. Maxillary molars—type traits and other characteristics.

E. Mandibular molars—type traits and other characteristics.

In Figure 4-22, the relationship between the roots of the maxillary teeth and the sinus is important in root canal therapy, oral surgery, and sinus lift procedures for implants. The first and second maxillary molars are generally of particular interest, especially with alveolar extension of the maxillary sinus, because of the possibility of perforating the sinus membrane during tooth removal and during placement of implants. Perforation with root canal instrumentation is also a risk to be evaluated closely.

The position of the mandibular molars, especially the third molar, is important because of the proximity of the roots and impacted third molars to the inferior dental (mandibular) canal and the inferior alveolar nerve. Radiographic indicators of risk of exposure of the inferior alveolar nerve after mandibular third molar extraction includes darkening of roots, interruption of the white lines of the canal, diversion of the canal, and narrowing of the tooth root.

Table 4-3

Chronologies of Permanent Teeth

TOOTH		FIRST EVIDENCE OF CALCIFICATION	CROWN COMPLETED (YEARS)	EMERGENCE (ERUPTION) (YEARS)	ROOT COMPLETED (YEARS)
CI	8, 9	3-4 mo	4-5	7-8	10
LI	7, 10	10-12 mo	4-5	8-9	11
C	6, 11	4-5 mo	6-7	11-12	13-15
P1	5, 12	$1\frac{1}{4}$-$1\frac{3}{4}$ yr	5-6	10-11	12-13
P2	4, 13	2-$2\frac{1}{4}$ yr	6-7	10-12	12-14
M1	3, 14	At birth	$2\frac{1}{2}$-3	6-7	9-10
M2	2, 15	$2\frac{1}{2}$-3 yr	7-8	12-13	14-16
M3	1, 16	7-9 yr	12-16	17-21	18-25

Maxillary Teeth

Right 1 2 3 4 5 6 7 8 | 9 10 11 12 13 14 15 16 Left
       32 31 30 29 28 27 26 25 | 24 23 22 21 20 19 18 17

Mandibular Teeth

CI	24, 25	3-4 mo	4-5	6-7	9
LI	23, 26	3-4 mo	4-5	7-8	10
C	22, 27	4-5 mo	6-7	9-10	12-14
P1	21, 28	$1\frac{1}{4}$-2 yr	5-6	10-12	12-13
P2	20, 29	$2\frac{1}{4}$-$2\frac{1}{2}$ yr	6-7	11-12	13-14
M1	19, 30	At birth	$2\frac{1}{2}$-3	6-7	9-10
M2	18, 31	$2\frac{1}{2}$-3 yr	7-8	11-13	14-15
M3	17, 32	8-10 yr	12-16	17-21	18-25

After Ash MM, Nelson SJ: Wheeler's Dental Anatomy, Physiology, and Occlusion, ed 8. Philadelphia: WB Saunders, 2003.

Table 4-4

Dimensions of Permanent Teeth*

	CROWN LENGTH	ROOT LENGTH	MD CROWN DIAMETER	FL CROWN DIAMETER	CURVATURE M	CURVATURE D
Maxillary Teeth						
Central incisor	10.5	13.0	8.5	7.0	3.5	2.5
Lateral incisor	9.0	13.0	6.5	6.0	3.0	2.0
Canine	10.0	17.0	7.5	8.0	2.5	1.5
First premolar	8.5	14.0	7.0	9.0	1.0	0.0
Second premolar	8.5	14.0	7.0	9.0	1.0	0.0
First molar	7.5	B 12, L 13	10.0	11.0	1.0	0.0
Second molar	7.0	B 11 L 12	9.0	11.0	1.0	0.0
Third molar	6.5	11	8.5	10.0	1.0	0.0
Mandibular Teeth						
Central incisor	9.0	12.5	5.0	6.0	3.0	2.0
Lateral incisor	9.5	14.0	5.5	6.0	3.0	2.0
Canine	11.0	16.0	7.0	7.5	2.5	1.0
First premolar	8.5	14.0	7.0	7.5	1.0	0.0
Second premolar	8.0	14.5	7.0	8.0	1.0	0.0
First molar	7.5	14.0	11.0	10.5	1.0	0.0
Second molar	7.0	13.0	10.5	10.0	1.0	0.0
Third molar	7.0	11.0	10.5	9.5	1.0	0.0

Adapted from Ash MM, Nelson SJ: Wheeler's Dental Anatomy, Physiology, and Occlusion, ed 8. Philadelphia, Saunders, 2003.

FL, Faciolingual, buccolingual, labiolingual; *MD,* mesiodistal.

*Average measurements in millimeters.

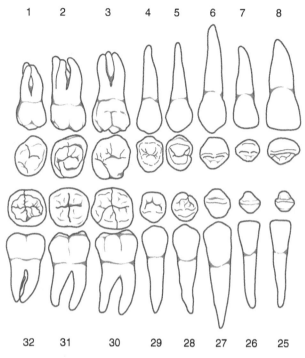

Figure 4-21 Schematic representations of the permanent teeth of the right side.

7.0 Development of Dental Occlusions

The development of occlusion involves three time frames (i.e., time of emergence and contacting of the primary teeth, period of the mixed dentition with emergence and contacting of permanent teeth, and time when the rest of the permanent teeth emerge and make occlusal contact). The factors that determine the size of the teeth and dimensions of the jaws and provide room for succedaneous teeth relate to the orderly transition from the primary dentition through the mixed dentition to the permanent dentition and its completion. For example, the chances for crowding in the permanent dentition based on the available spaces between the primary teeth (>6 mm) would be none; however, for 3 to 5 mm of spacing in the primary dentition, the chances of crowding are 1:5. If the primary teeth are crowded, there is a 1:1 chance of crowding of the permanent dentition. Among other factors, the availability of interdental spaces in the primary dentition depends on tooth size and dimension of the arches. The chance is small for crowding of the permanent dentition in the patient seen in Figure 4-23.

Table 4-5

Some Type and Arch Traits and Other Characteristics

	CI 8, 9	LI 7, 10	CI 24, 25	LI 23, 26
Pulp horns	Facial view, 3	Usually 2	1 or none	Variable
MI angle	Sharp right angle	Slight rounding	Sharp right angle	Some rounding
DI angle	Slight rounding	Distinct round	Sharp right angle	More rounded
Mesial profile	Straight	Slight rounding	Straight	Straight
Distal profile	Nearly round	Distinct round	Straight	Straight
Incisal outline	Straight	Straight	Straight	Slight DL twist
Proximal contacts				
Mesial	Incisal third	Incisal/middle third	Incisal third	Incisal third
Distal	Incisal/middle third	Middle third	Incisal third	Incisal third
Curve at CEJ				
Mesial	3.5 mm	3.0 mm	3.0 mm	3.0 mm
Distal	2.5 mm	2.0 mm	2.0 mm	2.0 mm
Contour height				
Facial/lingual	Cervical third	Cervical third	Cervical third	Cervical third
Pulp canal(s)	1	1	1, possibly 2	1
	CANINES 6, 11		**CANINES 22, 27**	
Pulp horns	1		1	
Facial aspect				
Proximal contacts				

Continued

Table 4-5

Some Type and Arch Traits and Other Characteristics—cont'd

	CANINES 6, 11	CANINES 22, 27
Mesial	Junction of incisal and middle third	Incisal third
Distal	Middle third	Middle third
Mesial aspect	Wider mesiodistally	Narrower, longer
Lingual aspect	Deeper lingual fossae	Flat lingual surface
Marginal ridges	Pronounced; 2 fossae	Parallel or slight convergence
Cingulum	Large; centered MD	Smaller; possibly off-center distally
Lingual pits/grooves	Common	None
Incisal aspect	Marked asymmetry < asymmetry Halves	Distal cusp mesial/distal Ridge rotated
Incisal/proximal	Cusp tip may be at or cusp tip lingual to root	Views labial to root axis line
CEJ curvature	2.5 mm (mesial)	1.0 mm (distal)
Contour height	0.5 mm	<0.5 mm
Facial/lingual	Cervical third	Cervical third

	FIRST PREMOLARS 5, 12	SECOND PREMOLARS 4, 13	FIRST PREMOLARS 21, 28	SECOND PREMOLARS 20, 29
Buccal/facial view				
Buccal cusps	Pointed	Obtuse	Pointed	More obtuse
Cusp tip	Tipped distally	Tipped mesially	Middle axis	Middle axis
Crown margins	Bulging	Narrow	Prominent	Prominent
Proximal contacts	MD, middle third	MD, middle third	MD, middle third	MD, middle third
Mesial BC ridge	Longer than D	Shorter than D	Shorter than D	M and D similar
Crown symmetry	Bilateral asymmetry	Symmetrical	Bilateral symmetry	Bilateral symmetry
Outline	Trapezoid	Trapezoid	Trapezoid	Trapezoid
Lingual view	All buccal crown profile visible	None of buccal profile visible	Most of buccal profile visible	None of buccal profile visible
Occlusal surface	Little visible	None visible	Mostly visible	Little visible
Mesial aspect	Transverse ridge	Transverse ridge	Transverse ridge	No transverse ridge
ML groove	None	None	Usually present	None
MM ridge groove	Usually present	Not present	Not present	Not present
MM ridge root(s)	Horizontal	Horizontal	Inclined apically	Horizontal
Usually 2, BL	Single	Single	Single	
Occlusal view				
Table outline	Trapezoidal (see Fig. 4-21)	Rectangular (see Fig. 4-21)	Triangle/diamond (see Fig. 4-21)	Square/round
Groove/pit pattern	Longer	Shorter	No central pit	Central pit
Y groove pattern	Absent	Present		
Supplemental grooves	Rare	Frequent		

	FIRST MOLARS 3, 14	SECOND MOLARS 2, 15	THIRD MOLARS 1, 16
Facial aspect	Widest of three	Intermediate width	Smallest width
DB cusp height	Same as MB cusp	DB slightly shorter	DB much shorter
MB root apex	In line with MB cusp	In line with center tip of crown	MB/DB fused, in line with crown center
Occlusal view			
Crown outline	Square/rhomboid (see Fig. 4-21)	More rhomboidal (see Fig. 4-21)	Triangle-/heart-shaped (see Fig. 4-21)

Table 4-5			
Some Type and Arch Traits and Other Characteristics—cont'd			
	FIRST MOLARS 3, 14	**SECOND MOLARS 2, 15**	**THIRD MOLARS 1, 16**
Lobes 5 4 3-4			
Lingual aspect			
DL cusp	Largest	Smaller width/height	Usually missing
Lingual root	Widest MD	Narrower	Narrowest
Dimensions			
	FIRST MOLARS 19, 30	**SECOND MOLARS 18, 31**	**THIRD MOLARS 17, 32**
Facial view			
Cusps	5-MB, DB, D, ML, DL	4-MB, DB, ML, DL	4-MB, DB,ML, DL
Buccal grooves	2	1	
Roots	Wide separation	Closer together, fused, short, marked relatively vertical distal inclination	
Lingual view	Visible buccal profiles/profiles/ surfaces	Profiles/surfaces proximal surfaces not visible	Not visible
Occlusal outline	Hex-/pentagonal-/rectangular- shaped	Heart-shaped/ovoid	
Groove(s)	Y pattern + 4 pattern	No pattern	

CI, Central incisor; *LI*, Lateral incisor; *CEJ*, Cementoenamel junction; *mm*, millimeters; *M*, mesial; *D*, distal; *B*, buccal; *L*, lingual

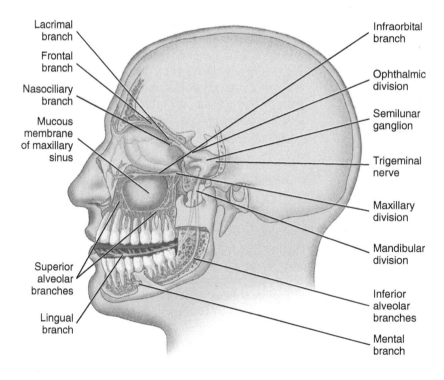

Figure 4-22 Distribution of the trigeminal nerve. *(From Nelson SJ, Ash MM: Wheeler's Dental Anatomy, Physiology, and Occlusion, ed 9. St. Louis, Saunders, 2010.)*

A. Development of primary occlusion.

The primary teeth should be in normal alignment and occlusion should occur shortly after the age of 2 years, with all the roots fully formed by the time the child is 3 years old. With the growth of the jaws, the anterior teeth separate, beginning between 4 and 5 years of age. The primary occlusion is also supported and made more efficient by the emergence of the first permanent molars (sometimes referred to as *6-year molars*) immediately distal to the primary second

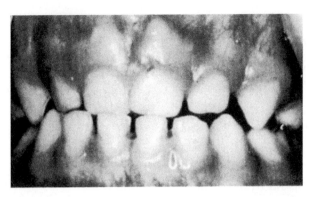

Figure 4-23 Primary dentition showing spacing that generally suggests a low probability of crowding in the permanent dentition. *(From Ash MM, Nelson SJ: Wheeler's Dental Anatomy, Physiology, and Occlusion, ed 8. Philadelphia, Saunders, 2003.)*

molars, as illustrated in the development of occlusion shown in Figure 4-24, *A* and *B*. The sequence of eruption (in months) is depicted in Figure 4-24, *C*. The completion of the primary occlusion and developing permanent dentition is shown in Figure 4-24, *D*.

B. Development of permanent occlusion.

The development of the permanent occlusion (Figure 4-25, *A*) begins with the emergence and contacts of the first permanent molars at about 6 years of age and, except for the third molar, is concluded at about 15 to 18 years of age. The emergence of the mandibular incisors (Figure 4-25, *B*) follows the 6-year molars at 6 to 7 years of age. The most favorable sequence of eruption or emergence of the permanent dentition for a normal occlusion is shown in Figure 4-25, *C*. The third molars emerge and come into occlusal contact later, usually by 25 years of age (Figure 4-25, *D*).

When the teeth are in ideal alignment so that proximal contacts and marginal ridges are in proper position (Figure 4-26), there is less of a chance of impaction of food into the interproximal areas, resulting in loss of periodontal attachment.

C. Tooth size, arch form, and arch dimensions.

Room for the development, eruption, and emergence of the permanent teeth during the mixed dentition period is influenced by the forward rotation of the maxillomandibular complex. An important part in the development of the occlusion of the permanent dentition is the premolar segment where the erupting premolars are significantly smaller in the mesiodistal diameter than the primary molars, which they replace (i.e., the mesiodistal diameters of the mandibular primary molars are greater than the mesiodistal diameters of the replacing premolars). This gain in space between the primary and permanent dentition in the dental arch is referred to as the *leeway space*. It has importance for the alignment of the mandibular incisors and for mandibular molar movement to correct

the end-to-end molar relationship in the mixed dentition period into a normal molar relationship in the permanent dentition (e.g., mesiobuccal cusp of the maxillary first molar occluding in the mesiobuccal developmental groove of the mandibular first molar, as shown in Figure 4-27, *A*, which is an angle class I molar relationship).

The arch form and width of the primary dentition generally is established for both the primary and the permanent dentitions by age 9 months. What does change is the increase in anterior-posterior dimensions of the jaws, which is necessary for the incorporation of the molars into the occlusion. The supporting alveolar bone and basal bone determine the shape of the dental arches.

There is a general relationship between the size of the teeth and the size of the dental arches; however, when a discrepancy is evident between the aggregate mesiodistal diameters of the crowns of the teeth and the size of the bony supporting arches, crowding or protrusion can occur. Arch width and perimeter dimensions can relate to differences between crowded and uncrowded dentitions.

In cases of restorative dentistry, the dimensions of the replacement teeth must be related to the size of the existing teeth and arch dimensions. For a maxillary arch length of 128 mm and a mandibular arch length of 126 mm, the sum of the mesiodistal diameter of all the mandibular teeth would have to be 126 mm, and the sum of the mesiodistal diameter of all the maxillary teeth would have to be 128 mm. Arch dimensions and tooth size vary considerably, and there is no template for any patient. The esthetics of tooth form, size, and color are important considerations in restoring teeth.

8.0 Occlusal Contact Relations and Mandibular Movements

The restorative dentist must preserve comfort and health throughout the functional (chewing) and parafunctional range of the patient's mandibular movements. Concepts of occlusion that incorporate principles of mandibular movement require a basic understanding of occlusal relations and potential influences on dental anatomy as a foundation. This section introduces occlusal contact relations that occur in maximum intercuspation of the teeth (centric positions) and the basic relations associated with mandibular movement (eccentric positions).

A. Static occlusal relationships.

In the generally accepted definition of normal occlusion, each mandibular tooth is positioned lingual to the maxillary counterpart. The mandibular teeth are positioned about one half of a tooth anterior to the maxillary counterpart, excluding the central incisors

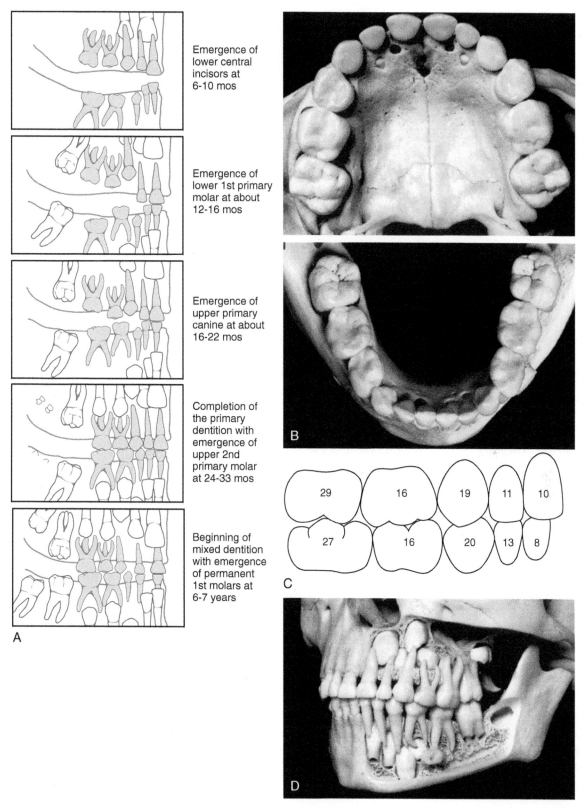

Emergence of lower central incisors at 6-10 mos

Emergence of lower 1st primary molar at about 12-16 mos

Emergence of upper primary canine at about 16-22 mos

Completion of the primary dentition with emergence of upper 2nd primary molar at 24-33 mos

Beginning of mixed dentition with emergence of permanent 1st molars at 6-7 years

Figure 4-24 Development of primary occlusion. **A,** Birth to mixed dentition. **B,** Mixed dentition with first permanent molar in position. **C,** Mean age of emergence (in months) of primary teeth. **D,** Anterior-lateral view of mixed dentition with first permanent molars in position and developing permanent dentition (empty crypt is a preparation artifact). *(A, From Schour L, Massler M: Studies in tooth development: the growth pattern of human teeth. Part II. J Am Dent Assoc 27:1918, 1940. D, From Ash MM, Ramfjord SP: Occlusion. Philadelphia, Saunders, 1995.)*

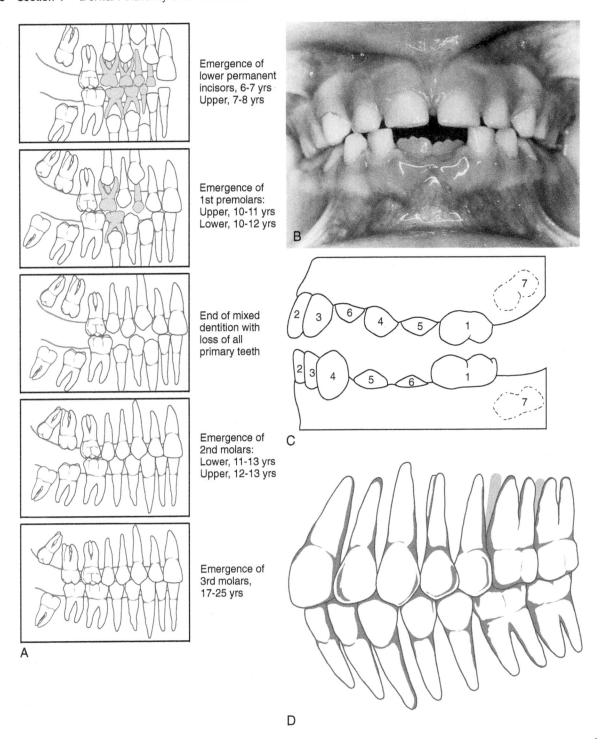

Figure 4-25 Development of permanent occlusion. A, Schematic representation of developing occlusion. **B,** Emergence of the mandibular central incisors. **C,** Sequence of eruption of the permanent teeth. **D,** Permanent dentition of 28 teeth at about 14 to 16 years of age. (**A,** *From Schour L, Massler M: The development of the human dentition. J Am Dent Assoc 28:1153, 1941.*)

(Figure 4-28). In this position, occlusal contacts may follow two primary forms (Figure 4-29). The following descriptions relate to so-called idealized contact relations—a concept that can be used as a basis for discussion as well as for developing occlusal contact relations in restorative dentistry and orthodontics.

Individuals often may show variations from the patterns as presented *without* having occlusal dysfunction.

1. Posterior cusp-fossa/cusp-embrasure occlusion, from an occlusal view (Figure 4-29, *A*)—the mandibular buccal cusps (mandibular supporting cusps) occlude as follows.

a. The first premolar cusp contacts the marginal ridges between the maxillary canine and first premolar.

b. The second premolar contacts marginal ridges between the first maxillary premolar and second maxillary premolar.

c. The mesiobuccal cusp of the first molar contacts the marginal ridges between the second maxillary premolar and first molar.

d. The distobuccal cusp of the first molar contacts the central fossa of the maxillary first molar (this is a key contact relationship to remember).

e. The distal cusp of the first molar contacts the distal fossa of the maxillary first molar.

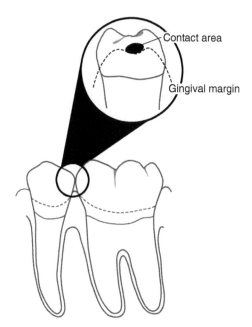

Figure 4-26 Schematic illustration of proximal contact areas and relationship to gingival margin.

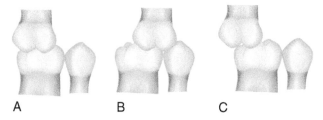

Figure 4-27 A, Angle class I molar relationship. **B,** Class II molar relationship. **C,** Class III molar relationship. *(From Nelson SJ, Ash MM: Wheeler's Dental Anatomy, Physiology, and Occlusion, ed 9. St. Louis, Saunders, 2010.)*

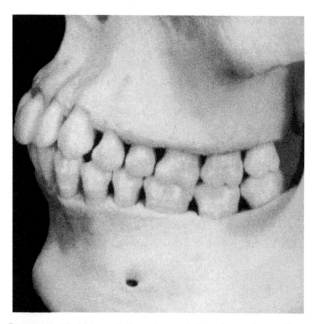

Figure 4-28 View of the step relationship of maxillary and mandibular teeth.

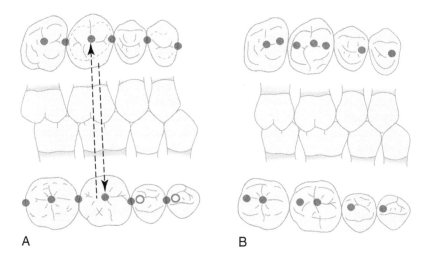

Figure 4-29 Example of idealized cusp-fossa relationship. **A,** Mesiolingual cusp of maxillary first molar occludes in the central fossa of the mandibular first molar. Distal buccal cusp of mandibular first molar occludes in the central fossa of the maxillary first molar. **B,** Concept of occlusion in which all supporting cusps occlude in fossae. *(From Nelson SJ, Ash MM: Wheeler's Dental Anatomy, Physiology, and Occlusion, ed 9. St. Louis, Saunders, 2010.)*

f. The mesiobuccal cusp of the second molar contacts the marginal ridges between the first and second maxillary molars.

g. The distobuccal cusp of the second molar contacts the central fossa of the maxillary second molar. As shown in Figure 4-29, *A*, the contact relations occurring with the *maxillary lingual cusps* (maxillary supporting cusps) follow a similar embrasure contact pattern, with the exception of the mesiolingual cusp of the first molar and the mesiolingual cusp of the second molar.

h. The mesiolingual cusp of the first molar contacts the central fossa of the mandibular first molar (this is a key contact relationship to remember).

i. The mesiolingual cusp of the second molar contacts the central fossa of the mandibular second molar.

2. Posterior cusp-fossa/cusp-fossa occlusion.

The cusp-fossa/cusp-fossa occlusion shares the same relationship as the embrasure form when considering the mesiolingual cusps of the maxillary molars and the distobuccal cusps of the mandibular molars. The supporting cusps contact the central fossae of the opposing counterparts in maximum intercuspation. The contact relations for the right mandibular supporting cusps and incisors are shown in Figure 4-29, *B*. The mandibular cusp pattern results in a fossa contact for each supporting cusp and results in a "one tooth contacting one tooth" relationship, as opposed to the mandibular teeth contacting the maxillary counterpart and the mesially occurring tooth as described for the cusp-embrasure occlusion (see Figure 4-29, *A*). The *mandibular supporting cusp* relations occur (see Figure 4-29, *B*) as follows.

a. The first premolar contacts the mesial triangular fossa of the maxillary first premolar.

b. The second premolar contacts the mesial triangular fossa of the maxillary second premolar.

c. The mesiobuccal cusp of the first molar contacts the mesial triangular fossa of the maxillary first molar.

d. The distobuccal cusp of the first molar contacts the central fossa of the maxillary first molar.

e. The distal cusp of the first molar contacts the distal triangular fossa of the maxillary first molar.

f. The mesiobuccal cusp of the second molar contacts the mesial triangular fossa of the maxillary second molar.

g. The distobuccal cusp of the second molar contacts the central fossa of the maxillary second molar.

As shown in Figure 4-29, *B*, the maxillary supporting cusp relationships follow a similar contact relationship with the mandibular counterparts. With the exception of the mesiolingual cusps of the maxillary molars, the remaining contacts in maximum intercuspation occur in the distal fossa of the mandibular counterparts.

B. Border movements of the mandible.

Primary movements of the TMJ involve some degree of rotation (hinge movement) and translation (sliding movements) of both joints. Although the TMJ is discussed separately, basic mandibular movements may be better understood by studying the border movements of the mandible. Border movements are the limits to which the mandible can move, whereas the functional movements generally occur within the border positions. Plane diagrams may be helpful to visualize the various positions and movements. Sagittal and horizontal plane diagrams of border movements are shown in Figure 4-30. Unassisted maximum opening for a normal person is considered to be about 40+ mm. Unassisted normal maximum lateral movements are considered to be about 10 to 12 mm. Maximum protrusion from incisal edge contact (IEC) is normally about 4 to 5+ mm. Chewing function takes place usually within a few millimeters of the intercuspal position (ICP) or centric occlusion (CO), which are terms used to define maximum intercuspation of the teeth.

1. Mandibular movements viewed from the frontal/or coronal plane.

Healthy individuals are able to move their mandibles laterally to both the left and the right. Chewing generally occurs on the side to which the mandible moves, as shown in Figure 4-31.

When the mandible moves to the right, the right side movement is termed *laterotrusive movement* (right working movement). The left side moves medially and protrusively to result in a *mediotrusive movement* (balancing or nonworking movement) (Figure 4-32, *A* and *B*). The laterotrusive movements and mediotrusive movements reverse sides when the mandible moves to the left.

From the basic contact relations occurring in maximum intercuspation, potential tooth contacts occurring when the mandible moves laterally and protrusively can be described.

2. Mandibular movements viewed from the horizontal plane.

When viewed in the horizontal plane, the paths for the mesiolingual cusp of the maxillary first molar and the distobuccal cusp of the mandibular first molar are shown in Figure 4-33.

a. In a normal alignment of the dentition, the mesiolingual cusp of the maxillary first molar opposes the central fossa of the mandibular first molar.

b. From this position, the cusp passes through the lingual groove when a laterotrusive (working) movement occurs.

c. During a mediotrusive movement (nonworking or balancing), the same cusp opposes the distobuccal groove.

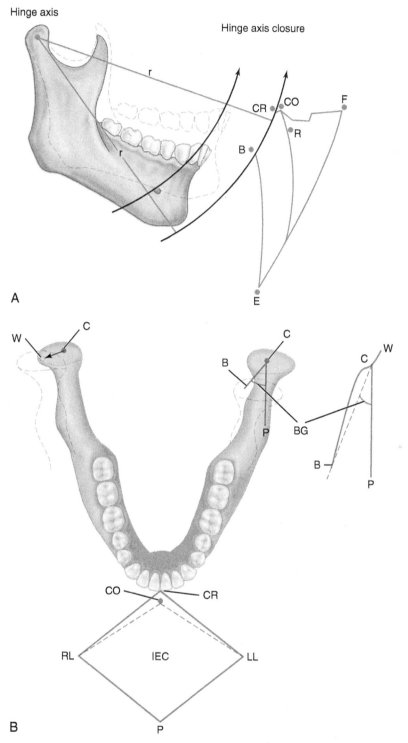

Figure 4-30 A, Schematic representation of mandibular movement envelope in the sagittal plane. **B,** Right mandibular movement with schematic representation of movement at the incisal point in the horizontal plane (*CR, LL, P, RL*) and at the condyle (*W, C, B, P*) made by a pantograph. Teeth are not in occlusion. On the right side, the condyle moves from centric (*C*) to right working (*W*). On the balancing side, the left condyle moves from *C* along line *B* and makes an angle *BG*, called the *Bennett angle*. *B* to *CR*, Opening and closing on hinge axis with no change in radius (*r*); *C* to *P*, Straight protrusive movement; *CO*, centric occlusion; *CR*, centric relation; *E*, maximum opening; *F*, maximum protrusion; *IEC*, incisal edge contact; *LL*, left lateral; *P*, protrusive; *R*, rest position; *RL*, right lateral. (*From Nelson SJ, Ash MM: Wheeler's Dental Anatomy, Physiology, and Occlusion, ed 9. St. Louis, Saunders, 2010.*)

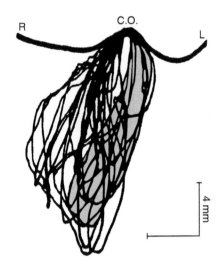

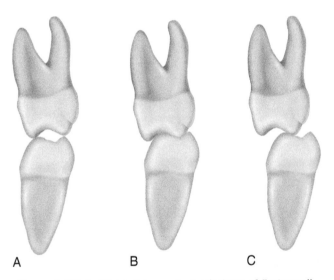

Figure 4-31 Mandibular movements during the process of chewing naturally. Incisor point movement is seen in the frontal plane. *C.O.*, Centric occlusion; *L*, left; *R*, right. *(From Nelson SJ, Ash MM: Wheeler's Dental Anatomy, Physiology, and Occlusion, ed 9. St. Louis, Saunders, 2010.)*

Figure 4-32 A, Right side contact relations of first maxillary and mandibular molars in right working (laterotrusive) position. **B,** Centric occlusion (intercuspal position). **C,** Nonworking side. *(From Nelson SJ, Ash MM: Wheeler's Dental Anatomy, Physiology, and Occlusion, ed 9. St. Louis, Saunders, 2010.)*

d. Mandibular protrusion results in the mesiolingual cusp passing through the central groove toward the distal marginal ridge of the mandibular molar.

e. Retrusive movement of the mandible results in the potential for contacts mesial to the intercuspal contacts on mandibular posterior teeth.

3. A similar pattern exists for mandibular movements as related to the anatomy of maxillary posterior teeth.

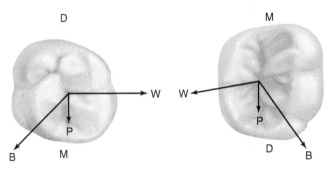

Figure 4-33 Projected protrusive (*P*), working (*W*), and balancing (*B*) side paths on maxillary and mandibular first molars made by supporting cusps. Mesiolingual cusp of the maxillary molar projected on the mandibular molar and distobuccal cusp of the mandibular molar on the maxillary molar. *D*, Distal; *M*, mesial. *(From Nelson SJ, Ash MM: Wheeler's Dental Anatomy, Physiology, and Occlusion, ed 9. St. Louis, Saunders, 2010.)*

a. The distobuccal cusps of the mandibular first molars oppose the central fossa of the maxillary first molars.

b. During a laterotrusive movement, the cusp passes through the buccal groove of the maxillary molar.

c. A mediotrusive movement opposes the maxillary mesiolingual cusp.

d. The maxillary supporting cusps and the mandibular supporting cusps oppose each other during mediotrusive movements (see Figure 4-33).

e. Protrusive movements result in the mandibular distobuccal cusp passing through the maxillary central groove toward the mesial marginal ridge.

f. Occlusal contacts occurring during retrusive movements occur distal to the contacts in maximal intercuspation on maxillary teeth.

What has just been described uses the first molars only; however, a similar pattern is generated for each supporting cusp.

Examining eccentric occlusal contact relations again from the frontal view, occlusal contact is possible along three primary anatomic areas of the posterior teeth.

g. During a right working movement, the right side molar teeth may contact along the lingual inclines of the maxillary buccal cusps and the buccal inclines of the mandibular buccal cusps (see Figure 4-32, *A*). Likewise, the lingual inclines of the maxillary lingual cusps may contact the buccal inclines of the mandibular lingual cusps. This relationship is sometimes called a *cross-tooth balance.*

h. When examining the mediotrusive side (left side nonworking), contact is also possible along the buccal inclines of the left maxillary lingual cusps and the lingual inclines of the left mandibular buccal cusps. Note: this relationship of bilateral occlusal contact during lateral excursions is sometimes referred to as a *balanced* or *cross-arch-balanced relationship.*

The above description has been based on a right side working and left side nonworking movement. A left working movement would produce a similar but reversed contact relationship between the right and left sides.

Three occlusal relationships for working movements considered acceptable restorative concepts for the natural dentition are described as follows.

i. If contact occurs only on the cuspid teeth during working movements, the relationship is sometimes referred to as a *canine-guided, canine rise,* or *cuspid-protected occlusion.* In this relationship, contact of the maxillary and mandibular canine teeth occurs to the extent that all posterior teeth are separated on the working and nonworking sides.

j. If the canine and the buccal cusps of the posterior teeth contact simultaneously during the working movement, to the extent that the nonworking side teeth are separated, the relationship may be referred to as a *group function occlusion.*

k. As the mandible slides into a protrusive position, contact generally occurs along the lingual surface of the maxillary anterior teeth and the facial surface or incisal edge of the mandibular anterior teeth. Most restorative concepts of occlusion for the natural dentition recommend that anterior contacts separate the posterior teeth during protrusive movement. This relationship is referred to as *anterior guidance* or *incisal guidance.* Although these descriptions may be generally accepted, posterior tooth contact in protrusive movement as well as posterior contact on the nonworking side does occur naturally. The dentist may choose to apply these contact relationships during certain prosthodontics procedures.

9.0 Anatomy, Physiology, and Function of the Temporomandibular Joint

The TMJ is a complex joint that allows a wide degree of freedom for many possible movements. Actions of the joints may have a profound effect on restorative dentistry and a person's ability to function normally. Understanding the anatomy of the TMJ and functional movements is a prerequisite to comprehensive diagnosis and treatment in the dental clinic.

A. TMJ anatomy.

The primary anatomic features of the TMJ are reviewed in diagrams showing a sagittal view of the joint, capsule, and TMJ ligament (oblique and horizontal bands) (Figure 4-34). The disc is attached to the medial and lateral poles of the condyle by discal ligaments. These ligaments limit movement within the lower joint space to rotation. The glenoid fossa and the condyle are covered by dense fibrous connective tissue (Figure 4-35). The articular meniscus (disc) is a biconcave structure composed of dense collagenous (hyaline) connective tissue. The central areas are primarily avascular and noninnervated in the adult. The anterior band aspect of the meniscus (disc and meniscus) inserts into the superior belly of the lateral pterygoid muscle (see Figure 4-35). These areas are innervated and vascular. The posterior discal attachment is called the *bilaminar zone* or *retrodiscal lamina* (Figure 4-36). This area is both vascularized and innervated. Elastic fibers are found in the superior lamina and collagen fibers inferiorly.

B. TMJ innervation.

The sensory innervation (not shown) for the TMJ is provided primarily by the auriculotemporal nerve (posterior and lateral TMJ). Anterior and medial innervation occurs through branches from the posterior deep temporal and masseteric nerves.

C. Ligaments.

Three primary ligaments and two accessory ligaments support the TMJ. Primary ligaments include the lateral and medial capsular ligament, the discal ligaments (also called collateral ligaments), and a very strong TMJ ligament (see Figure 4-34). The TMJ ligament consists of an inner layer of horizontal fibers and an outer portion of oblique fibers. The stylomandibular and sphenomandibular ligaments (Figure 4-37) make up the accessory ligaments, which function with the primary ligaments to limit excessive movement of the joint. The dense collagenous connective tissue in these ligaments does not stretch; however, the ligaments and masticatory muscles act like a hammock to suspend the condyle within the joint. This arrangement of structures enables complex movements, such as chewing.

D. Synovial joint.

The TMJ is a synovial joint in that the upper and lower joint spaces are lined by synovial cells (see Figure 4-35). Synovial fluid moistens these surfaces and provides lubrication and perhaps nutritional or metabolic functions.

E. Joint actions.

The TMJ is often referred to as a *ginglymoarthrodial joint,* referring to hinge and glide actions. The TMJ is also capable of free movement or diarthrosis. As the mandible articulates with both left and right TMJs, mandibular movement results in actions of both joints simultaneously. Hinge (rotation) occurs in the lower joint space. Glide (translation) occurs in the upper joint space. Each TMJ is able to rotate in three separate planes or axes (Figure 4-38).

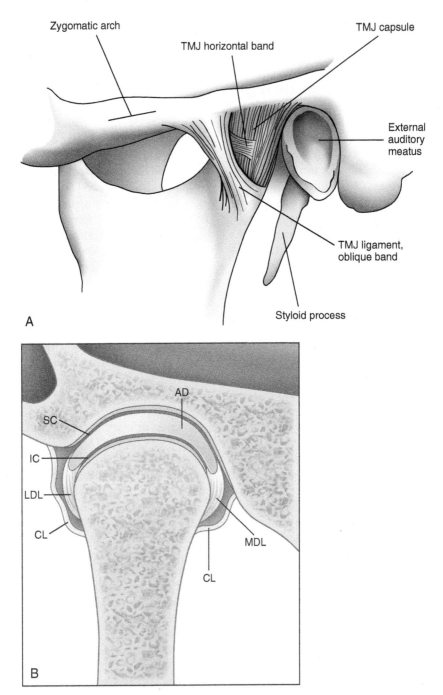

Figure 4-34 **A,** TMJ capsule and TMJ ligaments. **B,** TMJ (anterior view). *AD,* Articular disc; *CL,* capsular ligament; *IC,* inferior joint cavity; *LDL,* lateral discal ligament; *MDL,* medial discal ligament; *SC,* superior joint cavity. (**B,** *From Okeson JP: Management of Temporomandibular Disorders and Occlusion, ed 7. St. Louis, Mosby, 2013.)*

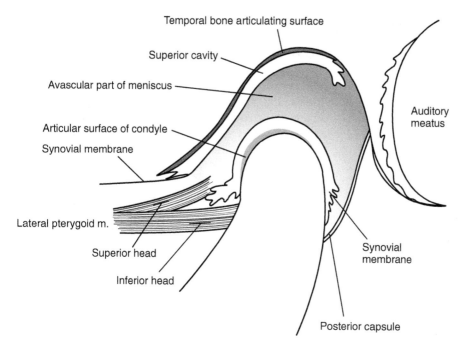

Figure 4-35 Schematic representation of the TMJ.

Temporal bone articulating surface
Superior cavity
Avascular part of meniscus
Articular surface of condyle
Synovial membrane
Lateral pterygoid m.
Superior head
Inferior head
Auditory meatus
Synovial membrane
Posterior capsule

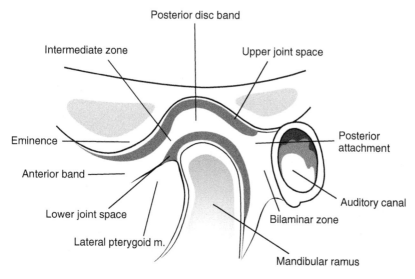

Figure 4-36 Articular disc of the TMJ. *(From Ash MM, Ramfjord SP: Occlusion. Philadelphia, Saunders, 1995; redrawn from Dolwick MF, Sanders B: Internal Derangement and Arthrosis. St. Louis, Mosby, 1985.)*

Posterior disc band
Intermediate zone
Upper joint space
Eminence
Anterior band
Lower joint space
Lateral pterygoid m.
Posterior attachment
Auditory canal
Bilaminar zone
Mandibular ramus

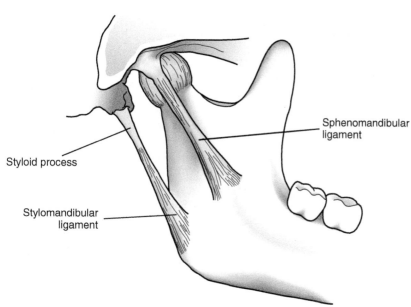

Figure 4-37 Accessory ligaments of the TMJ.

Sphenomandibular ligament
Styloid process
Stylomandibular ligament

An action or rotation that occurs in one joint may produce a different action in the other (i.e., while the working condyle rotates in the frontal [vertical] axis, the nonworking condyle translates). In any event, maximum opening equals the maximum rotation and maximum translation of both condyles.

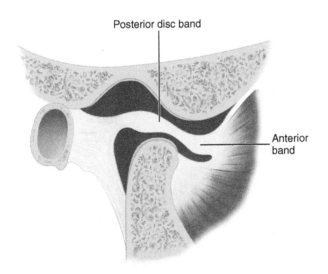

Figure 4-38 Articular disc—jaw in open position. *(From Nelson SJ, Ash MM: Wheeler's Dental Anatomy, Physiology, and Occlusion, ed 9. St. Louis, Saunders, 2010.)*

10.0 Masticatory Muscles

This section describes the basic musculature involved with mastication. This section serves only as a basic review. As in previous sections, the reader is directed to more detailed anatomic works for further study. At a minimum, the reader should be knowledgeable about the origin, insertion, innervation, and action of the basic muscles of mastication as related to the basic mandibular movements.

A. Masseter muscles (Figure 4-39).
   1. Superficial layer of masseter muscle.
      a. Origin—lower border of the zygomatic arch, the lateral surface of the ascending ramus, and body of the mandible.
      b. Insertion—mandibular angle extending from the lateral surface of the mandible near the second molar to the posterior lateral surface of the ramus.
      c. Innervation—cranial nerve (CN) V_3 (masseter nerve branch).
      d. Function—a powerful mandibular elevator muscle.
   2. Deep layer masseter muscle or zygomaticomandibular muscle.
      a. Origin—tendinous attachment of this muscle originates on the lower lateral border of the zygomatic arch and lateral surface of the mandibular ramus.

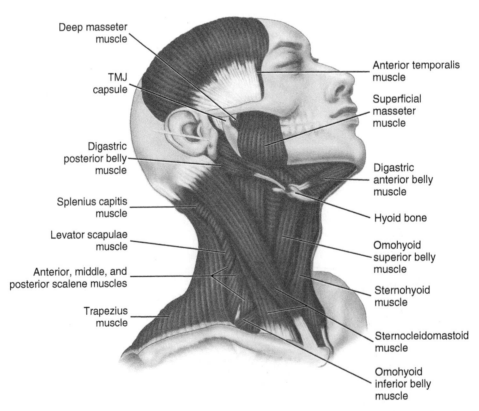

Figure 4-39 Muscles of the neck. *(From Nelson SJ, Ash MM: Wheeler's Dental Anatomy, Physiology, and Occlusion, ed 9. St. Louis, Saunders, 2010.)*

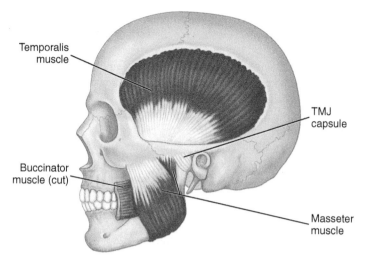

Figure 4-40 Masticatory muscles including the temporalis and masseter muscles. The deep masseter is attached to the zygoma. *(From Nelson SJ, Ash MM: Wheeler's Dental Anatomy, Physiology, and Occlusion, ed 9. St. Louis, Saunders, 2010.)*

b. Insertion—its insertion is concurrent with the superficial layer at the level of the mandibular angle.

c. Function—aids in retrusive mandibular movements.

B. Temporalis muscle (Figure 4-40).

1. Fan-shaped muscle located on the lateral side of the skull.

a. Origin—temporal fossa and fascia.

b. Insertion—tendinous attachment to the anterior border and mesial surface of the coronoid process and ascending mandibular ramus.

c. Innervation—temporal branches of the mandibular division of CN V.

d. Function—anterior and intermediate bundles of this muscle assist in mandibular elevation. The posterior bundle, owing to its horizontal orientation, retrudes the mandible.

C. Pterygoid muscles (Figure 4-41).

1. Medial pterygoid muscle—intraoral muscle located medial to the ascending ramus of the mandible. The medial pterygoid is orientated almost parallel to the masseter muscle.

a. Origin—medial surface of the lateral pterygoid plate, pyramidal process of the palatine bone.

b. Insertion—on the internal surface of the mandibular ramus and angle of the mandible.

c. Innervation—branch from the mandibular division of CN V.

d. Function—mandibular elevation and lateral positioning.

2. Lateral pterygoid muscle—superior head of lateral pterygoid (SHLP) and inferior head of lateral pterygoid (IHLP).

a. Origin—superior head origin is the greater sphenoid wing. The origin occurs on the lateral surface of the pterygoid plate.

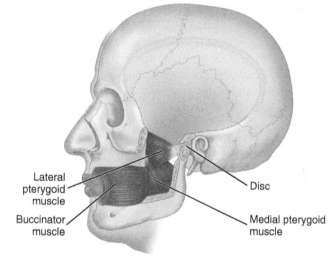

Figure 4-41 Positions of the lateral and medial pterygoid muscles shown with cutaway sections of bone. *(From Nelson SJ, Ash MM: Wheeler's Dental Anatomy, Physiology, and Occlusion, ed 9. St. Louis, Saunders, 2010.)*

b. Insertion—insertion of the tendinous process of the superior head is part of the anterior border of the condyle, articular disc, and joint capsule. The insertion of the lower head is to the condylar capsule and pterygoid fovea on the anterior surface of the neck of the condyle.

c. Innervation—CN V.

d. Function—although reports vary, the SHLP is thought to be responsible for the stabilization of the condylar head and disc against the articular eminence during closing or clenching. Hypothetically, both the SHLP and the IHLP can be regarded as parts of one muscle, with distribution of activities according to the biomechanical demands of the task. The IHLP plays a major role in the generation and fine control of horizontal forces, especially in the contralateral direction, which is required in masticatory and parafunctional activities.

3. Digastric muscle—anterior and posterior parts (see Figure 4-39).

   a. Attachments (anterior belly)—the attachment of this muscle is at the digastric fossa on the inner surface of the mandibular body near the midline. From this attachment, the muscle moves in a lateral, posterior, and inferior direction where it joins with the tendinous insertion of the posterior belly of the digastric muscle on the same side of the head. Both tendons pass through a fibrous loop of the hyoid bone.

   b. Attachments (posterior belly)—the origin of this muscle is at the mastoid notch of the temporal bone. From this origin, the muscle is oriented in a forward, medial, and inferior direction to join with the tendon of the anterior belly.

   c. Innervation—anterior part is a branch from the nerve to the mylohyoid, mandibular division of CN V. The posterior part is innervated by the digastric branch of the facial nerve.

   d. Function—this pair of muscles is an important depressor of the mandible.

11.0 Masticatory System and Role of Occlusion

Occlusion relates to the study of oral motor function and behavior. This complex system involves the peripheral and central nervous systems, the head and neck musculature, the TMJs, the periodontal tissues, and the teeth. These individual components all act together during the performance of daily functional activities such as chewing, sucking, swallowing, speaking, breathing, and (perhaps a daily activity) kissing. In addition, these systems are involved in activities not routinely recognized as functional. Aggressive clenching or grinding of the teeth (bruxism) and habits such as biting fingernails are generally considered parafunctional.

As an introductory study of a masticatory action, the process is simplified into three basic phases. The masticatory activity is first initiated with actions that are responses to need, including hunger or thirst. A person may make a conscious decision to eat or drink something, initiating an action. The second phase is very complex and involves neuromuscular programming before actually performing the task. An example would be opening one's mouth wide enough to insert a candy bar and then knowing how hard to bite on the candy bar to incise or chew it. The programming phase involves many things, such as one's previous experience with the food type and hardness as well as input from sensory receptors of the periodontal tissues and oral

soft tissues (e.g., lips and tongue). The third and final phase of the process is to execute the action. The current belief is that cyclical actions such as chewing probably involve neural activity of a so-called brainstem pattern generator. This pattern generator allows complex coordinated movement without much conscious input from the higher brain centers. However, these preprogrammed actions can be stopped at any time from any part of the system providing sensory feedback. For example, chewing is stopped quickly when one unexpectedly bites the cheek or tongue, and it can be hard to swallow an unwanted raw fish delicacy.

Basically, the masticatory system is remarkably adaptable, which is why clinical dentistry can be performed with such high success. The masticatory system tends to reach a state of homeostasis (stability). This state is achieved when forces exerted by the lips and cheeks, tongue, and occlusal forces and the support provided by the periodontal tissues act together to maintain tooth position within the dental arches. The health of the masticatory muscles and TMJs also influences the homeostasis or stability by influencing jaw position and occlusal forces.

As age, wear, and disease affect the masticatory system, a process of adaptation generally occurs. Functional adaptation occurs when jaw position changes because of pain, drifted teeth, or high restorations. If a high restoration prevents intercuspation in the normal jaw position, a patient may search to find a new position for the teeth. Adaptation may also occur structurally. In structural adaptation, changes occur to anatomic structures, such as tooth attrition, resorption, mobility, or migration. Structural adaptation may occur with excessive force or function resulting in resorption or deposition of bone. A third adaptive process may also occur. Humans may respond or adapt by changing their behavior. The adage "If it hurts, don't do it" is an example of behavioral adaptation. Behavioral adaptation also relates to patients' perceptions of suffering; this is an emotional condition relating to how pleasant or unpleasant the adaptation is to the patient. This is sometimes referred to as a person's *affect*.

All of these factors influence function of the masticatory system. The system tends to balance the effects of disease, aging, and restorative treatment through adaptive processes. Because there is no way to predict how well an individual will be able to adapt to disease or influences from restorative treatment, the challenge for the dentist is to prevent disease and provide treatment that minimizes a patient's need to adapt. In other words, a dentist telling a patient "You will get used to it" may be correct given enough time, but this is never considered sound dental practice.

Acknowledgment

The section editor acknowledges Dr. Major Ash (1921-2007) for his contributions as author and editor of the

Dental Anatomy and Occlusion section of the first edition. His outstanding efforts provided the foundation for this revision.

Bibliography

American Dental Association, Committee on Nomenclature: Committee adopts official method for the symbolic designation of teeth. *J Am Dent Assoc* 34:647, 1947.

American Dental Association, Committee on Dental Education and Hospitals: Tooth numbering and radiographic mounting. *Am Dent Assoc Trans* 109:25, 109:247, 1968.

Arulmozhi DK, et al: Migraine: current concepts and emerging therapies. *Vasc Pharmacol* 43:176, 2005.

Ash MM, Nelson SJ: *Wheeler's Dental Anatomy, Physiology and Occlusion*, ed 8. Philadelphia, Saunders, 2003.

Ash MM, Ramfjord SP: *An Introduction to Functional Occlusion*. Philadelphia, Saunders, 1982.

Ash MM, Ramfjord SP: *Occlusion*, ed 4. Philadelphia, Saunders, 1995.

Bader G, Lavigne G: Sleep bruxism: an overview of an oromandibular sleep movement disorder. *Sleep Med Rev* 4:27, 2000.

Black GV: *Descriptive Anatomy of the Human Teeth*, ed 4. Philadelphia, SS White Dental Manufacturing, 1897.

Carlsen O: *Dental Morphology*. Copenhagen, Munksgaard, 1987.

Charlick RE, et al: *Dental Anatomy*. Ann Arbor, MI, University of Michigan, 1974.

De Moor RJG, et al. The radix entomolaris in mandibular first molars: an endodontic challenge. *Int Endod J* 37:789, 2004.

Devlin TM (ed): *Textbook of Biochemistry with Clinical Correlations*, ed 5. New York, John Wiley (Wiley-Liss), 2002.

Dolwick MF, Sanders B: *Internal Derangement and Arthrosis*. St. Louis, Mosby, 1985.

dos Santos J: *Occlusion: Principles and Concepts*. St. Louis, Ishiyaki EuroAmerica, 1985.

Ellison JA, Stanziani P: SSRI-associated bruxism in four patients. *J Clin Psychiatry* 54:432, 1993.

Fédération Dentaire Internationale: Two-digit system of designating teeth. *Int Dent J* 21:104, 1971.

Fuller JL, Denehy GE: *Concise Dental Anatomy and Morphology*, ed 2. Chicago, Year Book, 1984.

Gay T, Piecuch JF: An electromyographic analysis of jaw movements. *Electromyogr Clin Neurophysiol* 26:365, 1986.

Gear RW: Neural control of oral behavior and its impact on occlusion. In: McNeill C (ed): *Science and Practice of Occlusion*. Chicago, Quintessence, 1997.

Gerber PB, Lynd LD: Selective serotonin-reuptake inhibitor-induced movement disorders. *Ann Pharmacother* 32:692, 1998.

Goadsby PJ, et al: Migraine: current understanding and treatment. *N Engl J Med* 346:257, 2002.

Goodman P: A universal system for identifying permanent and primary teeth. *J Dent Child* 34:312, 1987.

Gülekon N, et al: Variations in the anatomy of the auriculotemporal nerve. *Clin Anat* 18:15, 2005.

Haderup V: Dental nomenklatur og stenograft. *Dansk Tandl Tidskr* 3:3, 1891.

Hannam AG: Jaw muscle structure and function. In: McNeill C (ed): *Science and Practice of Occlusion*. Chicago, Quintessence, 1997.

Hannam AG, McMillan AS: Internal organization in the human jaw muscles. *Crit Rev Oral Biol Med* 5:55, 1994.

Hirsh J, et al: Oral anticoagulants: mechanism of action, clinical effectiveness, and optimal therapeutic range. *Chest* 108:231, 1995.

Ismail AI, Bandekar RR: Fluoride supplements and fluorosis: a meta-analysis. *Community Dent Oral Epidemiol* 27:48, 1999.

Kato T, et al: Topical review: sleep bruxism and the role of periphery sensory influences. *J Orofac Pain* 17:191, 2003.

Knott J, Meredith HV: Statistics on the eruption of the permanent dentition from serial data from North American white children. *Angle Orthod* 36:68, 1966.

Kraus BS, Jordon RE: *The Human Dentition Before Birth*. Philadelphia, Lea & Febiger, 1965.

Kraus BS, et al: *Dental Anatomy and Occlusion*. Baltimore, Williams & Wilkins, 1969.

Kronfeld R, Schour I: Neonatal dental hypoplasia. *J Am Dent Assoc* 26:18, 1939.

Lavigne GJ, et al: Neurobiological mechanisms involved in sleep bruxism. *Crit Rev Oral Biol Med* 14:30, 2003.

Lobbezoo F, Naeije M: Bruxism is mainly regulated centrally, not peripherally. *J Oral Rehabil* 8:1085, 2001.

Logan WHG, Kronfeld R: Development of the human jaws and surrounding structures from birth to age fifteen. *J Am Dent Assoc* 20:379, 1933.

Lunt RC, Law DB: A review of the chronology of deciduous teeth. *J Am Dent Assoc* 89:87, 1974.

Lyons H: Committee adopts official method for the symbolic designation of teeth. *J Am Dent Assoc* 34:647, 1947.

Lysell L, et al: Time and order of eruption of the primary teeth: a longitudinal study. *Odont Rev* 13:21, 1962.

Masters DH, Hoskins SW: Projection of cervical enamel into molar furcations. *J Periodontol* 35:49, 1964.

McCauley HB: Anatomic characteristics important in radiodontic interpretation. *Dent Radiogr Photogr* 18:1, 1945.

Mignogna MD, et al: Oral tuberculosis: a clinical evaluation of 42 cases. *Oral Dis* 6:25, 2000.

Milosevic A, et al: The occurrence of tooth wear in users of Ecstasy (3,4-methylenedioxymethamphetamine). *Community Dent Oral Epidemiol* 27:283, 1999.

Montgomery R, et al: *Biochemistry. A Case-Orientated Approach*, ed 6. St. Louis, Mosby, 1996.

Nomata N: A chronological study on the crown formation of the human deciduous dentition. *Bull Tokyo Med Dent Univ* 11:55, 1964.

Okeson JP: *Management of Temporomandibular Disorders and Occlusion*, ed 7. St. Louis, Mosby, 2013.

Orban B: *Oral Histology and Embryology*, ed 2. St. Louis, Mosby, 1981.

Palmer C: Palmer's dental notation. *Dental Cosmos* 33:194, 1981.

Peck S, Peck L: A time for change of tooth numbering systems. *J Dent Educ* 57:643, 1993.

Pelletier CE: *Pharmacology*. New York, Lange Medical Books, 2003.

Pindborg JJ: *Pathology of the Dental Hard Tissue*. Philadelphia, Saunders, 1970.

Rees LA: The structure and function of the temporomandibular joint. *Br Dent J* 96:125, 1954.

Regezi JA, Sciubba JJ: *Oral Pathology. Clinical Pathological Correlations*, ed 3. Philadelphia, Saunders, 1999.

Richardson AS, Castaldi CR: Dental development during the first two years of life. *J Can Dent Assoc* 33:418, 1967.

Romanelli F, et al: Possible paroxetine-induced bruxism. *Ann Pharmacother* 30:1246, 1996.

Ruangsri S, et al: Functional activity of superior head of human lateral pterygoid muscle during isometric force. *J Dent Res* 84:548, 2005.

Samaranayake LP: *Essential Microbiology for Dentistry*. New York, Churchill Livingstone, 1996.

Scapino RP: Morphology and mechanism of the jaw joint. In: McNeill C (ed): *Science and Practice of Occlusion*. Chicago, Quintessence, 1997.

Scheid R, Weiss G: *Woelfel's Dental Anatomy*. Philadelphia, Lippincott Williams & Wilkins, 2012.

Schour L, Massler M: Studies in tooth development: the growth pattern of human teeth. Part II. *J Am Dent Assoc* 27:1918, 1940.

Schour L, Massler M: The development of the human dentition. *J Am Dent Assoc* 28:1153, 1941.

Shafer WG, et al: *A Textbook of Oral Pathology*. Philadelphia, Saunders, 1983.

Sowter JW (ed): *Dental Laboratory Technology: Dental Anatomy*. Chapel Hill, NC, University of North Carolina, 1972.

Su WJ: Recent advances in molecular diagnosis of tuberculosis. *J Microbiol Immunol Infect* 35:209, 2002.

Tortora GJ: *Atlas of the Human Skeleton*. New York, John Wiley & Sons, 2000.

Turner II CG, Nichol CR, Scott GR: Scoring procedures for key morphological traits of the permanent dentition: The Arizona State University Dental Anthropology System. In: Kelley MA, Larsen CS (eds): *Advances in Dental Anthropology*. New York, Wiley-Liss, 1991.

Widmalm S, Lillie J, Ash M: Anatomical and electromyographic studies of the lateral pterygoid muscle. *J Oral Rehabil* 14:429, 1987.

Woelfel JB, Scheid RC: *Dental Anatomy: Its Relevance to Dentistry*, ed 6. Philadelphia, Lippincott Williams & Wilkins, 2003.

World Health Organization: *Oral Health Surveys: Basic Methods*, ed 3. Geneva, World Health Organization, 1987.

Zsigmondy A: Ghrundzüge einer praktischen Methode zur raschen und genauen, Vonnerkung der zahnartzlichen Beobachtungen und Operationen. *Dtsch Vjschr Zahnhk* 1:209, 1861.

Zsigmondy A: A practical method for rapidly noting dental observations and operations. *Br J Dent Sci* 17:580, 1874.

Sample Questions

1. There are several tooth numbering systems; some are used more than others, and some are used by dental specialties or by special organizations. The so-called universal system consists of _____.
   A. 2-digit sets of numbers for each tooth in each arch quadrant (e.g., 18 to 11)
   B. A single sequential number for teeth repeated in each quadrant (e.g., 8 to 1)
   C. A sequential alphabet letter for each tooth in an entire dentition (e.g., A to T)
   D. Different symbols for each numbered tooth in each quadrant (e.g., 8| to 1|)

2. From the occlusal perspective, which tooth in the primary dentition varies the *most* in form as compared to the permanent counterpart?
   A. Maxillary first primary molar
   B. Maxillary second primary molar
   C. Mandibular first primary molar
   D. Mandibular second primary molar

3. The primary maxillary first molar has which of the following characteristics?
   A. Larger in all dimensions than the primary maxillary second molar
   B. All three roots can be seen from mesial perspective
   C. Bifurcation of roots begins almost immediately at the site of the cervical line (CEJ)
   D. Mesial root is considerably shorter than the distal root

4. From a mesial perspective, the crown of the primary maxillary first molar has which of the following characteristics?
   A. Pronounced convexity on the buccal outline of the cervical third
   B. Cervical line mesially shows some curvature in an apical direction
   C. Dimension at the occlusal third is the same as at the cervical third
   D. Mesiobuccal cusp is longer and sharper than mesiolingual cusp

5. From the lingual perspective, the crown of the primary maxillary second molar has which of the following characteristics?

A. Small, well-developed mesiolingual cusp

B. Distolingual cusp smaller than the maxillary primary first molar distolingual cusp

C. No supplemental cusp apical to the mesiolingual cusp

D. Developmental groove separating mesiolingual and distolingual cusps

6. The primary mandibular first molar has which of the following characteristics?

A. Resembles other primary and permanent teeth

B. From the occlusal perspective, has a heart-shaped outline

C. Mesiobuccal cusp is smaller than the distobuccal cusp

D. No developmental groove evident between the buccal cusps

7. A comparison occlusally between the primary mandibular second molar and the permanent mandibular first molar shows which of the following differences?

A. Mesiobuccal, distobuccal, and distal cusps of the primary molar are almost equal in size; the distal cusp of the permanent molar is smaller than the other two cusps

B. Primary molar crown is wider buccolingually (compared with its mesiodistal measurement) than the permanent molar

C. Primary molar outline is hexagonal; permanent molar is rhomboidal

D. Ratio of crown/root length of both molars is the same

8. Comparison of permanent and primary teeth shows which of the following differences?

A. Crowns of anterior primary teeth are narrower mesiodistally (compared with their crown length) than the permanent teeth

B. Roots of primary anterior teeth are narrower and longer

C. Cervical ridges of enamel of primary anterior teeth are less prominent

D. Buccal and lingual surfaces of primary molars are less flat above the cervical curvature than surfaces of permanent molars

9. The overall length of the primary teeth that are given here are the average range of dimensions with one *exception*. Which range for what tooth is *not* correct?

A. Maxillary central incisor—16 to 17 mm

B. Mandibular central incisor—16 to 17 mm

C. Maxillary lateral incisor—16 to 17 mm

D. Mandibular lateral incisor—15 to 17 mm

10. For each type of tooth, the primary teeth consistently show which of the following characteristics?

A. Greater mesiodistal diameter relative to crown height than permanent teeth

B. Elongated appearance of primary crowns and roots

C. Crowns that are translucent white in color

D. Root trunk length is one half of crown height

11. Which primary tooth is generally accepted as the first to erupt and at about what mean age does eruption occur?

A. Maxillary central incisor, 8 to 12 months

B. Maxillary central incisor, 7 to 9 months

C. Mandibular central incisor, 6 to 10 months

D. Mandibular central incisor, 8 to 10 months

12. Which of the following is the most favorable sequence of eruption for the permanent dentition (right side)? (Eruption sequence indicated by numbers in parentheses.)

A. (1) 3, 30; (2) 8, 25; (3) 7, 26; (4) 27, 5; (5) 28, 4; (6) 29, 6; (7) 31, 2

B. (1) 3, 30; (2) 8, 25; (3) 26, 7; (4) 27, 6; (5) 28, 5; (6) 29, 4; (7) 31, 2

C. (1) 30, 3; (2) 25, 8; (3) 26, 7; (4) 27, 5; (5) 28, 4; (6) 29, 6; (7) 31, 2

D. (1) 30, 3; (2) 25, 8; (3) 26, 7; (4) 27, 6; (5) 28, 5; (6) 29, 4; (7) 2, 31

13. Which primary tooth generally erupts last?

A. Mandibular second molar

B. Maxillary second molar

C. Maxillary canine

D. Mandibular canine

14. Comparing the overall length of primary central incisors (E|F) with permanent maxillary central incisors (8|9), what is the correct ratio expressed as a percentage?

A. About 50%

B. About 60%

C. About 70%

D. About 80%

15. At what time is the crown completed for the tooth indicated?

A. Primary maxillary central incisor—3 weeks

B. Permanent maxillary central incisor—2 to 3 years

C. Primary maxillary lateral incisor—2 to 3 months

D. Permanent maxillary lateral incisor—2 to 3 years

16. When are the crowns of the primary maxillary second molars completed?

A. 11 months

B. 10 months

C. 9 months

D. 8 months

17. Which of the following is *not* a type trait of the permanent maxillary second premolar?

A. Buccal view: narrow shoulders (margins of crown; mesio-occlusal and disto-occlusal angles)

B. Occlusal table outline: ovoid

C. Mesiomarginal groove interrupts mesial marginal ridge

D. Lingual view: buccal profile is not visible

18. Which of the following are *not* type traits of permanent maxillary molars?

	First Molar	Second Molar	Third Molar
A. Buccal view:	Widest molar	Intermediate width	Smallest molar
B. Distolingual cusp:	Same size as M_2	Same size as M_1	Smallest size
C. Occlusal view:	Square/ rhomboid	More rhomboidal	Triangle- or heart-shaped
D. Mesiobuccal root apex:	In line with cusp tip	In line with crown center	Roots displaced

19. Which of the following is *not* an arch trait of the maxillary canine?
    A. In same dentition, crown is larger than the mandibular canine
    B. Incisal margin of the crown occupies at least one third to one half of crown height
    C. Labial aspect: mesial and distal marginal ridges converge toward cervix
    D. Marked symmetry of mesial and distal halves when viewed from incisal perspective

20. Which morphologic characteristic is representative of all posterior maxillary teeth?
    A. Marked mesial concavity on crowns and roots
    B. Tips of cusps well within the confines of the root trunks
    C. From mesial and distal aspect, crowns are rhomboidal in shape
    D. From mesial and distal aspect, all maxillary posterior crowns are trapezoidal with shortest uneven side toward occlusal surface

21. In terms of vertical dimension, where is the mental foramen found most frequently?
    A. At apices of the premolars
    B. Coronal to the apices
    C. Below the apices
    D. No particular location predominates

22. A major anatomic variant of the two-rooted mandibular molar is a tooth with an additional distolingual and third root. What is the prevalence of these three-rooted mandibular first molars?
    A. May exceed 10% in whites
    B. Less than 1% in Eurasian and Asian populations
    C. Greater than 5% (up to 40%) in populations with Mongolian traits
    D. Greater than 8% in African populations

23. Which of the following jaw activities does *not* involve one of the following muscles?
    A. Clenching, superior heads of lateral pterygoid muscles
    B. Clenching, inferior heads of lateral pterygoid muscles
    C. Ipsilateral jaw movements, inferior heads of lateral pterygoid muscles
    D. Simple jaw opening, deep masseter muscle

24. If jaw opening is divided into phases, and it is assumed that the surfaces of the articulating bones and disc are associated throughout jaw opening, what is the relationship of the disc and condyle in the following phases?
    A. In earliest phase, the condyle moves forward before the disc
    B. In early phase, the disc and condyle move anteriorly in concert
    C. In intermediate phase, the condyle moves forward at a slower rate
    D. In final phase, the disc moves forward at a faster rate

25. Occlusal interferences can be defined by *all* of the following *except* one. Which one is the *exception*?
    A. Occlusal contact relations that interfere with function
    B. Interference to jaw closure into the intercuspal position
    C. Interferences to laterotrusive movements
    D. Interferences to jaw opening

26. If posterior teeth on the left side contact occlusally during a right lateral excursion of the mandible, the left side occlusal contact would be referred to as _____.
    A. Laterotrusive contact
    B. Protrusive contact
    C. Mediotrusive contact
    D. Centric relation

27. Which one of the following is considered a primary ligament of the TMJ?
    A. Stylomandibular
    B. Sphenomandibular
    C. Stylohyoid
    D. Temporomandibular

28. Mandibular movement resulting from occlusal contacts of the teeth from retruded contact position (centric relation contact) to intercuspal position (slide in centric) may show all *except* one of the following directional components when viewed only in the horizontal plane. Which one is the *exception*?
    A. Vertical component
    B. Horizontal component
    C. Lateral component
    D. Protrusive component

29. Where is the height of contour located relative to the following teeth (viewed from the mesial)?
    A. Facial surfaces of all molars, middle third
    B. Lingual surfaces of all premolars and molars, cervical third
    C. Lingual surfaces of molars and premolars, cervical or middle third
    D. Anterior teeth, cervical or middle third

30. The occlusal surface of a primary mandibular first molar often has a prominent faciolingual ridge. This transverse ridge connects which two cusps?

A. Buccal and distolingual
B. Mesiolingual and distobuccal
C. Mesiobuccal and mesiolingual
D. Distobuccal and distolingual

31. Which premolar would be the *most* likely to have a single pulp horn?
    A. Maxillary first
    B. Mandibular first
    C. Mandibular second
    D. Maxillary second

32. Which one of the following is *not* a normal anatomic feature of mandibular incisors?
    A. Bifurcated roots
    B. Inconspicuous cingula
    C. Four developmental lobes
    D. Incisal edges placed slightly lingually

33. The heights of contour of the distal surfaces of permanent mandibular central incisors are located in which coronal third?
    A. Middle
    B. Cervical
    C. Occlusal
    D. Incisal

34. On average, approximately what is the dimension of the permanent maxillary canine at the widest mesio-distal diameter of the crown?
    A. 5.5 mm
    B. 6.5 mm
    C. 7.5 mm
    D. 8.5 mm

35. Which one of the following is found on the crown of permanent mandibular first molars but is not found on the crowns of mandibular second molars?
    A. Mesiobuccal cusp
    B. Distobuccal groove
    C. Lingual groove
    D. Distobuccal cusp

36. The Y-shaped central developmental groove is most likely found on which of the following premolars?
    A. Maxillary first
    B. Mandibular first
    C. Maxillary second
    D. Mandibular second

37. In a cusp-embrasure relationship, the maxillary first premolar is most likely to articulate with which of the following mandibular teeth?
    A. First premolar only
    B. First molar only
    C. Canine and first premolar
    D. First and second premolars

38. Equal contracture of the lateral pterygoid muscle bilaterally produces which of the following mandibular movements?
    A. Retrusive
    B. Elevation

C. Protrusive
D. Lateral

Test items 39-51 relate to the following scenario.

A 35-year-old woman presents with a painful limitation of jaw opening (28 mm), a painful tooth on the right side, and swelling at the angle of the jaw. She has a history of TMJ disease and conservative treatment. The medical history reveals that the patient is being treated for tuberculosis with combination antituberculosis drugs including rifampin (Rifadin). She is also being treated with warfarin (Coumadin), an anticoagulant; a low dose of aspirin; and paroxetine (Paxil) for depression. The intraoral examination shows extensive teeth wear from bruxism, diagnosed by a sleep specialist as sleep bruxism. Tooth 32 has a deep carious lesion and, on radiographic examination, a periapical radiolucency.

39. The incidence of tuberculosis is increasing as a result of an association with AIDS. Oral infections of tuberculosis occur but are uncommon. Diagnosis of oral lesions may present several challenges, as set forth in all of the following statements *except* one. Which one of the following statements is *false*?
    A. Lesions secondary to HIV may be present.
    B. Isolation of *Mycobacterium tuberculosis* by culture requires 4 to 6 weeks or longer.
    C. Mycobacteria can be demonstrated by special stains in only 27% to 60% of cases.
    D. Molecular tests (e.g., polymerase chain reaction) have slow turnaround times.

40. All the following side effects have been reported to be related to the use of rifampin *except* one. Which one is the *exception*?
    A. Green bodily fluids—sweat, tears, urine
    B. Hepatotoxicity
    C. Thrombocytopenia
    D. Rashes

41. Which of the following modes of action does *not* relate to rifampin?
    A. Inhibits RNA synthesis
    B. Binds tightly to eukaryotic RNA polymerase
    C. Tuberculocidal to intracellular and extracellular organisms
    D. Reduces activity of hepatic mixed-function oxidases

42. Exacerbation of bruxism has been reported to occur with all the following agents *except* one. Which one is the *exception*?
    A. Paroxetine
    B. Selective serotonin reuptake inhibitors
    C. Naproxen (Naprosyn)
    D. Amphetamine derivative ("Ecstasy")

43. Migraine headache is currently thought to be best understood on the basis of all of the following *except* one. Which one is the *exception*?

A. As a dysfunction of brainstem pathways or diencephalic nuclei
B. As a primary disorder of the brain
C. As similar in mechanism to tension headaches
D. As a neurovascular headache

44. Three key factors in the pathogenesis of pain in migraine are usually considered. Which of the following is *not* considered to be a key factor?
    A. Cranial blood vessels
    B. β-Amyloid-containing plaques in the brain
    C. Trigeminal innervation of the vessels
    D. Reflex connection of trigeminal system with cranial parasympathetic outflow

45. Treatment with low-dose aspirin is prescribed for which of the following reasons?
    A. To reduce the likelihood of platelet aggregation
    B. To stimulate cyclooxygenase in the platelets
    C. To increase the formation of thromboxane
    D. To cause platelets to regenerate cyclooxygenase

46. When there is a pulpal-periodontal infection of a mandibular third molar, which of the following listed facial and cervical spaces is most likely to have become infected when there is swelling at the angle of the jaw?
    A. Retromolar space
    B. Submaxillary space
    C. Submasseteric space
    D. Parotid space

47. Lymphatic drainage from tooth 32 would first involve which of the following node groups?
    A. Lateral upper deep cervical node
    B. Medial upper deep cervical node
    C. Lateral lower deep cervical node
    D. Submaxillary node

48. All of the following are considerations relevant to the diagnosis and treatment of tuberculosis *except* one. Which one is the *exception*?
    A. Increase in the prevalence of tuberculosis
    B. Oral tuberculosis lesions occur most frequently on the gingiva
    C. Emergence of multidrug-resistant strains
    D. High risk of *M. tuberculosis* infection in patients with HIV infection

49. Extraction of tooth 32 revealed attached soft tissue. Which of the following is *most* important for a presumptive diagnosis of tuberculosis?
    A. Caseous necrotic areas
    B. Acid-fast bacilli
    C. Epithelioid histiocytes
    D. Langerhans' giant cells

50. Which one of the following disorders is the *least* likely to be a differential diagnostic factor in the patient's limited jaw opening?
    A. Exacerbation of TMJ disease
    B. Trismus secondary to TMJ pain

C. Myalgia secondary to TMJ disease
D. Myositis secondary to bruxing

51. The patient is on an anticoagulant drug (e.g., warfarin) as well as rifampin. What is the effect of rifampin on the anticoagulation effect of warfarin?
    A. Increases anticoagulant effect of warfarin
    B. Increases cyclic conversion of vitamin K epoxide reductase
    C. Anticoagulation effect is inhibited
    D. Decreases metabolic clearance by inducing activity of hepatic oxidases

52. A transverse ridge is _____.
    A. The combination name for joining oblique and triangular ridges
    B. A combination name for joining buccal and lingual cusp triangular ridges
    C. Characteristically found on all primary and permanent molars
    D. Found occasionally on the primary maxillary first molar

53. From the occlusal aspect, the primary maxillary first molar has which of the following characteristics?
    A. Crown outline diverges lingually and distally
    B. Small traverse ridge frequently present called an oblique ridge
    C. Four cusps are present
    D. Mesial marginal ridge is thin and poorly developed

54. From the lingual perspective, the primary maxillary first molar has which of the following characteristics?
    A. Distolingual cusp is the most prominent cusp
    B. Mesiolingual cusp is poorly defined
    C. Distobuccal cusp cannot be seen from lingual aspect
    D. Crown converges considerably in a lingual direction

55. The primary maxillary second molar has which of the following characteristics?
    A. Does not have a well-defined mesial triangular fossa
    B. Oblique ridge absent or not well developed
    C. Development (central) groove is well defined
    D. Tubercle of Carabelli (supplementary cusp) is well developed

56. From the occlusal aspect, the primary maxillary second molar has which of the following characteristics?
    A. Rhomboidal in form
    B. Three well-developed cusps
    C. Two supplemental cusps, including tubercle of Carabelli
    D. Poorly defined mesial triangular fossa

57. From the occlusal aspect, the primary mandibular second molar has which of the following characteristics?

A. Rectangular in form

B. Outline of the crown converges mesially

C. Three buccal cusps are dissimilar in size

D. Cusps do not have well-defined triangular ridges

58. A comparison of the pulp chambers and root canals of maxillary primary and permanent second molars shows which of the following?

A. Enamel cap of primary tooth is thick but less consistent in depth

B. Comparatively less thickness of dentin at the occlusal fossa of primary molars

C. Pulp chambers are proportionally larger in primary molars

D. Pulp horns are lower in primary molars, especially distal horns

59. In a comparison of maxillary primary and permanent second molars, which of the following differences are noted?

A. Enamel rods at the cervix slope gingivally in the primary molar

B. Enamel rods at the cervix slope occlusally in the permanent molar

C. Buccal cervical ridges are less pronounced in the primary molar

D. Roots of primary teeth are longer and more slender compared with crown size than those of permanent teeth

60. Based on average mesiodistal diameters of the crowns of primary teeth, the range for average overall length of the primary maxillary arch is about what dimension?

A. 60 to 65 mm

B. 68 to 77 mm

C. 79 to 84 mm

D. 86 to 92 mm

61. What is the average height of curvature of the cervical line (CEJ) on the mesial and distal of the permanent maxillary and mandibular incisors?

A. About 3.5 mm on the mesial of the maxillary central incisor

B. About 1.5 mm on the distal of the maxillary central incisor

C. About 2.0 mm on the mesial of the mandibular central incisor

D. About 1.0 mm on the distal of the mandibular central incisor

62. Considering the period of $2\frac{1}{2}$ months to about 6 years of age, which of the following statements is true?

A. Not all the primary teeth have attained their occlusal level.

B. Parts of both jaws containing primary teeth change noticeably in size.

C. A significant increase in intercanine width occurs shortly before and during the time the primary teeth are lost and the permanent teeth emerge.

D. The dental arch form is more or less constant, and practically no dimensional changes take place in depth or width after 9 months of age.

63. Which sequence of eruption of permanent teeth occurs most often? (8-7-6-5-4-3-2-1 = M_3-M_2-M_1-P_2-P_1-C-LI-CI). First #, #'s in each series is considered to be the first to erupt.

A. 6-1-2-4-3-5-7-8 (maxilla)

B. 6-1-2-3-4-5-7-8 (maxilla)

C. 6-1-2-4-3-5-7-8 (mandible)

D. 1-6-2-4-5-3-7-8 (mandible)

64. The first evidence of calcification (weeks in utero) in the primary dentition occurs in which of the following teeth at about what age?

A. Maxillary central incisor—14 (13 to 16) weeks

B. Mandibular central incisor—12 (10 to 13) weeks

C. Maxillary lateral incisor—14 (13 to 16) weeks

D. Mandibular lateral incisor—14 (13 to 15) weeks

65. The *most* characteristic feature of the primary maxillary central incisor is which of the following?

A. Faciolingual breadth of the crown

B. Mesiodistal width of the crown

C. Mesial and distal margin outlines in line with profiles of root

D. Root/crown ratio

66. When is the crown of the permanent mandibular second molar completed?

A. About 7 to 8 years

B. About 8 to 9 years

C. About 9 to 10 years

D. About 10 to 11 years

67. Which of the following is *not* a type trait of the permanent maxillary first premolar?

A. Occlusal table outline, trapezoidal

B. Generally two roots—mesial and distal

C. Central groove is long

D. Supplementary grooves are rare

68. Which of the following are *not* type traits of permanent mandibular first and second premolars?

	First Premolar	Second Premolar
A. Buccal view:	Crown bilaterally asymmetrical	Bilaterally symmetrical
B. Lingual aspect:	Entire buccal profile visible	Buccal profile not seen
C. Lingual aspect:	Most of occlusal surface visible	Little, if any, seen
D. Lingual aspect:	Contour height—middle third	Cervical third

69. Which of the following are *not* arch traits of the canines?

	Maxillary Canine (6)	Mandibular Canine (27)
A. Crown size	Larger (same dentition)	Smaller (same dentition)
B. Lingual pits and grooves	Common	None
C. Labiolingual diameter	Near cervix same as 27	Near cervix same as 6
D. Incisal view, mesial and distal halves	Symmetrical	Marked asymmetry

70. Which of the following are *not* type traits of the permanent maxillary central and lateral incisors?

	Central Incisor	Lateral Incisor
A. Labial view: mesial contact	Incisal third	Junction incisal and middle third
B. Labial view: distal contact	Junction incisal and middle third	Middle third
C. Mesial view: contacts	Within incisal third	Junction incisal and middle third
D. Labial: mesioincisal angle	Slightly rounded	Sharp right angle

71. Which position of the mental foramen relative to the mandibular premolars and first molar occurs most frequently?
    A. Between first and second premolars
    B. In line with second premolar
    C. Distal to second premolar
    D. In line with mesial root of first molar

72. The maxillary sinus overlies the alveolar processes in particular in what teeth?
    A. First and second maxillary molars
    B. All maxillary molars
    C. First and second premolars
    D. First and second premolars and first and second molars

73. The masseter muscle, which has a complex of internal components, includes all of the following *except* one. Which one is the *exception*?
    A. Pennation
    B. Structural composition permitting regional activation
    C. Multiple internal aponeuroses
    D. Internal aponeuroses that do not move or deform

74. Sleep bruxism can be characterized by which of the following?
    A. Episodes of massive, bilateral clenching
    B. Tooth grinding that may last for 20 minutes
    C. Often coincides with passage from lighter to deeper sleep
    D. Occurs approximately every 20 minutes in the sleep cycle

75. More recent focus on causative factors in bruxism includes all of the following *except* one. Which one is the *exception*?
    A. Occlusal interferences
    B. Part of a sleep arousal response
    C. Pathophysiologic factors
    D. Neurotransmitters in the central nervous system

76. All of the following are supporting cusps *except* one. Which one is the *exception*?
    A. Buccal cusp of tooth #29
    B. Lingual cusp of tooth #4
    C. Mesiolingual cusp of tooth #3
    D. Mesiolingual cusp of tooth #19

77. Horizontal overlap (overjet) of the teeth is easily measured by which of the following methods?
    A. Measure from the facial surface of a mandibular incisor to the facial surface of a maxillary incisor with the subject in intercuspal position
    B. With the subject in intercuspal position, mark the position of the maxillary incisal edge on the facial surface of the mandibular incisor with a pencil. Then have the subject open the mouth and measure from the mark that you made to the incisal edge of the mandibular incisor
    C. Measure from the midline between the maxillary central incisors to the midline of the mandibular central incisors
    D. Measure from the incisal edge of a maxillary incisor to the incisal edge of a mandibular incisor with the mandible in the maximum open position

78. In a cusp-fossa occlusal relationship, the maxillary second premolar is most likely to articulate with which of the following mandibular teeth?
    A. First premolar only
    B. Second premolar only
    C. Canine and first premolar
    D. First and second premolars

79. Which of the following contributes primary sensory innervation to the TMJ?
    A. Auriculotemporal nerve
    B. Infraorbital nerve
    C. Branch of the lingual nerve
    D. Facial nerve

80. The smallest cusp on the crown of a five-lobed mandibular second premolar is the _____.
    A. Buccal cusp
    B. Distobuccal cusp
    C. Distal cusp
    D. Distolingual cusp

81. How many pulp horns does a typical primary mandibular first molar have?

A. One
B. Two
C. Three
D. Four

82. Rest position is defined as _____.
    A. Any position of the mandible that lacks contact of the teeth
    B. The centric relation position of the condyles with the teeth apart
    C. A mandibular position with masticatory muscles at complete rest
    D. A clinical mandibular position in relation to the interocclusal space

83. What is the point angle that represents the junction of the cutting edge of an incisor with the surface that is toward the tongue and the surface that is away from the midline?
    A. Distoproximoincisal
    B. Distolabioincisal
    C. Distolinguoincisal
    D. Labioincisolingual

84. Root bifurcation would be a more likely finding in which of the following permanent teeth?
    A. Maxillary canine
    B. Mandibular canine
    C. Maxillary central incisor
    D. Mandibular lateral incisor

85. What is the correct schematic outline of the following teeth?
    A. Mandibular premolars, viewed from occlusal, rhomboidal
    B. Maxillary central incisors, viewed from facial, triangle-shaped
    C. Maxillary lateral incisors, viewed from mesial, trapezoidal
    D. All mandibular posterior teeth, distal aspect, rhomboidal

86. A distinct central developmental groove, prominent buccal triangular ridge, two cusps, and distinct mesial and distal occlusal pits would be *most* characteristic of _____.
    A. Mandibular first premolars
    B. Primary mandibular first molars
    C. Primary mandibular second molars
    D. Mandibular second premolars

87. From the incisal view, a greater mesiodistal measurement than faciolingual measurement can be seen in which of the following permanent anterior crowns?
    A. Maxillary central incisor
    B. Maxillary canine
    C. Mandibular canine
    D. Mandibular central incisor

88. Maximum rotation and translation of both condyles occurs at _____.
    A. Maximum opening
    B. Maximum protrusive

C. Right and left lateral excursive movements
D. Hinge movement

Questions 89-100 relate to the following scenario.

A mother brings her 12-year-old boy to the dentist to ask about her son grinding his teeth and about some white "spots" located on the smooth-surfaced enamel of several of his anterior teeth and premolars. Among other questions about the cause of the defects, the mother asks when a systemic disturbance occurred that may have caused the "spots." The patient has excessive tooth wear from bruxing and clenching. The dentist measures the cervical-incisal length of the permanent maxillary central incisor (10.5 mm). The dentist also measures the distance from the CEJ to the midpoint of the defect (5.5 mm). Given that the crown is completed over 4 to 5 years, it is possible to estimate the age at which the hypoplasia occurred using 6 months or yearly periods in the following formula:

$$ADF = ACF - (\text{years of formation/crown height} \times \text{distance of defect from CEJ})$$

where *ADF* is age of defect formation and *ACF* is age of crown formation.

89. Using an average age of crown formation of both 4 and 5 years, the age of defect formation is estimated to be about what time?
    A. 7 to 9 months in utero
    B. 0 to 1 year old
    C. 1 to 2 years old
    D. 2 to 3 years old

90. The increase of fluorosis of permanent teeth in both populations with no fluoridation and populations with optimal fluoridation points to the need for dentists to caution parents with children about potential causes of fluorosis in children. Which of the following cautions about fluoride is correct, but the age or implied age is *not* correct?
    A. Excess (>1 ppm) fluoride in the drinking water during enamel formation
    B. Excessive (more than a pea-sized amount) use of fluoride toothpaste in children younger than 6 years old
    C. Use of fluoride toothpaste in children younger than 4 years old
    D. Use of a 1.1% sodium fluoride toothpaste or gel by children only when 6 years old or older

91. Systemic etiologic factors that are said to be associated with enamel defects such as hypoplasia occur generally during what time period?
    A. Before birth
    B. Generally after birth and before age 6 years
    C. During the first year postpartum for Hutchinson's incisors
    D. During birth

92. The differential diagnosis of white "spots" of the enamel of primary and permanent teeth should

include disorders that have a substantiated cause. Which of the following do *not* have an evidence-based causal relationship with enamel hypoplasia?

A. Rickets
B. Congenital syphilis
C. Measles
D. Fluorosis

93. Clenching and grinding of teeth involves contraction of skeletal-type muscles. Several types of myofilaments are present in the contractile elements of skeletal muscles. Which of the following statements about muscle filaments is *not* true?

A. Myosin forms the thick filament of muscle.
B. Actin is a major protein of thin filaments.
C. Titin is a protein of elastic filament.
D. Connectin is a protein of intermediate filament.

94. The clinical examination of the patient reveals extensive wear of the right canines and less wear of the lateral incisors. Also, there is tenderness of the jaw-closing muscles, particularly on the right side. Which of the following masticatory muscles would be involved primarily in providing *most* of the force for anterior tooth clenching?

A. Inferior lateral pterygoid muscle
B. Superior lateral pterygoid muscle
C. Anterior temporalis muscle
D. Masseter muscle

95. Sleep bruxism is defined by all of the following characteristics *except* one. Which one is the *exception*?

A. Stereotypic movement disorder
B. Grinding and clenching of the teeth during sleep
C. More frequent in children
D. Individuals who brux during the daytime inevitably brux at night

96. More recent physiologic evidence suggests that central or autonomic nervous system rather than peripheral sensory factors play a dominant role in the genesis of sleep bruxism. Which of the following statements about the central genesis of sleep bruxism is *not* true?

A. During sleep, the mouth is usually open because of motor repression.
B. Tooth contact most likely occurs in association with sleep arousal.
C. Some peripheral sensory factors may exert an influence on sleep bruxism through their interaction with sleep-awake mechanisms.
D. Sequential change from autonomic (cardiac) or brain cortical activities follows sleep bruxism–related jaw motor activity.

97. Aggravation of bruxism has been suggested to occur secondarily to all of the following occlusal relationships *except* one. Which one is the *exception*?

A. Occlusal interferences in centric relation
B. Occlusal interferences in the intercuspal position

C. Iatrogenic occlusal relations that interfere with bruxism
D. Angle class III malocclusion (prognathism)

98. The differential diagnosis of enamel hypoplasia should take into account suggested differences between nonfluoride and fluoride opacities. Which of the following statements does *not* suggest a basis for a diagnosis of nonfluoride enamel hypoplasia?

A. Levels of fluoride in drinking water that range from 0.2 to 0.34 ppm have been reported to be associated with prevalences of nonfluoride enamel opacities ranging from 22% to 35%.
B. At a level of 1 to 1.5 ppm of fluoride in drinking water, only a few fluoride opacities occur.
C. Most nonfluoride enamel opacities appear as white, opaque spots in smooth surface enamel; areas of mild dental fluorosis are lusterless, opaque white patches.
D. Fluorosis and nonfluoride opacities are clinically significantly different.

99. During muscle contraction, what physical change does *not* occur relative to muscle fiber contraction?

A. Sarcomeres—shorten
B. Thick and thin filaments—shorten
C. I band—shortens
D. H zone—shortens

100. Regarding SHLP and IHLP, which of the following statements is *not* true?

A. Hypothetically, SHLP and IHLP can be considered to be parts of one muscle.
B. Distributions of SHLP and IHLP activities are shaded according to biomechanical demands of tasks.
C. SHLP stabilizes the condyle and disc against the articular eminence in a wide range of jaw movements and forces.
D. IHLP plays a major role in the generation and fine control of horizontal forces.

101. From the following list, select four items most frequently associated with the primary mandibular first molar.

A. Three roots—mesiobuccal, distobuccal, and lingual
B. Transverse ridge is commonly present
C. Highly curved CEJ on buccal
D. Prominent buccal cervical ridge
E. Rhomboidal occlusal outline
F. Generally two or three cusps
G. Smallest primary molar mesiodistally

102. From the following list, select four items that are characteristic of primary teeth compared with permanent teeth.

A. Smaller in overall size
B. Thinner enamel covering crowns
C. Darker in color
D. Comparatively larger pulp chambers

E. Molars have more fused roots

F. Prominent cervical ridges

103. From the following list, select three items considered primary ligaments of the TMJ.
     A. Stylomandibular
     B. Discal
     C. Sphenomandibular
     D. Temporomandibular
     E. Capsular
     F. Discomalleolar

104. From the following list, select five items associated with the temporalis muscle.
     A. Intraoral
     B. Insertion on the angle of the mandible
     C. Innervation: mandibular division CN V
     D. Function: mandibular elevation
     E. Function: mandibular retrusion
     F. Origin: temporal fossa and fascia
     G. Fan-shaped muscle

105. From the following list, select four items associated with the deep masseter muscle.
     A. Zygomaticomandibular muscle
     B. Origin: lower lateral border of zygomatic arch
     C. Origin: lateral surface of mandibular ramus
     D. Innervation: CN VII
     E. Action: retrudes mandible
     F. Runs parallel with medial pterygoid muscle
     G. Protrudes mandible

106. Assuming a cusp/fossa/cusp fossa occlusal contact relationship, for each numbered centric stop, select the corresponding supporting cusp (using universal numbering system).

     1. Central fossa #2 _____   A. DB #31
     2. Central fossa #3 _____   B. MB #31
     3. Central fossa #30 _____   C. DB #30
     4. Central fossa #31 _____   D. MB #30
     5. Distal triangular fossa #29 _____   E. B #29
     6. Mesial triangular fossa #5 _____   F. B #28
     7. Distal triangular fossa #30 _____   G. DL #2
                                        H. ML #2
                                        I. DL #3
                                        J. ML #3
                                        K. L #4
                                        L. L #5

107. Assuming a cusp/fossa/cusp embrasure occlusal contact relationship, for each numbered centric stop,

select the corresponding supporting cusp (using universal numbering system).

     1. Central fossa #2 _____   A. DB #31
     2. Central fossa #3 _____   B. MB #31
     3. Central fossa #30 _____   C. DB #30
     4. Central fossa #31 _____   D. MB #30
     5. Distal marginal ridge #29 _____   E. B #29
     6. Mesial marginal ridge # 5 _____   F. B #28
     7. Distal marginal ridge #30 _____   G. DL #2
                                        H. ML #2
                                        I. DL #3
                                        J. ML #3
                                        K. L #4
                                        L. L #5

108. Considering emergence of primary teeth, match each tooth (universal system) with its proper sequence number.

     1. _____   Tooth A
     2. _____   Tooth B
     3. _____   Tooth C
     4. _____   Tooth D
     5. _____   Tooth E
     6. _____   Tooth P
     7. _____   Tooth Q
     8. _____   Tooth R
     9. _____   Tooth S
     10. _____   Tooth T

109. Considering emergence of permanent teeth, match each tooth (FDI system) with its proper sequence number.

     1. _____   Tooth #11
     2. _____   Tooth #12
     3. _____   Tooth #13
     4. _____   Tooth #14
     5. _____   Tooth #15
     6. _____   Tooth #16
     7. _____   Tooth #17
     8. _____   Tooth #18

110. For pattern of mandibular movement, select the most closely linked TMJ action pair (hint: each pair may be used once, more than once, or not at all).

1. Maximum opening _____
2. Maximum protrusive _____
3. Right laterotrusive _____
4. Left laterotrusive _____
5. Right mediotrusive _____
6. Left mediotrusive _____
7. Jaw deflects to right on maximum opening _____
8. Jaw deflects to left on maximum opening _____

A. Maximum translation, anteriorly, maximum rotation horizontal axis both TMJs
B. Restricted translation anteriorly right TMJ
C. Restricted translation anteriorly left TMJ
D. Right TMJ translates anteriorly, left TMJ rotates on vertical axis
E. Right TMJ rotates on vertical axis, left TMJ translates anteriorly
F. Minimum horizontal axis rotation, maximum translation anteriorly both TMJs

111. Using the list of border positions in the sagittal plane (Posselt's diagram), sequence the mandibular positions from 1 (occurring first) to 4 (occurring fourth). Follow the diagram starting from the hinge axis position and move anteriorly.

1. _____
2. _____
3. _____
4. _____

A. Maximum opening
B. Maximum intercuspation
C. Centric relation contact
D. Incisal edge contact
E. Maximum protrusive
F. Rest position

112. A junction of three surfaces of a tooth forms a _____.
   A. Line angle
   B. CEJ
   C. Point angle
   D. Sulcus
   E. Triangular ridge

113. Using the list of TMJ structures, sequence those occurring from posterior (1) to anterior (6).

1. _____
2. _____
3. _____
4. _____
5. _____
6. _____

A. Posterior attachment
B. SHLP
C. Anterior band
D. Bilaminar zone
E. Posterior band
F. Intermediate zone

114. From the following list, select the teeth that frequently have two roots.
   A. Permanent maxillary central incisor
   B. Permanent mandibular central incisor
   C. Maxillary cuspid
   D. Permanent mandibular first molar
   E. Primary mandibular first molar
   F. Maxillary first premolar
   G. Maxillary second premolar

115. The dental formula of I 2/2 C 1/1 M 2/2 is representative of which of the following dentitions?
   A. Collie dog
   B. Human child
   C. Human adult
   D. Ape
   E. None of the above

116. Sequence the order of emergence of maxillary permanent teeth from earliest (1) to last to emerge (7).

1. _____
2. _____
3. _____
4. _____
5. _____
6. _____
7. _____

A. Central incisor
B. Lateral incisor
C. Canine
D. First premolar
E. Second premolar
F. First molar
G. Second molar

117. Sequence the order of emergence of mandibular permanent teeth from earliest (1) to last to emerge (7).

1. _____
2. _____
3. _____
4. _____
5. _____
6. _____
7. _____

A. Central incisor
B. Lateral incisor
C. Canine
D. First premolar
E. Second premolar
F. First molar
G. Second molar

118. Match the list of occlusal conditions with the appropriate class.

1. Class 1 _____
2. Class 2 _____
3. Class 3 _____

A. Normal
B. Retrognathism
C. Prognathism

119. Examples of structural adaptation include which of the following?
   A. Attrition of the teeth
   B. Tooth migration
   C. Tooth mobility
   D. Tooth resorption
   E. All of the above

120. Concerning the TMJ, synonyms for the term *ginglymoarthrodial* could include which of the following?
   A. Hinge
   B. Glide
   C. Rotation
   D. Translation
   E. All of the above

Sample Examination

1. All of the following are supporting cusps *except* one. Which one is the *exception*?
   - A. Buccal cusp of tooth #29
   - B. Lingual cusp of tooth #4
   - C. Mesiolingual cusp of tooth #3
   - D. Mesiolingual cusp of tooth #19

2. The lateral pterygoid muscle attaches to which of the following?
   - A. Lateral surface of the lateral pterygoid plate
   - B. Medial surface of the lateral pterygoid plate
   - C. Lateral surface of the medial pterygoid plate
   - D. Medial surface of the medial pterygoid plate
   - E. Pyramidal process of palatine bone

3. A transverse ridge is _____.
   - A. A combination name for joining oblique and triangular ridges
   - B. A combination name for joining buccal and lingual cusp triangular ridges
   - C. Characteristically found on all primary and permanent molars
   - D. Found occasionally on maxillary primary first molar

4. Bronchogenic carcinoma is a complication *most* characteristic of which of the following conditions?
   - A. Silicosis
   - B. Asbestosis
   - C. Anthracosis
   - D. Sarcoidosis
   - E. Bronchiectasis

5. Which of the following statements regarding tubular reabsorption is *true*?
   - A. Most calcium filtered is passively reabsorbed and not regulated under any conditions.
   - B. Most urea is reabsorbed passively and is unaffected by regulatory mechanisms.
   - C. Glucose is reabsorbed by secondary active transport and facilitated diffusion.
   - D. Most filtered phosphate is reabsorbed in the collecting ducts and is unaffected by regulatory mechanisms.

6. The class of antibodies that plays an important role in type I hypersensitivity reactions is _____.
   - A. IgA
   - B. IgD
   - C. IgE
   - D. IgG
   - E. IgM

7. The amount of cytosine is equal to the amount of guanine in which of the following molecules?
   - A. DNA
   - B. RNA
   - C. DNA and RNA
   - D. Messenger RNA

8. The branchial arches disappear when the _____ branchial arch grows down to contact the _____.
   - A. Second; third branchial arch
   - B. Second; fifth branchial arch
   - C. Third; fifth branchial arch
   - D. First; first branchial groove
   - E. First; sixth branchial groove

9. Glucagon decreases which of the following?
   - A. Glycogenolysis
   - B. Gluconeogenesis
   - C. Glycogenesis
   - D. Blood glucose

10. When an enzyme is competitively inhibited, which of the following changes occur?
    - A. Apparent K_m is unchanged
    - B. Apparent K_m is decreased
    - C. V_{max} is decreased
    - D. V_{max} is unchanged

11. A typical primary mandibular first molar has how many pulp horns?
    - A. One
    - B. Two
    - C. Three
    - D. Four

Test items 12-14 refer to the following scenario.
A 3-year-old African girl presents in the emergency department with a palpable mass in her lower right mandible. She is in the United States visiting relatives with her parents. Her mother claims that a few days ago she noticed a growing mass in her daughter's jaw. There appears to be slight swelling around the area, although it is painless and not tender to the touch. After further examination, a biopsy specimen was taken, and the diagnosis of Burkitt's lymphoma was made.

12. Burkitt's lymphoma is a malignancy that affects which of the following cells?
    - A. Macrophages
    - B. T lymphocytes
    - C. B lymphocytes
    - D. Neutrophils
    - E. Keratinocytes

13. The pathology report reveals a characteristic pattern of tumor cells that is classically associated with Burkitt's lymphoma. Which of the following describes this histopathologic pattern?
    A. Honeycomb
    B. Cobweb
    C. Cotton wool
    D. Sun ray
    E. Starry sky

14. The African form of Burkitt's lymphoma has been linked to Epstein-Barr virus. This virus is also responsible for which of the following diseases?
    A. Mononucleosis
    B. Shingles
    C. Chickenpox
    D. Kaposi's sarcoma
    E. Herpangina

15. Measurement of horizontal overlap (overjet) of the teeth is easily done by which of the following methods?
    A. Measure from the facial surface of a mandibular incisor to the facial surface of a maxillary incisor with the subject in intercuspal position.
    B. With the subject intercuspal position, mark the position of the maxillary incisal edge on the facial surface of the mandibular incisor with a pencil. Have the subject open the mouth, and measure from the mark that you made to the incisal edge of the mandibular incisor.
    C. Measure from the midline between the maxillary central incisors to the midline of the mandibular central incisors.
    D. Measure from the incisal edge of a maxillary incisor to the incisal edge of a mandibular incisor with the mandible in the maximum open position.

16. Increasing the radius of arterioles increases which of the following?
    A. Systolic blood pressure
    B. Diastolic blood pressure
    C. Viscosity of the blood
    D. Capillary blood flow

17. Which of the following nerves supplies taste sensation to the anterior two thirds of the tongue?
    A. Hypoglossal
    B. Glossopharyngeal
    C. Lingual
    D. Facial
    E. Mental

18. Which of the following are *not* arch traits of the canines?

	Maxillary Canine (6)	Mandibular Canine (27)
A. Crown size	Larger (same dentition)	Smaller (same dentition)
B. Lingual pits or grooves	Common	None
C. Labiolingual diameter	Near cervix same as 27	Near cervix same as 6
D. Incisal view, mesial and distal halves	Symmetrical	Marked asymmetry

19. Which of the following statements regarding the regulation of gastrointestinal motility is *true*?
    A. Sympathetic stimulation inhibits motility.
    B. Parasympathetic stimulation inhibits motility.
    C. Gastrointestinal motility is not influenced by the central nervous system.
    D. Gastrointestinal motility is not influenced by hormones.

20. Which of the following structures is the *most* common site for oral cancer?
    A. Soft palate
    B. Lateral border of the tongue
    C. Lower lip
    D. Floor of mouth
    E. Buccal mucosa

21. Mandibular movement resulting from occlusal contacts of the teeth from retruded contact position (centric relation contact) to intercuspal position (slide in centric) may show all of the following directional components when viewed only in the horizontal plane *except* one. Which one is the *exception*?
    A. Vertical component
    B. Horizontal component
    C. Lateral component
    D. Protrusive component

22. Which of the following muscles is responsible for the formation of the posterior tonsillar pillar?
    A. Stylopharyngeus
    B. Tensor veli palatini
    C. Palatoglossus
    D. Palatopharyngeus
    E. Levator veli palatini

23. Which of the following does *not* occur to compensate for a decrease in blood pressure less than normal values?
    A. Increased cardiac output
    B. Increased stroke volume
    C. Increased heart rate
    D. Decreased total peripheral resistance

24. Relative or absolute lack of insulin in humans would result in which one of the following reactions in the liver?
    A. Increased glycogen synthesis
    B. Increased gluconeogenesis
    C. Decreased glycogen breakdown
    D. Increased amino acid uptake

25. In 2% glutaraldehyde, which of the following times is minimally sufficient for achieving sterilization?
    A. 15 minutes
    B. 1 to 2 hours

C. 6 hours

D. 12 hours

26. Which of the following bones is part of the superior wall (roof) of the orbit?

A. Zygomatic

B. Lacrimal

C. Sphenoid

D. Maxilla

E. Ethmoid

27. On average, approximately what is the dimension of the permanent maxillary canine at the widest mesio-distal diameter of the crown?

A. 5.5 mm

B. 6.5 mm

C. 7.5 mm

D. 8.5 mm

28. Both active transport and facilitated diffusion are characterized by which of the following?

A. Transport in one direction only

B. Hydrolysis of adenosine triphosphate

C. Transport against a concentration gradient

D. Competitive inhibition

29. Which of the following bacteria would be expected to colonize first onto plaque?

A. *Streptococcus*

B. *Bacteroides*

C. *Fusobacterium*

D. *Actinomyces*

E. *Prevotella*

30. Cell membranes typically contain all of the following compounds *except* one. Which one is the *exception*?

A. Phospholipids

B. Proteins

C. Cholesterols

D. Triacylglycerols

E. Sphingolipids

31. Which of the following muscles adducts the vocal cords?

A. Lateral cricoarytenoid

B. Posterior cricoarytenoid

C. Cricothyroid

D. Vocalis

E. Tensor veli palatini

32. Which of the following *best* describes anaplastic cells that have not invaded the basement membrane and are confined within their epithelium of origin?

A. Dysplasia

B. Hyperplasia

C. Metaplasia

D. Sarcoma

E. Carcinoma in situ

33. Which muscle of the anterolateral abdominal wall is described as being beltlike or straplike?

A. External oblique muscle

B. Internal oblique muscle

C. Transversus abdominis muscle

D. Rectus abdominis muscle

E. Quadratus lumborum muscle

34. In a comparison of maxillary primary and permanent second molars, which of the following differences are noted?

A. Enamel rods at the cervix slope gingivally in the primary molar.

B. Enamel rods at the cervix slope occlusally in the permanent molar.

C. Buccal cervical ridges are less pronounced in the primary molar.

D. Roots of primary teeth are longer and more slender compared with crown size than roots of permanent teeth.

Test items 35-37 refer to the following scenario.

A mother brings her 6-year-old daughter in for an examination because she noticed brown macules on her daughter's leg. The macules have jagged edges but do not appear raised. The mother is worried that her daughter may have a malignancy. After further evaluation and tests, the macules are identified as café au lait spots.

35. Café au lait spots are seen in conjunction with polyostotic fibrous dysplasia and endocrine abnormalities in which of the following disorders?

A. McCune-Albright syndrome

B. Stevens-Johnson syndrome

C. Marfan's syndrome

D. Gorlin-Goltz syndrome

E. Peutz-Jeghers syndrome

36. The patient's radiographs could be described as having what type of characteristic appearance?

A. Cotton-wool

B. Ground-glass

C. Cobweb

D. Soap bubble

E. Starry sky

37. A bone biopsy specimen was taken from the patient. Which of the following would *most* likely be observed under the microscope?

A. Dense inflammatory infiltrate

B. Fibrous tissue

C. Pleomorphic cells

D. Metastatic calcifications

E. Giant cells

38. The following overall lengths of the primary teeth that are listed all are the average range of dimensions *except* one. Which one is the *exception*?

A. Maxillary central incisor, 16 to 17 mm

B. Mandibular central incisor, 16 to 17 mm

C. Maxillary lateral incisor, 16 to 17 mm

D. Mandibular lateral incisor, 15 to 17 mm

39. Fibrotic and thickened heart valves that result in a reduction of blood flow through the valve characterize which of the following?

A. Stenosis
B. Regurgitation
C. Insufficiency
D. Prolapse
E. Ischemia

40. From the occlusal aspect, the primary maxillary second molar has which of the following characteristics?
    A. Rhomboidal in form
    B. Three well-developed cusps
    C. Two supplemental cusps, including tubercle of Carabelli
    D. Poorly defined mesial triangular fossa

41. All of the following local chemical factors would cause vasodilation of the arterioles *except* one. Which one is the *exception*?
    A. Decreased potassium
    B. Increased carbon dioxide
    C. Nitric oxide
    D. Decreased oxygen
    E. Histamine release

42. The inferior aspect of the diaphragm is supplied with blood by which of the following arteries?
    A. Median sacral artery
    B. Lumbar arteries
    C. Inferior phrenic arteries
    D. Celiac trunk
    E. Superior mesenteric artery

43. The coenzyme essential for normal amino acid metabolism is _____.
    A. Biotin
    B. Tetrahydrofolate
    C. Pyridoxal phosphate
    D. Niacin

44. Equal contracture of the lateral pterygoid muscle bilaterally produces which of the following mandibular movements?
    A. Retrusive
    B. Elevation
    C. Protrusive
    D. Lateral

45. Which of the following cells forms the myelin sheath around myelinated nerves in the central nervous system?
    A. Schwann's cells
    B. Astrocytes
    C. Microglia
    D. Oligodendrocytes
    E. Amphicytes

46. Which of the following mineralized tissues have the greatest percentage of inorganic material?
    A. Enamel
    B. Dentin
    C. Bone
    D. Calculus

47. Which of the following is *not* a feature of poststreptococcal glomerulonephritis?

A. Hematuria
B. Hypertension
C. Edema
D. Polyuria

48. In a cusp-embrasure relationship, the maxillary first premolar is *most* likely to articulate with which of the following mandibular teeth?
    A. First premolar only
    B. First molar only
    C. Canine and first premolar
    D. First and second premolars

49. There are several tooth numbering systems; some are used more than others, and some are used by dental specialties or by special organizations. The so-called universal system consists of _____.
    A. 2-digit sets of numbers for each tooth in each arch quadrant (e.g., 18 to 11)
    B. Single sequential number for teeth repeated in each quadrant (e.g., 8 to 1)
    C. A sequential alphabet letter for each tooth in an entire dentition (e.g., A to T)
    D. Different symbols for each numbered tooth in each quadrant (e.g., 8| to 1|)

Test items 50-55 refer to the following scenario.
A 24-year-old man presents to the office for an emergency visit after being hit on the left side of his face with a soccer ball. He complains that his "tooth got knocked out" and that his jaw feels "out of place." He has no other medical conditions.

50. During intraoral examination, you find that the patient's lower second premolar is missing. Which type of alveolodental fibers was *least* involved in resisting the force that pulled this patient's tooth out of its socket?
    A. Apical
    B. Oblique
    C. Alveolar crest
    D. Interradicular

51. A cusp of the patient's mandibular second molar has fractured off and dentin is exposed. If this patient were to drink something cold, what would he sense?
    A. Pain
    B. Pressure
    C. Vibration
    D. Temperature

52. You decide to take a radiograph of the fractured tooth. On the first film, you miss the apex of the tooth, so you decide to take another radiograph. Relaxation of which of the patient's muscles would help you in taking the second film?
    A. Geniohyoid
    B. Stylohyoid
    C. Mylohyoid
    D. Levator veli palatine
    E. Palatopharyngeus

53. On further examination, you determine that the articular disc of the patient's temporomandibular joint has been displaced. If the patient contracts his lateral pterygoid muscle, the disc will move _____.
    A. Posteriorly and medially
    B. Anteriorly and medially
    C. Posteriorly and laterally
    D. Anteriorly and laterally

54. During the examination, the patient observes that he cannot feel it when you touch part of his cheek and his upper lip. Which of the following nerves was probably damaged during the accident?
    A. Lingual
    B. Maxillary
    C. Long buccal
    D. Superior alveolar
    E. Inferior alveolar

55. You decide to restore the missing cusp on the patient's molar. During administration of the inferior alveolar nerve block, which of the following ligaments is *most* likely damaged?
    A. Sphenomandibular
    B. Stylomandibular
    C. Temporomandibular
    D. Interdental

56. Polycystic kidney disease is most commonly associated with _____.
    A. Renal cell carcinoma
    B. Peripheral neuropathy
    C. Urolithiasis
    D. Berry aneurysm
    E. Non-Hodgkin's lymphoma

57. Which of the following types of epithelium lines the oropharynx?
    A. Simple squamous
    B. Stratified squamous
    C. Simple cuboidal
    D. Simple columnar
    E. Pseudostratified columnar

58. A scientist has discovered a new peptide hormone. He thinks it acts through the second messenger system, which uses cyclic adenosine monophosphate (cAMP). If this is true, which of the following substances should decrease the response of this new peptide hormone in cells?
    A. Adenylate cyclase
    B. Monoamine oxidase inhibitors
    C. Phosphodiesterase
    D. Aspirin

59. From the occlusal perspective, which tooth in the primary dentition varies the most in form from that of any tooth in the permanent dentition?
    A. Maxillary first primary molar
    B. Maxillary second primary molar
    C. Mandibular first primary molar
    D. Mandibular primary second molar

60. The *most* common cause of osteomyelitis is _____.
    A. *Streptococcus pyogenes*
    B. *Staphylococcus aureus*
    C. *Lactobacillus casei*
    D. *Pseudomonas aeruginosa*
    E. *Escherichia coli*

61. The muscle that is found in the walls of the heart is characterized by _____.
    A. A peripherally placed nucleus
    B. Multiple nuclei
    C. Intercalated discs
    D. Fibers with spindle-shaped cells

62. The smallest cusp on the crown of a five-lobed mandibular second premolar is the _____.
    A. Buccal cusp
    B. Distobuccal cusp
    C. Distal cusp
    D. Distolingual cusp

63. Which of the following is *not* involved in the process of mineralization?
    A. Matrix vesicles
    B. Amelogenins
    C. Fluoride
    D. Phosphoryns

64. T-cell lymphoma is most likely to occur in a patient with which of the following conditions?
    A. Chronic granulomatous disease
    B. Myasthenia gravis
    C. Osteochondroma
    D. Wilson's disease
    E. Celiac sprue

65. For which of the following substances would you expect the renal clearance to be the lowest under normal conditions?
    A. Urea
    B. Creatinine
    C. Sodium
    D. Water
    E. Glucose

66. DiGeorge's syndrome is characterized by a deficiency of _____.
    A. B lymphocytes
    B. T lymphocytes
    C. Both B and T lymphocytes
    D. Antibodies
    E. Complement inhibitor

67. Which of the following phrases *best* describes restriction enzymes?
    A. Site-specific endonucleases
    B. Enzymes that regulate RNA
    C. Nonspecific endonucleases
    D. Topoisomerases

68. The gallbladder arises from the _____.
    A. Common hepatic duct
    B. Common bile duct
    C. Left hepatic duct

D. Cystic duct

E. Bile canaliculi

69. Which one of the following disorders is the *least* likely to be a differential diagnostic factor in limited jaw opening in a patient?

A. Exacerbation of temporomandibular joint (TMJ) and temporomandibular disorder

B. Trismus secondary to TMJ pain

C. Myalgia secondary to temporomandibular disorder

D. Myositis secondary to bruxing

70. The superior and inferior ophthalmic veins drain into the _____.

A. Internal jugular vein

B. Pterygoid plexus

C. Frontal vein

D. Infraorbital vein

E. Facial vein

Test items 71-74 refer to the following scenario.

A 6-year-old boy presents with a history of severe epistaxis. For the past 3 years, the patient has experienced these nosebleeds, often without any apparent cause. The patient is otherwise in good health, but his mother has noticed that he "bruises easily." Laboratory tests are ordered.

71. The laboratory test results show a normal prothrombin time (PT) but a prolonged partial thromboplastin time (PTT). A prolonged PTT suggests that the patient has an abnormality affecting which component of the coagulation cascade?

A. Activation of platelets

B. Activation of thromboplastin

C. Activation of plasminogen

D. Intrinsic pathway

E. Extrinsic pathway

72. The diagnosis of hemophilia A is made. This disease is caused by a deficiency of _____.

A. Factor V

B. Factor VII

C. Factor VIII

D. Factor IX

E. Factor X

73. Which of the following describes the hereditary transmission of this disease?

A. Autosomal dominant

B. Autosomal recessive

C. X-linked

D. It is not genetically transmitted

74. The clinical presentation of hemophilia B is indistinguishable from hemophilia A. Which of the following *best* describes the laboratory method needed to distinguish these two conditions?

A. Bleeding time

B. Assay of coagulation factor levels

C. Assay of von Willebrand's factor

D. Blood smear

E. Platelet count

75. Hydrolysis of which of the following compounds yields urea?

A. Ornithine

B. Argininosuccinate

C. Aspartate

D. Citrulline

76. The median pharyngeal raphe serves as the attachment site for which of the following muscles?

A. Lateral pterygoid muscle

B. Palatopharyngeus muscle

C. Levator veli palatini muscle

D. Salpingopharyngeus

E. Superior constrictor muscle

77. Which of the following is the *most* favorable sequence of eruption for the permanent dentition (right side)? (Eruption sequence given by numbers in parentheses.)

A. (1) 3, 30; (2) 8, 25; (3) 7, 26; (4) 27, 5; (5) 28, 4; (6) 29, 6; (7) 31, 2

B. (1) 3, 30; (2) 8, 25; (3) 26, 7; (4) 27, 6; (5) 28, 5; (6) 29, 4; (7) 31, 2

C. (1) 30, 3; (2) 25, 8; (3) 26, 7; (4) 27, 5; (5) 28, 4; (6) 29, 6; (7) 31, 2

D. (1) 30, 3; (2) 25, 8; (3) 26, 7; (4) 27, 6; (5) 28, 5; (6) 29, 4; (7) 2, 31

78. Which of the following metabolic activities is increased 1 hour after a meal (during the absorptive state)?

A. Glycogenolysis

B. Oxidation of free fatty acids

C. Glucagon release

D. Glycolysis

79. The *most* prominent mechanism of spread of the hepatitis A virus is by which of the following routes?

A. Oral-anal

B. Respiratory

C. Sexual contact

D. Perinatal

E. Insect vectors

80. If the molar percentage of guanine in a human DNA molecule is 30%, what is the molar percentage of adenine in that molecule?

A. 10%

B. 20%

C. 30%

D. 40%

E. 50%

81. The muscularis externa has a third layer in the _____.

A. Esophagus

B. Stomach

C. Liver

D. Small intestine

E. Large intestine

82. An infection by which of the following bacteria may result in the formation of gummas?
    A. *Mycobacterium tuberculosis*
    B. *Neisseria gonorrhoeae*
    C. *Treponema pallidum*
    D. *Bordetella pertussis*
    E. *Streptococcus pyogenes*

83. Hassall's corpuscles are found in the medulla of which of the following glands?
    A. Thymus
    B. Thyroid
    C. Parathyroid
    D. Pineal
    E. Suprarenal

84. The masseter originates from the _____.
    A. Condyle of the mandible
    B. Infratemporal crest of the sphenoid bone
    C. Inferior border of the zygomatic arch
    D. Pyramidal process of the palatine bone
    E. Mastoid process of temporal bone

85. Which of the following statements regarding the period of 2 ½ months to about 6 years of age is *true*?
    A. Not all the primary teeth have attained their occlusal level.
    B. Parts of both jaws containing primary teeth change noticeably in size.
    C. A significant increase in intercanine width occurs shortly before and during the time the primary teeth are lost and the permanent teeth emerge.
    D. Dental arch form is more or less constant and practically no dimensional changes occur in depth or width after 9 months of age.

86. The primary factor determining the percent of hemoglobin saturation is _____.
    A. Blood partial pressure of oxygen (Po_2)
    B. Blood partial pressure of carbon dioxide (Pco_2)
    C. Diphosphoglycerate concentration
    D. The temperature of the blood
    E. The acidity of the blood

87. What is the average height of curvature of the cervical line (cementoenamel junction) on the mesial and distal of the permanent maxillary and mandibular incisors?
    A. About 3.5 mm on the mesial of the maxillary central incisor
    B. About 1.5 mm on the distal of the maxillary central incisor
    C. About 2.0 mm on the mesial of the mandibular central incisor
    D. About 1.0 mm on the distal of the mandibular central incisor

88. Which of the following describes cells that are abnormal in appearance and may become premalignant?
    A. Aplasia
    B. Dysplasia
    C. Karyomegaly
    D. Pleomorphism
    E. Metaplasia

89. Which jaw activity does *not* involve one of the following muscles?
    A. Clenching—superior heads of lateral pterygoid muscles (LPM)
    B. Clenching—inferior heads of LPM
    C. Ipsilateral jaw movements—inferior heads of LPM
    D. Simple jaw opening—deep masseter muscle

90. Hemorrhagic infarction and tissue necrosis suggest which of the following?
    A. Aspergillosis
    B. Blastomycosis
    C. Histoplasmosis
    D. Mucormycosis
    E. Toxoplasmosis

91. Which of the following ribs cannot be palpated?
    A. First
    B. Second
    C. Third
    D. First and second

92. Which of the following is released by mast cells after antigen binding?
    A. IgE
    B. Lysozyme
    C. Interleukin-4
    D. Leukotriene
    E. Interferon

93. Where are the temperature control centers located?
    A. Cerebellum
    B. Hypothalamus
    C. Medulla
    D. Cerebral cortex

94. Which of the following is a major complication of chronic bronchitis?
    A. Myxedema
    B. Pneumothorax
    C. Emphysema
    D. Pernicious anemia
    E. Malignant transformation

95. A comparison occlusally between the primary mandibular second molar and the permanent mandibular first molar shows which of the following differences?
    A. The mesiobuccal, distobuccal, and distal cusps of the primary molar are almost equal in size; the distal cusp of the permanent molar is smaller than the other two cusps.
    B. The primary molar crown is wider buccolingually (compared with its mesiodistal measurement) than the permanent molar.
    C. The primary molar outline is hexagonal; the permanent molar is rhomboidal.
    D. The ratio of the crown/root length of both molars is the same.

96. Calcium binds to which of the following for contraction in smooth muscle?
    A. Troponin C
    B. Calmodulin
    C. Myosin
    D. Actin
    E. Desmosomes

97. The effects of which one of the following hormones are *not* mediated through cyclic adenosine monophosphate (cAMP)?
    A. Estrogen
    B. Glucagon
    C. Epinephrine
    D. Norepinephrine

Test items 98-102 refer to the following scenario.

A 43-year-old man presents for an emergency dental appointment complaining of a burning sensation in his mouth. On examination, white plaques are observed along the oral mucosa. The patient otherwise appears healthy. There is no history of systemic illness, but the patient stated that he had a blood transfusion more than 10 years ago after a car accident. The dentist referred the patient to emergency department for further tests.

98. On further evaluation, the emergency physician requests HIV and hepatitis tests. The laboratory performed both an enzyme-linked immunosorbent assay (ELISA) test and Western blot, which revealed that the patient is HIV-positive. The Western blot is used to identify which of the following?
    A. Antibodies
    B. DNA
    C. RNA
    D. Proteins
    E. Plaque-forming units

99. Given the patient's history, if active hepatitis was diagnosed later, which of the following would *most* likely be the causative agent?
    A. Hepatitis A
    B. Hepatitis B
    C. Hepatitis C
    D. Hepatitis D
    E. Hepatitis E

100. Which of the following would the physician likely prescribe for the patient's intraoral infection?
    A. Amoxicillin
    B. Vancomycin
    C. Ciprofloxacin
    D. Nystatin
    E. Chlorhexidine

101. All of the following molecules may be found within the nucleocapsid of HIV *except* one. Which one is the *exception*?
    A. Reverse transcriptase
    B. Integrase
    C. Neuraminidase

D. Protease
E. RNA

102. The patient is referred to an infectious disease specialist and placed on triple therapy. The patient is admitted to the emergency department 2 years later with a dry cough and shortness of breath. His temperature is 101° F. The *most* likely cause of the patient's pneumonia is _____.
    A. *Staphylococcus aureus*
    B. *Haemophilus influenzae*
    C. *Pneumocystis jiroveci* (formerly *Pneumocystis carinii*)
    D. *Klebsiella pneumoniae*
    E. *Streptococcus pneumoniae*

103. The primary maxillary first molar has which of the following characteristics?
    A. It is larger in all dimensions than the primary maxillary second molar.
    B. All three roots can be seen from mesial perspective.
    C. Bifurcation of roots begins almost immediately at the site of the cervical line (cementoenamel junction).
    D. The mesial root is considerably shorter than the distal root.

104. Which of the following is the end product of purine degradation in humans?
    A. Urea
    B. Uric acid
    C. Adenosine
    D. Xanthine

105. Which of the following is an essential amino acid?
    A. Tyrosine
    B. Tryptophan
    C. Proline
    D. Serine
    E. Alanine

106. Which of the following are the *most* abundant in the fovea centralis of the eyeball?
    A. Rod cells
    B. Cone cells
    C. Rod and cone cells
    D. Amacrine cells

107. The middle trunk of the brachial plexus of nerves arises from _____.
    A. C5
    B. C6
    C. C7
    D. C8

108. Tinea pedis, commonly known as athlete's foot, is a fungal infection that is caused by which of the following dermatophytes?
    A. *Microsporum*
    B. *Trichophyton*
    C. *Epidermophyton*

D. Both A and B

E. Both B and C

109. In comparing permanent and primary teeth, which of the following differences are noted?

A. Crowns of anterior primary teeth are narrower mesiodistally (compared with their crown length) than the permanent teeth.

B. Comparatively, the roots of primary anterior teeth are narrower and longer.

C. Cervical ridges of enamel of the primary anterior teeth are less prominent.

D. Buccal and lingual surfaces of primary molars are less flat above the cervical curvature than buccal and lingual surfaces of permanent molars.

110. Cystic fibrosis is a hereditary disorder that results from defective _____.

A. Collagen

B. Lysosomal enzymes

C. Chloride channels

D. Fibrillin

E. Myelin

111. Which of the following strata of oral epithelium is engaged in mitosis?

A. Basale

B. Granulosum

C. Corneum

D. Spinosum

112. The class of antibodies that plays an important role in mucosal immunity is _____.

A. IgA

B. IgD

C. IgE

D. IgG

E. IgM

113. Which of the following cells are defective in chronic granulomatous disease?

A. Neutrophils

B. Lymphocytes

C. Plasma cells

D. Killer T cells

E. Macrophages

114. Which of the following coenzymes serves as an intermediate carrier of one-carbon units in the synthesis of nucleic acids?

A. Ascorbic acid

B. Tetrahydrofolic acid

C. Biotin

D. Pyridoxine

115. Which of the following genetic diseases results from a deficiency in the liver enzyme that converts phenylalanine to tyrosine?

A. Albinism

B. Homocystinuria

C. Porphyria

D. Phenylketonuria

Test items 116-127 relate to the following scenario.

A 35-year-old woman presents with a painful limitation of jaw opening (28 mm), a painful tooth on the right side, and swelling at the angle of the jaw. She has a history of temporomandibular disorder and conservative treatment. Medical history reveals that the patient is being treated for tuberculosis (TB) with combination antituberculosis drugs including rifampin (Rifadin). She is also being treated with an anticoagulant, warfarin (Coumadin); a low dose of aspirin; and paroxetine (Paxil) for depression. The intraoral examination shows extensive teeth wear from bruxism, diagnosed by a sleep specialist as sleep bruxism. Tooth #32 has a deep carious lesion and, on radiographic examination, a periapical radiolucency.

116. The incidence of TB is increasing as a result of an association with AIDS. Oral infections of TB occur but are uncommon. Diagnosis of oral lesions may present several challenges, as set forth in all of the following statements *except* one. Which one of the following statements is *false*?

A. Lesions secondary to HIV may be present.

B. Isolation of *Mycobacterium tuberculosis* by culture requires 4 to 6 weeks or longer.

C. Mycobacteria can be demonstrated by special stains in only 27% to 60% of cases.

D. Molecular tests (e.g., polymerase chain reaction) show slow turnaround times.

117. All of the following side effects have been reported to be related to the use of rifampin *except* one. Which is the *exception*?

A. Green bodily fluids—sweat, tears, urine

B. Hepatitis

C. Leukopenia

D. Nephrotoxicity

118. Which of the following modes of action does *not* relate to rifampin?

A. Inhibits RNA synthesis

B. Binds tightly to eukaryotic RNA polymerase

C. Tuberculocidal to intracellular and extracellular organisms

D. Reduces activity of hepatic mixed-function oxidases

119. Exacerbation of bruxism has been reported to occur with all of the following agents *except* one. Which one is the *exception*?

A. Paroxetine

B. Selective serotonin reuptake inhibitors

C. Naproxen (Naprosyn)

D. Amphetamine derivative ("Ecstasy")

120. Migraine headache is currently thought to be best understood on the basis of all of the following *except* one. Which one is the *exception*?

A. As a dysfunction of brainstem pathways or diencephalic nuclei

B. As a primary disorder of the brain

C. As similar in mechanism to tension headaches

D. As a neurovascular headache

121. Three key factors in the pathogenesis of pain in migraine are usually considered. Which of the following is *not* considered to be a key factor?
   A. Cranial blood vessels
   B. β-Amyloid–containing plaques in the brain
   C. Trigeminal innervation of the vessels
   D. Reflex connection of trigeminal system with cranial parasympathetic outflow.

122. Why is the patient receiving treatment with low-dose aspirin?
   A. To reduce the likelihood of platelet aggregation
   B. To stimulate cyclooxygenase in the platelets
   C. To increase the formation of thromboxane
   D. To cause platelets to regenerate cyclooxygenase

123. In the case of pulpal-periodontal infection of a mandibular third molar, which of the following listed facial and cervical spaces is *most* likely to have become infected when there is swelling at the angle of the jaw?
   A. Retromolar space
   B. Submaxillary space
   C. Submasseteric space
   D. Parotid space

124. Lymphatic drainage from tooth #32 would first involve which of the following node groups?
   A. Lateral upper deep cervical node
   B. Medial upper deep cervical node
   C. Lateral lower deep cervical node
   D. Submaxillary node

125. All of the following are considerations relevant to the diagnosis and treatment of TB *except* one. Which one is the *exception*?
   A. Increase in the prevalence of TB
   B. Oral TB lesions occur most frequently on the gingiva
   C. Emergence of multidrug-resistant strains
   D. High risk of *M. tuberculosis* infection in patients with HIV

126. Extraction of tooth #32 revealed attached soft tissue. Which of the following is *most* important for a presumptive diagnosis of TB?
   A. Caseous necrotic areas
   B. Acid-fast bacilli
   C. Epithelioid histiocytes
   D. Langerhans' giant cells

127. The patient is taking an anticoagulant drug (warfarin) and rifampin. What is the effect of rifampin on the anticoagulation effect of warfarin?
   A. Increases the anticoagulant effect of warfarin
   B. Increases the cyclic conversion of vitamin K epoxide reductase
   C. Anticoagulation effect is inhibited
   D. Decreases metabolic clearance warfarin by inducing activity of hepatic oxidases

128. Gut-associated lymphoid tissue (GALT) produces secretory _____.
   A. IgA
   B. IgD
   C. IgE
   D. IgG
   E. IgM

129. Antinuclear antibodies (ANAs) are seen in serum samples from patients with _____.
   A. Hypogammaglobulinemia
   B. Chronic granulomatous disease
   C. Systemic lupus erythematosus
   D. Multiple myeloma
   E. Pheochromocytoma

130. What is the correct general structure of the backbone of DNA and RNA?
   A. Sugar-base-sugar
   B. Bases linked through phosphodiester linkages
   C. Bases linked through hydrogen bonds
   D. Sugars linked through phosphodiester linkages

131. All of the following are found in the posterior triangle of the neck *except* one. Which one is the *exception*?
   A. External jugular vein
   B. Subclavian vein
   C. Hypoglossal nerve
   D. Phrenic nerve
   E. Brachial plexus

132. Which of the following amino acids is positioned at every third residue in the primary structure of the helical portion of the collagen-α chains?
   A. Glycine
   B. Glutamate
   C. Proline
   D. Lysine
   E. Hydroxyproline

133. Which of the following would result in decreased glomerular filtration rate?
   A. A decrease in plasma protein concentration
   B. An obstruction of the tubular system, which would increase capsular hydrostatic pressure
   C. Vasodilation of the afferent arterioles
   D. Inulin administration

134. The *most* common form of breast cancer is _____.
   A. Adenocarcinoma
   B. Teratoma
   C. Follicular lymphoma
   D. Sarcoma
   E. Carcinoma

135. Which of the following are *not* type traits of the permanent maxillary central and lateral incisors?

	Central Incisor	Lateral Incisor
A. Labial view:	Incisal third mesial contact	Junction of incisal and middle third

B. Labial view: Junction of distal contact incisal and middle third   Middle third

C. Mesial view: Within incisal contacts third   Junction of incisal and middle third

D. Labial: mesioincisal angle   Slightly rounded   Sharp right angle

136. The apex of a medullary pyramid in the kidney is called the _____.
A. Cortex
B. Medulla
C. Renal papilla
D. Major calyx
E. Minor calyx

137. All of the following conditions are commonly associated with a group A β-hemolytic streptococcal infection *except* one. Which one is the *exception*?
A. Scarlet fever
B. Toxic shock syndrome
C. Pharyngitis
D. Endocarditis
E. Impetigo

138. The auriculotemporal nerve encircles which of the following vessels?
A. Maxillary artery
B. Superficial temporal artery
C. Deep auricular artery
D. Middle meningeal artery
E. Anterior tympanic artery

Test items 139-143 refer to the following scenario.

A 55-year-old man presents with malaise and dyspnea. He has a low-grade fever and reports that his shortness of breath has increased steadily over the past week and a half. He has a history of rheumatic fever and denies ever using recreational drugs. He is currently being treated by a dentist for full mouth reconstruction.

139. On further examination, a heart murmur was detected. Given the patient's past medical history, which heart valve is most likely affected?
A. Mitral valve
B. Tricuspid valve
C. Aortic valve
D. Pulmonary valve

140. Before the patient developed rheumatic fever, he likely had which of the following conditions?
A. Cystitis
B. Pharyngitis
C. Food poisoning
D. Thrombocytopenia
E. Meningitis

141. After further evaluation and tests, subacute endocarditis is diagnosed. If the infecting microbe was cultured in the laboratory, the results would *most* likely show that this microbe is positive for _____.
A. α-Hemolysis
B. β-Hemolysis
C. γ-Hemolysis
D. Coagulase
E. Lecithinase

142. Which of the following is the *most* likely complication that may occur from the vegetations forming on the patient's defective heart valve?
A. Myocardial infarction
B. Hemorrhage
C. Petechiae
D. Cor pulmonale
E. Embolus

143. After the diagnosis is made, the patient is immediately placed on high-dose intravenous antibiotics. One of the antibiotics that is administered to the patient is streptomycin, an aminoglycoside. The antimicrobial effect of streptomycin is to inhibit the synthesis of _____.
A. The bacterial cell wall
B. Folate
C. Proteins
D. Nucleic acids
E. β-Lactamase

144. The conversion of information from DNA into messenger RNA is called _____.
A. Translation
B. Transcription
C. Transduction
D. Transformation

145. Maximum rotation and translation of both condyles occurs at _____.
A. Maximum opening
B. Maximum protrusion
C. Right and left lateral excursive movements
D. Hinge movement

146. The right subclavian artery arises from the _____, and the left subclavian artery arises from the _____.
A. Axillary artery; aortic arch
B. Brachiocephalic artery; aortic arch
C. Aortic arch; brachiocephalic artery
D. Brachiocephalic artery; axillary artery
E. Axillary artery; brachial artery

147. Rest position is defined as _____.
A. Any position of the mandible that does not involve contact of the teeth
B. The centric relation position of the condyles with the teeth apart
C. A mandibular position with masticatory muscles at complete rest
D. A clinical mandibular position in relation to the interocclusal space

148. Which of the following ions has a higher intracellular concentration compared with the extracellular fluid?

A. Na$^+$
B. K$^+$
C. Cl$^-$
D. HCO$_3^-$
E. Ca^{2+}

149. All of the following cells are associated with chronic inflammation *except* one. Which one is the *exception*?
    A. Macrophages
    B. Neutrophils
    C. T lymphocytes
    D. B lymphocytes
    E. Plasma cells

150. When is the crown of the permanent mandibular second molar completed?
    A. About 7 to 8 years
    B. About 8 to 9 years
    C. About 9 to 10 years
    D. About 10 to 11 years

151. Which of the following proteoglycans is present in extracellular space?
    A. Hyaluronic acid
    B. Keratan sulfate
    C. Chondroitin sulfate
    D. Dermatan sulfate
    E. Heparin

152. The pancreas is enveloped at its head by the _____.
    A. First part of the duodenum
    B. Second part of the duodenum
    C. Third part of the duodenum
    D. Fourth part of the duodenum
    E. First part of the jejunum

153. Mucopolysaccharidoses are hereditary disorders that are characterized by the accumulation of glycosaminoglycans in various tissues secondary to which of the following?
    A. Overproduction (synthesis) of proteoglycans
    B. Deficiency of one of the lysosomal hydrolytic enzymes normally involved in the degradation of one or more of the glycosaminoglycans
    C. The synthesis of abnormal proteoglycans
    D. The synthesis of highly branched glycosaminoglycan chains
    E. Arginine

154. A hormone acts to stimulate its neighboring cell to divide. This hormone would best be described as belonging to which category of hormones?
    A. Paracrine
    B. Autocrine
    C. Endocrine

155. The *most* common cause of pyelonephritis is _____.
    A. *Staphylococcus aureus*
    B. *Vibrio cholerae*
    C. *Escherichia coli*
    D. *Helicobacter pylori*
    E. *Bordetella pertussis*

156. Which of the following types of epithelium lines acinar units of salivary glands?
    A. Simple squamous
    B. Stratified squamous
    C. Simple cuboidal
    D. Simple columnar
    E. Pseudostratified columnar

157. The _____ is a component of the juxtaglomerular apparatus which functions in regulation of blood pressure.
    A. Proximal convoluted tubule
    B. Distal convoluted tubule
    C. Bowman's capsule
    D. Glomerulus
    E. Macula densa

158. The masseter muscle, which has a complex of internal components, includes all of the following *except* one. Which one is the *exception*?
    A. Pennation
    B. Structural composition permitting regional activation
    C. Multiple internal aponeuroses
    D. Internal aponeuroses that do not move or deform

159. The cricopharyngeus muscle of the esophagus _____.
    A. Is a parasympathetic stimulator of peristalsis
    B. Is a sympathetic inhibitor of peristalsis
    C. Prevents swallowing air at the pharyngeal end
    D. Prevents regurgitation of stomach contents at the abdominal end
    E. Controls the gag reflex

160. The *most* common cause of bacterial meningitis in newborns is _____.
    A. *Staphylococcus aureus*
    B. *Streptococcus pneumoniae*
    C. *Escherichia coli*
    D. *Haemophilus influenzae*
    E. *Listeria monocytogenes*

161. In which one of the following tissues is glucose transport into the cell unaffected by insulin?
    A. Skeletal muscle
    B. Liver
    C. Adipose tissue
    D. Smooth muscle

162. Deoxygenated blood from the transverse sinus drains into the _____.
    A. Inferior sagittal sinus
    B. Confluence of sinuses
    C. Sigmoid sinus
    D. Straight sinus
    E. Internal jugular vein

163. The primary maxillary second molar has which of the following characteristics?
    A. Does not have a well-defined mesial triangular fossa
    B. Oblique ridge absent or not well developed

C. Development (central) groove is well defined

D. A tubercle of Carabelli (supplementary cusp) is well developed

164. Facial nerves are derived from the _____ branchial arch.
    A. First
    B. Second
    C. Third
    D. Fourth
    E. Fifth and sixth

165. Analysis of DNA fragments (probing) is possible owing to which of the following properties of DNA?
    A. Phosphodiester bonds
    B. Complementary strands
    C. Protein binding
    D. Western blotting

166. From the occlusal aspect, the primary mandibular second molar has which of the following characteristics?
    A. Rectangular in form
    B. Outline of the crown converges mesially
    C. Three buccal cusps are dissimilar in size
    D. Cusps do not have well-defined triangular ridges

167. Which of the following are *not* type traits of permanent maxillary molars?

	First Molar	Second Molar	Third Molar
A. Buccal view:	Widest molar	Intermediate width	Smallest molar
B. Distolingual cusp:	Same size as M_2	Same size as M_1	Smallest size
C. Occlusal view:	Square or rhomboid	More rhomboidal	Triangle- or heart-shaped
D. Mesiobuccal root apex:	In line with cusp tip	In line with crown center	Roots displaced

168. A cotton-wool appearance describes the radiograph of a patient with _____.
    A. Osteopetrosis
    B. Osteitis deformans
    C. Peutz-Jeghers syndrome
    D. Seborrheic keratosis
    E. Osteogenesis imperfecta

169. The energy for skeletal muscle contraction is derived from which of the following processes?
    A. Calcium release from sarcoplasmic membranes and binding to troponin
    B. Cleavage of adenosine triphosphate by the myosin head
    C. Membrane Na^+,K^+-ATPase pump
    D. Sodium influx during the action potential

170. Which of the following is a property of C fibers?
    A. Have the slowest conduction velocity of any nerve fiber type
    B. Have the largest diameter of any nerve fiber type
    C. Are afferent nerves from muscle spindles
    D. Are afferent nerves from Golgi tendon organs
    E. Are preganglionic autonomic fibers

171. To which of the following bones is the tensor tympani attached?
    A. Incus
    B. Malleus
    C. Stapes
    D. Hyoid
    E. Mandible

172. An increase in alkaline phosphatase may be seen in all of the following conditions *except* one. Which one is the *exception*?
    A. Hyperparathyroidism
    B. Osteoporosis
    C. Osteitis deformans
    D. Adenocarcinoma of the prostate
    E. Multiple myeloma

173. The hereditary transmission of Peutz-Jeghers syndrome is _____.
    A. Autosomal dominant
    B. Autosomal recessive
    C. Sex-linked dominant
    D. Sex-linked recessive
    E. Not genetically transmitted

174. Which one of the following is considered a primary ligament of the temporomandibular joint (TMJ)?
    A. Stylomandibular
    B. Sphenomandibular
    C. Stylohyoid
    D. Temporomandibular

Test items 175-180 refer to the following scenario.
A 60-year-old homeless man who lives in a community shelter presents with history of coughing for the past 6 months. He has a slight fever, hemoptysis, and productive cough with a yellowish sputum discharge. After further examination and tests, active tuberculosis (TB) is diagnosed.

175. When the sputum samples were taken to the laboratory, what test did the physician order to help make the diagnosis?
    A. Gram stain
    B. Acid-fast stain
    C. Spore stain
    D. Purified protein derivative test (tuberculin test)
    E. Voges-Proskauer test

176. After 2 weeks, the bacterial cultures came back from the laboratory confirming the initial diagnosis, positively identifying the organism *Mycobacterium tuberculosis*. *M. tuberculosis* is known to infect which of the following cells?

A. Fibroblasts
B. Basal cells
C. Type I pneumocytes
D. Macrophages
E. Erythrocytes

177. Which of the following is a glycolipid found on the surface of *M. tuberculosis* that plays a role in its pathogenesis?
    A. Cord factor
    B. O antigen
    C. Protein A
    D. Exotoxin A
    E. Lecithinase

178. Because the patient was living in a homeless shelter, the tuberculin test was administered to all of the staff and residents living at the shelter. This test is based on a delayed-type hypersensitivity reaction that is mediated by _____.
    A. Only IgG
    B. IgG and IgM
    C. IgE
    D. T cells and macrophages
    E. Mast cells and basophils

179. Which of the following is the most appropriate drug used in combination therapy for TB to treat the patient?
    A. Amoxicillin
    B. Clindamycin
    C. Cephalosporin
    D. Tetracycline
    E. Rifampin

180. After 3 weeks, the patient was feeling "much better" and was discharged from the hospital, although he remained on drug therapy for another 6 months. Which of the following *best* describes the calcified scar that later formed in the affected lung parenchyma and hilar lymph node?
    A. Gumma
    B. Chancre
    C. Metastatic calcifications
    D. Tubercle
    E. Ghon complex

181. An infection in a mandibular incisor with an apex below the mylohyoid muscle drains into which of the following spaces?
    A. Sublingual space
    B. Submental space
    C. Submandibular space
    D. Parapharyngeal space

182. Phospholipase C is an enzyme that plays an important role in the production of second messengers, which produce intracellular responses. Which two second messengers are produced through the action of this enzyme?
    A. Cyclic adenosine monophosphate and tyrosine kinase

B. Acetylcholine and histidine
    C. Adenylate cyclase and protein kinase
    D. 1,2-Diacylglycerol and inositol 1,4,5-triphosphate

183. Which of the following cytokines stimulates B lymphocytes to differentiate into plasma cells?
    A. Interleukin (IL)-1
    B. IL-2
    C. IL-3
    D. IL-4
    E. IL-5

184. Which of the following statements regarding the parasympathetic nervous system is *true*?
    A. The third cranial nerve (oculomotor nerve) carries sympathetic fibers to the smooth muscles of the eye.
    B. The facial and the glossopharyngeal cranial nerves carry the parasympathetic preganglionic fibers for autonomic innervation to the salivary glands.
    C. The parasympathetic nervous system innervates primarily striated muscle in the body.
    D. The parasympathetic nervous system is organized for diffuse activation and responses.

185. From the incisal view, a greater mesiodistal measurement than faciolingual measurement can be seen in which of the following permanent anterior crowns?
    A. Maxillary central incisor
    B. Maxillary canine
    C. Mandibular canine
    D. Mandibular central incisor

186. The vestigial cleft of Rathke's pouch in the hypophysis is located between the _____.
    A. Anterior and posterior lobes
    B. Anterior lobe and hypothalamus
    C. Posterior lobe and hypothalamus
    D. Median eminence and the optic chiasm

187. A comparison of the pulp chambers and root canals of maxillary primary and permanent second molars shows which of the following?
    A. Enamel cap of primary tooth is thick but less consistent in depth
    B. Comparatively less thickness of dentin at the occlusal fossa of primary molars
    C. Pulp chambers are proportionally larger in primary molars
    D. Pulp horns are lower in primary molars, especially distal horns

188. The center that provides output to the respiratory muscles is located in the _____.
    A. Pons
    B. Medulla
    C. Cerebral cortex
    D. Cerebellum
    E. Hypothalamus

189. The brachial plexus of nerves arises from which of the following roots of the anterior primary rami of spinal nerves?

A. All cervical roots (C1–C8)
B. All thoracic roots (T1–T12)
C. C8 and T1
D. C5–C8 and T1
E. C5–C8 and T1–T4

190. Aschoff's bodies are observed in which of the following conditions?
    A. Acute myelogenous leukemia
    B. Pheochromocytoma
    C. Osteopetrosis
    D. Rheumatic fever
    E. Scleroderma

191. Nonsteroidal antiinflammatory drugs are pain-relieving and antiinflammatory medications. They are effective because they act to inhibit prostaglandin synthesis by _____.
    A. Inhibiting fatty acid lipooxygenase activity
    B. Inhibiting fatty acid–specific cyclooxygenase activity
    C. Inhibiting fatty acid–specific hydroperoxidase activity
    D. Inhibiting phospholipase A_2

192. Terminal bronchioles are characterized by _____ cells.
    A. Goblet
    B. Ciliated cuboidal
    C. Nonciliated cuboidal
    D. Ciliated squamous
    E. Nonciliated squamous

193. A major anatomic variant of the two-rooted mandibular molar is a tooth with an additional distolingual and third root. What is the prevalence of three-rooted mandibular first molars?
    A. May exceed 10% in white populations
    B. Less than 1% in Eurasian and Asian populations
    C. Greater than 5% (up to 40%) in populations with Mongolian traits.
    D. Greater than 8% in African populations

194. Which one of the following statements regarding the regulation of gastrointestinal function is *true*?
    A. The main sympathetic nerve supply to the digestive tract is the vagus.
    B. In general, sympathetic stimulation is excitatory to digestive activity.
    C. Salivary secretion is stimulated by both branches of the autonomic nervous system, although not to the same degree.
    D. Parasympathetic stimulation of the salivary glands produces a saliva rich in mucus.

195. The occlusal surface of a primary mandibular first molar often has a prominent faciolingual ridge. Which two cusps does this transverse ridge connect?
    A. Buccal and distolingual
    B. Mesiolingual and distobuccal
    C. Mesiobuccal and mesiolingual
    D. Distobuccal and distolingual

196. Which of the following disorders is *least* likely to be included in the differential diagnosis of a patient with jaundice?
    A. Hepatitis
    B. Hemolytic anemia
    C. Cholelithiasis
    D. Glomerulonephritis
    E. Carcinoma of the pancreas

197. Arteriovenous anastomoses in deeper skin are important in _____.
    A. Immunity
    B. Thermoregulation
    C. Controlling the arrector pili muscle
    D. Pigmentation
    E. Pain sensation

198. Complications of Barrett's esophagus include all of the following *except* one. Which one is the *exception*?
    A. Varices
    B. Stricture
    C. Hemorrhage
    D. Adenocarcinoma
    E. Ulceration

Test items 199-202 refer to the following scenario.

A 30-year-old woman comes to the office for a dental examination. She has not been to the dentist in 2 years. The patient has type 1 diabetes, which requires her to take insulin. She is otherwise in good health. On intraoral examination, you notice that the dorsum of her tongue has a thick, matted appearance and diagnose hairy tongue. You also find that the patient has deep caries in the upper second maxillary molar.

199. Which type of papillae is affected that causes the hair-like appearance of the tongue?
    A. Foliate
    B. Circumvallate
    C. Fungiform
    D. Filiform

200. On the patient's radiograph, you notice that the pulp chamber in the carious molar appears smaller than the surrounding teeth. This is most likely due to the deposition of which type of dentin?
    A. Secondary
    B. Tertiary
    C. Mantle
    D. Sclerotic

201. You decide to remove the caries and prepare the patient for anesthesia. Which nerve must be anesthetized to ensure adequate anesthesia for the patient?
    A. Nasopalatine nerve
    B. Greater palatine nerve
    C. Anterior superior alveolar nerve
    D. Middle superior alveolar nerve
    E. Posterior superior alveolar nerve

202. After administering the anesthetic, the patient complains that her "heart feels like it's racing." You explain

to her that it may be from the epinephrine in the anesthesia. Which of the following glands could *most* likely cause the same symptoms in the patient?

A. Hypophysis
B. Thyroid
C. Pineal
D. Suprarenal

203. Which of the following microbes is the *most* common cause of gastroenteritis in children?

A. Reoviruses
B. Picornaviruses
C. Togaviruses
D. Paramyxoviruses

204. Name the point angle which represents the junction of the cutting edge of an incisor with the surface that is toward the tongue and the surface that is away from the midline.

A. Distoproximoincisal
B. Distolabioincisal
C. Distolinguoincisal
D. Labioincisolingual

205. Ureters travel inferiorly just _____ the parietal peritoneum of the posterior body wall. They pass _____ to the common iliac arteries as they enter the pelvis.

A. Above; posterior
B. Above; anterior
C. Below; posterior
D. Below; anterior
E. Above; superior

206. Aspartame contains aspartic acid and which of the following amino acids?

A. Phenylalanine
B. Leucine
C. Isoleucine
D. Lysine
E. Proline

207. Injury to which of the following nerves would affect abduction of the eyeball?

A. Optic nerve
B. Oculomotor
C. Trochlear
D. Trigeminal
E. Abducens

208. Which of the following statements regarding tubular secretion in the kidney is *true*?

A. The secretion of K^+ increases when a person has acidosis.
B. The secretion of H^+ increases when a person has alkalosis.
C. It is a process that transports substances from the filtrate to the capillary blood.
D. It accounts for most of the K^+ in the urine.

209. _____ marks the end of growth in length of long bones.

A. Diaphyseal closure
B. Epiphyseal closure
C. Ossification
D. Formation of periosteum
E. Cessation of bone remodeling

210. The presence of M-protein antibodies suggests immunity to infection by which type of bacteria?

A. *Streptococcus pyogenes*
B. Viridans streptococcus
C. *Streptococcus sanguis*
D. *Staphylococcus aureus*
E. *Lactobacillus casei*

211. The synthesis of all steroid hormones involves which of the following compounds?

A. Pregnenolone
B. Progesterone
C. Aldosterone
D. Cortisone
E. Testosterone

Questions 212-223 relate to the following scenario.

A mother brings her 12-year-old boy to the dentist to ask about her son grinding his teeth and about some white "spots" located on the smooth-surfaced enamel of several of his anterior teeth and premolars. Among other questions about the cause of the defects, the mother asks when a systemic disturbance occurred that may have caused the "spots." The patient has excessive tooth wear from bruxing and clenching. The dentist measures the cervical-incisal length of the permanent maxillary central incisor (10.5 mm). Also measured is the distance from the cementoenamel junction (CEJ) to the midpoint of the defect (5.5 mm). Given that the crown is completed over 4 to 5 years, it is possible to estimate the age at which the hypoplasia occurred using 6-month or yearly periods in the following formula:

$$ADF = ACF - (\text{years of formation/crown height} \times \text{distance of defect from CEJ})$$

where *ADF* is age of defect formation and *ACF* is age of crown formation.

212. Using an average age of crown formation of both 4 and 5 years, the age of defect formation is estimated to be about _____.

A. 7 to 9 months in utero
B. 0 to 1 year old
C. 1 to 2 years old
D. 2 to 3 years old

213. The increase of fluorosis of permanent teeth in both nonfluoridated and optimally fluoridated populations points to the need for dentists to caution parents about potential causes of fluorosis in children. Which of the following cautions about fluoride is correct, but the age or implied age is *not* correct?

A. Excess (>1 ppm) fluoride in the drinking water during enamel formation
B. Excessive (greater than pea-sized amount) use of fluoride toothpaste younger than 6 years old

C. Use of fluoride toothpaste only for children younger than 4 years old

D. Use of a 1.1% sodium fluoride toothpaste or gel by pediatric patients only when 6 years old and older

214. Systemic etiologic factors that are said to be associated with enamel defects such as hypoplasia occur generally in what period of time?

A. Before birth

B. Generally after birth and before age 6 years

C. During the first year postpartum for Hutchinson's incisors

D. During birth

215. The differential diagnosis of white "spots" of the enamel of primary and permanent teeth should include disorders that have a substantiated cause. Which of the following do *not* have an evidence-based causal relationship with enamel hypoplasia?

A. Rickets

B. Congenital syphilis

C. Measles

D. Fluorosis

216. Clenching and grinding of teeth involves contraction of skeletal-type muscles. Several types of myofilaments are present in the contractile elements of skeletal muscles. Which of the following statements about muscle filaments is *false*?

A. Myosin forms the thick filament of muscle.

B. Actin is a major protein of thin filaments.

C. Titin is a protein of elastic filament.

D. Connectin is a protein of intermediate filament.

217. The clinical examination of the patient reveals extensive wear of the right canines and less wear of the lateral incisors. Also, there is tenderness of the jaw-closing muscles, particularly on the right side. Which of the following masticatory muscles would be involved primarily in providing most of the force for anterior tooth clenching?

A. Inferior lateral pterygoid muscle

B. Superior lateral pterygoid muscle

C. Anterior temporalis muscle

D. Masseter muscle

218. Sleep bruxism is defined by all of the following characteristics *except* one. Which one is the *exception*?

A. Stereotypic movement disorder

B. Grinding and clenching of the teeth during sleep

C. More frequent in the younger generation

D. Individuals who brux during the daytime inevitably brux at night

219. Physiologic evidence suggests that central or autonomic nervous system factors rather than peripheral sensory factors play a dominant role in the genesis of sleep bruxism. Which of the following statements about the central genesis of sleep bruxism is *not* true?

A. During sleep, the mouth is usually open because of motor repression.

B. Tooth contact most likely occurs in association with sleep arousal.

C. Some peripheral sensory factors may exert an influence on sleep bruxism through their interaction with sleep-wake mechanisms.

D. Sequential change from autonomic (cardiac) or brain cortical activities follows sleep bruxism–related jaw motor activity.

220. Aggravation of bruxism has been suggested to occur secondary to all of the following occlusal relationships *except* one. Which one is the *exception*?

A. Occlusal interferences in centric relation

B. Occlusal interferences in the intercuspal position

C. Iatrogenic occlusal relations that *interfere* with bruxism

D. Angle class III malocclusion (prognathism)

221. The differential diagnosis of enamel hypoplasia should take into account suggested differences between nonfluoride and fluoride opacities. Which of the following statements does *not* suggest a basis for a diagnosis of nonfluoride enamel hypoplasia?

A. Levels of fluoride in drinking water that range from 0.2 to 0.34 ppm have been reported to be associated with prevalences of nonfluoride enamel opacities ranging from 22% to 35%.

B. At a level of 1 to 1.5 ppm of fluoride in drinking water, only a few fluoride opacities occur.

C. Most nonfluoride enamel opacities appear as white, opaque spots in smooth surface enamel; areas of mild dental fluorosis are lusterless, opaque white patches.

D. Fluorosis and nonfluoride opacities are clinically significantly different.

222. During muscle contraction, what physical change does *not* occur relative to muscle fiber contraction?

A. Sarcomeres—shorten

B. Thick and thin filaments—shorten

C. I band—shortens

D. H zone—shortens

223. Regarding the superior and inferior heads of the lateral pterygoid muscle (SHLP and IHLP), which of the following statements is *false*?

A. Hypothetically, SHLP and IHLP can be considered to be parts of one muscle.

B. Distributions of SHLP and IHLP activities are shaded according to biochemical demands of tasks.

C. SHLP stabilizes the condyle and disc against the articular eminence in a wide range of jaw movements and forces.

D. IHLP plays a major role in the generation and fine control of horizontal forces.

224. The process of active sodium transport in the ascending limb of the loop of Henle is essential for which of the following processes?

A. Regulation of chloride excretion
B. Regulation of pH in extracellular fluid
C. Regulation of aldosterone excretion
D. Regulation of water excretion

225. Hypertension (long-term) is compensated by which of the following renal mechanisms?
A. Increased circulating antidiuretic hormone (vasopressin)
B. Increased sympathetic activity
C. Decreased circulating aldosterone
D. Increased circulating angiotensin II

226. The most superficial layer of the epidermis is the stratum _____.
A. Spinosum
B. Basale
C. Granulosum
D. Lucidum
E. Corneum

227. Where are the cells that produce calcitonin located?
A. Red marrow
B. Adrenal gland
C. Parathyroid gland
D. Thyroid gland
E. Spleen

228. In mature dentin, the ratio of inorganic to organic matter is approximately _____.
A. 94:6
B. 50:50
C. 70:30
D. 80:20
E. 60:40

229. All of the following symptoms are mediated by antibodies *except* one. Which one is the *exception*?
A. Arthus reaction
B. Tuberculin reaction
C. Asthma
D. Erythroblastosis fetalis
E. Serum sickness

230. The pancreas produces enzymes that are responsible for the digestion of dietary compounds. Which of the following foods would *not* be digested by enzymes synthesized and secreted by the pancreas?
A. Carbohydrates
B. Lipids
C. Vitamins
D. Protein

231. The primary sensory neurons' nucleus of termination involved in the jaw jerk reflex is the _____.
A. Facial nucleus
B. Trochlear nucleus
C. Mesencephalic nucleus
D. Spinal trigeminal nucleus
E. Nucleus of solitary tract

232. Aldosterone _____.
A. Stimulates sodium reabsorption in the distal and collecting ducts
B. Is secreted by the juxtaglomerular apparatus
C. Stimulates potassium absorption in the distal tubule
D. Stimulates bicarbonate reabsorption in the proximal tubule

233. The first evidence of calcification (weeks in utero) in the primary dentition occurs in which of the following teeth at about what age?
A. Maxillary central incisor—14 (13 to 16) weeks
B. Mandibular central incisor—12 (10 to 13) weeks
C. Maxillary lateral incisor—14 (13 to 16) weeks
D. Mandibular lateral incisor—14 (13 to 15) weeks

234. From the lingual perspective, the crown of the primary maxillary second molar shows which of the following?
A. Small, well-developed mesiolingual cusp
B. Distolingual cusp smaller than maxillary primary first molar distolingual cusp
C. There is no supplemental cusp apical to the mesiolingual cusp
D. Developmental groove separating the mesiolingual and distolingual cusps

235. An 8-year-old boy presents with macroglossia and delayed eruption of his primary teeth. Which of the following conditions does he *most* likely have?
A. Plummer's disease
B. Osteochondroses
C. Cretinism
D. Wilson's disease
E. Mallory-Weiss syndrome

236. A major function of surfactant is to increase which of the following?
A. Pulmonary compliance
B. Alveolar surface tension
C. The work of breathing
D. The tendency of the lungs to collapse

237. Red pulp in the spleen consists of _____.
A. Fibroblasts
B. T lymphocytes
C. B lymphocytes
D. Macrophages
E. Chromaffin cells

238. The velocity of blood flow _____.
A. Is higher in the capillaries than in the arterioles
B. Is higher in the veins than in the venules
C. Is higher in the veins than in the arteries
D. Falls to zero in the descending aorta during diastole

239. Neuraminidase is produced by _____.
A. Influenza virus
B. Hepatitis C viruses
C. HIV
D. Measles virus
E. Rubella virus

240. Which sequence of eruption of permanent teeth occurs most often? (8-7-6-5-4-3-2-1 = M3-M2-M1-P2-P1-C-LI-CI). First #, #'s in each series is considered to be the first to erupt.
    A. 6-1-2-4-3-5-7-8 (maxilla)
    B. 6-1-2-3-4-5-7-8 (maxilla)
    C. (6-1)-2-4-3-5-7-8 (mandible)
    D. 1-6-2-4-5-3-7-8 (mandible)

241. All of the following are histopathologic features of malignant cells *except* one. Which one is the *exception*?
    A. Anaplasia
    B. Pleomorphism
    C. Aneuploidy
    D. Large nuclei
    E. Low nuclear-to-cytoplasmic ratio

242. The vertebral artery meets with the basilar artery at the lower border of the _____.
    A. Midbrain
    B. Pons
    C. Medulla
    D. Temporal lobe
    E. C1

243. Which of the following is *not* involved in the process of gene cloning?
    A. DNA polymerase
    B. RNA ligase
    C. RNA polymerase
    D. Restriction endonuclease

244. Which of the following is the *most* significant stimulant of the respiratory center?
    A. Decreased blood oxygen (O_2) tension
    B. Increased blood H^+ concentration
    C. Decreased blood H^+ concentration
    D. Increased blood carbon dioxide (CO_2) tension

245. The infraorbital nerve is a branch of the _____.
    A. Optic nerve
    B. Oculomotor nerve
    C. Ophthalmic nerve
    D. Maxillary nerve
    E. Mandibular nerve

246. Root bifurcation would be a more likely finding in which of the following permanent teeth?
    A. Maxillary canine
    B. Mandibular canine
    C. Maxillary central incisor
    D. Mandibular lateral incisor

247. Which one of the following carbohydrates is a ketose sugar?
    A. Galactose
    B. Fructose
    C. Glucose
    D. Mannose
    E. Glyceraldehydes

248. Which of the following antimicrobials is bacteriostatic and inhibits protein synthesis in bacteria?
    A. Streptomycin
    B. Penicillin V
    C. Ciprofloxacin
    D. Cephalexin
    E. Tetracycline

249. The auricular hillocks are derived from the _____.
    A. First branchial arch
    B. Second branchial arch
    C. First and second branchial arches
    D. Lateral nasal process
    E. Medial nasal process

250. Comparing the overall length of primary central incisors (E|F) with permanent maxillary central incisors (8|9), which is the correct ratio expressed as a percentage?
    A. About 50%
    B. About 60%
    C. About 70%
    D. About 80%

251. Ehlers-Danlos syndrome is a disease affecting _____.
    A. Bone
    B. Connective tissue
    C. Muscle
    D. Joints
    E. Glycogen synthesis

252. Which of the following participate in both fatty acid biosynthesis and β-oxidation of fatty acids?
    A. Malonyl coenzyme A (CoA)
    B. Flavin adenine dinucleotide (FAD)
    C. Acetyl CoA
    D. Nicotinamide adenine dinucleotide (NAD)

253. Insulin produces which of the following changes in mammalian cells?
    A. Increase in liver glycogen production
    B. Increase in blood glucose concentration
    C. Decrease in transport of glucose into muscle
    D. Increase in transport of glucose into the brain.

254. Osteocytes are found in _____ in mature bone.
    A. Trabeculae
    B. Lacunae
    C. The central canal
    D. Canaliculi
    E. Spicules

255. Which one of the following morphologic characteristics is representative of all posterior maxillary teeth?
    A. Marked mesial concavity on crowns and roots
    B. Tips of cusps are well within the confines of the root trunks
    C. From mesiodistal aspect, crowns are rhomboidal in shape
    D. From mesiodistal aspect, all maxillary posterior crowns are trapezoidal with shortest uneven side toward occlusal surface

256. Nephrolithiasis is *most* likely to be associated with which of the following conditions?

A. Hyperparathyroidism
B. Myxedema
C. Pyelonephritis
D. Wilson's disease
E. Thrombocytopenia

257. The rate-limiting enzyme in glycolysis is which of the following?
    A. Fructose-bisphosphatase
    B. Phosphofructokinase
    C. Phosphoglucose isomerase
    D. Glucokinase

258. Which type of collagen is characteristically found in cartilage?
    A. Type I
    B. Type II
    C. Type III
    D. Type IV

259. Which of the following is the *most* characteristic feature of the primary maxillary central incisor?
    A. Faciolingual breadth of the crown
    B. Mesiodistal width of the crown
    C. Mesial and distal margin outlines in line with profiles of root
    D. Root/crown ratio

260. The spread of an odontogenic infection to which of the following spaces would *most* likely be considered life-threatening?
    A. Submandibular space
    B. Sublingual space
    C. Parapharyngeal space
    D. Retropharyngeal space
    E. Pterygomandibular space

261. The most common mutation accounting for the pathogenesis of trisomy 21 is _____.
    A. Chromosome translocation
    B. Meiotic nondisjunction
    C. Mitotic nondisjunction
    D. Single deletion
    E. X-linked inheritance

262. What type of collagen is found in cementum?
    A. Type I collagen
    B. Type II collagen
    C. Type III collagen
    D. Type IV collagen
    E. Type V collagen

263. What happens to net filtration (ultrafiltration) in the glomerulus when plasma protein concentration is decreased?
    A. Net filtration increases
    B. Net filtration decreases
    C. Net filtration remains unchanged
    D. Net filtration ceases

264. The presence of Auer rods in a peripheral blood smear suggests which of the following conditions?
    A. Acute lymphocytic leukemia
    B. Acute lymphoblastic leukemia
    C. Acute myelogenous leukemia
    D. Chronic lymphocytic leukemia
    E. Hodgkin's lymphoma

265. Which of the following hormones are secreted by the posterior pituitary gland?
    A. Prolactin
    B. Follicle-stimulating hormone
    C. Luteinizing hormone
    D. Vasopressin

266. Which of the following is the predominant immunoglobulin in whole saliva?
    A. Secretory IgA
    B. Secretory IgG
    C. Secretory IgM
    D. Secretory IgB

267. Which of the following is *not* an arch trait of the maxillary canine?
    A. In the same dentition, the crown is larger than the mandibular canine
    B. The incisal margin of the crown occupies at least one third to one half of crown height
    C. Labial aspect: mesial and distal marginal ridges converge toward cervix
    D. Marked symmetry of mesial and distal halves when viewed from incisal

268. During exercise, which of the following is decreased?
    A. Oxidation of fatty acids
    B. Glucagon release
    C. Glycogenolysis
    D. Lipogenesis

269. Involution of the thymus would occur following which year in a healthy individual?
    A. 0 years (at birth)
    B. 12th year
    C. 20th year
    D. 60th year

270. Monoamine oxidase (MAO) _____.
    A. Inactivates reduced steroid derivatives
    B. Is activated by MAO inhibitors
    C. Inactivates catecholamines by oxidative deamination
    D. Is located in the synapse where it inactivates the neurotransmitter acetylcholine

271. Sleep bruxism can be characterized by which of the following?
    A. Episodes of massive, bilateral clenching
    B. Tooth grinding that may last for 20 minutes
    C. Often coincides with passage from lighter to deeper sleep
    D. Occurs approximately every 20 minutes in the sleep cycle

272. _____ is an endocrine disorder that causes an early loss of primary teeth and the early eruption of secondary teeth.
    A. Myxedema
    B. Hashimoto's thyroiditis

C. DiGeorge's syndrome

D. Plummer's disease

E. Dwarfism

273. Which of the following factors do *not* influence the rate at which a meal leaves the stomach?

A. Acidification of the duodenum

B. Increasing the tonicity of the intestine

C. Saline in the duodenum

D. Lipid in the intestine

274. Occlusal interferences can be defined by all of the following *except* one. Which one is the *exception*?

A. Occlusal contact relations that interfere with function

B. Interference to jaw closure into the intercuspal position

C. Interferences to laterotrusive movements

D. Interferences to jaw opening

275. The olecranon fossa is located on the _____ surface of the _____.

A. Superior; radius

B. Anterior; humerus

C. Posterior; humerus

D. Anterior; radius

276. Which of the following is usually *least* malignant?

A. Acute lymphoblastic leukemia

B. Acute lymphocytic leukemia

C. Acute myelogenous leukemia

D. Chronic lymphocytic leukemia

E. Chronic myelogenous leukemia

277. Each of the following describes collagen *except* one. Which one is the *exception*?

A. Most abundant protein in the body

B. Modifications to procollagen occur in the extra-cellular matrix

C. Incorporates hydroxyproline into the molecule by transfer RNA

D. Hydroxylation of proline requires vitamin C and molecular oxygen

278. Which position of the mental foramen relative to the mandibular premolars and first molar occurs *most* frequently?

A. Between the first and second premolars

B. In line with the second premolar

C. Distal to the second premolar

D. In line with the mesial root of the first molar

279. From the lingual perspective, the primary maxillary first molar has which of the following characteristics?

A. Distolingual cusp is the most prominent cusp

B. Mesiolingual cusp is poorly defined

C. Distobuccal cusp cannot be seen from lingual aspect

D. Crown converges considerably in a lingual direction

280. In addition to the esophagus itself, which of the following structures passes through the diaphragm through the esophageal opening?

A. Aorta

B. Inferior vena cava

C. Azygos vein

D. Posterior and anterior vagal trunks

E. Splanchnic nerves

281. Which one of the following does *not* release acetylcholine?

A. Sympathetic preganglionic fibers

B. Sympathetic postganglionic fibers that innervate the heart

C. Parasympathetic postganglionic fibers to effector organs

D. Parasympathetic preganglionic fibers

282. An infant with a diagnosis of osteopetrosis has dysfunctional _____.

A. Chondrocytes

B. Osteoblasts

C. Osteoclasts

D. Fibroblasts

E. Lymphocytes

283. Langerhans' cells are located primarily in stratum _____.

A. Corneum

B. Lucidum

C. Granulosum

D. Spinosum

E. Basale

284. Which of the following would be expected to increase blood pressure?

A. A drug that inhibits the angiotensin-converting enzyme and the production of angiotensin II (i.e., angiotensin-converting enzyme inhibitors)

B. A drug that inhibits the synthesis of nitric oxide

C. A drug that blocks vasopressin receptors

D. Increased stimulation of the carotid baroreceptor

285. At what age are the crowns of the primary maxillary second molars completed?

A. 11 months

B. 10 months

C. 9 months

D. 8 months

286. Which of the following processes is *not* a true component of swallowing?

A. Closure of the glottis

B. Involuntary relaxation of the upper esophageal sphincter

C. Involuntary movements of the tongue against the palate

D. Esophageal peristalsis

287. Which of the following receptors are recognized by CD8 lymphocytes?

A. Class I major histocompatibility complex (MHC) molecules

B. Class II MHC molecules

C. Surface IgE

D. Surface IgM

E. Histamine receptor

288. Which one of the following is *not* a normal anatomic feature of mandibular incisors?

A. Bifurcated roots

B. Inconspicuous cingula

C. Four developmental lobes

D. Incisal edges placed slightly lingually

289. The _____ differentiates into ameloblasts.

A. Stellate reticulum

B. Inner enamel epithelium in the cap stage

C. Inner enamel epithelium in the bell stage

D. Outer enamel epithelium in the cap stage

E. Outer enamel epithelium in the bell stage

290. Which of the following statements regarding the histology of the trachea is *true*?

A. The mucosa is covered with oral epithelium.

B. Elastic cartilage rings lie deep to the submucosa.

C. The cartilage is ring-shaped; the open end of the ring faces anterior.

D. The cartilage is covered by a perichondrium.

E. Skeletal muscle extends across the open end of each cartilage.

291. In pemphigus, autoantibodies are directed against which of the following structures?

A. Acetylcholine receptor

B. Sarcomere

C. Epidermis

D. Thyroid follicle

E. Lysosomes

292. Which one of the following is elevated in plasma during the absorptive period (compared with the postabsorptive state)?

A. Chylomicrons

B. Acetoacetate

C. Lactate

D. Glucagon

293. The more recent focus on causative factors in bruxism includes all of the following *except* one. Which one is the *exception*?

A. Occlusal interferences

B. Part of a sleep arousal response

C. Pathophysiologic factors

D. Neurotransmitters in the central nervous system

294. A distinct central developmental groove, prominent buccal triangular ridge, two cusps, and distinct mesial and distal occlusal pits would be *most* characteristic of _____.

A. Mandibular first premolars

B. Primary mandibular first molars

C. Primary mandibular second molars

D. Mandibular second premolars

295. An autoclave sterilizes dental instruments by causing which of the following?

A. Coagulation of proteins

B. Denaturing of proteins

C. Precipitation of nucleic acids

D. Disruption of cell membranes

E. Dissolution of lipids

296. Porphyrins use which amino acid in their synthesis?

A. Alanine

B. Phenylalanine

C. Cysteine

D. Glycine

297. The dental lamina arises from _____.

A. Somites

B. Neural crest cells

C. The first branchial arch

D. The second branchial arch

E. The buccopharyngeal membrane

298. Karyotyping can be used to diagnose which of the following diseases?

A. Klinefelter's syndrome

B. Multiple myeloma

C. Niemann-Pick disease

D. Pemphigus

E. Peutz-Jeghers syndrome

299. Muscle spindle stretching when the patellar tendon is tapped produces which of the following responses?

A. Muscle contraction within muscle where the spindles are located

B. Increased sympathetic stimulation of the spindles

C. Reduction in the number of afferent impulses entering the spinal cord

D. Inhibition of the stretch reflex

300. In terms of vertical dimension, where is the mental foramen found *most* frequently?

A. At the apices of the premolars

B. Coronal to the apices

C. Below the apices

D. No particular location predominates

301. Urinary filtrate is most hypotonic in the _____.

A. Proximal convoluted tubule

B. Descending limb of Henle's loop

C. Thin segment of Henle's loop

D. Thick ascending segment of Henle's loop

E. Distal convoluted tubule

302. There are _____ pairs of true ribs.

A. 4

B. 5

C. 7

D. 11

E. 12

303. Based on average mesiodistal diameters of the crowns of primary teeth, what is the approximate range for average overall length of the primary maxillary arch?

A. 60 to 68 mm

B. 68 to 76 mm

C. 76 to 84 mm

D. 84 to 92 mm

304. Symptoms of a myocardial infarction include all of the following *except* one. Which one is the *exception*?

A. Angina

B. Diaphoresis

C. Fever

D. Vomiting

E. Dyspnea

305. Which process transports amino acids across the luminal surface of the epithelia that lines the small intestine?

A. Simple diffusion

B. Primary active transport

C. Cotransport with Na^+

D. Cotransport with Cl^-

306. Which of the following cells are capable of mitosis?

A. Smooth muscle

B. Skeletal muscle

C. Cardiac muscle

D. Type I pneumocytes

E. Neurons

307. Vitamin K serves as a coenzyme for _____.

A. The enzymatic hydroxylation of proline to 4-hydroxyproline

B. The carboxylation of inactive prothrombin to form active prothrombin

C. The synthesis of nucleic acids

D. Protein synthesis

308. Squamous cell carcinoma is the most common oral cancer. It is a tumor of _____.

A. Melanocytes

B. Basal cells

C. Fibroblasts

D. Keratinocytes

E. Macrophages

309. Which of the following is *not* a type trait of the permanent maxillary first premolar?

A. Occlusal table outline, trapezoidal

B. Generally two roots—mesial and distal

C. Central groove is long

D. Supplementary grooves are rare

310. Which of the following skin lesions is *most* likely premalignant?

A. Verruca vulgaris

B. Keloids

C. Seborrheic keratosis

D. Actinic keratosis

E. Compound nevus

311. Which of the following statements regarding the hormone secretin is *true*?

A. It is responsible for activating chymotrypsinogen.

B. It stimulates the release of pancreatic secretion rich in bicarbonate.

C. It stimulates the release of pancreatic enzymes.

D. It stimulates the contraction of the gallbladder to release bile.

312. Which primary tooth generally erupts last?

A. Mandibular second molar

B. Maxillary second molar

C. Maxillary canine

D. Mandibular canine

313. The latissimus dorsi muscle is supplied by the _____.

A. Medial pectoral nerve

B. Eleventh cranial nerve

C. Dorsal scapular nerve

D. Thoracodorsal nerve

314. Which of the following responses is due to the stimulation of α-adrenergic receptors?

A. Slowing of heart rate

B. Constriction of blood vessels in skin

C. Increased gastrointestinal motility

D. Increased renal blood flow

315. Which of the following contributes primary sensory innervation to the temporomandibular joint (TMJ)?

A. Auriculotemporal nerve

B. Infraorbital nerve

C. Branch of the lingual nerve

D. Facial nerve

316. All of the following arteries are branches of the mandibular division of the maxillary artery *except* one. Which one is the *exception*?

A. Incisive artery

B. Submental artery

C. Middle meningeal artery

D. Mylohyoid artery

E. Deep auricular artery

317. Rheumatoid arthritis is characterized by inflammation of the _____.

A. Articular capsule

B. Articular cartilage

C. Cortical bone

D. Perichondrium

E. Synovium

318. Which of the following are *not* type traits of permanent mandibular first and second premolars?

		First Premolar	**Second Premolar**
A.	Buccal view:	Crown bilaterally asymmetrical	Bilaterally symmetrical
B.	Lingual aspect:	Entire buccal profile visible	Buccal profile not seen
C.	Lingual aspect:	Most of occlusal surface visible	Little, if any, seen
D.	Lingual aspect:	Contour height: middle third	Cervical third

319. Which of the following muscles of the back is supplied by the eleventh cranial nerve?

A. Levator scapulae

B. Latissimus dorsi

C. Trapezius

D. Major rhomboid

E. Minor rhomboid

320. A positive quelling reaction can be observed in bacteria with a _____.

A. Thick peptidoglycan layer
B. Capsule
C. Flagella
D. Cell wall that contains teichoic acid
E. Glycocalyx coating

321. In which of the following might arterial blood pressure be abnormally high?
A. Ventricular fibrillation
B. Heart failure
C. Anaphylactic shock
D. Increased intracranial pressure

322. All of the following can be found in the cell wall of a gram-negative bacterium *except* one. Which one is the *exception*?
A. Endotoxin
B. A thin peptidoglycan layer
C. Lipopolysaccharide
D. Teichoic acid
E. O antigen

323. The articulating surfaces of the temporomandibular joint (TMJ) are covered with _____.
A. Fibrocartilage
B. Hyaline cartilage
C. Articular cartilage
D. Elastic cartilage
E. Perichondrium

324. The binding of epinephrine or glucagon to the corresponding membrane receptor has which of the following effects on glycogen metabolism?
A. Net synthesis of glycogen is increased
B. Glycogen phosphorylase is activated, whereas glycogen synthase is inactivated
C. Glycogen phosphorylase is inactivated, whereas glycogen synthase is activated
D. Both glycogen synthase and phosphorylase are activated
E. Both glycogen synthase and phosphorylase are inactivated

325. If posterior teeth on the left side contact occlusally during a right lateral excursion of the mandible, the left side occlusal contact would be referred to as _____.
A. Laterotrusive contact
B. Protrusive contact
C. Mediotrusive contact
D. Centric relation

326. Blood from the internal carotid artery reaches the posterior cerebral artery by the _____.
A. Anterior cerebral artery
B. Anterior communicating artery
C. Posterior communicating artery
D. Posterior superior cerebellar artery
E. Basilar artery

327. Adenosine triphosphate (ATP) is used directly for each of the following processes *except* one. Which one is the *exception*?

A. Accumulation of Ca^{2+} by the sarcoplasmic reticulum
B. Transport of Na^+ from intracellular to extracellular fluid
C. Transport of K^+ from extracellular to intracellular fluid
D. Transport of H^+ from parietal cells into the lumen of the stomach
E. Transport of glucose into muscle cells

328. All of the following microbes are associated with infections secondary to HIV infection *except* one. Which one is the *exception*?
A. *Pneumocystis jiroveci* (formerly *Pneumocystis carinii*)
B. Epstein-Barr virus
C. Coxsackievirus
D. *Mycobacterium tuberculosis*
E. *Candida albicans*

329. Which of the following is *not* a type trait of the permanent maxillary second premolar?
A. Buccal view: narrow shoulders (margins of crown; mesio-occlusal and disto-occlusal angles)
B. Occlusal table outline: ovoid
C. Mesiomarginal groove interrupts mesial marginal ridge
D. Lingual view: buccal profile is not visible

330. What is the correct schematic outline of the following teeth?
A. Mandibular premolars, viewed from occlusal, rhomboidal.
B. Maxillary central incisors, viewed from facial, triangles.
C. Maxillary lateral incisors, viewed from mesial, trapezoidal.
D. All mandibular posterior teeth, distal aspect, rhomboidal.

331. Which of the following consists of glucose molecules linked together that act as the structural component of plaque?
A. Fructose
B. Sucrose
C. Levans
D. Dextrans
E. Fructans

332. Hydroxyapatite _____.
A. Is weakened if fluoride is substituted for some of the hydroxyl ions
B. Is a noncrystalline structure
C. If containing carbonate ion becomes more soluble
D. Is composed of calcium and phosphate in a 1:1 ratio

333. Tooth enamel is derived from _____.
A. Endoderm
B. Mesoderm

C. Ectoderm

D. Endoderm and mesoderm

E. Ectoderm and mesoderm

334. Which portion of uriniferous tubules contains squamous epithelial cells?

A. Proximal convoluted tubule

B. Thick descending limb of Henle's loop

C. Thin segment of Henle's loop

D. Thick ascending segment of Henle's loop

E. Distal convoluted tubule

335. Which of the following enzymes found in the liver is involved in gluconeogenesis during the postabsorptive state?

A. Glucose-6-phosphate dehydrogenase

B. Phosphogluconate dehydrogenase

C. Glucose-6-phosphatase

D. Glucokinase

336. The heights of contour of the distal surfaces of permanent mandibular central incisors are located in which coronal third?

A. Middle

B. Cervical

C. Occlusal

D. Incisal

337. Accumulation of fluid in the pericardium occurs *most* often with which of the following conditions?

A. Unstable angina

B. Cardiomyopathy

C. Myocarditis

D. Acute pericarditis

E. Tamponade

338. The correct order of tooth formation is _____.

A. Ameloblasts form, odontoblasts form, ameloblasts start to form enamel, odontoblasts start to form dentin

B. Ameloblasts form, odontoblasts form, odontoblasts start to form dentin, ameloblasts start to form enamel

C. Odontoblasts form, odontoblasts start to form dentin, ameloblasts form, ameloblasts start to form enamel

D. Ameloblasts form, ameloblasts start to form enamel, odontoblasts form, odontoblasts start to form dentin

E. Odontoblasts form, ameloblasts form, odontoblasts start to form dentin, ameloblasts start to form enamel

339. Reduction division occurs during the _____.

A. First stage of mitosis

B. Second stage of mitosis

C. First stage of meiosis

D. Second stage of meiosis

E. Third stage of meiosis

340. All of the following factors play a role in the virulence of the microbe that causes whooping cough *except* one. Which one is the *exception*?

A. IgA protease

B. Hemagglutinin

C. Exotoxin

D. Capsule

E. Pili

341. The minimum volume of air that remains in the lungs after a maximal expiration is termed the _____.

A. Tidal volume

B. Functional residual capacity

C. Residual volume

D. Vital capacity

342. From a mesial perspective, the primary maxillary first molar has which of the following characteristics?

A. Pronounced convexity on the buccal outline of the cervical third

B. The cervical line mesially shows some curvature in an apical direction

C. The dimension at the occlusal third is the same as at the cervical third

D. The mesiobuccal cusp is longer and sharper than the mesiolingual cusp

343. The embryo develops from the _____.

A. The entire blastocyst

B. The entire trophoblast

C. The embryonic disc

D. The extraembryonic coelom

E. The morula

344. Which primary tooth is generally accepted as the first to erupt, and at about what mean age does it erupt?

A. Maxillary central incisor; 8 to 12 months

B. Maxillary central incisor; 7 to 9 months

C. Mandibular central incisor; 6 to 10 months

D. Mandibular central incisor; 8 to 10 months

345. Blood levels of progesterone are highest during _____.

A. The follicular phase of the ovarian cycle

B. The luteal phase of the ovarian cycle

C. Ovulation

D. Menstruation

346. The _____ of the heart is also known as the mitral valve.

A. Right atrioventricular valve

B. Left atrioventricular valve

C. Pulmonary valve

D. Aortic valve

E. Tricuspid valve

347. The most common cause of death in diabetic patients is _____.

A. Peripheral neuropathy

B. Pancreatic cancer

C. Cardiovascular disease

D. Kidney failure

E. Opportunistic infections

348. For the tooth indicated, at what time is the crown completed?

A. Primary maxillary central incisor; 3 weeks
B. Permanent maxillary central incisor; 2 to 3 years
C. Primary maxillary lateral incisor; 2 to 3 months
D. Permanent maxillary lateral incisor; 2 to 3 years

349. The Y-shaped central developmental groove is most likely found on which of the following premolars?
A. Maxillary first
B. Mandibular first
C. Maxillary second
D. Mandibular second

350. The sternal angle between the manubrium and the sternum marks the position of the _____ rib.
A. First
B. Second
C. Third
D. Fourth
E. Fifth

351. Which compound is produced in the hexose monophosphate (pentose phosphate) pathway?
A. Adenosine triphosphate (ATP)
B. Nicotinamide adenine dinucleotide (NADH)
C. Nicotinamide adenine dinucleotide phosphate (NADPH)
D. Fructose-1,6-bisphosphate
E. Phospho*enol*pyruvate

352. Which of the following is the *most* common cause of subacute endocarditis?
A. *Staphylococcus aureus*
B. *Staphylococcus epidermidis*
C. Viridans streptococcus
D. *Streptococcus pyogenes*
E. *Streptococcus pneumoniae*

353. From the occlusal aspect, the primary maxillary first molar has which of the following characteristics? (Choose all that apply.)
A. Crown outline diverges lingually and distally
B. Small transverse ridge frequently present called an *oblique ridge*
C. Four cusps are present
D. Thin and poorly developed mesial marginal ridge

354. Lymph from the mandibular incisors drains chiefly into _____.
A. Submandibular nodes
B. Submental nodes
C. Superficial parotid nodes
D. Deep cervical nodes
E. Occipital nodes

355. Which of the following may be observed in a child with a diagnosis of rickets?
A. Dark pigmentation on the oral mucosa
B. Early eruption of teeth
C. Hutchinson's incisors
D. Abnormal dentin
E. Macroglossia

356. Which of the following coenzymes are involved in the metabolism of pyruvate to acetyl coenzyme A (CoA)?

A. Thiamine pyrophosphate, lipoic acid, flavin adenine dinucleotide (FAD), nicotinamide adenine dinucleotide (NAD), and CoA
B. NAD, tetrahydrofolate, lipoic acid, FAD, and vitamin B_{12}
C. Mg^2, FAD, NAD, and biotin
D. CoA, niacin, FAD, and ascorbic acid

357. The primary mandibular first molar has which of the following characteristics?
A. Resembles other primary and permanent teeth
B. Has a heart-shaped outline from the occlusal perspective
C. Mesiobuccal cusp is smaller than distobuccal cusp
D. No developmental groove is evident between buccal cusps

358. Which of the following muscles attaches to the anterior end of the articular disc of the temporomandibular joint?
A. Superficial head of the medial pterygoid muscle
B. Deep head of the medial pterygoid muscle
C. Superior head of the lateral pterygoid muscle
D. Inferior head of the lateral pterygoid muscle

359. In a cusp-fossa occlusal relationship, the maxillary second premolar is most likely to articulate with which of the following mandibular teeth?
A. First premolar only
B. Second premolar only
C. Canine and first premolar
D. First and second premolars

360. The presence of which of the following in a patient's serum indicates that the patient is a highly infectious hepatitis B carrier?
A. Hepatitis B surface antigen (HBsAg)
B. Hepatitis B surface antibody (HBsAb)
C. Hepatitis B core antigen (HBcAg)
D. Hepatitis B e antigen (HBeAg)
E. Hepatitis B e antibody (HBeAb)

361. Which of the following statements regarding salivary secretion is *true*?
A. In general, saliva is more hypertonic than plasma.
B. As salivary flow increases, bicarbonate concentration decreases.
C. As salivary flow increases, ionic concentration increases.
D. Salivary secretion is regulated primarily by hormonal stimulation.

362. The pulmonary vein of the lung carries _____.
A. Unoxygenated blood from the lungs to the heart
B. Oxygenated blood from the lungs to the heart
C. Unoxygenated blood to the lungs from the heart
D. Oxygenated blood to the lungs from the heart
E. Oxygenated blood from the heart to the lungs

363. _____ vertebrae are characterized by a heart-shaped body.
A. Cervical
B. Thoracic

C. Lumbar

D. Sacral

E. Coccygeal

364. Lipid micelles are stabilized by which of the following?

A. Hydrophobic interactions

B. Hydrophilic interactions

C. Interactions of lipid and water

D. Interaction of hydrophobic lipid tails with hydrophobic domains of proteins

365. HIV binds directly to the surface receptors of CD4 lymphocytes with _____.

A. Reverse transcriptase

B. Integrase

C. Hemagglutinin

D. gp120

E. Protease

366. The maxillary sinus overlies the alveolar processes in particular in what teeth?

A. First and second maxillary molars

B. All maxillary molars

C. First and second premolars

D. First and second premolars and first and second molars

367. If jaw opening is divided into phases, and it is assumed that the surfaces of the articulating bones and disc are associated throughout jaw opening, what is the relationship of the disc and condyle in the following phases?

A. In the earliest phase, the condyle moves forward before the disc.

B. In the early phase, the disc and condyle move anteriorly in concert.

C. In an intermediate phase, the condyle moves forward at a slower rate.

D. In the final phase, the disc moves forward at a faster rate.

368. Endotoxin consists of _____.

A. Lipopolysaccharide

B. M protein

C. Hyaluronidase

D. Lactic acid

E. Coagulase

369. The trochlea of the humerus bone articulates with the _____.

A. Ulna of the forearm

B. Radius of the forearm

C. Coronoid process of the ulna of the forearm

D. Olecranon of the ulna of the forearm

E. Medial epicondyle

370. Increased formation of ketone bodies during fasting is a result of which of the following?

A. Increased oxidation of fatty acids as a source of fuel

B. Decreased formation of acetyl coenzyme A (CoA) in the liver

C. Decreased levels of glucagon

D. Increased glycogenesis in muscle

371. Nucleus ambiguus contains the cell bodies of which of the following cranial nerves?

A. III, IV, and V

B. VII, IX, and X

C. VII, IX, and XI

D. IX, X, and XI

E. IX, X, and XII

372. The participation of calcium in the contraction of skeletal muscle is facilitated or associated with which of the following?

A. Calcium release from sarcoplasmic reticulum

B. Calcium binding to the myosin heads

C. Active transport of calcium out of longitudinal tubules

D. Uptake of calcium by T-tubules

373. What type of vaccine is used for *Clostridium tetani*?

A. Capsular polysaccharides

B. Toxoids

C. Killed bacteria

D. Immunoglobulins

E. No vaccine is available

374. Where is the height of contour located relative to the following teeth (viewed from the mesial)?

A. Facial surfaces of all molars—middle third

B. Lingual surfaces of all premolars and molars—cervical third

C. Lingual surfaces of molars and premolars—cervical or middle third

D. Anterior teeth—cervical or middle third

375. The γ motoneurons control which of the following?

A. Muscle spindles

B. Iris of the eye

C. Voluntary muscle fibers

D. Pyloric sphincter

376. Which of the following organelles is surrounded by a double membrane?

A. Ribosome

B. Golgi apparatus

C. Lysosome

D. Cytoplasmic inclusion

E. Mitochondria

F. Ganglion cells

377. Calcium that enters the cell during smooth muscle excitation binds with which of the following?

A. Calmodulin

B. Inactive myosin kinase

C. Troponin

D. Myosin

E. Actin

378. The lumen of the gastrointestinal tract is lined with _____.

A. Mucosa

B. Submucosa

C. Muscularis externa

D. Fibrosa

E. Adventitia

379. Which one of the following is found on the crown of permanent mandibular first molars but is not found on the crowns of mandibular second molars?

A. Mesiobuccal cusp

B. Distobuccal groove

C. Lingual groove

D. Distobuccal cusp

380. Which of the following mediators aid in the killing of intracellular bacteria?

A. Histamine

B. Interleukin-2

C. Catalase

D. IgG

E. Lysozyme

381. Chromosomes line up at a cell's equator during which phase of mitosis?

A. Telophase

B. Metaphase

C. Interphase

D. Anaphase

E. Prophase

382. Following the production of Okazaki fragments, _____ is required to close the gap between the fragments.

A. DNA ligase

B. DNA polymerase

C. RNA polymerase

D. Reverse transcriptase

383. The maxillary nerve passes through which of the following?

A. Superior orbital fissure

B. Internal acoustic meatus

C. Foramen ovale

D. Foramen rotundum

E. Foramen spinosum

384. A productive cough may be seen in all of the following conditions *except* one. Which one is the *exception*?

A. Pneumonia

B. Lung abscess

C. Bronchiectasis

D. Asthma

E. Bronchogenic carcinoma

385. For each type of tooth, the primary teeth consistently show which of the following characteristics?

A. Greater mesiodistal diameter relative to crown height than permanent teeth

B. Elongated appearance of the primary crowns and roots

C. Crowns that are translucent white in color

D. Root trunk one half of crown height

386. All of the following are rotator cuff muscles except *one*. Which one is the *exception*?

A. Supraspinatous muscle

B. Infraspinatous muscle

C. Teres minor muscle

D. Teres major muscle

E. Subscapularis muscle

387. Which of the following does *not* affect the muscle tension produced during contraction?

A. Extent of motor unit recruitment

B. Proportion of each single motor unit that is stimulated to contract

C. Number of muscle fibers contracting

D. Frequency of stimulation

388. Cytochrome P-450 enzymes may be found in which of the following cellular organelles?

A. Mitochondria

B. Golgi apparatus

C. Lysosome

D. Ribosome

E. Endoplasmic reticulum

389. A patient has a heart rate of 70 beats/min. End-diastolic volume is 140 mL. End-systolic volume is 30 mL. Calculate the cardiac output of this individual.

A. 9800 mL

B. 2100 mL

C. 7700 mL

D. 15,400 mL

390. Which premolar would be the *most* likely to have a single pulp horn?

A. Maxillary first

B. Mandibular first

C. Mandibular second

D. Maxillary second

391. Which of the following microorganisms produce dipicolinic acid?

A. *Actinomycetes*

B. *Histoplasma*

C. *Streptococcus*

D. *Staphylococcus*

E. *Clostridium*

392. Which of the following describes the function of RNA polymerase?

A. Translates DNA into protein

B. Terminates transcription

C. Removes introns during transcription

D. Synthesizes RNA 5′ → 3′

393. Which of the following bones is formed by intramembranous ossification?

A. Humerus

B. Lumbar vertebrae

C. Frontal bone of the skull

D. Ribs

E. Clavicle

394. The pressure in a capillary in skeletal muscle is 37 mm Hg at the arteriolar end and 16 mm Hg at the venular end. The interstitial pressure is 0 mm Hg. The

colloid osmotic pressure is 26 mm Hg in the capillary and 1 mm Hg in the interstitial fluid. The net force producing fluid movement across the capillary wall is which of the following?
A. 1 mm Hg out of the capillary
B. 3 mm Hg out of the capillary
C. 12 mm Hg out of the capillary
D. 3 mm Hg into the capillary

395. Which of the following forms of thyroid hormone is most readily found in the circulation?
A. Triiodothyronine (T_3)
B. Thyroxine (T_4)
C. Thyroglobulin
D. Thyroid-stimulating hormone (TSH)

396. Dust cells can be found in the _____.
A. Brain
B. Heart
C. Lungs
D. Liver
E. Spleen

397. The lateral thoracic wall of the axilla is covered by which of the following muscles?
A. Pectoralis major
B. Pectoralis minor
C. Serratus anterior
D. Subscapularis
E. Latissimus dorsi

398. Carbon dioxide (CO_2) generated in the tissues is carried in venous blood primarily in which form?
A. CO_2 in the plasma
B. H_2CO_3 in the plasma
C. HCO_3^- in the plasma
D. CO_2 in the red blood cells
E. Carboxyhemoglobin in the red blood cells

399. Oral epithelium is composed of _____ epithelium.
A. Keratinized simple squamous
B. Keratinized stratified squamous
C. Nonkeratinized simple squamous
D. Nonkeratinized stratified squamous
E. Nonkeratinized stratified columnar

400. Chondroitin sulfate is a major component of which of the following?
A. Bacterial cell walls
B. Mucin
C. IgA
D. Cartilage
E. Hair

401. The left subclavian artery arises _____.
A. Directly from the arch of the aorta
B. From the brachiocephalic trunk
C. From the common carotid artery
D. From the external carotid artery
E. From the internal carotid artery

402. The superior sagittal sinus is the site of reabsorption of what fluid?
A. Thoracic duct fluid
B. Exocrine pancreas fluid
C. Cerebrospinal fluid
D. Primary submandibular gland fluid
E. Common bile duct fluid

403. To what nerve does the chorda tympani join before it enters the submandibular gland?
A. Greater petrosal
B. Inferior alveolar
C. Tensor veli palatini
D. Lingual
E. Auriculotemporal

404. The pterygomandibular space is the site of what injection?
A. Inferior alveolar nerve block
B. Mental nerve block
C. Infraorbital nerve block
D. Greater palatine nerve block
E. Nasopalatine nerve block

405. The squamosal suture joins what two bones?
A. Zygoma and frontal
B. Parietal and temporal
C. Sphenoid and frontal
D. Occipital and parietal
E. Right parietal and left parietal

406. The anterior border of trapezius muscle forms which anatomic site?
A. The posterior border of the anterior triangle of the neck
B. The posterior border of the posterior triangle of the neck
C. The anterior border of the posterior triangle of the neck
D. The anterior border of the posterior triangle of the neck
E. None of the above

407. The twelfth cranial nerve (hypoglossal) supplies motor innervations to which muscle or muscles?
A. Heart
B. Masseter
C. Muscles of the tongue
D. Brachialis
E. Orbicularis oris

408. Which vein of the arm is the preferred site for venipuncture for purposes of a long-term venous drip?
A. Cephalic vein
B. Median antebrachial vein
C. Median cubital vein
D. Basilic vein
E. Dorsal venous arch

409. What type of collagen is found in teeth?
A. I
B. II
C. III
D. IV
E. None of the above

410. Which of the following nerves passes through the parotid gland?
    A. Superior alveolar
    B. Inferior alveolar
    C. Hypoglossal
    D. Glossopharyngeal
    E. Facial

411. In the citric acid cycle beginning with oxaloacetate, which of the following is produced last?
    A. α-Ketoglutarate
    B. Malate
    C. Citrate
    D. Succinate
    E. Fumarate
    F. Isocitrate

412. Pernicious anemia and neurologic degeneration are characteristic of lack of _____.
    A. Vitamin C
    B. Vitamin K
    C. Vitamin B_{12}
    D. Vitamin B_1
    E. Vitamin D

413. From the following list, select the secretions produced by cells other than those from the pancreas. (Choose all that apply.)
    A. Hydrogen chloride
    B. HCO_3^-
    C. Pepsinogen
    D. Lipase
    E. Amylase
    F. Chymotrypsinogen
    G. Enterokinase

414. From the following categories of taste flavors, which have been identified as acting via closing of ion channels? (Choose all that apply.)
    A. Bitter
    B. Sweet
    C. Sour
    D. Salty
    E. Umami

415. Identify all of the following that are *not* part of the cytosol. (Choose all that apply.)
    A. Nucleolus
    B. Aqueous area between the plasma membrane and endoplasmic reticulum
    C. Aqueous content of the endoplasmic reticulum
    D. Catalytic enzyme–rich fluid of the lysozyme

416. Which one of the following sites is characteristic of rough endoplasmic reticulum?
    A. Site of lipid synthesis
    B. Site of calcium storage
    C. Site of protein synthesis
    D. Site of drug detoxification

417. Which chemical is produced in mitochondria as a result of oxidative phosphorylation?

A. Adenosine monophosphate (AMP)
B. Lysozyme
C. Adenosine diphosphate (ADP)
D. Adenosine triphosphate (ATP)
E. Adenosine

418. Which of the following are characteristics of adenosine triphosphate (ATP)? (Choose all that apply.)
    A. Metabolized to cyclic adenosine monophosphate (cAMP)
    B. Metabolized to guanosine triphosphate (GTP)
    C. The universal currency of biochemical energy
    D. Involved in kinase reactions
    E. Is an enzyme

419. From Z-disk to Z-disk defines _____.
    A. The length of the Golgi apparatus
    B. A T tubule
    C. The length of a thin filament
    D. A sarcomere

420. Which one of the following lipoprotein particles is responsible for transporting excess cholesterol back to the liver?
    A. Very-low-density lipoprotein
    B. Low-density lipoprotein
    C. High-density lipoprotein
    D. Chylomicron

421. The presence of the injectisome or injectosome system in some bacteria is considered to facilitate virulence and invasion of the host. Why?
    A. Microbes use this method of export to secrete the quorum-sensing autoinducer into the surrounding environment, facilitating host cell death.
    B. Microbes use this system to insert bacterial proteins into the eukaryotic cell, facilitating an invasion.
    C. Microbes use this system to facilitate global regulation of bacterial processes through the export of quorum-sensing molecules.
    D. Microbes use this system to facilitate global regulation of the microbiome of the host.

422. What substance is commonly associated with mucosal surfaces, whose primary mode of activity is to protect the host by preventing the microbe or pathogen from adhering to the mucosal surfaces?
    A. IgA
    B. IgG
    C. IgM
    D. Interleukin-1

423. Which of the following characteristics apply to chlorhexidine? (Choose all that apply.)
    A. Effective against several gram-positive and gram-negative bacteria
    B. Has a persistent antimicrobial effect
    C. Has a sporicidal effect after 10 minutes

D. Can be used in oral rinses

E. Is the most effective cold disinfectant agent for dental instruments

424. Which term applies to a malignant neoplasm of bone?

A. Adenocarcinoma

B. Melanoma

C. Astrocytoma

D. Osteosarcoma

E. Myeloma

425. What are characteristics of squamous papilloma? (Choose all that apply.)

A. Often leads to squamous cell carcinoma

B. Has fingerlike projections

C. Invades underlying tissue

D. May be pedunculated

E. A benign neoplasm

426. A platelet count of 15,000 platelets/μL would have what effect in a patient? (Choose all that apply.)

A. Normal prothrombin time (PT)

B. Normal partial thromboplastin time (PTT)

C. Normal bleeding tendency

D. Likelihood of petechiae

E. A slightly above normal platelet count

427. What are characteristics of plasma cell myeloma (multiple myeloma)? (Choose all that apply.)

A. Malignant condition

B. Produces functional immunoglobulins

C. Bence-Jones proteins are found in the urine

D. Radiographic findings include "punched-out" radiolucencies in bones

E. Usually arises in the bone marrow

428. An adult patient has the following signs and symptoms: weight gain, enlarged face and tongue, mental and physical slowness, decreased heart rate, and sensitivity to cold temperatures. What is the most likely disorder associated with these conditions?

A. Hyperthyroidism

B. Diabetes insipidus

C. Hereditary hypercholesterolemia

D. Asthma

E. Myxedema

429. Myasthenia gravis is a disorder that is usually caused by _____.

A. Trauma to a specific skeletal muscle

B. Trauma to the central nervous system

C. Autoimmune factors

D. Excessive sympathetic stimulation

E. Trauma to a nerve or nerves to skeletal muscle

430. Wickham's striae and saw-tooth rete ridges are observed in which condition?

A. Pemphigoid of the mucous membrane

B. Lichen planus

C. Erythema multiforme

D. Peutz-Jeghers syndrome

E. Psoriasis

431. Assuming a cusp/fossa/cusp fossa occlusal contact relationship, the distal buccal cusp of tooth #31 supports which centric stop?

A. Central fossa #2

B. Central fossa #3

C. Central fossa #30

D. Central fossa #31

E. Distal triangular fossa #29

432. Assuming a cusp/fossa/cusp fossa occlusal contact relationship, the distal lingual cusp of tooth #3 supports which centric stop?

A. Central fossa #30

B. Central fossa #31

C. Distal triangular fossa #29

D. Mesial triangular fossa #5

E. Distal triangular fossa #30

433. Regarding emergence of primary teeth, which tooth's (universal system) normal emergence is last?

A. Tooth A

B. Tooth B

C. Tooth C

D. Tooth D

E. Tooth E

F. Tooth P

G. Tooth Q

H. Tooth R

I. Tooth S

J. Tooth T

434. Regarding temporomandibular joint (TMJ) action, minimum horizontal axis rotation with maximum translation anteriorly for both left and right TMJs would lead to what mandibular movement or position?

A. Maximum opening

B. Right laterotrusive

C. Left laterotrusive

D. Maximum protrusive

E. Centric relation contact

435. The junction of mesial, buccal, and occlusal tooth surfaces is an example of _____.

A. Line angle

B. Cementoenamel junction

C. Point angle

D. Sulcus

E. Triangular ridge

436. Identify the structure in the temporomandibular joint that is located most anteriorly.

A. Posterior attachment

B. Superior head of lateral pterygoid muscle

C. Anterior band

D. Bilaminar zone

E. Posterior band

F. Intermediate zone

437. Which of the following are characteristics of primary teeth compared with permanent teeth? (Choose all that apply.)

A. Smaller in overall size and crown dimensions
B. Darker in color
C. Molar roots more widely flared
D. Smaller pulp chambers
E. More prominent cervical ridges

438. The first evidence of calcification of permanent tooth #3 typically occurs at what age?
A. At birth
B. 3 to 4 months
C. 4 to 5 months
D. $1\frac{1}{2}$ to $1\frac{3}{4}$ years
E. 2 to $2\frac{1}{4}$ years

439. What is the largest cusp of the primary first maxillary molar?
A. Mesiolingual
B. Distolingual
C. Mesiobuccal
D. Distobuccal

440. Which muscle is located deep to and almost parallel to the masseter muscle?
A. Temporalis
B. Buccinator
C. Medial pterygoid
D. Lateral pterygoid

Answer Key for Section 1

1. **A.** The inferior head of the lateral pterygoid muscle attaches to the lateral surface of the lateral pterygoid plate of the sphenoid bone. Its superior head attaches to the infratemporal crest of the greater wing of the sphenoid bone. The deep fibers of the medial pterygoid muscle attach to the medial surface of the lateral pterygoid plate.

2. **D.** The palatopharyngeus forms the posterior tonsillar pillar. It also functions to close off the nasopharynx and larynx during swallowing. The anterior tonsillar pillar is formed by the palatoglossus.

3. **E.** The superior and inferior ophthalmic veins drain into the facial vein and cavernous sinus.

4. **C.** The masseter originates from the inferior border of the zygomatic arch; specifically, its superficial head and deep head originate from the anterior two thirds and posterior one third of the inferior border, respectively. Its superficial head inserts into the lateral surface of the angle of the mandible; its deep head inserts into the ramus and body of the mandible.

5. **A.** Lateral cricoarytenoid. The oblique and transverse arytenoids and thyroarytenoid also adduct the vocal folds. The posterior cricoarytenoid abducts the vocal cords. The cricothyroid muscle raises the cricoid cartilage and tenses the vocal cords.

6. **A.** The site of cell division (mitosis) occurs in the stratum basale (basal layer, stratum germinativum) of oral epithelium.

7. **D.** After branching from the mandibular nerve (CN V_3), the auriculotemporal nerve travels posteriorly and encircles the middle meningeal artery, remaining posterior and medial to the condyle. It continues up toward the TMJ, external ear, and temporal region, passing through the parotid gland and traveling with the superficial temporal artery and vein.

8. **C.** Intercalated discs are found only in cardiac muscle. Multiple, peripherally positioned nuclei are found in the fibers of skeletal muscle. Smooth muscle cells are spindle-shaped.

9. **C.** The hypoglossal nerve (CN XII) is not found in the posterior triangle; however, it is present in the submandibular triangle. Contents of the posterior triangle include the external jugular and subclavian veins and their tributaries, the subclavian artery and its branches, branches of the cervical plexus, CN XI, nerves to the upper limb and muscles of the triangle floor, the phrenic nerve, and the brachial plexus.

10. **C.** Deoxygenated blood from the transverse sinus drains to the sigmoid sinus, which empties into the internal jugular veins. The transverse sinuses receive blood from the confluence of sinuses, which is located in the posterior cranium.

11. **A.** The vestigial cleft of Rathke's pouch is located between the anterior and posterior lobes—specifically, between the pars intermedia and anterior lobe. It consists of cystlike spaces (Rathke's cysts) and represents the vestigial lumen of Rathke's pouch.

12. **B.** The thymus is active at birth and increases in size until puberty (around age 12), after which it gradually atrophies and is replaced by fatty tissue.

13. **C.** The internal carotid artery is joined to the posterior cerebral artery via the posterior communicating artery, which is part of the circle of Willis.

14. **D.** It is a branch of the maxillary nerve (CN V_2). The maxillary nerve branches from the trigeminal ganglion and exits the skull through the foramen rotundum. When it reaches the pterygopalatine ganglion, it terminates as the infraorbital and zygomatic nerves.

15. **A.** Of the cell types listed, only smooth muscle cells are capable of cell division.

16. **C.** The acinar units of salivary glands are lined by simple cuboidal epithelium. This type of epithelium also lines the bronchioles, thyroid gland, and ovary capsule.

17. **B.** The tendon of the tensor tympani is attached to the handle of the malleus in the middle ear. Loud sounds cause the tensor tympani to contract, pulling the malleus and tympanic membrane inward to reduce vibrations and prevent damage.

18. **C.** The ratio of inorganic to organic matter in mature dentin is approximately $70:30$. In enamel and cementum, it is approximately $96:4$ and $50:50$, respectively.

19. **D.** Oligodendrocytes produce the myelin sheath around myelinated axons in the CNS. Schwann's cells make up the myelin sheath around myelinated axons in the autonomic nervous system.

20. **D.** The facial nerve supplies taste sensation to the anterior two thirds of the tongue, via one of its branches, the chorda tympani (see Figure 1-8).

The chorda tympani branches from the facial nerve, carrying both sensory fibers for taste and preganglionic parasympathetic fibers. It exits from of the temporal bone to join the lingual nerve (a branch of CN V_3) as it courses inferiorly toward the submandibular ganglion. Postganglionic parasympathetic fibers emerge from the ganglion and continue toward the sublingual and submandibular glands. Sensory fibers also branch from the nerve and provide taste sensation to the anterior two thirds of the tongue.

21. **B.** Oblique alveolodental fibers resist occlusal forces that occur along the long axis of the tooth. The rest of the alveolodental (PDL) fibers listed provide resistance against forces that pull the tooth in an occlusal direction (i.e., forces that try to pull the tooth from its socket).

22. **A.** When pulpal nerves are stimulated, they can transmit only one signal: pain.

23. **C.** The mylohyoid muscle forms the floor of the mouth. Relaxation of this muscle would help the dentist push the film down, to help ensure that the apical root is captured on the radiograph.

24. **B.** Fibers of the lateral pterygoid muscle are attached to the anterior end of the disc. Contraction of this muscle pulls the disc in an anterior and medial direction.

25. **B.** The sensory distribution for the maxillary nerve (CN V_2) includes the cheek, upper lip, lower eyelid, nasopharynx, tonsils, palate, and maxillary teeth. The sensory distribution for the long buccal also includes the (lower) cheek; however, it does not include the upper lip. The long buccal is a branch of the mandibular nerve (CN V_3) and provides sensory nerves to the cheek, buccal gingiva of the posterior mandibular teeth, and buccal mucosa.

26. **A.** The IAN courses between the sphenomandibular ligament and the ramus of the mandible before entering the mandibular foramen. The sphenomandibular ligament may be damaged during the administration of an IAN block.

27. **C.** The lateral thoracic wall of the axilla is covered by the serratus anterior muscle. The anterior wall is covered by pectoralis major and pectoralis minor. Latissimus dorsi contributes to the inferior aspect of the posterior wall.

28. **A.** The trochlea of the humerus articulates with the ulna of the forearm. The capitulum of the humerus bone articulates with the radius of the forearm. The coronoid fossa, located just superior to the trochlea, fits the coronoid process of the ulna of the forearm. The olecranon fossa of the humerus fits the olecranon of the ulna of the forearm. The medial epicondyle is on the humerus itself and serves as an attachment site for muscles.

29. **C.** The trapezius muscle is supplied by CN XI. The latissimus dorsi is supplied by the thoracodorsal nerve, the levator scapulae is supplied by the dorsal scapular nerve, and the major and minor rhomboid muscles are supplied by the dorsal scapular nerve.

30. **C.** There are seven pairs of true ribs, meaning they attach directly to the sternum via costal cartilages. The remaining five pairs are called false ribs because they attach indirectly to the sternum via costal cartilages. The last pair does not attach at all.

31. **B.** Thoracic vertebrae are characterized by a heart-shaped body.

32. **B.** The sternal angle between the manubrium and the sternum marks the position of the second rib. From this location, ribs can be counted externally. This is important because the first rib cannot be palpated.

33. **D.** The rectus abdominis muscle of the anterolateral abdominal wall is described as being beltlike or straplike. The remaining three muscles of the anterolateral abdominal wall (external oblique muscle, internal oblique muscle, and transversus abdominis muscle) all are described as sheetlike. The quadratus lumborum muscle is part of the posterior abdominal wall.

34. **D.** The posterior and anterior vagal trunks pass through the diaphragm through the esophageal opening. The aorta enters the diaphragm through the median arch, the inferior vena cava through its own opening in the central tendon, the azygos vein through the right crus, and the splanchnic nerves through the crura.

35. **C.** The inferior aspect of the diaphragm is supplied with blood by the inferior phrenic arteries. The median sacral artery supplies the anterior aspect of the sacral area, and the lumbar arteries supply the lower abdominal wall. The celiac trunk and superior mesenteric arteries are unpaired branches to the gut and associated glands.

36. **D.** Oral epithelium is composed of nonkeratinized, stratified, squamous epithelium.

37. **D.** The cartilage of the trachea is covered by a perichondrium. The mucosa is covered with respiratory epithelium. Hyaline cartilage rings lie deep to the submucosa. The open end of the cartilage faces the posterior. Smooth muscle extends across the open end of each cartilage.

38. **B.** Terminal bronchioles are characterized by ciliated cuboidal cells.

39. **E.** The most superficial layer of the epidermis is the stratum corneum. From deep to superficial, the layers are basale, spinosum, granulosum, lucidum, and corneum.

40. **D.** Langerhans' cells are located primarily in stratum spinosum.

41. B. Arteriovenous anastomoses in deeper skin are important in thermoregulation.

42. C. The frontal bone of the skull is formed by intramembranous ossification. The humerus, vertebrae, ribs, and clavicle all are formed by endochondral ossification.

43. B. Osteocytes are found in lacunae in mature bone.

44. B. Epiphyseal closure marks the end of growth in length of long bones.

45. B. The branchial arches disappear when the second arch grows down to contact the fifth branchial arch.

46. B. Facial nerves are derived from the second branchial arch. The trigeminal nerve is derived from the first branchial arch.

47. E. In the liver, smooth endoplasmic reticulum is involved in glycogen metabolism and detoxification of various drugs and alcohols; it contains P450 enzymes, which are cytochromes that are important in the detoxification process.

48. A. Type I collagen is the predominant collagen found in cementum. Type III collagen may be present during the formation of cementum, but it is largely reduced during maturation.

49. B. In smooth muscle, the binding of calcium to calmodulin activates the enzyme myosin light chain kinase. This enzyme phosphorylates myosin, allowing it to bind to actin, and the muscle contracts. For contraction in skeletal and cardiac muscle, calcium binds to troponin C.

50. B. The mandibular incisors as well as the lower lip, floor of the mouth, tip of the tongue, and chin primarily drain into the submental nodes. The rest of the mandibular teeth (premolars and molars) mainly drain into the submandibular nodes.

51. C. Fibers of the superior head of the lateral pterygoid muscle attach to the anterior end of the disc, which helps to balance and stabilize the disc during mouth closure.

52. B. The submental artery is a branch of the facial artery. Branches of the mandibular division of the maxillary artery include the inferior alveolar, deep auricular, anterior tympanic, mylohyoid, incisive, mental, and middle meningeal arteries.

53. D. The maxillary nerve (CN V_2) exits the skull through the foramen rotundum. It passes through the pterygopalatine fossa, where it communicates with the pterygopalatine ganglion. Contents of the superior orbital fissure include CN III, CN IV, CN V_1, and CN VI and the ophthalmic veins. CN VII and CN VIII pass through the internal acoustic meatus, and CN V_3 (mandibular nerve) passes through the foramen ovale. The foramen spinosum is not associated with any cranial nerves; it contains the middle meningeal vessels.

54. E. The abducens nerve (CN VI) provides innervation to the lateral rectus muscle, which moves the eyeball laterally (i.e., abducts the eye). The medial rectus muscle, which is innervated by the oculomotor nerve (CN III), is responsible for adduction of the eyeball.

55. D. The nucleus ambiguus is found in the medulla of the brainstem. It contains the cell bodies of motor neurons for CN IX, CN X, and CN XI. The cell bodies of sensory neurons of CN VII, CN IX, and CN X are contained in the nucleus of the solitary tract.

56. A. The articulating surfaces of the TMJ are covered with fibrocartilage, directly overlying periosteum. The nonarticulating surfaces of the TMJ are covered with periosteum. The articulating surfaces of diarthrodial joints are covered with hyaline cartilage.

57. C. The mesencephalic nucleus contains the nuclei of the trigeminal sensory nerves (CN V) involved in proprioception and the jaw jerk reflex, including PDL fibers involved in the reflex. It is located in the midbrain and pons.

58. D. The red pulp of the spleen consists of cords, containing numerous macrophages, and venous sinusoids. It is the site of blood filtration. The white pulp of the spleen contains numerous T and B lymphocytes.

59. B. The two vertebral arteries join together at the border of the pons to form the basilar artery. Branches of the basilar provide blood supply to the pons.

60. D. Calcitonin is secreted by parafollicular cells (clear cells) that are located at the periphery of thyroid follicles in the thyroid gland. Calcitonin plays an important role in the regulation of calcium and phosphates. It suppresses bone reabsorption, resulting in decreased calcium and phosphate release.

61. B. During metaphase, mitotic spindles form. Chromosomes attach to these spindles, with their centromeres aligned with the equator of the cell.

62. B. The oropharynx is lined by stratified squamous epithelium. This type of epithelium also lines the oral cavity, laryngopharynx, esophagus, vaginal canal, and anal canal.

63. E. Mitochondria are surrounded by a double (inner and outer) membrane. The nuclear membrane (not listed), which surrounds the nucleus, also consists of a double (inner and outer) membrane.

64. A. The medulla of the thymus contains Hassall's corpuscles, which consist of epithelial cells with keratohyaline granules. The medulla is the lighter staining (less dense) central area of the gland, where maturation of T cells occurs.

65. **B.** The fovea centralis contains only cone cells. It is located approximately 2.5 mm lateral to the optic disc in a yellow-pigmented area (macula luna). Vision is most acute from this area.

66. **C.** The roof of the orbit consists of the lesser wing of the sphenoid bone and the orbital plate of the frontal bone (not listed).

67. **D.** The elongation and overgrowth of filiform papillae results in hairy tongue. Filiform papillae are thin, pointy projections that make up the most numerous papillae and gives the tongue's dorsal surface its characteristic rough texture. Note: a loss of filiform papillae results in glossitis.

68. **B.** Tertiary dentin, or reactive or reparative dentin, is dentin that is formed in localized areas in response to trauma or other stimuli, such as caries, tooth wear, or dental work. Histologically, its consistency and organization vary; it has no defined dentinal tubule pattern.

69. **E.** Innervation to the maxillary second molar as well as the palatal and distobuccal root of the maxillary first molar and the maxillary sinus is provided by the posterior superior alveolar nerve. The nerve is a branch of the maxillary nerve (CN V_2).

70. **D.** The suprarenal glands secrete epinephrine. Specifically, chromaffin cells of the adrenal medulla, which act as modified postganglionic sympathetic neurons that synthesize, store, and secrete catecholamines, produce epinephrine. It also produces norepinephrine.

71. **D.** The teres major muscle is a shoulder muscle; however, it is not a rotator muscle. All of the other options listed in this question are rotator cuff muscles.

72. **D.** The brachial plexus of nerves arises from five roots from the anterior primary rami of spinal nerves C5 through C8 and T1.

73. **B.** The right subclavian artery arises from the brachiocephalic artery, and the left subclavian artery arises from the aortic arch. The subclavian artery becomes the axillary artery on crossing the first rib. The axillary artery becomes the brachial artery when it leaves the axilla.

74. **B.** The pulmonary vein of the lung carries oxygenated blood from the lungs to the left atrium of the heart. The pulmonary artery carries unoxygenated blood from the right ventricle of the heart to the lungs.

75. **B.** The left atrioventricular valve of the heart is also known as the mitral valve. The right atrioventricular valve of the heart is also known as the tricuspid valve. The aortic valve prevents regurgitation of blood from the aorta back into the left ventricle, and the pulmonary valve prevents regurgitation of blood from the pulmonary artery back into the right ventricle.

76. **C.** The cricopharyngeus muscle prevents swallowing air at the pharyngeal end of the esophagus.

77. **A.** The pancreas is enveloped at its head by the first part of the duodenum.

78. **A.** The bile canaliculi drain bile to interlobular ducts. The interlobular ducts form right and left hepatic ducts. These ducts join to form the common hepatic duct. The gallbladder arises from the common hepatic duct.

79. **C.** The apex of a medullary pyramid in the kidney is called the renal papilla. The cortex is the outer layer of the kidney. The medulla is the inner layer. Minor calyces receive secretions from the renal papillae. Several minor calyces join to form a major calyx.

80. **D.** Ureters travel inferiorly just below the parietal peritoneum of the posterior body wall. They pass anterior to the common iliac arteries as they enter the pelvis.

81. **A.** The lumen of the gastrointestinal tract is lined with mucosa. The rest of the choices are in order from lumen out. Fibrosa and adventitia are synonymous.

82. **A.** GALT produces secretory IgA.

83. **B.** The muscularis externa has a third layer in the stomach. It is an inner oblique layer of smooth muscle. In the rest of the digestive tract, the muscularis externa has two layers, an inner circular layer and an outer longitudinal layer.

84. **C.** The thin segment of Henle's loop contains squamous epithelial cells. The proximal convoluted tubule (also known as the thick descending limb of Henle's loop), the thick ascending segment of Henle's loop, and the distal convoluted tubule all consist of cuboidal epithelial cells.

85. **E.** The macula densa is a component of the juxtaglomerular apparatus that functions in regulation of blood pressure. The proximal convoluted tubule, distal convoluted tubule, Bowman's capsule, and glomerulus all function in the production of urine.

86. **E.** Urinary filtrate is most hypotonic in the distal convoluted tubule. It is isotonic in the proximal convoluted tubule and thick descending limb of Henle's loop. It becomes hypertonic as it passes through the thin descending limb of Henle's loop and becomes hypotonic as it passes through the thick ascending segment of Henle's loop. Finally, it becomes increasingly hypotonic as it passes through the distal convoluted tubule.

87. **C.** The inner enamel epithelium in the bell stage differentiates into ameloblasts.

88. **B.** The dental lamina arises from neural crest cells.

89. **B.** The correct order of tooth formation is ameloblasts form, odontoblasts form, odontoblasts start to form dentin, ameloblasts start to form enamel.

90. C. The auricular hillocks are derived from the first and second branchial arches.

91. C. Reduction division occurs during the first stage of meiosis. The second stage mirrors mitosis. There is no third stage of meiosis.

92. C. The embryo develops from the embryonic disc. The morula, blastocyst, and trophoblast all include structures of the extraembryonic coelom that lead to development of the amnion, vitelline sac, and chorion.

93. C. Tooth enamel is derived from ectoderm. Dentin and pulp are derived from mesoderm.

94. C. The olecranon fossa is located on the posterior surface of the humerus.

95. D. The latissimus dorsi muscle is supplied by the thoracodorsal nerve.

96. C. The middle trunk of the brachial plexus of nerves arises from C7.

97. A. The first rib cannot be palpated.

98. B. Odontogenic infections of a mandibular incisor with an apex below the mylohyoid muscle have the potential to spread to the submental space. If the apex is above the mylohyoid muscle, the infection would spread to the sublingual space. Both of these spaces communicate with the submandibular space.

99. D. From the retropharyngeal space (i.e., "danger space"), odontogenic infections can quickly spread down this space into the thorax (posterior mediastinum) and cause possible death.

100. E. The superior, middle, and inferior constrictor muscles all insert into the median pharyngeal raphe (the superior constrictor muscle was the only one listed); however, their origins differ.

101. B. The brachiocephalic trunk branches off from the aorta and bifurcates into the right subclavian and right common carotid arteries. The left common carotid artery and left subclavian artery branch off separately from the arch of the aorta.

102. C. Cerebrospinal fluid is drained via resorption into the superior sagittal sinus. A narrow canal with cerebrospinal fluid runs the length of the spinal cord. It is continuous with the ventricular system of the brain and is a remnant of the lumen of the embryonic neural tube.

103. C. The juguloomohyoid lymph node along with the jugulodigastric and other lymph nodes of the cervical chain is part of the deep cervical vertical chain of lymph nodes. The entire chain receives afferents from the superficial horizontal ring of lymph nodes, including submental and submandibular nodes, and the deep horizontal ring, including retropharyngeal, paratracheal, pretracheal, prelaryngeal, and infrahyoid nodes.

104. D. The chorda tympani nerve arises from the descending part of the facial nerve (CN VII) and courses forward to enter the middle ear. It crosses anteriorly, over the medial aspect of the tympanic membrane and passes over the medial aspect of the handle of the malleus. It leaves the middle ear through the petrotympanic fissure and enters the infratemporal region below the skull and joins the lingual nerve.

105. B. The masticator space includes the temporal space, infratemporal space, submasseteric space, and pterygomandibular space. The pterygomandibular space is located between the medial pterygoid muscle and mandibular ramus and contains the inferior alveolar nerve, artery, and vein; lingual nerve; and chorda tympani.

106. B. The squamosal suture joins the parietal and temporal bones. The parietal bone articulates with the opposite parietal bone, occipital bone, temporal bone, frontal bone, and greater wing of the sphenoid bone. The temporal bone articulates with the occipital bone, greater wing and body of the sphenoid bone, parietal bone, and zygomatic bone.

107. D. The posterior triangle of the neck is limited posteriorly by the anterior border of the trapezius muscle. The borders are formed by the posterior border of the sternocleidomastoid muscle, anterior border of trapezius muscle, and clavicle.

108. E. The hypoglossal nerve (CN XII) provides motor innervation for all intrinsic and extrinsic muscles of the tongue. It exits from the medulla through the hypoglossal canal and descends in the neck superficial to the carotid sheath. The nerve curves anteriorly and disappears deep to the mylohyoid muscle to enter the floor of the mouth, where it branches to supply the musculature of the tongue.

109. A. The suprascapular nerve arises from the upper trunk of the brachial plexus and passes through the suprascapular notch of the scapula. It is sensory to the shoulder joint.

110. C. In most cases, the median cubital vein is chosen. The dorsal venous arch on the back of the hand is the preferred site for long-term intravenous drips.

111. C. The anterior interventricular artery supplies the interventricular septum. Occlusion of this artery can lead to an infarct that could damage the atrioventricular bundle and cut one or both ventricles from the conducting system. If this happens, the ventricles continue to beat at a reduced rate, a condition known as heart block. Heart block is treatable with surgical placement of a subcutaneous pacemaker.

112. C. The descending aorta descends from vertebral level T4. It turns slightly to the right and comes to lie anterior to the vertebral bodies within the posterior mediastinum. It descends through the posterior mediastinum. The thoracic aorta ends by passing through the diaphragm at T12 to become the abdominal aorta.

113. **E.** The phrenic nerve arises from the neck from spinal nerves C3, C4, and C5. It descends along the anterior surface of the scalenus anterior muscle and enters the thoracic inlet anterior to the subclavian artery. It then descends along the lateral aspect of the mediastinum to the diaphragm.

114. **C.** The quadrate lobe lies between the gallbladder, the ligamentum teres, and the porta hepatis. The left lobe lies to the left of the ligamentum teres and the ligamentum venosum. The right lobe lies to the right of the inferior vena cava and the gallbladder. The caudate lobe lies between the inferior vena cava, the ligamentum venosum, and the porta hepatis.

115. **B.** Type II collagen is found in hyaline cartilage. Type I collagen is found in connective tissues, tendons, ligaments, bone, teeth, and dermis of skin. Type III collagen is found in reticulin fibers. Type IV collagen is found in basement membranes. Collagen fibers are high-molecular-weight proteins that vary in diameter and usually are arranged in bundles.

116. **B.** Cortical bone contains osteons with concentric lamellae accentuated by lacunae, which contain osteocytes.

117. **C.** Polymorphonuclear leukocytes make up about 70% of the circulating leukocytes. Polymorphonuclear leukocytes phagocytize microorganisms and contain granules filled with enzymes such as collagenase or elastase. These enzymes are released and cause tissue destruction when the polymorphonuclear leukocyte cells degranulate.

118. **C.** Because dentin forms before enamel, the odontoblastic process occasionally penetrates the DEJ. These tubules may contain the living process of the odontoblast, which may contribute to the vitality of the DEJ. Enamel spindles are shorter than enamel tufts.

119. **C.** Transseptal fibers extend from the cementum of one tooth to the corresponding area of cementum of the adjacent tooth. This fiber group functions in resistance to the separation of each tooth. Transseptal fibers are found in the mesiodistal plane and are not present in the buccolingual plane.

120. **A.** Fibers of the superior head of the lateral pterygoid muscle originate as fibers from the inferior aspect of the greater wing of the sphenoid. They attach to the anterior portion of the articular disc and anterior aspect of the condylar neck. Most inserting fibers blend with the tendon of the inferior head to insert into the pterygoid fovea of the condylar neck. A smaller number of deeper and more medial fibers insert into the medial aspect of the capsule and disc.

Answer Key for Section 2

1. **B.** Cyclooxygenase includes isoenzymes of prostaglandin endoperoxidase synthase, which is required for the first step in the synthesis of prostaglandins from arachidonic acid. Phospholipase A_2, which is involved in the synthesis of arachidonic acid, is inhibited by nonsteroidal antiinflammatory agents.

2. **A.** The initial rate-limiting reaction involves the removal of six carbons from cholesterol and hydroxylation of the steroid nucleus to produce pregnenolone. Pregnenolone can be further isomerized and oxidized to produce the other steroid hormones.

3. **A.** A micelle is a globular structure that forms when the polar heads of an amphipathic molecule (fatty acids) interact with the aqueous external environment and the nonpolar hydrocarbon tails are clustered inside.

4. **B.** A ketose sugar is one that contains a keto group. Glyceraldehyde, mannose, glucose, and galactose all are aldoses because they contain an aldehyde group.

5. **B.** Individuals with mucopolysaccharidoses have normal production of proteoglycans and glycosaminoglycans but, owing to genetic defects, lack the enzymes that degrade mucopolysaccharides.

6. **E.** Arginine is an amino acid that is deaminated to form ornithine primarily in the liver as part of the urea cycle. Ornithine, argininosuccinate, aspartate, and citrulline are generated in the urea cycle but do not provide free ammonia for urea synthesis.

7. **B.** Both epinephrine and glucagons result in activities that serve to increase (maintain) blood glucose. Activation of glycogen phosphorylase results in glycogen degradation, ultimately providing a source of glucose. Glycogen synthase inhibition results in decreased synthesis of glycogen.

8. **D.** In contrast to noncompetitive inhibition, the inhibitor competes for the same site as the substrate. It is possible (with increased amounts of substrate) to reach the V_{max}. Apparent K_m is increased because more substrate is required to reach $\frac{1}{2} V_{max}$ (the definition of K_m).

9. **C.** NADPH is required as a reducing agent for the synthesis of fatty acids. The hexose monophosphate pathway also produces ribose 5-phosphate for nucleotide synthesis. No ATP or NADH is produced in the pathway. Fructose 1,6-bisphosphate is produced during glycolysis.

10. **D.** Oxidation of fatty acids, glucagon release, and glycogenolysis all are increased to provide energy sources for exercising muscle. The synthesis of lipid (lipogenesis) would be decreased during periods of exercise.

11. **A.** During a fast, catabolism is increased to provide additional sources of energy; this is characterized by increased use of fatty acids. When the production of acetyl CoA (produced by enhanced β-oxidation) exceeds the oxidative capacity of the citric acid cycle, ketone bodies are formed. During fasting conditions, glucagon concentrations are increased, and glycogenesis is inhibited because of limited energy availability. Acetyl CoA production in the liver is increased because of enhanced β-oxidation.

12. **C.** Glucose 6-phosphate dehydrogenase and 6-phosphogluconate dehydrogenase are irreversible enzymes in the pentose phosphate pathway. Glucokinase is involved with phosphorylation of glucose when hepatic concentrations of glucose are high. Glucose 6-phosphatase hydrolyzes glucose 6-phosphate to form free glucose as the final step in gluconeogenesis.

13. **B.** Glucose transport in muscle and adipose tissue is under the influence of insulin-sensitive glucose transporters. Although several metabolic pathways are influenced by insulin, glucose uptake into the liver is not affected by insulin.

14. **D.** Phenylketonuria is an inherited disorder of amino acid metabolism in which the affected individual lacks enzymes to metabolize phenylalanine. Albinism is a condition that results in a defect in tyrosine metabolism and the inability to produce melanin. Porphyria is an inherited disorder involving defects in heme synthesis. Homocystinuria is a disorder in the metabolism of homocysteine resulting in high levels of homocysteine and methionine in plasma and urine.

15. **B.** Guanine base pairs with cytosine, which, on a molar basis, also equals 30% of the DNA. If guanine and cytosine constitute a total of 60% of DNA, the remaining percentage (40%) must be equally divided between the base pairs of adenine and thymine (20% + 20%).

16. **A.** Restriction enzymes are also known as restriction endonucleases. These enzymes cleave DNA at

367

specific sites to release fragments of DNA for further analysis and characterization by complementary probes.

17. **B.** Tetrahydrofolic acid is the coenzyme form of folic acid required for the synthesis of nucleic acids and normal cell division and replication.

18. **A.** DNA ligase is required to ligate the fragments together. DNA and RNA polymerases are catalysts that synthesize DNA and RNA in a continuous process. Reverse transcriptase is an enzyme found in viruses that makes DNA by using viral RNA.

19. **C.** RNA synthesis is not required for genetic cloning. All the other enzymes are required to synthesize and splice DNA.

20. **B.** Vitamin K is involved with the posttranslational modification of glutamic acid to form γ-carboxyglutamic acid. This carboxylation permits prothrombin to interact with platelets and ions in the process of clot formation. Hydroxylation of proline requires ascorbic acid and iron.

21. **D.** Chondroitin sulfate is a glucosaminoglycan found in ligaments, tendons, and cartilage. It is the most abundant glucosaminoglycan in the body.

22. **A.** The α chains are polypeptides that characterize the collagen molecule. The most abundant amino acids in collagen are proline and glycine. Proline (owing to its imino ring structure), interrupts the α chain, resulting in the bending and twisting of the peptide. Glycine (owing to its small size) fits into the smaller spaces of the peptide and is positioned at every third position in the chain.

23. **C.** Although fluoride may be incorporated in mineralized tissues, it is not required for the mineralization process. Matrix vesicles produced by osteoblasts are considered to be the initial site of mineralization. Amelogenins are matrix proteins in enamel that regulate crystallite growth. Phosphoryns are initiator proteins that bind minerals to facilitate nucleation and crystal growth.

24. **E.** The transport of glucose into muscle (and fat) cells is due to the activity of glucose transporters (GLUT-4), which does not require ATP and is independent of any ionic concentration gradient. ATP is required for the activity of all other transport mechanisms listed.

25. **D.** Facilitated diffusion does not require energy and moves down a concentration gradient. Active transport, in addition to using energy, is often coupled to transport ions in both directions across the membrane. Both active transport and facilitated diffusion are carrier-mediated and are influenced by competitive inhibition.

26. **B.** The salivary glands are influenced by both the sympathetic and the parasympathetic (glossopharyngeal and facial) branches of the ANS. The

oculomotor nerve (third cranial nerve) carries parasympathetic fibers to the eye, which, when stimulated, produce constriction of the pupil. The parasympathetic system innervates primarily smooth and cardiac muscle, resulting in specific activation and responses.

27. **B.** Regulation of blood flow to skin is under the control of factors acting locally (metabolites) and α-adrenergic receptors. Slowing of the heart and activation of GI motility are mediated through the cholinergic system. α-Adrenergic receptors produce decreased renal blood flow.

28. **A.** C fibers are the smallest of the sensory and motor fibers. They are postganglionic, are unmyelinated, and have the slowest conduction velocity.

29. **A.** Calcium is stored and released from the sarcoplasmic reticulum during excitation-contraction coupling. This provides an extensive reservoir of calcium, while permitting intracellular free Ca^{2+} to be low when the muscle fiber is at rest. The release of calcium is due to conformational changes that open Ca^{2+} channels in the sarcoplasmic reticulum.

30. **A.** Calmodulin is a calcium-binding protein in smooth muscle, which, when bound to myosin, initiates contraction. Calmodulin activates myosin kinase, which results in myosin-actin cross-linking and contraction of smooth muscle.

31. **B.** A motor unit is composed of a single motoneuron and the muscle fibers it innervates. Because the motoneuron stimulates all muscle fibers it innervates, "fractions" of a motor unit cannot be stimulated. The number of motor units recruited, the number of muscle fibers contracting, and the frequency of stimulation all affect the degree of muscle tension produced.

32. **B.** The sum total of the pressures moving fluid *out* of the capillary is P_c (37 mm Hg) and π_{if} (1 mm Hg) at the arteriolar end and P_c (16 mm Hg) and π_{if} (1 mm Hg) at the venular end. The sum total of the pressures moving *into* the capillary is P_{if} (0 mm Hg) and π_p (26 mm Hg). The net exchange pressure on the arteriolar end leads to ultrafiltration (12 mm Hg). On the venular end, reabsorption occurs (9 mm Hg). Overall net exchange results in 3 mm Hg of fluid loss out of the capillary.

33. **C.** CO is the volume of blood pumped per minute by each ventricle. The CO is influenced by cardiac rate and stroke volume (EDV − ESV). The CO for this patient is 70×110 mL, or 7700 mL/min.

34. **B.** The velocity of blood flow is the rate of displacement of blood per unit time. Velocity changes inversely with cross-sectional area (cm^2). The greater the area in the vessels, the lower the velocity. Because blood is always flowing secondary to

the distensibility of the arterial tree, velocity is never zero.

35. **D.** Decreasing TPR would produce greater reductions in blood pressure. Owing to the baroreceptor reflex, cardiac heart rate would increase. Increased stroke volume (owing to increased venous return and sympathetic stimulation of cardiac muscle) would also occur. Increased CO would occur because of increased heart rate and stroke volume.

36. **C.** Although some CO_2 is transported unchanged in the plasma and in the RBCs as carbaminohemoglobin, most is transported in the form of HCO_3^- in the plasma.

37. **D.** The most potent stimulant of the respiratory center that increases the rate of breathing (hyperventilation) is increased CO_2 tension. CO_2 is permeable to the blood-brain barrier and ultimately produces an increase in H^+ of the cerebrospinal fluid. However, plasma H^+ and HCO_3^- are not permeable and have little direct effect on the respiratory center. The respiratory center is not sensitive to O_2 tension, in contrast to peripheral chemoreceptors.

38. **A.** Hemoglobin is a globular protein responsible for transporting most of the O_2 in the blood. The percent saturation of hemoglobin is a function of the Po_2 of the blood. The relationship of Po_2 and hemoglobin saturation is not linear but rather sigmoid in shape. Percent saturation increases greatly at low Po_2 and less at higher Po_2. Increased Pco_2, temperature, diphosphoglycerate, and H^+ decrease the affinity of hemoglobin for O_2 but do not alter the characteristic sigmoid nature of the saturation curve.

39. **E.** Renal clearance is the volume of plasma completely cleared of a substance by the kidneys per unit of time. The renal clearance of glucose is usually 0 because, although it is filtered, it is completely reabsorbed when the plasma glucose concentration is normal. In an uncontrolled diabetic, plasma glucose levels exceed the reabsorptive capacity (T_m), and glucose appears in the urine. Urea is filtered and passively reabsorbed to a slight degree. Creatinine is both freely filtered and secreted to a slight extent. Sodium and water are filtered and reabsorbed to various degrees secondary to physiologic regulation of aldosterone and ADH.

40. **D.** In the ascending (distal) loop of Henle, active sodium absorption results in an increased osmolarity of the interstitial fluid, which plays a role in the retention of water under conditions of dehydration.

41. **C.** Under conditions of expansion of extracellular volume (long-term hypertension), renin release

and aldosterone secretion are reduced. Increasing ADH, angiotensin II, and increasing sympathetic activity would result in an increase in blood pressure.

42. **D.** Potassium is passively (via the cotransport system) secreted from the plasma into the distal and collecting tubules. Under conditions of acidosis, an individual may become hyperkalemic because the kidneys retain K^+ and secrete H^+. Under conditions of alkalosis, K^+ secretion is increased, and H^+ secretion is reduced.

43. **C.** Saliva is formed by a process that first involves the formation of a solution by the acinar cells, which is subsequently modified by the ductile cells to produce a more hypotonic solution (compared with plasma). The modification primarily involves the reabsorption of sodium and chloride and secretion of potassium and bicarbonate. As salivary flow increases, the ductile cells have less time to modify the composition of saliva, which results in greater concentrations of sodium and chloride ions. Bicarbonate concentration increases as salivary flow increases as a result of the selective stimulation of bicarbonate by the parasympathetic system. The salivary glands are primarily under the regulation of both branches of the ANS.

44. **A.** Secretory IgA is an immunoglobulin that is unique to the oral cavity. The secretory component is synthesized by salivary epithelial cells and complexes with IgA to form secretory IgA.

45. **C.** Vitamins are not digested by enzymes from the pancreas; however, digestion of carbohydrates, fats, and proteins may be required to make vitamins available for absorption. The pancreas produces amylase for carbohydrate digestion, lipase for lipid digestion, and several proteolytic enzymes (trypsinogen, chymotrypsinogen, and procarboxypeptidase) for the digestion of protein.

46. **B.** Secretin stimulates bicarbonate secretion from the pancreatic ducts. CCK is responsible for stimulating pancreatic enzyme secretion and contraction of the gallbladder. Chymotrypsinogen is activated by trypsin in the intestine.

47. **D.** Phospholipase C, activated by a component of the G protein ($G\alpha$) complexed with GTP, catalyzes the production of diacylglycerol and IP_3. Diacylglycerol activates protein kinases, which phosphorylate proteins, and IP_3 produces increased release of calcium from intracellular stores.

48. **D.** Vasopressin, also known as ADH, is a peptide secreted from the posterior pituitary in response to an increase in serum osmolarity. The other hormones listed are synthesized and secreted from the anterior pituitary.

49. **A.** Estrogen is a steroid hormone and does not require a membrane receptor and the second

messenger cAMP. Steroid hormones directly enter the cell and stimulate intracellular receptors. Peptide hormones and hormones derived from single amino acids are not readily lipid-soluble (characteristic of membranes) and require membrane receptors and a second messenger system (e.g., cAMP, IP_3). Many of the effects of epinephrine and norepinephrine and all of the effects of glucagon are mediated by cAMP.

50. **C.** Phosphodiesterases are intracellular enzymes that degrade cyclic nucleotides, catalyzing the hydrolysis of cAMP to a metabolite, 5′ AMP, which lacks the second messenger properties of cAMP. Adenylate cyclase is an enzyme that catalyzes the conversion of ATP to cAMP. MAO is an enzyme located in presynaptic nerve terminals that degrades dopamine, norepinephrine, and epinephrine to inactive substances. Aspirin inhibits prostaglandin synthesis by inhibiting the cyclooxygenase enzyme.

51. **E.** Heparin, an anticoagulant, is different from the other glycosaminoglycans because it is an extracellular compound. Hyaluronic acid is found in synovial fluid; keratan sulfate is found in loose connective tissue such as cornea, chondroitin sulfate in cartilage, ligaments and tendons; and dermatan sulfate is found in skin and blood vessels.

52. **D.** In the initial step of the synthesis of porphyrin, succinyl CoA and glycine are condensed in a rate-limiting step in the liver.

53. **B.** An essential amino acid is one that cannot be synthesized by humans, and humans need to acquire them in the diet from plant or bacterial sources. All of the other amino acids can be synthesized by humans from other compounds and are not classified as "essential."

54. **A.** Aspartame is a peptide derivative composed of aspartic acid and phenylalanine.

55. **B.** Cells degrade purine nucleotides to uric acid. Xanthine is an intermediate in a series of reactions, but the final product in humans is uric acid, which is excreted in the urine. Urea is the degradation product of compounds containing amino groups (amino acids).

56. **C.** Malonyl CoA is produced after carboxylation of acetyl CoA in the synthetic process of fatty acids. FAD and NAD^+ are involved in fatty acid oxidation, but NADPH is the source of reducing agents in the synthesis of fatty acids.

57. **B.** This enzyme catalyzes the phosphorylation of fructose 6-phosphate to fructose 1,6-bisphosphate. This irreversible reaction is inhibited by ATP and citrate (indicators of energy abundance within the cell). The reaction is stimulated by AMP.

58. **C.** Pyridoxal phosphate is the active coenzyme of pyridoxine, which is involved in many enzyme systems essential for normal amino acid metabolism. Biotin is required for carboxylation reactions. Tetrahydrofolate, the coenzyme form of folic acid, is required for the synthesis of nucleic acids and porphyrin. Niacin participates in energy metabolism (oxidation-reduction reactions).

59. **D.** Energy sources are high immediately after a meal. Glycogenolysis (glycogen breakdown) is reduced. Lipolysis and oxidation of free fatty acids are also unnecessary during this time. Glucagon release is inhibited because of elevated glucose. Glycolysis is increased because of elevated intracellular glucose.

60. **A.** In the irreversible oxidative decarboxylation of pyruvate to acetyl CoA by pyruvate dehydrogenase, the five coenzymes listed are required.

61. **B.** Insulin is a polypeptide hormone that promotes energy storage when it is readily available. The lack of insulin would interfere with this process. Under conditions of reduced insulin, hyperglycemia would result owing to increased gluconeogenesis in the liver. Glycogen breakdown would be enhanced, and glycogen synthesis would be decreased. Because insulin promotes amino acid uptake in the liver, lack of insulin would result in decreased uptake.

62. **A.** After a meal, chylomicrons are synthesized in the intestine to transport lipid to the liver. Acetoacetate (ketone body) is found under conditions of increased β oxidation (fasting). Glucagon is secreted in response to reduced blood sugar, which usually is not present after a meal. Lactate, a product of anaerobic glycolysis, is not elevated under conditions of elevated energy sources in the postabsorptive state.

63. **A.** Insulin is a hormone that is secreted under conditions of increased sources of energy (glucose) and results in increased uptake and storage of glucose in the form of glycogen. In the process, blood glucose is decreased. The transport of glucose into the brain is not affected by the hormone.

64. **D.** RNA polymerase is an enzyme that transcribes DNA into RNA chains. Synthesis is similar to DNA reproduction because it is synthesized 5′ → 3′.

65. **B.** A probe is a single strand of DNA synthesized with a radioisotope that is complementary to a segment of DNA of interest. The radiolabeled complex can be analyzed subsequently on a gel by a technique known as a Southern blot.

66. **A.** Because DNA is a double-stranded molecule, cytosine is always base paired to guanine and guanine to cytosine. There would be equal amounts of these compounds. It is unlikely that RNA or mRNA, being a single-stranded molecule, would have equal amounts of these bases.

67. D. The backbone of DNA and RNA is composed of sugars (deoxyribose or ribose) joined $3' \rightarrow 5'$.

68. B. Translation is the conversion of information from mRNA into a protein. Transduction is the incorporation of genetic information carried by a virus into bacteria.

69. A. Inorganic mineral accounts for 95% of enamel, compared with 84% of calculus, 70% of dentin, and 60% of bone.

70. C. tRNA is not required for the hydroxylation of collagen because the process occurs after translation of mRNA and synthesis of collagen. Ascorbic acid is required to modify the collagen molecule by hydroxylating proline to permit cross-linking among collagen in tissues.

71. C. Substitution of most ions (with the exception of fluoride) increases the solubility of the crystal structure. The ratio of calcium and phosphate in hydroxyapatite is $1.67:1$.

72. B. Type II collagen is one of the fibril-forming collagens found in cartilaginous structures. Type I is characterized as having high tensile strength and is found in skin, tendon, bone, and dentin. Type III collagen is characteristically more distensible and is found in large blood vessels. Type IV is found in basement membranes.

73. C. Amino acids are transported across the luminal surface of the intestine by Na^+ amino acid cotransporters in the apical membrane; this is facilitated by the Na^+ gradient established in the intestinal cells.

74. D. Triacylglycerol is not commonly a component of cell membranes because it serves primarily as a molecule for storage and transport of fatty acids. Phospholipids are abundant because they form the bilayer structure characteristic of membranes. Proteins are present and serve various functions as enzymes, receptors, and transporters and carriers. Cholesterol stabilizes the membrane and is responsible for the maintenance of fluidity. Sphingolipids are components of myelin, which insulates membranes in neurons.

75. C. MAO is an enzyme located in the presynaptic nerve terminal, which degrades dopamine, norepinephrine, and epinephrine to inactive substances.

76. B. The sympathetic postganglionic fibers innervating the heart release norepinephrine. Acetylcholine is a neurotransmitter in sympathetic preganglionic fibers, parasympathetic postganglionic fibers, and parasympathetic preganglionic fibers.

77. B. The hypothalamus coordinates many activities mediated by the ANS, including food intake, thirst, and temperature regulation. The cerebellum functions to regulate movement and posture.

The medulla is responsible for coordinating respiration. The cerebral cortex performs functions of perception, cognition, higher motor functions, memory, and emotion.

78. B. In the process of muscle contraction, ATP bound to myosin is cleaved to form ADP and P_i. Myosin is released to bind to a new actin site producing a force-generating stroke. Sodium influx and calcium binding are involved in the excitation-contraction coupling process but do not serve as a source of energy.

79. A. Stretching of muscle spindles results in a reflex that is intended to adjust the muscle to its resting length by contracting the muscle in which it is found. The stretching of the spindle increases afferent impulses to the spinal cord and through a monosynaptic reflex stimulates muscle contraction via an α motoneuron.

80. A. Muscles are innervated by two types of motoneurons (α and γ). The α motoneurons innervate voluntary muscle fibers (extrafusal skeletal muscles). The γ motoneurons innervate the muscle spindles (intrafusal muscle fibers). The muscles of the iris are controlled by both sympathetic innervation (dilation) and parasympathetic innervation (constriction). The pyloric sphincter in the stomach is regulated primarily by the enteric nervous system and regulatory hormones in the GI tract.

81. B. Nitric oxide is a molecule produced in endothelial cells that acts directly on smooth muscle to produce relaxation and vasodilation. Inhibition of its synthesis would be expected to increase blood pressure. Inhibitors of angiotensin II synthesis should reduce blood pressure because angiotensin II stimulates aldosterone synthesis resulting in increased fluid retention. Angiotensin II is also a potent vasoconstrictor. Blocking vasopressin (also a potent vasoconstrictor) receptors would reduce blood pressure. Stimulation of the baroreceptor would produce a reflex that would reduce CO and peripheral sympathetic tone.

82. B. The concentration of K^+ within cells is approximately 30 times greater than in the ECF; the other ions have greater concentrations in ECF compared with concentrations within the cell.

83. A. All the other factors produce vasodilation and hyperemia to increase the exchange of metabolites in the tissue.

84. D. Capillary blood flow is proportional to changes in the radius (r^4) of the vessel. Decreasing the radius would produce increased vascular pressure. Viscosity of the blood depends primarily on the hematocrit (percentage of RBCs) and would not be changed by changes in the radius of the vessels.

85. D. Under conditions of increased intracranial pressure, the vasomotor regions of the medulla are stimulated owing to localized ischemia resulting in an increase in systemic blood pressure. Ventricular fibrillation refers to irregular, rapid, uncoordinated contractions of the ventricle that are ineffective in pumping blood. Anaphylactic shock is caused by severe allergic reactions, widespread release of histamine, and subsequent vasodilation.

86. A. Surfactant is synthesized by alveolar cells and functions to reduce the surface tension of the alveoli. This reduction of surface tension increases pulmonary compliance and decreases the work of breathing. It also decreases the tendency of the lungs to collapse. Lack of surfactant results in neonatal respiratory distress syndrome.

87. C. Residual volume is the volume of air remaining after a maximal forced expiration. Tidal volume is the amount of air exchanged (expiration and inspiration) during normal quiet breathing. FRC is a combination of the expired reserve volume (forced expiration) plus the residual volume. Vital capacity is the volume of air expired after maximal inspiration.

88. B. The regulatory centers for respiration are in the brainstem—specifically, the medulla. The medulla contains three groups of neurons (medullary respiratory center, apneustic center, and pneumotaxic center). The cerebral cortex may influence the medullary centers but does not totally control respiration.

89. A. Aldosterone secretion is mediated through the renin-angiotensin system. Angiotensin II stimulates the synthesis and release of aldosterone from the adrenal gland. It acts on the distal tubule and collecting ducts to increase sodium reabsorption and potassium secretion.

90. A. Net filtration depends on the hydrostatic pressures in the glomerular capillary, the hydrostatic pressures in Bowman's space, and the oncotic pressures in the capillary and Bowman's capsule. Reducing the plasma protein (reducing the oncotic pressure) lowers the tendency to retain fluid in the capillary; this results in a net increase in filtration.

91. B. Increasing the hydrostatic pressure within the glomerulus would decrease the net ultrafiltration pressure. Reduced plasma protein concentration decreases the oncotic pressure in the plasma, which would increase filtration. Vasodilation of the afferent arterioles would increase capillary pressure resulting in increased filtration. Inulin, although used to measure glomerular filtration, does not affect GFR.

92. C. Under normal conditions, all glucose is reabsorbed by both secondary active transport systems and facilitated diffusion using GLUT 1 and 2 carriers. Calcium is passively reabsorbed, but its reabsorption is also regulated by PTH in the distal tubule. Not all urea is reabsorbed, but about half is excreted. Its permeability is altered by changes in vasopressin. Phosphate reabsorption is also regulated by PTH.

93. C. The movement of the tongue against the palate is the only voluntary process among the four possible answers.

94. A. The GI tract is regulated by both the sympathetic and the parasympathetic branches of the ANS. The parasympathetic system is stimulatory, and the sympathetic system is inhibitory. The CNS influences motility and secretory activity through the ANS. Numerous endocrine factors (e.g., secretin, gastrin, CCK) are also involved with the regulation of GI activity.

95. C. The salivary glands are under the influence of both the sympathetic and the parasympathetic nervous system. Parasympathetic stimulation results in a more watery secretion compared with sympathetic stimulation, which produces increased amounts of protein with reduced volume. The vagus is parasympathetic, which in general is stimulatory to the GI tract. Sympathetics generally are inhibitory to the GI tract. (The exceptions are salivary glands.)

96. C. Fat in the intestine, low pH, and increased osmolarity of intestinal contents reduce gastric emptying. This reflex is mediated through neuronal and endocrine factors comprising the enterogastric reflex. Saline in the intestine does not affect gastric emptying.

97. B. T_4 and T_3 are formed by the cleavage of thyroglobulin after stimulation by TSH. Most T_4 is converted to T_3 in liver and kidney. Thyroglobulin is the storage form of thyroid hormone. TSH is produced in the anterior pituitary. It is not a hormone secreted from the thyroid but acts to stimulate the synthesis and secretion of thyroid hormones.

98. A. The terminology used is a classic descriptor of the relationship between the hormone source and target tissue. Paracrine refers to the target tissue as a cell in close proximity to the secreting tissue. Autocrine stimulation refers to a cell that releases a factor (hormone) that stimulates the cell from which it was released. Endocrine factors are hormones that have an effect at a distal site in the body.

99. B. Progesterone concentration in blood is highest after the surge of LH following ovulation. During ovulation, estrogen surges as a result of positive feedback during the follicular phase. During menstruation, there are sharp declines in estrogen and progesterone secondary to reduced secretion of LH and FSH.

100. **C.** Glucagon is secreted from the pancreas in response to reduced plasma glucose secondary to fasting and exercise. It functions to mobilize energy stores (glucose) and return blood glucose to normal levels. Glycogen synthesis (glycogenesis) does not occur in response to glucagon.

101. **C, F, A, D, E, B** is the correct order of the tricarboxylic acid cycle enzymes. Citrate synthase catalyzes the reaction of forming citrate from oxaloacetate, and acetyl CoA is the first step of the cycle. Isocitrate is converted to α-ketoglutarate by isocitrate dehydrogenase, and the conversion of α-ketoglutarate to succinyl CoA by α-ketoglutarate dehydrogenase follows. The enzyme for the conversion of succinyl CoA to succinate (succinyl-CoA synthase) was not listed. Succinate dehydrogenase converts succinate to fumarate. Fumerase was not listed for the production of malate, and malate dehydrogenase converts malate back to oxaloacetate.

102. **C and E.** Night blindness can result from a deficiency of vitamin A, and rickets is due to a deficiency of vitamin D. Scurvy results from a deficiency of vitamin C. Both pernicious anemia and neurologic degeneration can result from a deficiency of vitamin B_{12}.

103. **B, D, E, F.** HCl and pepsinogen are gastric secretions. HCO_3^- is the bicarbonate secretion of the pancreas. Both pancreatic amylase and lipase are secreted by the pancreas as well as the proenzyme form of the proteolytic enzyme chymotrypsin. Enterokinase is secreted by Brunner's glands in the duodenum.

104. **C and D.** Secretin inhibits gastric acid secretion. CCK stimulates contraction of the gallbladder and increases pancreatic HCO_3^- production, so it does not inhibit HCO_3^- production.

105. **C.** All are polysaccharides with the exception of acetylglucosamine, which is a monosaccharide derivative of glucose.

106. **A.** In skeletal muscle, the electrical impulse traversing through the T-tubules causes a mechanical conformational change of the dihydropyridine receptor to release calcium from the SR. In cardiac muscle, the electrical impulse causes the dihydropyridine receptor to influx a small amount of Ca^{2+}, which triggers more Ca^{2+} release from the SR. This calcium-triggered calcium release is called electrochemical coupling. In smooth muscle, hormones and neurotransmitters may produce an

additional increase in intracellular calcium (pharmacomechanical coupling).

107. **A, B, E.** Bitter flavors activate G proteins to produce IP_3 and Ca^{2+}. Sweet receptors activate G proteins and the second messenger cAMP. Umami, the taste sensation from L-glutamate and aspartate, also occurs via G proteins. Sour and salty flavors are sensed via the closing of K^+ and Na^+ channels, respectively.

108. **A.** As the stimulated flow of saliva increases, the Na^+ concentration more closely resembles the concentration in plasma; the increased flow rate allows less time for the ductal modification of the Na^+ concentration.

109. **D.** Chylomicrons transport dietary triglycerides, whereas VLDL transports endogenously synthesized triglycerides. LDL is responsible for delivering cholesterol to the peripheral tissues after the triglycerides have been hydrolyzed. HDL is responsible for transporting excess cholesterol back to the liver.

110. **B.** The term *cytosol* refers to the aqueous area between the plasma membrane and the membrane-bound organelles. The term *cytoplasm* refers to all of the area outside of the nucleus.

111. **C.** The smooth endoplasmic reticulum is associated with lipid synthesis, calcium storage, and drug detoxification. The rough endoplasmic reticulum is associated with protein synthesis.

112. **A.** The mitochondria contain the enzyme responsible for the generation of ATP via oxidative phosphorylation.

113. **D.** CoA transfers acyl groups between molecules. ATP transfers phosphate groups. Biotin transfers CO_2, and tetrahydrofolate transfers one-carbon units. NADPH transfers electrons.

114. **D.** rRNA is transcribed and assembled in the nucleolus.

115. **B.** Blood and bone are specialized forms of connective tissue.

116. **C.** The universal carrier of biochemical energy is ATP, which with the ATP-ADP cycle can act as both a phosphate donor and phosphate acceptor.

117. **D.** The basic unit of muscle contraction is the sarcomere, which spans from Z-disc to Z-disc.

118. **B.** Cardiac muscle fibers may be binucleate, they are connected by intercalated discs, and the fibers can branch. However, the terminal cisternae of the SR is located at the Z-disc, not the A-band to I-band junction.

119. **C.** Fibrous proteins are usually structural proteins, whereas globular proteins are usually enzymes, hormones, and antibodies.

120. **B.** The net result of the glycolytic pathway is two ATP, two NADH, and two pyruvate.

Answer Key for Section 3

1. **B.** Neutrophils are quick to arrive to the site of infection or injury and are associated with acute inflammation. All of the other cells listed are mediators of chronic inflammation.

2. **C.** Dust cells, along with heart failure cells, are macrophages that are found in the lungs. They are part of the reticuloendothelial system.

3. **E.** Bacteria that are phagocytosed by macrophages are kept in membrane-bound vacuoles called *phagosomes*. A phagosome fuses with a lysosome, which contains many degradative enzymes, including lysozyme.

4. **C.** Although IgE is the least prevalent immunoglobulin in the body, it is the major antibody mediator of type I hypersensitivity reactions. These reactions are caused primarily by prior sensitization and the accumulation of IgE to a specific allergen.

5. **B.** DiGeorge's syndrome is characterized by a deficiency of T cells. It is caused by the failure of the third and fourth branchial pouches to develop normally, resulting in a lack of thymus and parathyroid development.

6. **E.** Intraoral *Streptococcus viridans, a member of the* viridans streptococci is the most common cause of subacute endocarditis. *Staphylococcus aureus, often colonizing the nares and sinus cavity* is the most common cause of acute endocarditis.

7. **D.** Aschoff bodies are the classic lesions observed in rheumatic fever. They are areas of focal necrosis surrounded by a dense inflammatory infiltrate and may be observed in heart tissues.

8. **C.** Endotoxin or lipopolysaccharide is found in the cell walls of Gram-negative bacteria.

9. **D.** Endocarditis is most commonly caused by group B, α-hemolytic streptococci, such as *S. viridans, S. mutans, S. sanguis,* and *S. salivarius.* All of the other conditions are associated with group A β-hemolytic streptococcal infections, such as *S. pyogenes.*

10. **A.** The only disease listed that is related to an abnormal number of chromosomes is Klinefelter's syndrome. This disease is characterized by two or more X chromosomes and one or more Y chromosomes. Typically, affected individuals have 47 chromosomes with a karyotype of XXY.

11. **C.** Pemphigus is an autoimmune disease wherein autoantibodies against epidermis cells are produced. Histologically, a phenomenon called *acantholysis,* in which epidermal cells appear to detach and separate from each other, is observed.

12. **E.** Chronic bronchitis predisposes affected individuals to squamous neoplasia of the bronchial epithelium (i.e., bronchogenic carcinoma).

13. **A.** Chronic granulomatosis results from neutrophils with a defective reduced nicotinamide adenine dinucleotide phosphate oxidase system. This defect affects their ability to kill microorganisms because they are unable to produce superoxide radicals.

14. **B.** Dysplastic cells are abnormal in appearance and organization. The potential to develop into a malignant tumor is present; however, this risk varies.

15. **D.** The HIV envelope contains two glycoproteins, gp120 and gp41. gp120 binds specifically with CD4 surface receptors.

16. **A.** The most common cause of gastroenteritis in children is the rotavirus. It is a reovirus.

17. **B.** A radiographic finding of a cotton-wool appearance is common in patients with a diagnosis of osteitis deformans or Paget's disease.

18. **B.** Autoclaves function by denaturing proteins. They are effective against spores.

19. **B.** Ehlers-Danlos syndrome is characterized by defects in collagen (i.e., connective tissues).

20. **B.** Increased levels of alkaline phosphatase may be observed in diseases that display extensive bone loss. Osteoporosis is characterized by a decrease in bone mass. There are either normal or decreased levels of alkaline phosphatase in patients with this disease.

21. **C.** The leading cause of death for diabetic patients is cardiovascular disease. Other complications include retinopathy, nephropathy, and peripheral neuropathy.

22. **A.** Neuraminidase is found on the surface envelope of influenza viruses. It functions to attach the virus to the host cell.

23. **D.** Actinic keratosis produces dry, scaly plaques with an erythematous base. They may be premalignant. Both compound and intraepidermal nevi are benign.

24. **A.** Hepatitis A is spread via oral-anal/fecal contamination. The other hepatitis viruses can be transmitted through blood, sexual contact, or perinatally.

25. E. Cardiac tamponade is a serious condition caused by accumulation of fluid in the pericardium. This fluid accumulation can result in impaired ventricular filling and can rapidly lead to decreased cardiac output and death.

26. C. Pyelonephritis is usually caused by Gram-negative, rod-shaped bacteria that are part of the normal flora of the enteric tract. It is most commonly caused by *Escherichia coli*, followed by members of the following genera *Proteus*, *Klebsiella*, and *Enterobacter*.

27. D. Polycystic kidney disease is characterized by the formation of cysts in the kidneys. It is commonly associated with berry aneurysms.

28. D. Squamous cell carcinoma is the most common oral cancer, accounting for 90% of all cases. It is a cancer of squamous epithelium, specifically a malignant tumor of keratinocytes.

29. E. Both *Epidermophyton* and *Trichophyton* can cause tinea pedis.

30. A. Stenosis describes fibrotic and thickened valves, resulting in reduced blood flow through the valve.

31. C. Cystic fibrosis results from an abnormal chloride channel that affects all exocrine glands.

32. B. Trisomy 21, which is also known as *Down syndrome*, is a disorder affecting autosomes. It is generally caused by meiotic nondisjunction in the mother, which results in an extra copy of chromosome 21 (trisomy 21).

33. D. These oral findings can be observed in patients with hyperthyroidism. The only endocrine disorder listed that is related to hyperthyroidism is Plummer's disease. It is caused by a nodular growth or adenoma of the thyroid.

34. D. Poststreptococcal glomerulonephritis is a classic example of nephritic syndrome, which occurs after a *Streptococcus* infection (e.g., strep throat). It is characterized by all of the symptoms listed except polyuria. A decrease in urination is usually observed.

35. B. Osteomyelitis, or an infection of bone, is most commonly caused by *Staphylococcus aureus*. Symptoms include pain and systemic signs of infection (i.e., fever, malaise).

36. E. All of the features listed are commonly observed in malignant cells except a low nuclear-to-cytoplasmic ratio. Because of the large nuclei present, there is usually a high nuclear-to-cytoplasmic ratio.

37. E. Although the cells have not yet invaded the basement membrane, the likelihood of invasive growth is presumed to be high.

38. D. The Western blot tests for HIV proteins. The ELISA tests for HIV antibodies. When these two tests are used together, an accuracy rate of 99% is achieved.

39. C. Because 90% of blood transfusion–related hepatitis cases are caused by hepatitis C, and the patient has a history of having had a blood transfusion, hepatitis C is the most likely causative agent.

40. D. Opportunistic infections are a serious problem in patients infected with HIV. This patient's intraoral thrush, which is caused by *C. albicans*, is such an infection. Treatment for candidiasis includes nystatin.

41. C. HIV is an RNA virus that contains three enzymes: reverse transcriptase, integrase, and protease. Neuraminidase is a protein found on the surface of the influenza virus.

42. C. Although all of the microbes listed cause pneumonia, the most common cause of pneumonia in patients with AIDS is *P. jiroveci*.

43. A. McCune-Albright syndrome is a type of fibrous dysplasia that manifests with a triad of symptoms including polyostotic fibrous dysplasia, café au lait spots, and endocrine abnormalities.

44. B. Fibrous dysplasia is caused by replacement of normal bone with irregular bone containing fibrous connective tissue; this gives the radiographs a characteristic ground-glass appearance.

45. B. Fibrous dysplasia is caused by replacement of normal bone with irregular bone and fibrous connective tissue. The pathology report usually describes abnormally shaped trabeculae in loosely arranged fibrous tissue.

46. D. PTT measures the intrinsic and common pathways of the coagulation cascade. A prolonged PTT could result from a deficiency of factor V, VIII, IX, X, XI, or XII or of prothrombin or fibrinogen.

47. C. Hemophilia A is caused by a deficiency of factor VIII (antihemophilic factor).

48. C. Hemophilia A is a hereditary disorder that is X-linked; it affects only males. However, females can be carriers.

49. B. The only way to distinguish hemophilia A from hemophilia B is to assay the levels of coagulation factors. Hemophilia A is caused by a deficiency of factor VIII, whereas hemophilia B is caused by a deficiency of factor IX.

50. C. Gummas are granulomas that may be seen in tertiary syphilis, and syphilis is caused by *Treponema pallidum*. Granulomas may also be seen in tuberculosis, an infection caused by *Mycobacterium tuberculosis*; however, in this disease, they are known as *tubercles*.

51. A. CD8 lymphocytes recognize class I MHC molecules on antigen-presenting cells. CD4 lymphocytes recognize class II MHC molecules on antigen-presenting cells.

52. E. IL-5 is released by helper T cells to stimulate B lymphocytes to differentiate into plasma cells. It also activates eosinophils and increases the production of IgA.

53. **B.** Tuberculin reaction (i.e., PPD skin test) is an example of a type IV delayed (cell-mediated) hypersensitivity reaction. Type IV reactions are the only type of hypersensitivity immune reactions that are not mediated by antibodies. They are mainly mediated by T cells.

54. **D.** Mast cells contain dense granules with inflammatory mediators, including histamine and SRS-A, which is a leukotriene.

55. **C.** Symptoms of a myocardial infarction include chest pain, shortness of breath, diaphoresis (sweating), clammy hands, nausea, and vomiting.

56. **B.** A quelling reaction occurs in a laboratory when the polysaccharide capsule of a bacterium swells after being treated with antiserum or antibodies.

57. **E.** Dipicolinic acid is found only in spores. *Clostridium* is the only spore-forming microorganism listed.

58. **D.** Dextrans consist of glucose molecules linked together. They not only act as the structural component of plaque, but they also they contribute to the retention of lactic acid near the tooth. Fructans or levans are also found in plaque; however, they contain fructose.

59. **C.** The most common cause of bacterial meningitis in newborns is *Escherichia coli*. *Haemophilus influenzae* and *Neisseria meningitidis* are the most common causes of bacterial meningitis in infants and children (*H. influenzae*) and young adults (*N. meningitidis*).

60. **D.** Teichoic acid may be found only in the cell walls of Gram-positive bacteria and contain antigenic properties. All of the other answers listed are found in the cell walls of Gram-negative bacteria.

61. **B.** The tetanus vaccine consists of tetanus toxoid. It is part of the DPT vaccine and should be given about every 10 years.

62. **A.** IgA is found in mucosal secretions of the genitourinary, intestinal, and respiratory tracts, including tears, saliva, and colostrums.

63. **D.** HBeAg is present when there is active viral replication and the carrier is highly infectious.

64. **C.** Opportunistic infections are seen in patients with AIDS. All of the microbes listed represent opportunistic organisms except coxsackievirus.

65. **E.** Rheumatoid arthritis is characterized by inflammation of the synovial membrane. Granulation tissue forms in the synovium and expands over the articular cartilage; this causes the destruction of the underlying cartilage and results in fibrotic changes or ankylosis.

66. **A.** The most common form of breast cancer is adenocarcinoma arising from the ductal epithelium.

67. **E.** Both tetracycline and streptomycin, an aminoglycoside, inhibit protein synthesis in bacteria. However, streptomycin is bactericidal, not bacteriostatic.

68. **D.** Rickets is a vitamin D deficiency seen in infants and children.

69. **D.** The minimal time required is 12 hours.

70. **C.** Cretinism is hypothyroidism in children. Oral findings include macroglossia, prolonged retention of primary teeth, and delayed eruption of permanent teeth.

71. **A.** In general, plaque is first colonized by Gram-positive cocci bacteria, such as streptococci, followed by Gram-negative, rod-shaped anaerobes, such as *Bacteroides*, *Fusobacterium*, *Porphyromonas*, *Prevotella*, and then filament-type bacteria, such as *Actinomyces*.

72. **A.** Peutz-Jeghers syndrome is a hereditary disease that is transmitted by autosomal dominance.

73. **B.** Although all of the structures listed are intraoral sites at which oral cancer may develop, more than 50% occur on the tongue.

74. **C.** Auer rods are observed in blast cells characteristic of acute myeloid leukemia.

75. **D.** The most significant complication of Barrett's esophagus is esophageal adenocarcinoma.

76. **A.** M-protein is an important virulence factor found in *S. pyogenes*. It has sufficient antigenic similarity to human cardiac myosin such that upon developing antibodies against M protein as the result of the first infection, subsequent exposure to *S. pyogenes* will result in the non-suppurative aspects associated with streptococcal disease where the host's own immunoglobulin will attack the heart leading to rheumatic manifestations.

77. **D.** An infection by molds, such as mucormycosis, results in the invasion of blood vessel endothelium; this leads to hemorrhagic infarction and tissue necrosis.

78. **D.** Chronic lymphocytic leukemia is characterized by the proliferation of B cells. It is both the most common and the least malignant type of leukemia.

79. **B.** Consequences of asbestosis include mesothelioma and bronchogenic carcinoma.

80. **D.** Jaundice is characterized by yellowness of tissues, including skin, eyes, and mucous membranes. It is caused by diseases that increase serum conjugated or unconjugated bilirubin. These conditions include liver disease, such as cirrhosis or hepatitis; hemolytic anemias; obstruction of the common bile duct, as caused by gallstones or cholelithiasis; and carcinoma involving the head of the pancreas.

81. **D.** Asthma is an obstructive lung disease caused by narrowing of the airways. Common symptoms

include dyspnea, wheezing on expiration, and a dry cough.

82. C. Systemic lupus erythematosus, also known as *lupus*, is considered an autoimmune disease, although the exact cause is unknown. It is characterized by the presence of ANAs. Common ANA findings include anti-DNA, anti-RNA, and anti-Sm antigen.

83. A. Because of the excessive levels of serum calcium, osseous changes, such as metastatic calcifications and kidney stones, occur in patients with hyperparathyroidism.

84. C. Osteopetrosis, also known as *Albers-Schönberg disease* or *marble bone disease*, is caused by abnormal osteoclasts. The lack of bone resorption results in defective bone remodeling and increased bone density, which may invade into the bone marrow space.

85. A. Whooping cough is caused by *Bordetella. pertussis*. All of the factors listed contribute to its virulence except IgA protease. This enzyme is produced by *Haemophilus influenzae*, another Gram-negative, rod-shaped bacteria.

86. E. Celiac sprue is characterized by malabsorption and mucosal lesions of the small intestines that are caused by an allergy to gluten. T-cell lymphoma is a complication of this disease.

87. B. TB is caused by the bacterium *Mycobacterium tuberculosis*. While this organism is considered to be Gram positive, the Gram stain is of limited value in their identification because of their waxy cell walls. To identify these bacteria, an acid-fast stain must be ordered.

88. D. *M. tuberculosis* infects macrophages, which are initially unable to kill the phagocytosed bacteria.

89. A. Cord factor is a glycolipid found on the surface of *M. tuberculosis*.

90. D. Type IV delayed type hypersensitivity reactions are the only type of hypersensitivity immune reactions that are not mediated by antibodies. They are mainly mediated by T cells.

91. E. Treatment for TB includes multidrug therapy. Rifampin, isoniazid, and ethambutol are three of the first-line drugs used. When treating this infection it is best to consult with the local public health department as to whether or not drug resistant variants of this microbe are resident within the community as this may require a change to drugs used to treat the patient.

92. E. Ghon complex describes the calcified scar that remains after the primary infection. It is usually found in the lung and includes the primary lesion and its regional lymph node.

93. A. Given the patient's history of rheumatic fever, the heart murmur is most likely from a dysfunctioning mitral valve. Rheumatic fever most commonly affects the mitral valve, resulting in mitral valve stenosis, regurgitation, or both.

94. B. Rheumatic fever is usually preceded by a group A streptococcal respiratory infection (e.g., strep throat or pharyngitis).

95. A. Viridans streptococci are the most common cause of subacute endocarditis. Viridans streptococci are α-hemolytic streptococci, representing incomplete lysis of sheep erythrocytes when grown on solid media.

96. E. During subacute endocarditis, vegetations, or thrombi, form on previously damaged heart valves. Complications can arise if the embolization of the thrombus occurs (i.e., when a fragment separates and enters the circulation), causing septic infarcts. Other complications include valvular dysfunction and abscess formation.

97. C. Aminoglycosides block the 30S ribosomal subunit to inhibit protein synthesis.

98. C. Burkitt's lymphoma is an aggressive lymphoma that affects B lymphocytes.

99. E. Histologic evaluation of Burkitt's lymphoma reveals a characteristic "starry-sky" appearance, which results from the lighter colored macrophages present.

100. A. Epstein-Barr virus (EBV) is responsible for causing mononucleosis, a disease that also affects B lymphocytes.

101. C. Pili aid in the attachment of bacteria to host cell surfaces. Attachment is often the first requirement for invasion of the host by the bacterium. Most often appreciated for its role in bacterial conjugation, pili also facilitate attachment to surfaces and aid in the development of biofilms.

102. B. The type III secretion system of Gram-negative bacteria also may be referred to as the injectisome or injectosome. The system codes for a protein appendage type that resembles a molecular syringe whose sole function is to facilitate the coordinated injection of proteins into the host cell.

103. C. This question is assessing whether or not you appreciate the mechanism of action of IgA, which is the principal immunoglobulin associated with mucosal surfaces. Choice C is correct because it accurately describes the activity. The other answers describe other aspects of the immune system that do not relate to how IgA serves to protect the host.

104. E. Mucormycosis, the condition mediated by fungi in the order Mucorales is an opportunistic infection that typically manifests with oral or cerebral presentations and almost always is found in patients with hyperglycemia and metabolic acidosis. Given the patient's history, your clinical observation, and the lack of other diagnostic information provided, an empiric assessment of mucormycosis is the best answer. The other mycoses described could result in lesions, but additional information would be required to make this determination.

105. **C.** Decolorization serves to remove the primary stain from Gram-negative cells. Consequently, the cells would appear purple—hence failure of the differential requirement intended by the protocol.

106. **C.** This question requires you to interpret the history of the patient given in the stem, appreciate the common symptoms associated with malaria, and recall the responsible microbe, *Plasmodium* parasite. It would be useful on completing your review of malaria also to review the symptoms caused by the other two parasites suggested as answers for choices **D** and **E**, the circumstances where complement might lyse erythrocytes.

107. **D.** Doxycycline and other members of the tetracycline class of antibiotics when consumed either by the mother during pregnancy or by the child during the development period of teeth result in a blue-gray or yellow-brown opalescent discoloration of teeth. This discoloration is often bilateral and affects the teeth within both arches. The level of discoloration may be continuous or in a stripe pattern and is related to the administration of the drug. The other antimicrobials listed also have side effects. Streptomycin affects the cranial nerves and leads to hearing loss. Chloramphenicol can result in the development of aplastic anemia. The administration of antibiotics can often lead to stomach upset, diarrhea, and abdominal pain.

108. **E.** The dental anatomy observed in the slide represents a Hutchinson's incisor, which is a direct consequence of the developing fetus being exposed to syphilis. The route of acquisition is transplacental. Infants with this condition have teeth that are smaller and more widely spaced than normal with notches on their biting surfaces. On reviewing this question, you may wish to review the other microbes within the TORCH complex, which is an abbreviation for perinatal infections. The microbes within the TORCH group can lead to severe fetal anomalies, stillbirth or septic abortion. The microbes within this group are *T. gondii*; other infections, which include the one associated with this question (coxsackievirus, syphilis, VZV, HIV, and parvovirus B19); rubella; CMV; and HSV 2.

109. **A.** From the patient's history, you appreciate that the pharyngitis caused by the β-hemolytic group A streptococcus resulted in the subsequent development of rheumatic diseases owing to the cross-reactivity of the streptococcal antigens with antigens of her heart. Consequently, the subsequent rheumatic fever damaged her valve, which predisposed her to develop subsequent bacterial endocarditis. Consequently, you need to recall that group A streptococcus is β-hemolytic on trypticase soy agar with sheep blood and is sensitive to bacitracin. Should the question have asked you the identity of the microbe responsible for the endocarditis, your answer would most likely have been one of the streptococci from the viridans group.

110. **E.** The patient's history provides sufficient information from which you can make an empiric determination of cause. The patient developed an aspiration pneumonia as a consequence of the introduction of foreign material into his lungs. The foreign material in this patient's case was the debris that he inhaled from the emesis episodes. The debris brought with it bacteria from his oral cavity rich in anaerobes and at sufficient concentrations ($>100^8$) to cause pneumonitis.

111. **C.** Bactericidal antibiotics result in the death of the microbe. In the figure, the concentration of viable cells is measured. The antibiotic that results in cell death is "C." The antibiotic identified by choice **A** is likely an antimetabolite antibiotic, such as trimethoprim, which would require the pools of folate to be diluted before its having an effect on activity, and the antibiotic type in choice **B** could be any of the inhibitors of protein synthesis whereupon dilution growth may resume.

112. **C.** The patient is presenting with the classic exanthem referred to as *impetigo*. The data within the stem require that you identify this as streptococcal impetigo rather than staphylococcal mediated impetigo. Should you not recall the catalase difference between the two organisms, you may recall that impetigo mediated by staphylococci rarely moves down the body, but this is quite common with streptococcal impetigo. As with rheumatic disease, group A streptococcus implicated in impetigo can have consequences through the deposition of immune complexes within the kidney resulting in glomerulonephritis.

113. **C.** *P. jiroveci* pneumonia (formerly *P. carinii* pneumonia) principally manifests with the symptoms described in the stem, with the hallmark symptom shortness of breath. The figure further reinforces the history with its classic image. The key is appreciate the size, which enables you to rule out the other choices.

114. **C.** The image on the right is representative of Koplik spots, which are a consequence of the prodromic viral enanthem of measles and typically erupt 2 days before the rash (exanthema). They typically

appear as white lesions on the buccal mucosa near each Stensen's duct. The lesions fade as the rash develops.

115. **A.** Rotavirus is the most common cause of severe diarrhea among infants and young children. The absence of inflammation and leukocytes in blood or stool strongly suggest a virus. The only two viruses available to select are the correct choice and choice E, which would not likely cause GI disease because it is described as an enveloped virus that would likely have been inactivated by the host before reaching the GI tract.

116. **B.** The patient's history reveals the offending agent is likely an opportunistic pathogen and requires that you be able to differentiate the causes of meningitis. However, the question is made simpler with the figure. The India ink stain reveals an encapsulated fungus. Of the two fungi available for selection, *C. neoformans* is the one most likely responsible for the symptoms.

117. **D.** The patient's history is remarkable in that she presents with weight loss and foul-smelling greasy stools, which is suggestive that the parasite has invaded the bile duct and is likely retarding the delivery of bile to the intestine. Based on the niche bias and figure, of the parasites listed, the one best answer is *G. lamblia*. The ameba associated with choices **A** through **C** may cause diarrhea but without the secondary sequelae described. *Naegleria fowleri* lives in warm fresh water ponds, lakes, and underchlorinated swimming pools. It can invade the nervous system of the host through the olfactory mucosa and cribriform plate of nasal tissues and result in a case mortality of greater than 98%.

118. **B.** The critical element to this question is to read that the effect must be persistent. Of the antiseptics listed, the only one with persistent activity is chlorhexidine gluconate.

119. **B.** The hormones associated with pregnancy result in numerous changes within the oral cavity that have as a net consequence the lowering of the ability of the gingival tissues to resist infection. Additionally, there is increasing evidence that the same hormones, progesterone and estrogen, can promote the growth of some oral anaerobes over the growth of the other microbes in residence. *Prevotella intermedia* is one such organism that blooms during pregnancy with its additional growth promoting inflammation of the gingiva.

120. **C.** The individual described has developed a urinary tract infection. Of the choices described, the two most likely microbes responsible for urinary tract infection are *E. coli* and *Proteus vulgaris*. Both are Gram-negative rods, but only *Proteus* is urease-positive. The other organisms described do not agree with the data presented within the stem.

121. **A.** 3. Benign neoplasm of fibrous tissue origin
B. 2. Malignant neoplasm of bone
C. 4. Variably sized mass of blood in the tissues, usually secondary to trauma
D. 5. Benign neoplasm of epithelial origin with fingerlike projections
E. 1. Benign or malignant tumor

122. 1. **B.** Epithelial dysplasia (mild, moderate, and severe) and carcinoma in situ are precancerous lesions (i.e., invasion has not occurred).
2. **C.** In primary SCC, tumor cells have invaded beyond the basement membrane into the underlying connective tissue.
3. **A.** Metastatic SCC is spread of the primary tumor to noncontiguous regions (e.g., regional lymph nodes or distant sites).

Answer Key for Section 4

1. **C.** Universal tooth numbering system for primary dentition, A though T.
2. **A.** Said to be the most atypical of human molars.
3. **C.** Choice **A,** smaller in all dimensions; choice **B,** all roots seen from buccal aspect; choice **D,** roots nearly the same length.
4. **D.** *Mesial aspect:* choice **A,** pronounced convexity present; choice **B,** curvature in an occlusal direction; choice **C,** cervical third greater occlusal third; choice **D,** mesiolingual cusp longer and sharper than mesiobuccal cusp.
5. **D.** *Lingual aspect:* choice **D,** Well-defined developmental groove separating mesiolingual and distolingual cusps; choice **A,** mesiolingual cusp large and well developed; choice **B,** distolingual cusp well developed, more so than that of the primary first molar; choice **C,** there is a supplemental cusp apical to the mesiolingual cusp but poorly developed.
6. **D.** A developmental depression but not a groove divides the two buccal cusps. Choice **A,** it does not resemble other primary teeth; choice **B,** it has a rhomboidal outline from the occlusal aspect; choice **C,** the mesiobuccal cusp is larger.
7. **A.** The mesiobuccal, distobuccal, and distal cusps are almost equal in size, whereas the distal cusp of the permanent molar is smaller. Choice **B,** the primary molar crown is *narrower,* not wider buccolingually; choice **C,** the primary molar outline is rectangular; choice **D,** the crown/root ratio is not the same.
8. **B.** Comparatively, roots of primary anterior teeth are narrower and longer. Choice **A,** crowns of anterior primary teeth are *wider,* not narrower; choice **C,** cervical ridges of primary anterior teeth *more* prominent; choice **D,** buccal and lingual surfaces are *more flat,* not less flat.
9. **B.** The overall average length of the primary mandibular central incisor is quoted as 14 mm (Black GV, cited by Ash and Nelson, 2003), 16 mm (Woelfel and Scheid, 2002), and 14 mm (Kraus et al., 1969). The correct answer is 14 to 16 mm, not 16 to 17 mm.
10. **A.** Greater mesiodistal diameter relative to crown height than permanent teeth. Choice **B,** squat appearance, not elongated appearance; choice **C,** crowns are a milky white, not translucent white; choice **D,** there is no root trunk.

11. **C.** Chronologies from textbooks vary so that age of eruption for the primary mandibular central incisor may be given as 6 months (Woelfel and Scheid, 2002), 6.5 months (Kraus et al., 1969), 7.5 months (Charlick et al., 1974), and 8 (6 to 10) months (Ash and Nelson, 2003).
12. **C.** The most favorable sequence for prevention of malocclusion.
13. **B.** Textbook chronologies indicate that the maxillary primary second molar is most commonly the last to erupt: 24 months (Woelfel and Scheid, 2002), 20 to 30 months (Kraus et al., 1969), and 25 to 33 months (Ash and Nelson, 2003).
14. **C.** The length of the primary maxillary central incisor is quoted as 16 mm (Black GV, cited by Ash and Nelson, 2003), 16 mm (Kraus et al., 1969), and 17.2 mm (Woelfel and Scheid, 2002). The permanent maxillary incisor is quoted as 23.6 mm (Ash and Nelson, 2003), 23.5 mm (Kraus et al., 1969), and 23.6 mm (Woelfel and Scheid, 2002). 16/23.5 = 0.68 or 68%; 17.2/23.6 = 0.73 or 73%. The answer is about 70%.
15. **C.** The correct answer for choice **A** would be about 1.5 months or 6 weeks; choice **B,** about 4 to 5 years; choice **C,** about 2.5 months or 10 weeks; choice **D,** about 4 to 5 years.
16. **A.** (Ash and Nelson, 2003; Woelfel and Scheid, 2002).
17. **C.** No, or almost never does the mesial marginal developmental groove cross the mesial marginal ridge.
18. **B.** M_1: distobuccal height equals mesiobuccal height; M_2: distobuccal cusp height slightly less than mesiobuccal cusp height; M_3: distobuccal cusp height much shorter than mesiobuccal cusp height.
19. **D.** Marked *asymmetry* of mesial and distal halves.
20. **D.** From mesial and distal aspect, all posterior teeth have a trapezoidal outline with the shortest uneven side toward the occlusal surface. Choice **A,** present primarily on first premolar; **B,** exceptions may be the distobuccal root of the maxillary second molar; **C,** from mesial and distal aspect, all posterior mandibular teeth, not maxillary posterior teeth, have a rhomboidal outline.
21. **C.** Below the apices, 63% of the time.
22. **C.** Greater than 5% (up to 40%) in populations with Mongolian traits. Choice **A,** does not exceed 4.2%

in whites; choice **B,** less than 5% in Eurasian and Asian populations; choice **D,** less than 3% in African populations.

23. **D.** Generally a jaw-closing muscle; may stabilize and act with lateral jaw movements.

24. **B.** In the earliest phase, the condyle moves forward *in concert* with the disc, *not before.*

25. **D.** Occlusal contact relations do *not* interfere with jaw opening, but TMJ and muscle disorders may.

26. **C.** Mediotrusive contact, but may be called a non-working (balancing) contact.

27. **D.** TMJ (Ash and Nelson, 2003); craniomandibular (Woelfel and Scheid, 2002).

28. **A.** Vertical component not seen on horizontal tracing.

29. **C.** Height of contour on lingual surfaces of molars and premolars is at the cervical or middle third.

30. **C.** Transverse ridge connecting mesiobuccal and mesiolingual cusps.

31. **B.** Mandibular first premolar is most likely to have a single pulp horn.

32. **A.** Bifurcated roots are not a normal feature of mandibular incisors.

33. **D.** Height of contour on distal surface of permanent mandibular central incisors is at the incisal third.

34. **C.** The dimension of the permanent maxillary canine at the widest mesiodistal diameter is 7.5 mm (7.5 mm [Ash and Nelson, 2003]; 7.6 mm [6.3 to 9.5 mm] [Woelfel and Scheid, 2002]).

35. **B.** Distobuccal developmental groove is *not* found on mandibular second molars.

36. **D.** Y-shaped central developmental groove is found on the mandibular second premolar.

37. **D.** In the cusp-embrasure occlusal relationship, the maxillary first premolar is most likely to articulate with the first and second premolars.

38. **C.** Equal bilateral contraction of the lateral pterygoid muscles results in protrusion of the mandible.

39. **D.** Molecular tests such as the polymerase chain reaction have a fast, not slow, turnaround time.

40. **A.** Rifampin causes orange, not green, urine, tears, and sweat.

41. **B.** The drug binds tightly only to *prokaryotic* RNA polymerase. Choice **D,** rifampin *induces* activity of hepatic mixed oxidases.

42. **C.** Naproxen has not been reported to exacerbate bruxism.

43. **C.** The mechanisms of the two types of headaches are quite different. Choices **A, B,** and **D** are considered true.

44. **B.** β-Amyloid deposits are a component of Alzheimer's disease but not of migraine headaches.

45. **A.** (Montgomery et al., 1996).

46. **B.** Considering the clinical findings, infection is most likely to involve the submaxillary space.

47. **A.** Given the clinical findings and the involved molar position, it is the lateral upper deep cervical node group that would most likely be the first involved with lymph drainage.

48. **B.** Oral tuberculosis most often involves the *tongue.*

49. **B.** Langerhans' giant cells, epithelioid cells, and caseous necrotic areas are highly suggestive of tuberculosis; however, special stains for acid-fast bacilli and isolation of *M. tuberculosis* may be necessary, keeping in mind that staining may not differentiate tuberculosis from other mycobacterial infections. Other molecular tests may be indicated.

50. **D.** There is no evidence of a connection between myositis and bruxing.

51. **C.** The anticoagulant effect of warfarin is inhibited by rifampin. Choice **A,** Rifampin *decreases* the anticoagulation effect of warfarin; choice **B,** rifampin *interferes* with cyclic conversion; choice **D,** rifampin *increases* the metabolic clearance.

52. **B.** Combination name for joining buccal and lingual cusp triangular ridges.

53. **B, C, D.** For choice **A,** the crown outline converges only *lingually*; choice **B,** the small transverse ridge has been called an oblique ridge.

54. **D.** Choice **A,** the *mesiolingual* cusp is most prominent; choice **B,** the *distolingual* cusp is poorly defined; choice **C,** the *distobuccal* cusp *may be seen* because it is longer.

55. **C.** The central groove is well defined. Choice **A,** the primary maxillary second molar *does* have a well-defined mesial triangular fossa; choice **B,** the oblique ridge is *prominent*; choice **D,** the supplementary cusp is *not* well-developed.

56. **A.** Choice **B,** it has *four* well-developed cusps; choice **C,** it has only *one* supplementary cusp; choice **D,** it has a *well-developed* mesial triangular fossa.

57. **A.** Choice **B,** the outline of the crown converges *distally*; choice **C,** the three buccal cusps are *similar* in size; choice **D,** *well-defined* triangular ridges extend from the cusp tips.

58. **C.** Choice **A,** Enamel cap *thinner* and *more* consistent in depth; choice **B,** comparatively *greater* thickness; choice **D,** pulp horns are *higher* in primary molars.

59. **D.** Choice **A,** Enamel rods slope *occlusally*, not gingivally, in the primary molars; choice **B,** enamel rods at cervix slope *gingivally*, not occlusally, in permanent molars; choice **C,** the buccal cervical ridge is *more* pronounced.

60. **B.** The total of average overall mesiodistal diameters of primary maxillary crowns is quoted as 68.2 mm (Black GV, cited by Ash and Nelson, 2003) and 76.8 mm (Woelfel and Scheid, 2002).

61. **A.** On average, the height of curvature is 3.5 mm on the mesial and 2.5 mm on the distal of the

maxillary central incisor; it is 3.0 mm on the mesial and 2.0 mm on the distal of the mandibular central incisor.

62. **D.** The width and depth of arch are more or less constant after 9 months of age. However, a substantial increase in the anterior-posterior distance occurs for permanent molars.

63. **C.** These are the most common sequences of eruption.

64. **A.** First evidence of the maxillary central incisor calcification is given as 14 (13 to 16) weeks (Kraus and Jordon, 1965; Ash and Nelson, 2003) and as 4 months (Woelfel and Scheid, 2002).

65. **B.** (Kraus et al., 1969).

66. **A.** The correct answer (7 to 8 years) is based on textbook chronologies (Ash and Nelson, 2003; Woelfel and Scheid, 2002), which are based on original chronologies by Schour and Massler (1940), modified for permanent dentition by Kronfeld (Bur) and by Kronfeld and Schour (1939) for deciduous teeth, as well as, with slight modifications, by McCall and Schour (cited by Orban, 1981).

67. **B.** The permanent maxillary first premolar usually has two roots, but they are buccal and lingual, not mesial and distal.

68. **D.** (Ash and Nelson, 2003).

69. **C.** The labiolingual diameter of crown near the cervix is *greater* than in mandibular canine.

70. **D.** The labial, mesioincisal angle of tooth #8 and #9 (central incisors) is a sharp, right angle, not slightly rounded. The labial, mesioincisal angle of tooth #7 and #10 (lateral incisors) is slightly rounded, not a sharp right angle.

71. **C.** Distal to the second premolar, 56%.

72. **A.** (McCauley, 1945; Ash and Nelson, 2003).

73. **D.** Internal aponeuroses *do* move and deform.

74. **A.** Choice **B,** tooth grinding in sleep bruxism lasts 5 minutes, not 20 minutes; choice **C,** sleep bruxism often coincides with passage from deep to lighter sleep, not lighter to deep sleep; choice **D,** sleep bruxism occurs approximately every 90 minutes, not every 20 minutes in the sleep cycle.

75. **A.** Bruxism is now thought to be mainly regulated centrally, not peripherally.

76. **D.** Mandibular supporting cusps are buccal cusps.

77. **A.** To measure horizontal overlap, measure from labial of mandibular central incisor to labial of maxillary central incisor.

78. **B.** (Ash and Nelson, 2003).

79. **A.** The auriculotemporal nerve provides primary innervation to the TMJ.

80. **D.** The distolabial cusp is smallest on a five-lobed mandibular second premolar.

81. **D.** The primary mandibular first molar typically has four pulp horns.

82. **D.** Clinically in relation to interocclusal space.

83. **C.** (Ash and Nelson, 2003).

84. **B.** Root bifurcation is more likely in the mandibular canine.

85. **D.** All posterior teeth viewed from distal aspect have a rhomboidal outline.

86. **A.** A distinct developmental groove, prominent buccal triangular ridge, two cusps, and distinct mesial and distal occlusal pits are most characteristic of the mandibular first premolar.

87. **A.** From the incisal aspect, the maxillary central incisor has a greater mesiodistal diameter (8.5 mm) than faciolingual diameter (7.0 mm). Choice **B,** the mesiodistal diameter is 7.5 mm, and the faciolingual diameter is 8.0 mm; choice **C,** the mesiodistal diameter is 7.0 mm, and the faciolingual diameter is 7.5 mm; choice **D,** the mesiodistal diameter is 5.5 mm, and the faciolingual diameter is 6.0 mm.

88. **A.** Maximum condylar rotation occurs with maximum jaw opening.

89. **D.** Use of the formula indicates on the basis of ±6 months that the age of defect formation is 2 to 3 years.

90. **C.** Choices **A** and **B** are correct. Choice **D** is per the product manufacturer's recommendations.

91. **B.** Systemic etiologic factors for hypoplasia are thought to occur possibly after birth and before 6 years of age.

92. **C.** Measles is not known to cause enamel hypoplasia.

93. **D.** Intermediate filament is a smooth muscle filament. Connectin is another name for titin. Choices **A, B,** and **C** statements are true and refer to *skeletal* muscle filaments.

94. **D.** Masseter muscles provide most of the force between molar teeth with clenching in the intercuspal position.

95. **D.** Individuals who brux during the day do not necessarily brux at night.

96. **D.** Sequential changes from autonomic cardiac or brain cortical activities *precede* sleep bruxism–related jaw motor activity.

97. **D.** Malocclusion has not been suggested as causing or aggravating bruxism.

98. **D.** Fluorosis versus nonfluoride opacities may be difficult to diagnose clinically.

99. **B.** Thick and thin filaments do not change in length.

100. **C.** SHLP helps stabilize the head and condyle against the eminence in clenching; choices **A, B,** and **D** are true.

101. **B, C, D, E.** See Figures 4-13 through 4-20.

102. **A, B, D,** and **F.** See Ch. Identification characteristics of primary teeth.

103. **B, D,** and **E.** See section on TMJ ligaments.

104. **C, D, E, F,** and **G.** See section on temporalis muscle. Note: the anterior and middle bundles of this

muscle elevate the mandible, whereas the posterior bundles retrude the mandible.

105. **A, B, C,** and **E.** See section on deep layer masseter muscle.

106. 1—A, 2—C, 3—J, 4—H, 5—K, 6—F, 7—I. See Figure 4-29.

107. 1—A, 2—C, 3—J, 4—H, 5—K, 6—F, 7—I. See Figure 4-29.

108. 1—P, 2—E, 3—D, 4—Q, 5—S, 6—B, 7—C, 8—R, 9—T, 10—A. See Table 4-1; although similar in average emergence age, mandibular first molars tend to develop slightly earlier than the maxillary first molars.

109. 1—16, 2—11, 3—12, 4—14, 5—15, 6—13, 7—17, 8—18. See Table 4-3; right maxillary 1—first molar, 2—central incisor, 3—lateral incisor, 4—first premolar, 5—second premolar, 6—cuspid, 7—second molar, 8—third molar.

110. 1—A, 2—F, 3—E, 4—D, 5—D, 6—E, 7—B, 8—C.

111. 1—C, 2—B, 3—D, 4—E. See Figure 4-30.

112. **C.** A point angle is a junction of three tooth surfaces. An example is the mesiobucco-occlusal point angle.

113. Proper sequence posterior to anterior is 1—posterior attachment, 2—bilaminar zone, 3—posterior band, 4—intermediate zone, 5—anterior band, 6—SHLP. See Figure 4-36.

114. **D, E, F.** Two roots are a common feature of the permanent and primary mandibular molars and maxillary first premolars.

115. **B.** Adult human and ape dentitions include premolars.

116. 1—F, 2—A, 3—B, 4—D, 5—E, 6—C, 7—G. See Figure 4-25, C.

117. 1. F, 2. A, 3. B, 4. C, 5. D, 6. E, 7. G. See Figure 4-25, C.

118. 1—A, 2—B, 3—C. See Figure 4-27.

119. **E.** All of the above.

120. **E.** All of the above.

Answer Key for Sample Examination

1. **D.** Mandibular supporting cusps are buccal cusps.

2. **A.** The inferior head of the lateral pterygoid muscle attaches to the lateral surface of the lateral pterygoid plate of the sphenoid bone. Its superior head attaches to the infratemporal crest of the greater wing of the sphenoid bone. The deep fibers of the medial pterygoid muscle attaches to the medial surface of the lateral pterygoid plate.

3. **B.** A transverse ridge is a combination name for joining buccal and lingual cusp triangular ridges.

4. **B.** Consequences of asbestosis include mesothelioma and bronchogenic carcinoma.

5. **C.** Under normal conditions, all glucose is reabsorbed by both secondary active transport systems and facilitated diffusion using glucose transporters (GLUT1 and GLUT2). Calcium is passively reabsorbed, but its reabsorption is also regulated by parathyroid hormone in the distal tubule. Not all urea is reabsorbed; about half is excreted. Its permeability is altered by changes in vasopressin. Phosphate reabsorption is also regulated by parathyroid hormone.

6. **C.** Although IgE is the least prevalent immunoglobulin in the body, it is the major antibody mediator of type I hypersensitivity reactions. These reactions are caused primarily by prior sensitization and the accumulation of IgE to a specific allergen.

7. **A.** Because DNA is a double-stranded molecule, cytosine is always base paired to guanine, and guanine is always base paired to cytosine. There are equal amounts of these compounds. It is unlikely that RNA or mRNA, being a single-stranded molecule, would have equal amounts of these bases.

8. **B.** The branchial arches disappear when the second arch grows down to contact the fifth branchial arch.

9. **C.** Glucagon is secreted from the pancreas in response to reduced plasma glucose secondary to fasting and exercise. It functions to mobilize energy stores (glucose) and return blood glucose to normal levels. Glycogen synthesis (glycogenesis) does not occur in response to glucagon.

10. **D.** In contrast to in noncompetitive inhibition, the inhibitor competes for the same site as the substrate. It is possible (with increased amounts of substrate) to reach the V_{max}. Apparent K_m is increased because more substrate is required to reach $\frac{1}{2} V_{max}$ (the definition of K_m).

11. **D.** The primary mandibular first molar typically has four pulp horns.

12. **C.** Burkitt's lymphoma is an aggressive lymphoma that affects B lymphocytes.

13. **E.** Histologic evaluation of Burkitt's lymphoma reveals a characteristic starry sky appearance, which results from the lighter colored macrophages present.

14. **A.** Epstein-Barr virus is responsible for causing mononucleosis, a disease that also affects B lymphocytes.

15. **A.** To measure horizontal overlap, measure from labial of mandibular central incisor to labial of maxillary central incisor (Ash and Nelson, 2003; Woelfel and Scheid, 2002).

16. **D.** Capillary blood flow is proportional to changes in the radius (r4) of the vessel. Decreasing the radius would produce increased vascular pressure. Viscosity of the blood depends primarily on the hematocrit (percentage of red blood cells) and would not be changed by changes in the radius of the vessels.

17. **D.** The facial nerve supplies special sensory (taste) to the anterior two thirds of the tongue, via one of its branches, the chorda tympani. The chorda tympani branches from the facial nerve, carrying both sensory fibers for taste and preganglionic parasympathetic fibers. It exits from the temporal bone to join the lingual nerve (a branch of CN V3) as it courses inferiorly toward the submandibular ganglion (see Figure 1-7). Postganglionic parasympathetic fibers emerge from the ganglion and continue toward the sublingual and submandibular glands (see Figure 1-8). Sensory fibers also branch from the nerve and provide taste sensation to the anterior two thirds of the tongue.

18. **C.** The labiolingual diameter of the crown near the cervix is *greater* than in the mandibular canine (Kraus et al., 1969).

19. **A.** The gastrointestinal tract is regulated by both the sympathetic and the parasympathetic branches of the autonomic nervous system. The parasympathetic system is stimulatory, and the sympathetic system is inhibitory. The central nervous system influences motility and secretory activity through the autonomic nervous system. Numerous endocrine factors (e.g., secretin, gastrin, cholecystokinin) are also involved with the regulation of gastrointestinal activity.

20. **C.** Although all of the structures listed are common sites for oral cancer, the lower vermilion border of the lip is the most common oral site.

21. **A.** The vertical component is not seen on the horizontal tracing.

22. **D.** The palatopharyngeus forms the posterior tonsillar pillar. It also functions to close off the nasopharynx and larynx during swallowing. The anterior tonsillar pillar is formed by the palatoglossus.

23. **D.** Decreasing total peripheral resistance would produce greater reductions in blood pressure. As a result of the baroreceptor reflex, cardiac heart rate would increase. Increased stroke volume (owing to increased venous return and sympathetic stimulation of cardiac muscle) would also occur. Increased cardiac output would occur secondary to increased heart rate and stroke volume.

24. **B.** Insulin is a polypeptide hormone that promotes energy storage when it is readily available. The lack of insulin would interfere with this process. Under conditions of reduced insulin, hyperglycemia would result owing to increased gluconeogenesis in the liver. Glycogen breakdown would be enhanced, and glycogen synthesis would be decreased. Because insulin promotes amino acid uptake in the liver, lack of insulin would result in decreased uptake.

25. **D.** A minimum of 12 hours is required.

26. **C.** The roof of the orbit consists of the lesser wing of the sphenoid bone and the orbital plate of the frontal bone (not listed).

27. **C.** The dimension of the permanent maxillary canine at the widest mesiodistal diameter is 7.5 mm (7.5 mm, Ash and Nelson, 2003; 7.6 mm [6.3 to 9.5 mm] Woelfel and Scheid, 2002).

28. **D.** Facilitated diffusion does not require energy and moves down a concentration gradient. Active transport, in addition to using energy, is often coupled to transport ions in both directions across the membrane. Both active transport and facilitated diffusion are carrier-mediated and are influenced by competitive inhibition.

29. **A.** In general, plaque is first colonized by gram-positive cocci bacteria, such as *Streptococcus* species. They are followed by gram-negative, rod-shaped anaerobes, such as *Bacteroides, Fusobacterium, Porphyromonas*, and *Prevotella*, and then filament-type bacteria, such as *Actinomyces*.

30. **D.** Triacylglycerol is not commonly a component of cell membranes because it serves primarily as a molecule for storage and transport of fatty acids. Phospholipids are abundant because they form the bilayer structure characteristic of membranes. Proteins are present and serve various functions as enzymes, receptors, and transporters or carriers. Cholesterol stabilizes the membrane and is responsible for the maintenance of fluidity. Sphingolipids are components of myelin, which insulates membranes in neurons.

31. **A.** The lateral cricoarytenoid adducts the vocal cords. The oblique and transverse arytenoids and thyroarytenoid also adduct the vocal folds. The posterior cricoarytenoid abducts the vocal cords. The cricothyroid muscle raises the cricoid cartilage and tenses the vocal cords.

32. **E.** Carcinoma in situ is the best term. Although the cells have not yet invaded the basement membrane, the likelihood of invasive growth is presumed to be high.

33. **D.** The rectus abdominis muscle of the anterolateral abdominal wall is described as being beltlike or straplike. The remaining three muscles of the anterolateral abdominal wall (external oblique muscle, internal oblique muscle, and transversus abdominis muscle) are described as sheetlike. The quadratus lumborum muscle is part of the posterior abdominal wall.

34. **D.** Roots of primary teeth are longer and more slender compared with crown size than roots of permanent teeth. For choice **A**, enamel rods slope *occlusally*, not gingivally, in the primary molars. For choice **B**, enamel rods at the cervix slope *gingivally*, not occlusally, in permanent molars. For choice **C**, the buccal cervical ridge is *more* pronounced.

35. **A.** McCune-Albright syndrome is a type of fibrous dysplasia that manifests with a triad of symptoms, including polyostotic fibrous dysplasia, café au lait spots, and endocrine abnormalities.

36. **B.** Fibrous dysplasia is caused by replacement of normal bone with an irregular bone containing fibrous connective tissue. This gives the radiographs a characteristic ground-glass appearance.

37. **B.** Fibrous dysplasia is caused by replacement of normal bone with irregular bone containing fibrous connective tissue. The pathology report usually describes abnormally shaped trabeculae in loosely arranged fibrous tissue.

38. **B.** The overall average length of the primary mandibular central incisor is 14 mm (Black GV, cited by Ash and Nelson, 2003); 16 mm (Woelfel and Scheid, 2002); 14 mm (Kraus et-al., 1969). The answer is 14 to 16 mm, not 16 to 17 mm.

39. **A.** Stenosis describes fibrotic and thickened valves, resulting in reduced blood flow through the valve.

40. **A.** The primary maxillary second molar is rhomboidal in form. For choice **B**, it has *four* well-developed cusps. For choice **C**, it has only *one* supplementary cusp. For choice **D**, it has a *well-developed* mesial triangular fossa.

41. **A.** All the other factors produce vasodilation and hyperemia to increase the exchange of metabolites in the tissue.

42. **C.** The inferior aspect of the diaphragm is supplied with blood by the inferior phrenic arteries. The median sacral artery supplies the anterior aspect of the sacral area, and the lumbar arteries supply the lower abdominal wall. The celiac trunk and superior mesenteric arteries are both unpaired branches to the gut and associated glands.

43. **C.** Pyridoxal phosphate is the active coenzyme of pyridoxine, which is involved in many enzyme systems essential for normal amino acid metabolism. Biotin is required for carboxylation reactions. Tetrahydrofolate, the coenzyme form of folic acid, is required for the synthesis of nucleic acids and porphyrin. Niacin participates in energy metabolism (oxidation-reduction reactions).

44. **C.** Equal bilateral contraction of the lateral pterygoid muscles results in protrusion of the mandible.

45. **D.** Oligodendrocytes produce the myelin sheath around myelinated axons in the central nervous system. Schwann's cells make up the myelin sheath around myelinated axons in the parasympathetic nervous system.

46. **A.** Inorganic mineral makes up 95% of enamel compared with 84% of calculus, 70% of dentin, and 60% of bone.

47. **D.** Poststreptococcal glomerulonephritis is a classic example of nephritic syndrome, which occurs after a *Streptococcus* infection (e.g., strep throat). It is characterized by all of the symptoms listed except polyuria. A decrease in urination is usually observed.

48. **D.** In the cusp-embrasure occlusal relationship, the maxillary first premolar is most likely to articulate with the first and second premolars.

49. **C.** The universal tooth numbering system for primary dentition uses a sequential alphabet letter for each tooth in an entire dentition—A though T.

50. **B.** Oblique alveolodental fibers resist occlusal forces that occur along the long axis of the tooth. The rest of the alveolodental (periodontal ligament) fibers listed provide resistance against forces that pull the tooth in an occlusal direction (i.e., forces that try to pull the tooth from its socket).

51. **A.** When pulpal nerves are stimulated, they can only transmit one signal: pain.

52. **C.** The mylohyoid muscle forms the floor of the mouth. Relaxation of this muscle would help the dentist push the film down, to help ensure that the apical root is captured on the radiograph.

53. **B.** Fibers of the lateral pterygoid muscle are attached to the anterior end of the disc. Contraction of this muscle pulls the disc in an anterior and medial direction.

54. **B.** The sensory distribution for the maxillary nerve (CN V2) includes the cheek and upper lip, lower eyelid, upper lip, nasopharynx, tonsils, palate, and maxillary teeth. The sensory distribution for the long buccal nerve also includes the (lower) cheek; however, it does not include the upper lip. The long buccal is a branch of the mandibular nerve (CN V3) and provides sensory nerves to the cheek, buccal gingiva of the posterior mandibular teeth, and buccal mucosa.

55. **A.** The inferior alveolar nerve courses between the sphenomandibular ligament and the ramus of the mandible before entering the mandibular foramen. The sphenomandibular ligament may be damaged during the administration of an inferior alveolar nerve block.

56. **D.** Polycystic kidney disease is characterized by the formation of cysts in kidney. It is commonly associated with berry aneurysms.

57. **B.** The oropharynx is lined by stratified squamous epithelium. This type of epithelium also lines the oral cavity, laryngopharynx, esophagus, vaginal canal, and anal canal.

58. **C.** Phosphodiesterases are intracellular enzymes that degrade cyclic nucleotides, catalyzing the hydrolysis of cAMP to a metabolite, adenosine 5′-monophosphate, which lacks the second messenger properties of cAMP. Adenylate cyclase is an enzyme that catalyzes the conversion of adenosine triphosphate to cAMP. Monoamine oxidase is an enzyme located in presynaptic nerve terminals that degrades dopamine, norepinephrine, and epinephrine to inactive substances. Aspirin inhibits prostaglandin synthesis by inhibiting the cyclooxygenase enzyme.

59. **A.** The maxillary first primary molar is said to be the most atypical of human molars.

60. **B.** Osteomyelitis, or an infection of bone, is most commonly caused by *S. aureus*. Symptoms include pain and systemic signs of infection (i.e., fever, malaise).

61. **C.** Intercalated discs are found only in cardiac muscle. Multiple, peripherally positioned nuclei are found in the fibers of skeletal muscle. Smooth muscle cells are spindle-shaped.

62. **D.** The distolingual cusp is smallest on a five-lobed mandibular second premolar.

63. **C.** Although fluoride may be incorporated in mineralized tissues, it is not required for the mineralization process. Matrix vesicles produced by osteoblasts are considered to be the initial site of mineralization. Amelogenins are matrix proteins in enamel that regulate crystallite growth. Phosphoryns are initiator proteins that bind minerals to facilitate nucleation and crystal growth.

64. **E.** Celiac sprue is characterized by malabsorption and mucosal lesions of the small intestines and is caused by an allergy to gluten. A complication of this disease includes T-cell lymphomas.

65. **E.** Renal clearance is the volume of plasma completely cleared of a substance by the kidneys per unit of time. The renal clearance of glucose is usually 0 because, although it is filtered, it is completely reabsorbed when the plasma glucose concentration is within normal levels. In a patient with uncontrolled diabetes, plasma glucose levels exceed the reabsorptive capacity, and glucose then appears in the urine. Urea is filtered and passively reabsorbed to a slight degree. Creatinine is both freely filtered and secreted to a slight extent. Sodium and water are filtered and reabsorbed to various degrees secondary to physiologic regulation of aldosterone and antidiuretic hormone.

66. **B.** DiGeorge's syndrome is characterized by a deficiency of T cells. It is caused by the failure of the third and fourth branchial pouches to develop normally, resulting in a lack of thymus and parathyroid development.

67. **A.** Restriction enzymes are also known as *restriction endonucleases*. These enzymes cleave DNA at specific sites to release fragments of DNA for further analysis and characterization by complementary probes.

68. **A.** The bile canaliculi drain bile to interlobular ducts. The interlobular ducts form right and left hepatic ducts. These ducts join to form the common hepatic duct. The gallbladder arises from the common hepatic duct.

69. **D.** There is no evidence of a connection between myositis and bruxing.

70. **E.** The superior and inferior ophthalmic veins drain into the facial vein and cavernous sinus.

71. **D.** PTT measures the intrinsic and common pathways of the coagulation cascade. A prolonged PTT could result from a deficiency of factor V, VIII, IX, X, XI, or XII or of prothrombin or fibrinogen.

72. **C.** Hemophilia A is caused by a deficiency of factor VIII (antihemophilic factor).

73. **C.** Hemophilia A is a hereditary disorder that is X-linked and affects only males. However, females can be carriers.

74. **B.** The only way to distinguish hemophilia A from hemophilia B is to assay the levels of coagulation factors. Hemophilia A is caused by a deficiency of factor VIII, whereas hemophilia B is caused by a deficiency of factor IX.

75. **E.** Arginine is an amino acid that is deaminated to form ornithine primarily in the liver as part of the urea cycle. Ornithine, argininosuccinate, aspartate, and citrulline are generated in the urea cycle but do not provide free ammonia for urea synthesis.

76. **E.** The superior, middle, and inferior constrictor muscles all insert into the median pharyngeal raphe (the superior constrictor muscle was the only one listed in the answer choices); however, their origins differ.

77. **C.** This is the most favorable sequence for prevention of malocclusion.

78. **D.** Immediately after a meal, energy sources are high. Glycogenolysis (glycogen breakdown) is reduced. Lipolysis and oxidation of free fatty acids are also unnecessary during this time. Glucagon release is inhibited secondary to elevated glucose. Glycolysis is increased secondary to elevated intracellular glucose.

79. **A.** Hepatitis A is spread via oral-anal or fecal contamination. The other hepatitis viruses can be transmitted through blood, sexual contact, or perinatally.

80. **B.** Guanine base pairs with cytosine, which, on a molar basis, also equals 30% of the DNA. If guanine and cytosine constitute 60% of DNA, the remaining percentage (40%) must be equally divided between the base pairs of adenine and thymine (20% + 20%).

81. **B.** The muscularis externa has a third layer in the stomach. It is an inner oblique layer of smooth muscle. In the rest of the digestive tract, the muscularis externa has two layers: an inner circular layer and an outer longitudinal layer.

82. **C.** Gummas are granulomas that may be seen in tertiary syphilis. Syphilis is caused by *T. pallidum*. Granulomas may also be seen in tuberculosis, an infection caused by *M. tuberculosis*; however, in this disease, they are known as *tubercles*.

83. **A.** The medulla of the thymus contains Hassall's corpuscles, which consist of epithelial cells with keratohyaline granules. The medulla is the lighter staining (less dense) central area of the gland, where T-cell maturation occurs.

84. **C.** The masseter originates from the inferior border of the zygomatic arch; specifically, its superficial head and deep head originate from the anterior two thirds and posterior one third of the inferior border, respectively. The superficial head inserts into the lateral surface of the angle of the mandible; the deep head inserts into the ramus and body of the mandible.

85. **D.** The width and depth of arch are more or less constant after 9 months of age. However, a substantial increase in the anterior-posterior distance occurs for permanent molars.

86. **A.** Hemoglobin is a globular protein responsible for transporting most of the oxygen in the blood. The

percent saturation of hemoglobin is a function of the P_{O_2} of the blood. The relationship of P_{O_2} and hemoglobin saturation is not linear but rather sigmoidal. Percent saturation increases greatly at low P_{O_2} and less at higher P_{O_2}. Increased P_{CO_2}, temperature, diphosphoglycerate, and H^+ decrease the affinity of hemoglobin for oxygen but do not alter the characteristic sigmoidal nature of the saturation curve.

87. **A.** On average, the height of curvature is 3.5 mm on the mesial and 2.5 mm on the distal of the maxillary central incisor; it is 3.0 mm on the mesial and 2.0 mm on the distal of the mandibular central incisor.

88. **B.** Dysplastic cells are abnormal in appearance and organization. The potential to develop into a malignant tumor is present; however, this risk varies.

89. **D.** The deep masseter muscle is generally a jaw-closing muscle. It may stabilize and act with lateral jaw movements.

90. **D.** An infection by molds, such as mucormycosis, results in the invasion of blood vessel endothelium. This leads to hemorrhagic infarction and tissue necrosis.

91. **A.** The first rib cannot be palpated.

92. **D.** Mast cells contain dense granules with inflammatory mediators, including histamine and slow-reacting substance of anaphylaxis (SRSA), which is a leukotriene.

93. **B.** The hypothalamus coordinates many activities mediated by the autonomic nervous system, including food intake, thirst, and temperature regulation. The cerebellum functions to regulate movement and posture. The medulla is responsible for coordinating respiration. The cerebral cortex performs functions of perception, cognition, higher motor functions, memory, and emotion.

94. **E.** Chronic bronchitis predisposes affected individuals to squamous neoplasia of the bronchial epithelium (i.e., bronchogenic carcinoma).

95. **A.** The mesiobuccal, distobuccal, and distal cusps are almost equal in size, whereas the distal cusp of the permanent molar is smaller. For choice **B**, the primary molar crown is *narrower*, not wider buccolingually. For choice **C**, the primary molar outline is rectangular. For choice **D**, the crown/root ratio is not the same.

96. **B.** In smooth muscle, the binding of calcium to calmodulin activates the enzyme myosin light chain kinase. This enzyme phosphorylates myosin, allowing it to bind to actin, and the muscle contracts. For contraction in skeletal and cardiac muscle, calcium binds to troponin C.

97. **A.** Estrogen is a steroid hormone and does not require a membrane receptor and the second messenger cAMP. Steroid hormones directly enter the cell and stimulate intracellular receptors. Peptide hormones and hormones derived from single amino acids are not readily lipid-soluble (characteristic of membranes) and require membrane receptors and a second messenger system (e.g., cAMP, inositol triphosphate). Many of the effects of epinephrine and norepinephrine and all of the effects of glucagon are mediated by cAMP.

98. **D.** The Western blot tests for HIV proteins. The ELISA tests for HIV antibodies. When these two tests are used together, a 99% accuracy rate is achieved.

99. **C.** Because 90% of blood transfusion–related hepatitis cases are caused by hepatitis C, and the patient has a history of having had a blood transfusion, hepatitis C is the correct answer.

100. **D.** Opportunistic infections are a serious problem in patients with HIV infection. This patient's intraoral thrush is an opportunistic infection that is caused by *Candida albicans*. Treatment for candidiasis includes nystatin.

101. **C.** HIV is an RNA virus that contains three enzymes: reverse transcriptase, integrase, and protease. Neuraminidase is a protein found on the surface of the influenza virus.

102. **C.** Although all of the microbes listed cause pneumonia, the most common cause of pneumonia in patients with AIDS is *P. jiroveci*.

103. **C.** Bifurcation of roots begins almost immediately at the site of the cervical line (cementoenamel junction). For choice **A**, it is smaller in all dimensions. For choice **B**, all roots are seen from the buccal aspect. For choice **D**, the roots are nearly the same length.

104. **B.** Cells degrade purine nucleotides to uric acid. Xanthine is an intermediate in a series of reactions, but the final product in humans is uric acid, which is excreted in the urine. Urea is the degradation product of compounds containing amino groups (amino acids).

105. **B.** An essential amino acid is one that cannot be synthesized by humans and must be obtained in the diet from plant or bacterial sources. All of the other amino acids can be synthesized by humans from other compounds and are not classified as "essential."

106. **B.** The fovea centralis contains only cone cells. It is located approximately 2.5 mm lateral to the optic disc in a yellow-pigmented area (macula luna). Vision is most acute from this area.

107. **C.** The middle trunk of the brachial plexus of nerves arises from C7.

108. **E.** Both *Epidermophyton* and *Trichophyton* can cause tinea pedis.

109. **B.** Comparatively, roots of primary anterior teeth are narrower and longer. For choice **A**, crowns of anterior primary teeth are *wider*, not narrower. For choice **C**, cervical ridges of primary anterior teeth are *more* prominent. For choice **D**, buccal and lingual surfaces are *more flat*, not less flat.

110. **C.** Cystic fibrosis results from an abnormal chloride channel that affects all exocrine glands.

111. **A.** The site of cell division (mitosis) occurs in the stratum basale (basal layer, stratum germinativum) of oral epithelium.

112. **A.** IgA is found in mucosal secretions of the genitourinary, intestinal, and respiratory tracts, including tears, saliva, and colostrum.

113. **A.** Chronic granulomatosis results from neutrophils with a defective nicotinamide adenine dinucleotide phosphate oxidase system. This affects their ability to kill microorganisms because they are unable to produce superoxide radicals.

114. **B.** Tetrahydrofolic acid is the coenzyme form of folic acid required for the synthesis of nucleic acids and normal cell division and replication.

115. **D.** Phenylketonuria is an inherited disorder of amino acid metabolism in which the affected individual lacks enzymes to metabolize phenylalanine. Albinism is a condition that results in a defect in tyrosine metabolism and the inability to produce melanin. Porphyria is an inherited disorder involving defects in heme synthesis. Homocystinuria is a disorder in the metabolism of homocysteine resulting in high levels of homocysteine and methionine in plasma and urine.

116. **D.** Molecular tests such as the polymerase chain reaction have a fast, not slow, turnaround time.

117. **A.** Rifampin causes orange, not green, urine, tears, and sweat.

118. **B.** The drug binds tightly only to *prokaryotic* RNA polymerase. Also, rifampin *induces* activity of hepatic mixed oxidases.

119. **C.** Naproxen has not been reported to exacerbate bruxism. For A, refer to Romanelli et-al., 1996; B, Refer to Gerber and Lynd, 1998; D, Refer to Milosevic et-al., 1999.

120. **C.** The mechanisms of the two types of headaches are quite different. A, B, and D are considered true.

121. **B.** β-Amyloid deposits are a component of Alzheimer's disease but not of migraine headaches.

122. **A.** Low-dose aspirin reduces the likelihood of platelet aggregation. (Montgomery et-al., 1996).

123. **B.** Infection is most likely to involve the submaxillary space, considering the clinical findings.

124. **A.** Given the clinical findings and the involved molar position, the lateral upper deep cervical node group would most likely be the first involved with lymph drainage (Shafer et-al., 1983).

125. **B.** Oral TB most often involves the *tongue*.

126. **B.** Langerhans' giant cells, epithelioid cells, and caseous necrotic areas are highly suggestive of TB; however, special stains for acid-fast bacilli and isolation of *M. tuberculosis* may be necessary, keeping in mind that staining may not differentiate TB from other mycobacterial infections. Other molecular tests may be indicated.

127. **C.** The anticoagulant effect of warfarin is inhibited by rifampin. For choice **A**, rifampin *decreases* the anticoagulation effect of warfarin. For choice **B**, rifampin *interferes* with cyclic conversion. For choice **D**, rifampin *increases* the metabolic clearance.

128. **A.** GALT produces secretory IgA.

129. **C.** Systemic lupus erythematosus, also known as *lupus*, is considered an autoimmune disease, although the exact cause is unknown. It is characterized by the presence of ANAs. Common ANA findings include anti-DNA, anti-RNA, and anti-Sm antigen.

130. **D.** The backbone of DNA and RNA is composed of sugars (deoxyribose or ribose) joined $3' \rightarrow 5'$.

131. **C.** The hypoglossal (CN XII) nerve is not found in the posterior triangle; however, it is present in the submandibular triangle. Contents of the posterior triangle include the external jugular and subclavian veins and their tributaries, the subclavian artery and its branches, branches of the cervical plexus, CN XI, nerves to the upper limb and muscles of the triangle floor, the phrenic nerve, and the brachial plexus.

132. **A.** The α-chains are polypeptides that characterize the collagen molecule. The most abundant amino acids in collagen are proline and glycine. Proline (owing to its amino ring structure), interrupts the α-chain, resulting in the bending and twisting of the peptide. Glycine (owing to its small size) fits into the smaller spaces of the peptide and is positioned at every third position in the chain.

133. **B.** Increasing the hydrostatic pressure within the glomerulus would decrease the net ultrafiltration pressure. Reduced plasma protein concentration decreases the oncotic pressure in the plasma, which would increase filtration. Vasodilation of the afferent arterioles would increase capillary pressure resulting in increased filtration. Inulin, although used to measure glomerular filtration, does not affect glomerular filtration rate.

134. **A.** The most common form of breast cancer is adenocarcinoma arising from the ductal epithelium.

135. **D.** The labial mesioincisal angle of tooth #8 and #9 (central incisors) is a sharp, right angle, not slightly rounded. The labial mesioincisal angle of tooth #7 and #10 (lateral incisors) is slightly rounded, not a sharp right angle.

136. **C.** The apex of a medullary pyramid in the kidney is called the renal papilla. The cortex is the outer layer of the kidney. The medulla is the inner layer. Minor calyces receive secretions from the renal papillae. Several minor calyces join to form a major calyx.

137. **D.** Endocarditis is most commonly caused by group B α-hemolytic streptococci, such as viridans streptococcus, *Streptococcus mutans*, *Streptococcus sanguis*, and *Streptococcus salivarius*. All of the other conditions listed are associated with group A β-hemolytic streptococcal infections, such as *Streptococcus pyogenes*.

138. **D.** After branching from the mandibular nerve (CN V3), the auriculotemporal nerve travels posteriorly and encircles the middle meningeal artery, remaining posterior and medial to the condyle. It continues up toward the temporomandibular joint, external ear, and temporal region, passing through the parotid gland and traveling with the superficial temporal artery and vein.

139. **A.** Given the patient's history of rheumatic fever, the heart murmur is most likely from a dysfunctioning mitral valve. Rheumatic fever most commonly affects the mitral valve, resulting in mitral valve stenosis, regurgitation, or both.

140. **B.** Rheumatic fever is usually preceded by a group A streptococcus respiratory infection (e.g., strep throat or pharyngitis).

141. **A.** The most common cause of subacute endocarditis is viridans streptococcus. Viridans streptococci are α-hemolytic streptococci, representing incomplete lysis of red blood cells in laboratory cultures.

142. **E.** During subacute endocarditis, vegetations, or thrombi, form on previously damaged heart valves. Complications can arise if embolization of the thrombus occurs (i.e., when a fragment separates and enters the circulation), causing septic infarcts. Other complications include valvular dysfunction or abscess formation.

143. **C.** Aminoglycosides block the 30S ribosomal subunit to inhibit protein synthesis.

144. **B.** Translation is the conversion of information from mRNA into a protein. Transduction is the incorporation of genetic information carried by a virus into bacteria.

145. **A.** Maximum condylar rotation occurs with maximum jaw opening.

146. **B.** The right subclavian artery arises from the brachiocephalic artery, and the left subclavian artery arises from the aortic arch. The subclavian artery becomes the axillary artery on crossing the first rib. The axillary artery becomes the brachial artery when it leaves the axilla.

147. **D.** Rest position is defined clinically in relation to interocclusal space.

148. **B.** The concentration of K⁺ within cells is approximately 30 times greater compared with the extracellular fluid; the other ions are in greater concentrations in extracellular fluid compared with values within the cell.

149. **B.** Neutrophils are quick to arrive to the site of infection or injury and are associated with acute inflammation. All of the other cells listed are mediators of chronic inflammation.

150. **A.** The correct answer (7 to 8 years) is based on chronologies in Ash and Nelson, 2003 and Woelfel and Scheid, 2002, which are based on original chronologies by Schour and Massler, modified for permanent dentition by Kronfeld (Bur) and by Kronfeld and Schour (1939) for deciduous teeth. Also, with slight modifications, by McCall and Schour (cited by Orban, 1981).

151. **E.** Heparin, an anticoagulant, is different from the other glycosaminoglycans because it is an extracellular compound. Hyaluronic acid is found in synovial fluid; keratan sulfate is found in loose connective tissue such as cornea; chondroitin sulfate is found in cartilage, ligaments, and tendons; and dermatan sulfate is found in skin and blood vessels.

152. **A.** The pancreas is enveloped at its head by the first part of the duodenum.

153. **B.** Individuals with mucopolysaccharidoses have normal production of proteoglycans and glycosaminoglycans but, owing to genetic defects, lack the enzymes that degrade mucopolysaccharides.

154. **A.** The terminology used is a classic descriptor of the relationship between the hormone source and target tissue. *Paracrine* refers to the target tissue as a cell in close proximity to the secreting tissue. *Autocrine* stimulation refers to a cell that releases a factor (hormone) that stimulates the cell from which it was released. *Endocrine* factors are hormones that have an effect at a distal site in the body.

155. **C.** Pyelonephritis is usually caused by gram-negative, rod-shaped bacteria that are part of the normal flora of the enteric tract. It is most commonly caused by *E. coli*, followed by *Proteus*, *Klebsiella*, and *Enterobacter*.

156. **C.** The salivary glands are lined by simple cuboidal epithelium. This type of epithelium also lines the bronchioles, thyroid gland, and ovary capsule.

157. **E.** The macula densa is a component of the juxtaglomerular apparatus that functions in regulation of blood pressure. The proximal convoluted tubule, distal convoluted tubule, Bowman's capsule, and glomerulus all function in the production of urine.

158. **D.** Internal aponeuroses *do* move and deform.

159. **C.** The cricopharyngeus muscle prevents swallowing air at the pharyngeal end of the esophagus.

160. **C.** The most common cause of bacterial meningitis in newborns is *E. coli*. The most common cause of bacterial meningitis in infants and children is *H. influenzae* and in young adults is *Neisseria meningitidis*.

161. **B.** Glucose transport in muscle and adipose tissue is under the influence of insulin-sensitive glucose transporters. Although several metabolic pathways are influenced by insulin, glucose uptake into the liver is not affected by insulin.

162. **C.** Deoxygenated blood from the transverse sinus drains to the sigmoid sinus, which empties into the internal jugular veins. The transverse sinuses receive blood from the confluence of sinuses, which is located in the posterior cranium.

163. **C.** The central groove is well defined. For choice **A**, the primary maxillary second molar *does* have a well-defined mesial triangular fossa. For choice **B**, the oblique ridge is *prominent*. For choice **D**, the supplementary cusp is *not* well developed.

164. **B.** Facial nerves are derived from the second branchial arch. The trigeminal nerve is derived from the first branchial arch.

165. **B.** A probe is a single strand of DNA synthesized with a radioisotope that is complementary to a segment of DNA of interest. The radiolabeled complex can be analyzed subsequently on a gel by a technique known as a *Southern blot*.

166. **A.** The primary mandibular second molar is rectangular in form. For choice **B**, the outline of the crown converges *distally*. For choice **C**, the three buccal cusps are *similar* in size. For choice **D**, *well-defined* triangular ridges extend from the cusp tips.

167. **B.** For M_1, distobuccal height equals mesiobuccal height; for M_2, distobuccal cusp height is slightly less than mesiobuccal cusp height; for M_3, distobuccal cusp height is much shorter than mesiobuccal cusp height.

168. **B.** The radiographic finding of a cotton-wool appearance is common in patients with a diagnosis of osteitis deformans or Paget's disease.

169. **B.** In the process of muscle contraction, adenosine triphosphate bound to myosin is cleaved to form adenosine diphosphate and inorganic phosphate. Myosin is released to bind to a new actin site producing a force-generating stroke. Sodium influx and calcium binding are involved in the excitation-contraction coupling process but do not serve as a source of energy.

170. **A.** C fibers are the smallest of the sensory and motor fibers. They are postganglionic, are unmyelinated, and have the slowest conduction velocity.

171. **B.** The tendon of the tensor tympani is attached to the handle of the malleus in the middle ear. Loud sounds cause the tensor tympani to contract, pulling the malleus and tympanic membrane inward to reduce vibrations and prevent damage.

172. **B.** Increased levels of alkaline phosphatase may be observed in diseases that display extensive bone loss. Osteoporosis is characterized by a decrease in bone mass. There are either normal or decreased levels of alkaline phosphatase in patients with this disease.

173. **A.** Peutz-Jeghers syndrome is a hereditary disease that is transmitted by autosomal dominance.

174. **D.** The temporomandibular (TMJ) (Ash and Nelson, 2003); and craniomandibular (Woelfel and Scheid, 2002) are primary ligaments of the TMJ.

175. **B.** TB is caused by *M. tuberculosis*. Gram staining of these bacteria cannot be performed because of their waxy cell walls. To identify these bacteria, an acid-fast stain must be ordered.

176. **D.** *M. tuberculosis* infects macrophages, which are initially unable to kill the phagocytosed bacteria.

177. **A.** Cord factor is a glycolipid found on the surface of *M. tuberculosis*.

178. **D.** Type IV delayed-type hypersensitivity reactions are the only type of hypersensitivity immune reactions that are not mediated by antibodies. They are mainly mediated by T cells.

179. **E.** Treatment for TB includes a multidrug therapy. Rifampin, isoniazid, and ethambutol are three of the first-line drugs used.

180. **E.** Ghon complex describes the calcified scar that remains following the primary infection. It is usually found in the lung and includes the primary lesion and its regional lymph node.

181. **B.** Odontogenic infections of a mandibular incisor with an apex below the mylohyoid muscle have the potential to spread to the submental space. If the apex is above the mylohyoid muscle, the infection would spread to the sublingual space. Both of these spaces communicate with the submandibular space.

182. **D.** Phospholipase C, activated by a component of the G-protein (Gα) complexed with guanosine triphosphate, catalyzes the production of diacylglycerol and inositol triphosphate. Diacylglycerol activates protein kinases, which phosphorylates proteins, and inositol triphosphate produces increased release of calcium from intracellular stores.

183. **E.** IL-5 is released by helper T cells to stimulate B lymphocytes to differentiate into plasma cells. It also activates eosinophils and increases the production of IgA.

184. **B.** The salivary glands are influenced by both the sympathetic and the parasympathetic (glossopharyngeal and facial) branches of the autonomic nervous system. The oculomotor nerve (CN III)

carries parasympathetic fibers to the eye, which, when stimulated, produce constriction of the pupil. The parasympathetic system innervates primarily smooth and cardiac muscle, resulting in specific activation and responses.

185. **A.** From the incisal aspect, the maxillary central incisor has a greater mesiodistal diameter (8.5 mm) than faciolingual diameter (7.0 mm). For choice **B**, the mesiodistal diameter is 7.5 , and the faciolingual diameter is 8.0 mm. For choice **C**, the mesiodistal diameter is 7.0 mm, and the faciolingual diameter is 7.5 mm. For choice **D**, the mesiodistal diameter is 5.5 mm, and the faciolingual diameter is 6.0 mm.

186. **A.** The vestigial cleft of Rathke's pouch is located between the anterior and posterior lobes—specifically, between the pars intermedia and anterior lobe. It consists of cystlike spaces (Rathke's cysts) and represents the vestigial lumen of Rathke's pouch.

187. **C.** Pulp chambers are proportionally larger in primary molars. For choice **A**, the enamel cap is *thinner* and *more* consistent in depth. For choice **B**, there is comparatively *greater* thickness. For choice **D**, pulp horns are *higher* in primary molars.

188. **B.** The regulatory centers for respiration are in the brainstem—specifically, the medulla. The medulla contains three groups of neurons (medullary respiratory center, apneustic center, and pneumotaxic center). The cerebral cortex may influence the medullary centers but does not totally control respiration.

189. **D.** The brachial plexus of nerves arises from five roots from the anterior primary rami of spinal nerves C5–C8 and T1.

190. **D.** Aschoff's bodies are the classic lesions observed in rheumatic fever. They are areas of focal necrosis surrounded by a dense inflammatory infiltration and may be observed in heart tissues.

191. **B.** Cyclooxygenase includes isoenzymes of prostaglandin endoperoxidase synthase, which is required for the first step in the synthesis of prostaglandins from arachidonic acid. Phospholipase A_2, which is involved in the synthesis of arachidonic acid, is inhibited by steroidal antiinflammatory agents.

192. **B.** Terminal bronchioles are characterized by ciliated cuboidal cells.

193. **C.** Prevalence is greater than 5% (up to 40%) in populations with Mongolian traits. For choice **A**, prevalence does not exceed 4.2% in white. For choice **B**, prevalence is less than 5% in Eurasian and Asian populations. For choice **D**, prevalence is less than 3% in African populations.

194. **C.** The salivary glands are under the influence of both the sympathetic and the parasympathetic nervous system. Parasympathetic stimulation results in a more watery secretion compared with sympathetic stimulation, which produces increased amounts of protein with reduced volume. The vagus is parasympathetic, which in general is stimulatory to the gastrointestinal tract. In general, sympathetic nerves are inhibitory to the gastrointestinal tract. (The exceptions are salivary glands).

195. **C.** The transverse ridge connects mesiobuccal and mesiolingual cusps.

196. **D.** Jaundice is characterized by yellowness of tissues, including skin, eyes, and mucous membranes. It is caused by diseases that increase serum conjugated or unconjugated bilirubin. These conditions include liver disease, such as cirrhosis or hepatitis; hemolytic anemias; obstruction of the common bile duct, such as caused by gallstones or cholelithiasis; and carcinoma involving the head of the pancreas.

197. **B.** Arteriovenous anastomoses in deeper skin are important in thermoregulation.

198. **A.** Complications of Barrett's esophagus include adenocarcinoma, stricture formation, and hemorrhage (ulceration).

199. **D.** The elongation and overgrowth of filiform papillae result in hairy tongue. Filiform papillae are thin, pointy projections that make up the most numerous papillae and give the tongue's dorsal surface its characteristic rough texture. Note: a loss of filiform papillae results in glossitis.

200. **B.** Tertiary dentin, or reactive or reparative dentin, is dentin that is formed in localized areas in response to trauma or other stimuli, such as caries, tooth wear, or dental work. Histologically, consistency and organization vary; it has no defined dentinal tubule pattern.

201. **E.** Innervation to the maxillary second molar as well as the palatal and distobuccal root of the maxillary first molar and the maxillary sinus is provided by the posterior superior alveolar nerve. The nerve is a branch of the maxillary nerve (CN V2).

202. **D.** The suprarenal glands secrete epinephrine. Specifically, chromaffin cells of the adrenal medulla, which act as modified postganglionic sympathetic neurons that synthesize, store, and secrete catecholamines, produce epinephrine. It also produces norepinephrine.

203. **A.** The most common cause of gastroenteritis in children is the rotavirus. It is found in the reovirus family.

204. **C.** The answer is distolinguoincisal. (Ash and Nelson, 2003.)

205. **D.** Ureters travel inferiorly just below the parietal peritoneum of the posterior body wall. They pass

anterior to the common iliac arteries as they enter the pelvis.

206. **A.** Aspartame is a peptide derivative composed of aspartic acid and phenylalanine.

207. **E.** The abducens nerve (CN VI) provides innervation to the lateral rectus muscle, which moves the eyeball laterally (i.e., abducts the eye). The medial rectus muscle, which is innervated by the oculomotor nerve (CN III), is responsible for adduction of the eyeball.

208. **D.** K$^+$ is passively (via the cotransport system) secreted from the plasma into the distal and collecting tubules. Under conditions of acidosis, an individual may become hyperkalemic because the kidneys retain K$^+$ and secrete H$^+$. Under conditions of alkalosis, K$^+$ secretion is increased, and H$^+$ secretion is reduced.

209. **B.** Epiphyseal closure marks the end of growth in length of long bones.

210. **A.** M-protein is an important virulent factor found only in *S. pyogenes*.

211. **A.** The initial rate-limiting reaction involves the removal of six carbons from cholesterol and hydroxylation of the steroid nucleus to produce pregnenolone. Pregnenolone can be further isomerized and oxidized to produce the other steroid hormones.

212. **D.** Use of the formula indicates on the basis of ±6 months that the age of defect formation is 2 to 3 years.

213. **C.** The age is incorrect for use of fluoride toothpaste. Choices **A** and **B** are correct. Choice **D** is per the product manufacturer's recommendations.

214. **B.** Systemic etiologic factors for hypoplasia are thought to occur possibly after birth and before 6 years of age.

215. **C.** Measles is not known to cause enamel hypoplasia.

216. **D.** Intermediate filament is a smooth muscle filament. Connectin is another name for titin. Statements in choices **A**, **B**, and **C** are true and refer to *skeletal* muscle filaments.

217. **D.** Masseter muscles provide most of the force between molar teeth with clenching in the intercuspal position.

218. **D.** Individuals who brux during the day do not always brux at night.

219. **D.** Sequential changes from autonomic cardiac and brain cortical activities *precede* sleep bruxism–related jaw motor activity.

220. **D.** Malocclusion has not been suggested as causing or aggravating bruxism.

221. **D.** Fluorosis versus nonfluoride opacities may be difficult to diagnose clinically.

222. **B.** Thick and thin filaments do not change in length.

223. **C.** SHLP helps stabilize the head and condyle against the eminence in clenching. Choices **A**, **B**, and D are true.

224. **D.** In the ascending (distal) loop of Henle, active sodium absorption results in an increased osmolarity of the interstitial fluid, which plays a role in the retention of water under conditions of dehydration.

225. **C.** Under conditions of expansion of extracellular volume (long-term hypertension), renin release and aldosterone secretion are reduced. Increasing antidiuretic hormone, angiotensin II, and increasing sympathetic activity would result in an increase in blood pressure.

226. **E.** The most superficial layer of the epidermis is the stratum corneum. From deep to superficial, the layers are basale, spinosum, granulosum, lucidum, and corneum.

227. **D.** Calcitonin is secreted by parafollicular cells (clear cells) that are located at the periphery of thyroid follicles in the thyroid gland. Calcitonin plays an important role in the regulation of calcium and phosphates. It suppresses bone reabsorption, resulting in decreased calcium and phosphate release.

228. **C.** The ratio of inorganic to organic matter in mature dentin is approximately 70:30. In enamel and cementum, it is approximately 96:4 and 50:50, respectively.

229. **B.** Tuberculin reaction (i.e., purified protein derivative skin test) is an example of type IV delayed (cell-mediated) hypersensitivity. Type IV delayed-hypersensitivity reactions are the only type of hypersensitivity immune reactions that are not mediated by antibodies. They are mainly mediated by T cells.

230. **C.** Vitamins are not digested by enzymes from the pancreas; however, digestion of carbohydrates, fats, and proteins may be required to make vitamins available for absorption. The pancreas produces amylase for carbohydrate digestion, lipase for lipid digestion, and several proteolytic enzymes (trypsinogen, chymotrypsinogen, and procarboxypeptidase) for the digestion of protein.

231. **C.** The mesencephalic nucleus contains the nuclei of the trigeminal sensory nerves (CN V) involved in proprioception and the jaw jerk reflex, including periodontal ligament fibers involved in the reflex. It is located in the midbrain and pons.

232. **A.** Aldosterone secretion is mediated through the renin-angiotensin system. Angiotensin II stimulates the synthesis and release of aldosterone from the adrenal gland. It acts on the distal tubule and collecting ducts to increase sodium reabsorption and potassium secretion.

233. **A.** First evidence of the maxillary central incisor calcification is given as 14 (13 to 16) weeks by Kraus and Jordon, 1965, and by Ash and Nelson, 2003; this is given as 4 months by Woelfel and Scheid, 2003.

234. **D.** *Lingual aspect:* well-defined developmental groove separates mesiolingual and distolingual cusps. For choice **A**, mesiolingual cusp is large and well developed. For choice **B**, distolingual cusp is well developed, more so than that of the primary first molar. For choice **C**, there is a supplemental cusp apical to the mesiolingual cusp but poorly developed.

235. **B.** Cretinism is hypothyroidism in children. Oral findings include macroglossia, prolonged retention of primary teeth, and delayed eruption of permanent teeth.

236. **A.** Surfactant is synthesized by alveolar cells and functions to reduce the surface tension of the alveoli. This reduction of surface tension increases pulmonary compliance and decreases the work of breathing. It also decreases the tendency of the lungs to collapse. Lack of surfactant results in neonatal respiratory distress syndrome.

237. **D.** The red pulp of the spleen consists of cords, containing numerous macrophages, and venous sinusoids. It is the site of blood filtration. The white pulp of the spleen contains numerous T and B lymphocytes.

238. **B.** The velocity of blood flow is the rate of displacement of blood per unit time. Velocity changes inversely with cross-sectional area (cm^2). The greater the area in the vessels, the lower the velocity. Because blood is always flowing as a result of the distensibility of the arterial tree, velocity is never zero.

239. **A.** Neuraminidase is found on the surface envelope of influenza viruses. It functions to attach the virus to the host cell.

240. **C.** These are the most common sequences of eruption.

241. **E.** All of the features listed are commonly observed in malignant cells except a low nuclear-to-cytoplasmic ratio. Because of the large nuclei present, there is usually a high nuclear-to-cytoplasmic ratio.

242. **B.** The two vertebral arteries join together at the border of the pons to form the basilar artery. Branches of the basilar artery provide blood supply to the pons.

243. **C.** RNA synthesis is not required for genetic cloning. All the other enzymes are required to synthesize and splice DNA.

244. **D.** The most potent stimulant of the respiratory center that increases the rate of breathing (hyperventilation) is increased CO_2 tension. CO_2 is permeable to the blood-brain barrier and ultimately produces an increase in H^+ of the cerebrospinal fluid. However, plasma H^+ and HCO_3^- are not permeable and have little direct effect on the respiratory center. The respiratory center is not sensitive to O_2 tension, in contrast to peripheral chemoreceptors.

245. **D.** It is a branch of the maxillary nerve (CN V2). The maxillary nerve branches from the trigeminal ganglion and exits the skull through the foramen rotundum. When it reaches the pterygopalatine ganglion, it terminates as the infraorbital and zygomatic nerves.

246. **B.** Root bifurcation is more likely in the mandibular canine.

247. **B.** A ketose sugar is one that contains a keto group. Glyceraldehyde, mannose, glucose, and galactose all are aldoses because they contain an aldehyde group.

248. **E.** Both tetracycline and streptomycin, an aminoglycoside, inhibit protein synthesis in bacteria. However, streptomycin is bactericidal, not bacteriostatic.

249. **C.** The auricular hillocks are derived from the first and second branchial arches.

250. **C.** In the literature, the length of the primary maxillary central incisor is 16 mm (Black GV, cited in Ash and Nelson, 2003); 16 mm (Kraus et-al., 1969); or 17.2 mm (Woelfel and Scheid, 2002). The permanent maxillary incisor is 23.6 mm (Ash and Nelson, 2003); 23.5 mm (Kraus et-al., 1969); 23.6 mm (Woelfel and Scheid, 2002). 16/23.5 = 0.68 or 68%; 17.2/23.6 = 0.73 or 73%. The answer is about 70%.

251. **B.** Ehlers-Danlos syndrome is characterized by defects in collagen (i.e., connective tissues).

252. **C.** Malonyl CoA is produced after carboxylation of acetyl CoA in the synthetic process of fatty acids. FAD and NAD are involved in fatty acid oxidation, but nicotinamide adenine dinucleotide phosphate is the source of reducing agents in the synthesis of fatty acids.

253. **A.** Insulin is a hormone that is secreted under conditions of increased sources of energy (glucose) and results in increased uptake and storage of glucose in the form of glycogen. In the process, blood glucose is decreased. The transport of glucose into the brain is not affected by the hormone.

254. **B.** Osteocytes are found in lacunae in mature bone.

255. **D.** From the mesiodistal aspect, all posterior teeth have a trapezoidal outline with the shortest uneven side toward the occlusal surface. For choice **A**, marked mesial concavity is present primarily on first premolar. For choice **B**, exceptions may be the distobuccal root of the maxillary

second molar. For choice **C**, from the mesiodistal aspect, all posterior mandibular teeth, not maxillary posterior teeth, have a rhomboidal outline.

256. **A.** As a result of the excessive levels of serum calcium, osseous changes, such as metastatic calcifications and kidney stones, occur in patients with hyperparathyroidism.

257. **B.** This enzyme catalyzes the phosphorylation of fructose 6-phosphate to fructose 1,6-bisphosphate. This irreversible reaction is inhibited by adenosine triphosphate and citrate (indicators of energy abundance within the cell). The reaction is stimulated by adenosine monophosphate.

258. **B.** Type II collagen is a fibril-forming collagens found in cartilaginous structures. Type I is characterized as having high tensile strength and is found in skin, tendon, bone, and dentin. Type III collagen is characteristically more distensible and is found in large blood vessels. Type IV is found in basement membranes.

259. **B.** Mesiodistal width of the crown is the most characteristic feature. (Kraus et-al., 1969.)

260. **D.** From the retropharyngeal space (i.e., "danger space"), odontogenic infections can quickly spread down this space into the thorax (posterior mediastinum) and possibly cause death.

261. **B.** Trisomy 21, which is also known as *Down syndrome*, is a disorder affecting autosomes. It is generally caused by meiotic nondisjunction in the mother, which results in an extra copy of chromosome 21 (trisomy 21).

262. **A.** Type I collagen is the predominant collagen found in cementum. Type III collagen may be present during the formation of cementum, but it is largely reduced during maturation.

263. **A.** Net filtration depends on the hydrostatic pressures in the glomerular capillary, the hydrostatic pressures in Bowman's space, and the oncotic pressures in the capillary and Bowman's capsule. Reducing the plasma protein (reducing the oncotic pressure) lowers the tendency to retain fluid in the capillary. This would result in a net increase in filtration.

264. **C.** Auer rods are observed in blast cells characteristic of acute myelogenous leukemia.

265. **D.** Vasopressin, also known as *antidiuretic hormone*, is a peptide secreted from the posterior pituitary in response to an increase in serum osmolarity. The other hormones listed are synthesized and secreted from the anterior pituitary.

266. **A.** Secretory IgA is an immunoglobulin that is unique to the oral cavity. The secretory component is synthesized by salivary epithelial cells and complexes with IgA to form secretory IgA.

267. **D.** There is marked *asymmetry* of mesial and distal halves.

268. **D.** Oxidation of fatty acids, glucagon release, and glycogenolysis all are increased to provide energy sources for exercising muscle. The synthesis of lipid (lipogenesis) would be decreased during periods of exercise.

269. **B.** The thymus is active at birth and increases in size until puberty (around age 12), after which it gradually atrophies and is replaced by fatty tissue.

270. **C.** MAO is an enzyme located in the presynaptic nerve terminal, which degrades dopamine, norepinephrine, and epinephrine to inactive substances.

271. **A.** Sleep bruxism is characterized by episodes of massive, bilateral clenching. For choice **B**, tooth grinding in sleep bruxism lasts 5 minutes, not 20 minutes. For choice **C**, sleep bruxism often coincides with passage from deeper to lighter sleep, not lighter to deeper sleep. For choice **D**, sleep bruxism occurs approximately every 90 minutes, not every 20 minutes, in the sleep cycle.

272. **D.** These oral findings can be observed in patients with hyperthyroidism. The only endocrine disorder listed that is related to hyperthyroidism is Plummer's disease. It is caused by a nodular growth or adenoma of the thyroid.

273. **C.** Fat in the intestine, low pH, and increased osmolarity of intestinal contents reduce gastric emptying. This reflex is mediated through neuronal and endocrine factors comprising the enterogastric reflex. Saline in the intestine would not affect gastric emptying.

274. **D.** Occlusal contact relations do *not* interfere with jaw opening, but temporomandibular joint and muscle disorders may.

275. **C.** The olecranon fossa is located on the posterior surface of the humerus.

276. **D.** Chronic lymphocytic leukemia is characterized by the proliferation of B cells. It is both the most common and the least malignant type of leukemia.

277. **C.** tRNA is not required for the hydroxylation of collagen because the process occurs after translation of messenger RNA and synthesis of collagen. Ascorbic acid is required to modify the collagen molecule by hydroxylating proline to permit cross-linking among collagen in tissues.

278. **C.** Distal to the second premolar occurs 56% of the time.

279. **D.** Crown converges considerably in a lingual direction. For choice **A**, the *mesiolingual* cusp is most prominent. For choice **B**, the *distolingual* cusp is poorly defined. For choice **C**, the *distobuccal* cusp *may be seen* because it is longer.

280. **D.** The posterior and anterior vagal trunks pass through the diaphragm through the esophageal opening. The aorta enters the diaphragm through

the median arch; the inferior vena cava, through its own opening in the central tendon; the azygos vein, through the right crus; and the splanchnic nerves, through the crura.

281. **B.** The sympathetic postganglionic fibers innervating the heart release norepinephrine. Acetylcholine is a neurotransmitter in sympathetic preganglionic fibers, parasympathetic postganglionic fibers, and parasympathetic preganglionic fibers.

282. **C.** Osteopetrosis, also known as *Albers-Schönberg disease* or *marble bone disease*, is caused by abnormal osteoclasts. The lack of bone resorption results in defective bone remodeling and increased bone density, which may invade into the bone marrow space.

283. **D.** Langerhans' cells are located primarily in stratum spinosum.

284. **B.** Nitric oxide is a molecule produced in endothelial cells that acts directly on smooth muscle to produce relaxation and vasodilation. Inhibition of its synthesis would be expected to increase blood pressure. Inhibitors of angiotensin II synthesis should reduce blood pressure because angiotensin II stimulates aldosterone synthesis resulting in increased fluid retention. Angiotensin II is also a potent vasoconstrictor. Blocking vasopressin (also a potent vasoconstrictor) receptors would reduce blood pressure. Stimulation of the baroreceptor would produce a reflex that would reduce cardiac output and peripheral sympathetic tone.

285. **A.** The primary maxillary second molars are completed by age 11 months.(Ash and Nelson, 2003; Woelfel and Scheid, 2002.)

286. **C.** The movement of the tongue against the palate is the only voluntary process among the four possible answers.

287. **A.** CD8 lymphocytes recognize class I MHC molecules on antigen-presenting cells. CD4 lymphocytes recognize class II MHC molecules on antigen-presenting cells.

288. **A.** Bifurcated roots are not a normal feature of mandibular incisors.

289. **C.** The inner enamel epithelium in the bell stage differentiates into ameloblasts.

290. **D.** The cartilage of the trachea is covered by a perichondrium. The mucosa is covered with respiratory epithelium. Hyaline cartilage rings lie deep to the submucosa. The open end of the cartilage faces the posterior. Smooth muscle extends across the open end of each cartilage.

291. **C.** Pemphigus is an autoimmune disease wherein autoantibodies against epidermis cells are produced. Histologically, a phenomenon called *acantholysis*, wherein epidermal cells appear to detach and separate from each other, is observed.

292. **A.** After a meal, chylomicrons are synthesized in the intestine to transport lipid to the liver. Acetoacetate (ketone body) is found under conditions of increased β-oxidation (fasting). Glucagon is secreted in response to reduced blood sugar, which usually is not present after a meal. Lactate, a product of anaerobic glycolysis, is not elevated under conditions of elevated energy sources in the postabsorptive state.

293. **A.** Bruxism is now thought to be mainly regulated centrally, not peripherally.

294. **A.** A distinct developmental groove, prominent buccal triangular ridge, two cusps, and distinct mesial and distal occlusal pits are most characteristic of the mandibular first premolar.

295. **B.** Autoclaves function by denaturing proteins. The autoclave process is effective against spores.

296. **D.** In the initial step of the synthesis of porphyrin, succinyl coenzyme A and glycine are condensed in a rate-limiting step in the liver.

297. **B.** The dental lamina arises from neural crest cells.

298. **A.** The only disease listed that is related to an abnormal number of chromosomes is Klinefelter's syndrome. This disease is characterized by two or more X chromosomes and one or more Y chromosome. Typically, affected individuals have 47 chromosomes with a karyotype of XXY.

299. **A.** Stretching of muscle spindles results in a reflex that is intended to adjust the muscle to its resting length by contracting the muscle in which it is found. The stretching of the spindle increases afferent impulses to the spinal cord and through a monosynaptic reflex stimulates muscle contraction via an α motoneuron.

300. **C.** The mental foramen is found below the apices 63% of the time.

301. **E.** Urinary filtrate is most hypotonic in the distal convoluted tubule. It is isotonic in the proximal convoluted tubule and thick descending limb of Henle's loop. It becomes hypertonic as it passes through the thin descending limb of Henle's loop, and becomes hypotonic as it passes through the thick ascending segment of Henle's loop. Finally, it becomes increasingly hypotonic as it passes through the distal convoluted tubule.

302. **C.** There are seven pairs of true ribs, meaning they attach directly to the sternum via costal cartilages. The remaining five pairs are called *false ribs* because they attach indirectly to the sternum via costal cartilages. The last pair does not attach at all.

303. **B.** The total of average overall mesiodistal diameters of primary maxillary crowns is reported as 68.2 mm (Black GV, cited by Ash and Nelson, 2003); or 76.8 mm (Woelfel and Scheid, 2002).

304. **C.** Symptoms of a myocardial infarction include chest pain, shortness of breath, diaphoresis

(sweating), clammy hands, nausea, and vomiting.

305. **C.** Amino acids are transported across the luminal surface of the intestine by Na$^+$ amino acid cotransporters in the apical membrane. This is facilitated by the Na$^+$ gradient established in the intestinal cells.

306. **A.** Of the cell types listed, only smooth muscle cells are capable of cell division.

307. **B.** Vitamin K is involved with the posttranslational modification of glutamic acid to form γ-carboxyglutamic acid. This carboxylation permits prothrombin to interact with platelets and ions in the process of clot formation. Hydroxylation of proline requires ascorbic acid and iron.

308. **D.** Squamous cell carcinoma is the most common oral cancer, occurring in 90% of all cases. It is a cancer of squamous epithelium, specifically a tumor of keratinocytes.

309. **B.** The permanent maxillary first premolar usually has two roots, but they are buccal and lingual, not mesial and distal.

310. **D.** Actinic keratosis produces dry, scaly plaques with an erythematous base. They may be premalignant. Both compound and intraepidermal nevi are benign. Only junctional nevi are considered to be premalignant.

311. **B.** Secretin stimulates bicarbonate secretion from the pancreatic ducts. Cholecystokinin is responsible for stimulating pancreatic enzyme secretion and contraction of the gallbladder. Chymotrypsinogen is activated by trypsin in the intestine.

312. **B.** Textbook chronologies indicate that the maxillary primary second molar is most commonly the last to erupt: 24 months (Woelfel and Scheid, 2002), 20 to 30 months (Kraus et-al., 1969), or 25 to 33 months(Ash and Nelson, 2003).

313. **D.** The latissimus dorsi muscle is supplied by the thoracodorsal nerve.

314. **B.** Regulation of blood flow to skin is under the control of factors acting locally (metabolites) and α-adrenergic receptors. Slowing of the heart and activation of gastrointestinal motility are mediated through the cholinergic system. α-Adrenergic receptors produce decreased renal blood flow.

315. **A.** The auriculotemporal nerve provides primary innervation to the TMJ.

316. **B.** The submental artery is a branch of the facial artery. Branches of the mandibular division of the maxillary artery include the inferior alveolar, deep auricular, anterior tympanic, mylohyoid, incisive, mental, and middle meningeal arteries.

317. **E.** Rheumatoid arthritis is characterized by inflammation of the synovial membrane. Granulation tissue forms in the synovium and expands over the articular cartilage. This causes the destruction of the underlying cartilage and results in fibrotic changes or ankylosis.

318. **D.** (Ash and Nelson, 2003.)

319. **C.** The trapezius muscle is supplied by CN XI. The latissimus dorsi is supplied by the thoracodorsal nerve, the levator scapulae is supplied by the dorsal scapular nerve, and the major and minor rhomboid muscles are supplied by the dorsal scapular nerve.

320. **B.** A quelling reaction occurs in a laboratory when the polysaccharide capsule of a bacterium swells after being treated with antiserum or antibodies.

321. **D.** Under conditions of increased intracranial pressure, the vasomotor regions of the medulla are stimulated secondary to localized ischemia resulting in an increase in systemic blood pressure. Ventricular fibrillation refers to irregular, rapid, uncoordinated contractions of the ventricle that do not result in blood movement. Anaphylactic shock is caused by severe allergic reactions, widespread release of histamine, and subsequent vasodilation.

322. **D.** Teichoic acid may be found only in the cell walls of gram-positive bacteria and contain antigenic properties. All of the other answers listed are found in the cell walls of gram-negative bacteria.

323. **A.** The articulating surfaces of the TMJ are covered with fibrocartilage, directly overlying periosteum. The nonarticulating surfaces of the TMJ are covered with periosteum. The articulating surfaces of diarthrodial joints are covered with hyaline cartilage.

324. **B.** Both epinephrine and glucagons result in activities that serve to increase (maintain) blood glucose. Activation of glycogen phosphorylase results in glycogen degradation, ultimately providing a source of glucose. Glycogen synthase inhibition results in decreased synthesis of glycogen.

325. **C.** The left side occlusal contact would be referred to as mediotrusive contact but may be called a nonworking (balancing) contact.

326. **C.** The internal carotid artery is joined to the posterior cerebral artery via the posterior communicating artery, which is part of the circle of Willis.

327. **E.** The transport of glucose into muscle (and fat) cells is due to the activity of glucose transporters (GLUT-4), which does not require ATP and is independent of any ionic concentration gradient. ATP is required for the activity of all other transport mechanisms listed.

328. **C.** Opportunistic infections are seen in patients with AIDS. All of the microbes listed represent opportunistic organisms except coxsackievirus.

329. **C.** The mesial marginal developmental groove never or almost never crosses the mesial marginal ridge.

330. **D.** All posterior teeth viewed from the distal aspect have a rhomboidal outline.

331. **D.** Dextrans consist of glucose molecules linked together. They not only act as the structural component of plaque, but also they contribute to the retention of lactic acid near the tooth. Fructans or levans are also found in plaque; however, they contain fructose.

332. **C.** Substitution of most ions (with the exception of fluoride) increases the solubility of the crystal structure. The ratio of calcium and phosphate in hydroxyapatite is 1.67:1.

333. **C.** Tooth enamel is derived from ectoderm. Dentin and pulp are derived from mesoderm.

334. **C.** The thin segment of Henle's loop contains squamous epithelial cells. The proximal convoluted tubule (also known as the *thick descending limb of Henle's loop*), the thick ascending segment of Henle's loop, and the distal convoluted tubule all consist of cuboidal epithelial cells.

335. **C.** Glucose-6-phosphate dehydrogenase and phosphogluconate dehydrogenase are irreversible enzymes in the pentose phosphate pathway. Glucokinase is involved with phosphorylation of glucose when hepatic concentrations of glucose are high. Glucose-6-phosphatase hydrolyzes glucose-6-phosphate to form free glucose as the final step in gluconeogenesis.

336. **D.** Height of contour on the distal surface of permanent mandibular central incisors is at the incisal third.

337. **E.** Cardiac tamponade is a serious condition caused by accumulation of fluid in the pericardium. This can result in impaired ventricular filling and can rapidly lead to decreased cardiac output and death.

338. **B.** The correct order of tooth formation: ameloblasts form, odontoblasts form, odontoblasts start to form dentin, ameloblasts start to form enamel.

339. **C.** Reduction division occurs during the first stage of meiosis. The second stage mirrors mitosis. There is no third stage of meiosis.

340. **A.** Whooping cough is caused by *Bordetella pertussis*. All of the factors listed contribute to its virulence except IgA protease. This enzyme is produced by *Haemophilus influenzae*, another gram-negative, rod-shaped bacterium.

341. **C.** Residual volume is the volume of air remaining after a maximal forced expiration. Tidal volume is the amount of air exchanged (expiration and inspiration) during normal quiet breathing. Functional residual capacity is a combination of the expired reserve volume (forced expiration) plus the residual volume. Vital capacity is the volume of air expired after maximal inspiration.

342. **D.** *Mesial aspect:* The mesiobuccal cusp is longer and sharper than the mesiolingual cusp. for choice A,

Pronounced convexity is present (Ash and Nelson, 2003). For choice **B**, curvature is in an occlusal direction. For choice **C**, cervical third is greater than occlusal third.

343. **C.** The embryo develops from the embryonic disc. The morula, blastocyst, and trophoblast all include structures of the extraembryonic coelom that lead to development of the amnion, vitelline sac, and chorion.

344. **C.** Chronologies from textbooks vary so that age of eruption for the primary mandibular central incisor may be given as 6 months (Woelfel and Scheid, 2002);, 6.5 months (Kraus et-al., 1969);, 7.5 months (Charlick et-al.,);, or 8 (6 to 10) months (Ash and Nelson, 2003).

345. **B.** Progesterone concentration in blood is highest following the surge of luteinizing hormone after ovulation. During ovulation, estrogen surges as a result of positive feedback during the follicular phase. During menstruation, there are sharp declines in estrogen and progesterone secondary to reduced secretion of luteinizing hormone and follicle-stimulating hormone.

346. **B.** The left atrioventricular valve of the heart is also known as the *mitral valve*. The right atrioventricular valve of the heart is also known as the *tricuspid valve*. The aortic valve prevents regurgitation of blood from the aorta back into the left ventricle, and the pulmonary valve prevents regurgitation of blood from the pulmonary artery back into the right ventricle.

347. **C.** The leading cause of death for diabetic patients is cardiovascular disease. Other complications include retinopathy, nephropathy, and peripheral neuropathy.

348. **C.** The correct answer for choice **A** would be about *1.5 months or 6 weeks*; for choice **B**, about *4 to 5 years*; for choice **C**, about *2.5 months or 10 weeks* (2 to 3 months is listed in the question); and for choice **D**, about *4 to 5 years*.

349. **D.** The Y-shaped central developmental groove is found on the mandibular second premolar.

350. **B.** The sternal angle between the manubrium and the sternum marks the position of the second rib. From this location, ribs can be counted externally. This is important because the first rib cannot be palpated.

351. **C.** NADPH is required as a reducing agent for the synthesis of fatty acids. The hexose monophosphate pathway also produces ribose-5-phosphate for nucleotide synthesis. No ATP or NADH is produced in the pathway. Fructose-1,6-bisphosphate is produced during glycolysis.

352. **C.** Intraoral viridans streptococcus is the most common cause of subacute endocarditis. *S. aureus* is the most common cause of acute endocarditis.

353. **B, C, D.** For choice **A**, the crown outline converges only *lingually*.

354. **B.** The mandibular incisors as well as the lower lip, floor of the mouth, tip of the tongue, and chin, primarily drain into the submental nodes. The rest of the mandibular teeth (premolars and molars) mainly drain into the submandibular nodes.

355. **D.** Rickets is a vitamin D deficiency seen in infants and children. Oral findings include a delayed eruption of teeth and abnormal dentin.

356. **A.** In the irreversible oxidative decarboxylation of pyruvate to acetyl CoA by pyruvate dehydrogenase, the five coenzymes listed are required.

357. **D.** A developmental depression but not a groove divides the two buccal cusps. For choice **A**, it does not resemble other primary teeth. For choice **B**, it has a rhomboidal outline from the occlusal aspect. For choice **C**, the mesiobuccal cusp is larger.

358. **D.** Fibers of the superior head of the lateral pterygoid muscle attach to the anterior end of the disc, which helps to balance and stabilize the disc during mouth closure.

359. **B.** The maxillary second premolar is most likely to articulate with the second premolar only. (Ash and Nelson, 2003.)

360. **D.** HBeAg is present when there is active viral replication and the carrier is highly infectious.

361. **C.** Saliva is formed by a process that first involves the formation of a solution by the acinar cells, which is subsequently modified by the ductile cells to produce a more hypotonic solution (compared with plasma). The modification primarily involves the reabsorption of sodium and chloride and secretion of potassium and bicarbonate. As salivary flow increases, the ductile cells have less time to modify the composition of saliva, which results in greater concentrations of sodium and chloride ions. Bicarbonate concentration increases as salivary flow increases owing to the selective stimulation of bicarbonate by the parasympathetic system. The salivary glands are primarily under the regulation of both branches of the autonomic nervous system.

362. **B.** The pulmonary vein of the lung carries oxygenated blood from the lungs to the left atrium of the heart. The pulmonary artery carries unoxygenated blood from the right ventricle of the heart to the lungs.

363. **B.** Thoracic vertebrae are characterized by a heart-shaped body.

364. **A.** A micelle is a globular structure that forms when the polar heads of an amphipathic molecule (fatty acids) interact with the aqueous external environment and the nonpolar hydrocarbon tails are clustered inside.

365. **D.** The HIV envelope contains two glycoproteins, gp120 and gp41. gp120 binds specifically with CD4 surface receptors.

366. **A.** The answer is first and second maxillary molars. (McCauley, 1945; Ash and Nelson, 2003.)

367. **B.** In the earliest phase, the condyle moves forward *in concert* with the disc, *not before*.

368. **A.** Endotoxin or lipopolysaccharide is found in the cell walls of gram-negative bacteria.

369. **A.** The trochlea of the humerus articulates with the ulna of the forearm. The capitulum of the humerus bone articulates with the radius of the forearm. The coronoid fossa, located just superior to the trochlea, fits the coronoid process of the ulna of the forearm. The olecranon fossa of the humerus fits the olecranon of the ulna of the forearm. The medial epicondyle is on the humerus itself and serves as an attachment site for muscles.

370. **A.** During a fast, catabolism is increased to provide additional sources of energy. This is characterized by increased use of fatty acids. When the production of acetyl CoA (produced by enhanced β-oxidation) exceeds the oxidative capacity of the citric acid cycle, ketone bodies are formed. During fasting conditions, glucagon concentrations are increased, and glycogenesis is inhibited secondary to limited energy availability. Acetyl CoA production in the liver is increased because of enhanced β-oxidation.

371. **D.** The nucleus ambiguus is found in the medulla of the brainstem. It contains the cell bodies of motoneurons for CN IX, X, and XI. The cell bodies of sensory neurons of CN VII, IX, and X are contained in the nucleus of the solitary tract.

372. **A.** Calcium is stored and released from the sarcoplasmic reticulum during excitation-contraction coupling. This provides an extensive reservoir of calcium, while permitting intracellular free Ca^{2+} to be low when the muscle fiber is at rest. The release of calcium is due to conformational changes, which opens Ca^{2+} channels in the sarcoplasmic reticulum.

373. **B.** The tetanus vaccine consists of tetanus toxoid. It is part of the diphtheria, pertussis, tetanus (DPT) vaccine and should be given about every 10 years.

374. **C.** Height of contour on lingual surfaces of molars and premolars is at the cervical or middle third.

375. **A.** Muscles are innervated by two types of motoneurons (α and γ). The α motoneurons innervate voluntary muscle fibers (extrafusal skeletal muscles). The γ motoneurons innervate the muscle spindles (intrafusal muscle fibers). The muscles of the iris are controlled by both sympathetic innervation (dilation) and parasympathetic innervation (constriction). The pyloric sphincter in the stomach is regulated primarily by the

enteric nervous system and regulatory hormones in the gastrointestinal tract.

376. E. Mitochondria are surrounded by a double (inner and outer) membrane. The nuclear membrane (not listed), which surrounds the nucleus, also consists of a double (inner and outer) membrane.

377. A. Calmodulin is a calcium-binding protein in smooth muscle, which, when bound to myosin, initiates contraction. Calmodulin activates myosin kinase, which results in myosin-actin cross-linking and contraction of smooth muscle.

378. A. The lumen of the gastrointestinal tract is lined with mucosa. The rest of the choices are in order from lumen out. Fibrosa and adventitia are synonymous.

379. B. Distobuccal developmental groove is *not* found on mandibular second molars.

380. E. Bacteria that are phagocytosed by macrophages are kept in membrane-bound vacuoles called *phagosomes*. A phagosome fuses with a lysosome, which contains many degradative enzymes, including lysozyme.

381. B. During metaphase, mitotic spindles form. Chromosomes attach to these spindles, with their centromeres aligned with the equator of the cell.

382. A. DNA ligase is required to ligate the fragments together. DNA and RNA polymerases are catalysts that synthesize DNA and RNA in a continuous process. Reverse transcriptase is an enzyme found in viruses that makes DNA by using viral RNA.

383. D. The maxillary nerve (CN V2) exits the skull through the foramen rotundum. It then passes through the pterygopalatine fossa, where it communicates with the pterygopalatine ganglion. Contents of the superior orbital fissure include CN III, IV, V1, and VI and the ophthalmic veins. CN VII and VIII pass through the internal acoustic meatus, and CN V3 (mandibular nerve) passes through the foramen ovale. The foramen spinosum is not associated with any cranial nerves; it contains the middle meningeal vessels.

384. D. Asthma is an obstructive lung disease caused by narrowing of the airways. Common symptoms include dyspnea, wheezing on expiration, and a dry cough.

385. A. Greater mesiodistal diameter relative to crown height than permanent teeth is correct. For choice **B**, squat appearance, not elongated appearance, is correct. For choice **C**, crowns are a milky white, not translucent white. For choice **D**, there is no root trunk.

386. D. The teres major muscle is a shoulder muscle; however, it is not a rotator muscle. All of the other four muscles listed are rotator cuff muscles.

387. B. A motor unit is composed of a single motoneuron and the muscle fibers it innervates. Because the motoneuron stimulates all muscle fibers it innervates, "fractions" of a motor unit cannot be stimulated. The number of motor units recruited, the number of muscle fibers contracting, and the frequency of stimulation all affect the degree of muscle tension produced.

388. E. In the liver, smooth endoplasmic reticulum is involved in glycogen metabolism and detoxification of various drugs and alcohols; it contains cytochrome P-450 enzymes, which are cytochromes that are important in the detoxification process.

389. C. Cardiac output is the volume of blood pumped per minute by each ventricle. This is influenced by cardiac rate and stroke volume (end-diastolic volume—end-systolic volume). The cardiac output for this patient is 70×110 mL or 7700 mL per minute.

390. B. The mandibular first premolar is most likely to have a single pulp horn.

391. E. Dipicolinic acid is found only in spores. *Clostridium* is the only spore-forming microorganism listed.

392. D. RNA polymerase is an enzyme that transcribes DNA into RNA chains. Synthesis is similar to DNA reproduction because it is synthesized $5' \rightarrow 3'$.

393. C. The frontal bone of the skull is formed by intramembranous ossification. The humerus, vertebrae, ribs, and clavicle all are formed by endochondral ossification.

394. B. The sum total of the pressures moving fluid *out* of the capillary is P_c (37 mm Hg) and π_{if} (1 mm Hg) at the arteriolar end and P_c (16 mm Hg) and π_{if} (1 mm Hg) at the venular end. The sum total of the pressures moving *into* the capillary is P_{if} (0 mm Hg) and π_p (26 mm Hg). The net exchange pressure on the arteriolar end leads to ultrafiltration (12 mm Hg). On the venular end, reabsorption occurs (9 mm Hg). Overall net exchange results in 3 mm Hg of fluid loss out of the capillary.

395. B. T_4 and T_3 are formed by the cleavage of thyroglobulin after stimulation by TSH. Most T_4 is converted to T_3 in liver and kidney. Thyroglobulin is the storage form of thyroid hormone. TSH is produced in the anterior pituitary. It is not a hormone secreted from the thyroid but acts to stimulate the synthesis and secretion of thyroid hormones.

396. C. Dust cells, along with heart failure cells, are macrophages that are found in the lungs. They are part of the reticuloendothelial system.

397. C. The lateral thoracic wall of the axilla is covered by the serratus anterior muscle. The anterior wall is covered by pectoralis major and pectoralis minor. Latissimus dorsi contributes to the inferior aspect of the posterior wall.

398. **C.** Although some CO_2 is transported unchanged in the plasma and in the red blood cells as carbaminohemoglobin, most is transported in the form of HCO_3^- in the plasma.

399. **D.** Oral epithelium is composed of nonkeratinized, stratified, squamous epithelium.

400. **D.** Chondroitin sulfate is a glucosaminoglycan found in ligaments, tendons, and cartilage. It is the most abundant glucosaminoglycan in the body.

401. **A.** The left common carotid artery and left subclavian artery branch off separately from the arch of the aorta. The brachiocephalic trunk branches off from the aorta and bifurcates into the right subclavian and right common carotid arteries.

402. **C.** Cerebrospinal fluid is drained via resorption into the superior sagittal sinus. A narrow canal with cerebrospinal fluid runs the length of the spinal cord. It is continuous with the ventricular system of the brain and is a remnant of the lumen of the embryonic neural tube.

403. **D.** The chorda tympani nerve arises from the descending part of the facial nerve (CN VII) and courses forward to enter the middle ear. It crosses anteriorly over the medial aspect of the tympanic membrane and passes over the medial aspect of the handle of the malleus. It leaves the middle ear through the petrotympanic fissure and enters the infratemporal region below the skull and joins the lingual nerve.

404. **A.** The pterygomandibular space is located between the medial pterygoid muscle and mandibular ramus and contains the inferior alveolar nerve, artery, and vein; lingual nerve; and chorda tympani.

405. **B.** The squamosal suture joins the parietal and temporal bones. The parietal bone articulates with the opposite parietal bone at the sagittal suture. Other sutures of the skull include coronal (frontal and parietal bones), lambdoid (occipital and parietal bones), suture between the greater wing of the sphenoid and the frontal bone, and suture between the frontal bone and zygomatic bone.

406. **B.** The posterior triangle of the neck is limited posteriorly by the anterior border of the trapezius muscle. The borders are formed by the posterior border of the sternocleidomastoid muscle, anterior border of trapezius muscle, and the clavicle.

407. **C.** The hypoglossal nerve (CN XII) provides motor innervation for all intrinsic and extrinsic muscles of the tongue. It exits from the medulla through the hypoglossal canal and descends in the neck superficial to the carotid sheath. The nerve curves anteriorly and disappears deep to the mylohyoid muscle to enter the floor of the mouth, where it branches to supply the musculature of the tongue.

408. **E.** The dorsal venous arch on the back of the hand is the preferred site for long-term intravenous drips. This is a convenient site to maintain, in part because bending the elbow does not interfere with flow. In most cases, the median cubital vein is chosen for blood draws.

409. **A.** Type I collagen is found in connective tissues, tendons, ligaments, bone, teeth, and the dermis of skin. Type II collagen is found in hyaline cartilage. Type III collagen is found in reticulin fibers. Type IV collagen is found in basement membranes. Collagen fibers are high-molecular-weight proteins that vary in diameter and usually are arranged in bundles.

410. **E.** The facial nerve emerges through the stylomastoid foramen giving rise to the posterior auricular nerve and twigs to the digastric and stylohyoid muscles before entering the parotid gland. It then divides into branches supplying several muscles, including the muscles of facial expression.

411. **B.** Citrate synthase catalyzes the reaction of forming citrate from oxaloacetate and acetyl coenzyme A (CoA) as the first step of the cycle. Isocitrate is converted to α-ketoglutarate by isocitrate dehydrogenase, followed by the conversion of α-ketoglutarate to succinyl CoA by α-ketoglutarate dehydrogenase. Succinyl CoA is converted to succinate. Succinate dehydrogenase converts succinate to fumarate. Fumarase catalyzes the conversion of fumarate to malate, and malate dehydrogenase converts malate back to oxaloacetate.

412. **C.** Night blindness can result from a deficiency of vitamin A, and rickets can result from a deficiency of vitamin D. Scurvy results from a deficiency of vitamin C. Both pernicious anemia and neurologic degeneration can result from a deficiency of vitamin B_{12}.

413. **A, C, G.** Hydrogen chloride and pepsinogen are gastric secretions. Enterokinase is secreted by the glands of Brunner in the duodenum. HCO_3^- is the bicarbonate secretion of the pancreas. Both pancreatic amylase and lipase are secreted by the pancreas and the proenzyme form of the proteolytic enzyme chymotrypsin.

414. **C, D.** Sour and salty flavors are sensed via the closing of K^+ and Na^+ channels, respectively. Bitter flavors activate G-proteins to produce inositol triphosphate and Ca^{2+}. Sweet receptors activate G-proteins and the second messenger cyclic adenosine monophosphate. Umami, the taste sensation from L-glutamate and aspartate, also occurs via G proteins.

415. A, C, D. The cytosol refers to the aqueous area between the plasma membrane and the membrane-bound organelles. The term *cytoplasm* refers to all of the area outside of the nucleus. The nucleolus is within the substance of the nucleus.

416. C. The rough endoplasmic reticulum is associated with protein synthesis. The smooth endoplasmic reticulum is associated with lipid synthesis, calcium storage, and drug detoxification.

417. D. The mitochondria contain the enzyme responsible for the generation of ATP via oxidative phosphorylation.

418. A, C, D. ATP is metabolized to adenosine diphosphate (ADP) in many reactions, including kinase reactions. It is converted to cAMP by adenylyl cyclase. ATP is the universal currency of biochemical energy. It is not directly metabolized to guanosine or GTP. It is not an enzyme. Most enzymes end in "ase."

419. D. The basic unit of muscle contraction is the sarcomere which spans from Z-disk to Z-disk.

420. C. High-density lipoprotein is responsible for transporting excess cholesterol back to the liver. Chylomicrons transport dietary triglycerides, whereas very-low-density lipoprotein transports endogenously synthesized triglycerides. Low-density lipoprotein is responsible for delivering cholesterol to the peripheral tissues when the triglycerides have been hydrolyzed.

421. B. The injectisome or injectosome of gram-negative bacteria is also referred to as the *type III secretion system*. The system codes for a protein appendage type that resembles a molecular syringe whose sole function is to facilitate the coordinated injection of proteins into the host cell. Choice **A** is incorrect because the autoinducers of quorum system are chromosomally encoded and secreted via a different system. Choice **C** is incorrect because microbes respond to environmental stimuli that result in the expression of various proteins exported by the machine. Choice **D** is incorrect because the secretion apparatus is used to inject regulatory molecules into the host and not bacteria. The microbiome is composed of bacteria.

422. A. This question is assessing whether or not you appreciate the mechanism of action of IgA, which is the principal immunoglobulin associated with mucosal surfaces.

423. A, B, D. Chlorhexidine is known to inhibit many bacteria but is not effective against bacterial spores. It is also known to persist in the mouth when used as a mouthwash. It is much less effective as a disinfectant of inanimate objects compared with other substances, such as glutaraldehyde.

424. D. "Osteo" indicates bone. Sarcoma refers to a malignancy of mesenchymal origin.

425. B, D, E. Squamous papilloma is a benign neoplasm that does not lead to squamous cell carcinoma. It is characterized by exophytic growth rather than invasion of tissue and has fingerlike projections at its base. It can be pedunculated or sessile.

426. A, B, D. Normal platelet counts range from 150,000 to 450,000 platelets/μL. Thrombocytopenia applies generally to platelet counts less than 100,000 platelets/μL. Spontaneous bleeding usually occurs at platelet counts less than 20,000 platelets/μL. The platelet count mentioned in the question is extremely low making spontaneous bleeding and petechiae likely. PT and PTT are normal, unless other abnormalities are present. The causes of thrombocytopenia are as follows:
a. Decreased platelet production, which may be due to reduced marrow output.
b. Decreased platelet survival, which may be due to autoantibodies or disseminated intravascular coagulation and thrombotic microangiopathies.
c. Sequestration, which can result from an enlarged spleen.
d. Dilution, which is due to large transfusions because prolonged blood storage reduces viable platelets.

427. A, C, D, E. Plasma cells originate in the bone marrow, and if they become neoplastic, they tend to crowd out other cells of the bone marrow. Although they produce antibodies, the antibodies are nonfunctional. Bone radiolucencies and Bence-Jones proteinuria are characteristic.

428. E. This adult patient has myxedema or hypothyroidism. Hyperthyroidism would result in very different symptoms, many of which are opposite to those of hypothyroidism. Hypercholesterolemia often has very subtle symptoms, although weight gain is often associated with it. Diabetes insipidus is characterized by excessive urination and resulting thirst. Asthma symptoms are related to the airway.

429. C. Myasthenia gravis is an autoimmune disease caused by autoantibodies to acetylcholine receptors at the neuromuscular junctions. It is characterized by muscle weakness.

430. B. Lichen planus can have both skin and oral manifestations There are two types of oral lichen planus. Reticular lichen planus is characterized by intersecting white lines known as *Wickham's striae*, which are most often seen along the buccal mucosa. Erosive lichen planus is less common and exhibits erythematous, ulcerated areas. On the gingiva, this appearance is termed *desquamative gingivitis*. Histologically, lichen planus is characterized by saw-tooth rete ridges and the presence of Civatte bodies.

431. A. The correct answer is central fossa #2.

432. E. The correct answer is distal triangular fossa #30.

433. A. Although similar in average emergence age, the mandibular molars tend to develop slightly earlier than the maxillary molars.

434. D. The movement at the TMJ would lead to little opening but maximum movement protrusively.

435. C. A point angle is a junction of three tooth surfaces, of which the mesiobucco-occlusal point angle is an example.

436. B. The proper sequence poster to anterior is (1) posterior attachment, (2) bilaminar zone, (3) posterior band, (4) intermediate zone, (5) anterior band, (6) SHLP.

437. A, C, E. Primary teeth are smaller in overall size and crown dimensions, with molar roots more widely flared and more prominent cervical ridges.

438. A. The first molars are the first permanent teeth to erupt and have the earliest evidence of calcification.

439. C. The mesiobuccal cusp is the largest and the distolingual cusp is the smallest. Often, the distolingual cusp is missing.

440. C. The medial pterygoid muscle is located medial to the mandibular ramus. Its origin is the medial surface of the lateral pterygoid plate and pyramidal process of the palatine bone. Its insertion is the internal surface of the mandibular ramus and angle of the mandible. The temporalis muscle is fan-shaped and lies above and mostly posterior to the masseter. The buccinator muscle lies perpendicular to the masseter. The lateral pterygoid muscle also lies mostly perpendicular to the masseter muscle.

Index

Page numbers followed by "f" indicate figures, "t" indicate tables, and "b" indicate boxes.